Attention and Time

Attention and Time

Edited by

Anna C. Nobre

Jennifer T. Coull

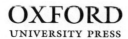

OXFORD
UNIVERSITY PRESS

OXFORD
UNIVERSITY PRESS

Great Clarendon Street, Oxford ox2 6DP

Oxford University Press is a department of the University of Oxford.
It furthers the University's objective of excellence in research, scholarship,
and education by publishing worldwide in

Oxford New York

Auckland Cape Town Dar es Salaam Hong Kong Karachi
Kuala Lumpur Madrid Melbourne Mexico City Nairobi
New Delhi Shanghai Taipei Toronto

With offices in

Argentina Austria Brazil Chile Czech Republic France Greece
Guatemala Hungary Italy Japan Poland Portugal Singapore
South Korea Switzerland Thailand Turkey Ukraine Vietnam

Oxford is a registered trade mark of Oxford University Press
in the UK and in certain other countries

Published in the United States
by Oxford University Press Inc., New York

© Oxford University Press, 2010

The moral rights of the authors have been asserted
Database right Oxford University Press (maker)

First published 2010

British Library Cataloguing in Publication Data

Data available

Library of Congress Cataloging in Publication Data

Data available

Typeset in Minion
by Glyph International, Bangalore, India
Printed in UK
on acid-free paper by
CPI Litho

ISBN 978-0-19-956345-6

10 9 8 7 6 5 4 3 2 1

To Ben and Rosie (JTC)
To Luciano (ACN)

Contents

List of Contributors

Britt Anderson
Department of Psychology
and Centre for Theoretical Neuroscience
University of Waterloo
Waterloo, ON, Canada

Scott W. Brown
Department of Psychology
University of Southern Maine
Portland, ME, USA

Marc J. Buehner
School of Psychology
Cardiff University
Cardiff, Wales, UK

Boris Burle
Laboratoire de Neurobiologie de la Cognition
Universite de Provence
Marseille, France

David Burr
1. Stella Maris Foundation
Calambrone, Pisa
2. Department of Psychology
University of Florence, Florence
3. Istituto di Neuroscienze del CNR
Pisa, Italy

Ángel Correa
Departamento de Psicología
Experimental y Fisiología del
Comportamiento,
Universidad de Granada
Granada, Spain

Jennifer T. Coull
Laboratoire de Neurobiologie de la Cognition
Universite de Provence and CNRS
Marseille, France

David M. Eagleman
Department of Neuroscience and
Department of Psychiatry
Baylor College of Medicine
Houston, TX, USA

Christopher D. Fiorillo
Department of Bio and Brain Engineering
Korea Advanced Institute of Science and
Technology
Daejeon, South Korea

Thierry Hasbroucq
Laboratoire de Neurobiologie
de la Cognition
Universite de Provence
Marseille, France

Joachim Hoffmann
Department of Psychology
Julius-Maximilians University of Würzburg
Würzburg, Germany

Amelia R. Hunt
School of Psychology
University of Aberdeen
Aberdeen, UK

Alan Johnston
Department of Cognitive, Perceptual
and Brain Sciences
University College London
London, UK

Mari Riess Jones
1. Department of Psychology
The Ohio State University
2. University of California, Santa Barbara
Columbus, OH, USA

Bjørg Elisabeth Kilavik
Institut de Neurosciences Cognitives
de la Méditerranée
CNRS and Université Aix-Marseille 2,
Marseille, France

Alan Kingstone
Brain and Attention Research (BAR)
Laboratory
Department of Psychology
University of British Columbia
Vancouver, BC, Canada

Kathrin Lange
Department of Experimental Psychology
Heinrich Heine University
Düsseldorf, Germany

Sander A. Los
Department of Cognitive Psychology
Vrije Universiteit
Amsterdam, The Netherlands

Juan Lupiáñez
Departamento de Psicología
Experimental y Fisiología
del Comportamiento
Universidad de Granda
Granada, Spain

Concetta Morrone
1. Department of Physiological Sciences
University of Pisa
2. Stella Maris Foundation
Calambrone, Pisa, Italy

Anna Christina Nobre
Brain & Cognition Laboratory
Department of Experimental Psychology
University of Oxford
Oxford, UK

Redmond O'Connell
School of Psychology and Trinity College
Institute of Neuroscience
Trinity College Dublin
Dublin, Ireland

Christian N. L. Olivers
Department of Cognitive Psychology
Vrije Universiteit
Amsterdam, The Netherlands

Harold Pashler
Department of Psychology
University of California
San Diego, CA, USA

Micha Pfeuty
Laboratoire d'Imagerie Moléculaire
et Fonctionnelle
CNRS (UMR 5231)
Université Victor Segalen
Bordeaux, France

Viviane Pouthas
Unité de Neurosciences Cognitives
et Imagerie Cérébrale
CNRS (UPR 640) – LENA
Hôpital Pitié-Salpêtrière
Paris, France

Peter Praamstra
Behavioural Brain Sciences Centre
University of Birmingham
Birmingham, UK

Jane E. Raymond
Wolfson Centre for Clinical and Cognitive
Neuroscience
School of Psychology
Bangor University
Bangor, Wales, UK

Alexa Riehle
Institut de Neurosciences Cognitives
de la Méditerranée
CNRS and Université Aix-Marseille 2
Marseille, France

Ian H Robertson
School of Psychology and
Trinity College Institute of
Neuroscience
Trinity College Dublin
Dublin, Ireland

Brigitte Röder
Biological Psychology and Neuropsychology
University of Hamburg
Hamburg, Germany

Bettina Rolke
Department of Cognitive and
Biological Psychology
Psychological Institute
University of Tübingen
Tübingen, Germany

Eric Ruthruff
Department of Psychology
University of New Mexico
Albuquerque, NM, USA

Ricarda I. Schubotz
Motor Cognition Group
Max Planck Institute For
Neurological Research
Cologne, Germany

Kimron L. Shapiro
Wolfson Centre for Clinical and
Cognitive Neuroscience
School of Psychology
Bangor University
Bangor, Wales, UK

David L. Sheinberg
Dept. of Neuroscience
Brown University
Providence, RI, USA

Mariano Sigman
Laboratory of Integrative Neuroscience
Department of Physics
University of Buenos Aires
Buenos Aires, Argentina

Charles Spence
Crossmodal Research Laboratory
Department of Experimental
Psychology
University of Oxford
Oxford, UK

Christophe Tandonnet
Laboratoire de Psychologie
Cognitive
Universite de Provence
Marseille, France

Peter Ulric Tse
Department of Psychological and
Brain Sciences
Dartmouth College
Hanover, NH, USA

Rolf Ulrich
Department of Cognitive and
Biological Psychology
Psychological Institute
University of Tübingen
Tübingen, Germany

Antonino Vallesi
Rotman Research Institute at Baycrest
Toronto, ON, Canada

Annika Wagener
Department of Psychology
Julius-Maximilians University of Würzburg
Würzburg, Germany

Kielan Yarrow
Department of Psychology
City University London, UK

Wieske van Zoest
Faculty of Psychology & Education
Cognitive Psychology,
Vrije Universiteit
Amsterdam, The Netherlands

Introduction

Attention ___ Time: fill in the blank

This book is a freeze-frame of the many different but interrelated ongoing research efforts addressing the interplay between attention and time. Some topics have been with us for decades while others are just beginning to be addressed. Never have they all been brought together into a single volume. There is one aim and one hope. The aim is to synthesize and organize all of this material in a well structured way, so as to provide a functional map to the interested scholar and help avoid conflations and confusions while navigating the territory. The hope is that the book will spark interest in some of these fundamental but less trodden experimental issues and reveal points of synergy across lines of research.

The editors struggled with the function word between the two obvious nouns in the title of the book ('in', 'across', 'to', 'for' ...?). This is no wonder, since the point of the book is exactly to explore the multiple types of functional interrelationships between the two concepts—'time' and 'attention'. In the end we opted for a non-committal 'and', which should be read as a multi-purpose placeholder for more meaningful connectors.

Section 1 of the book is concerned with the basic notion that attentional selection operates *through* and is limited *in* time. To begin with, it is imperative to acknowledge that information processing itself takes time and that the very nature of representations constructed from the integration of incoming stimulus energy and endogenous signals related to our memories, goals, and expectations changes continually over time. The representations upon which selection operates may therefore depend on the task context, goals, and responses (Hunt, van Zoest, and Kingstone, Chapter 1). Furthermore, because the evolving analysis of any given stimulus occupies time, when two or more stimuli occur in close temporal proximity, their neural states interact. Whereas some stages of stimulus analysis can proceed largely unaffected by concurrent processing, other critical stages of analysis require effortful and dedicated processing so that any competing processing is delayed or degraded. Several phenomena of performance deficits relating to the temporal collision of salient or task-relevant events have been described. In most cases, despite the evocative labels given to these effects, the exact mechanisms underlying the performance deficits remain unresolved. Three examples of the limitations of attention over time are presented: 'inhibition of return' (Lupiáñez, Chapter 2), the 'attentional blink' (Shapiro and Raymond, Chapter 3; Olivers, Chapter 4), and the 'psychological refractory period' (Sigman, Chapter 5). Mechanisms are considered for each phenomenon in turn, but it is possible that some common fundamental principles of neural information processing contribute to temporal limitations across these different experimental situations. In contrast to these short-term temporal limits on attention, Chapter 6 (Robertson and O'Connell) explores the mechanisms and adaptive explanations for our well recognized limitation in sustaining a state of vigilant attention over prolonged periods of time. Finally, Section 1 concludes (Spence, Chapter 7) with the complementary consideration of whether the timing of information processing can itself come under attentional control so that analysis of expected, task-relevant events takes precedence, occurring earlier or more rapidly than the processing of other events ('prior entry'). Moreover, this chapter helps illustrate the important distinction between the perception of temporal order versus that of temporal duration, which often become conflated under the catch-all term 'timing'. Chapter 7 deals with the attentional modulation of temporal order, whereas the attentional modulation of duration perception is covered in the opening chapters of Section 2.

Section 2 is concerned with the modulatory effects of attention and related functions *over* time perception. Psychology has taught us that the intuition that our perceptual canvas captures a near-veridical picture of external reality is deeply misguided. The lesson also extends to our perception of the fourth dimension, which is subject to several deformations and illusions depending on ongoing task demands. Of main interest are the durations in the range relevant to controlling perception and action in ongoing cognitive tasks (hundreds of milliseconds to seconds, known as 'interval timing'). Accurate perception of these intervals is shown to depend on the allocation of attention and to be sensitive to interference by competing, secondary tasks. Interestingly, these modulatory effects vary not only as a function of the attentional demands of the secondary, distractor task (Brown, Chapter 8) but also the timing requirements of the primary, timing task (Ruthruff and Pashler, Chapter 9). These intriguing findings raise the possibility that multiple time-keeping mechanisms may exist, which are differentially sensitive to competing task demands, or that time-keeping mechanisms may be differentially available to different types of task-related processes. Furthermore, even in the absence of competing demands, the subjective duration of events still varies with the degree of attention: salient or task-relevant events seem to last longer. Two alternative possible mechanisms for this effect are considered in which processing is dilated per unit time for salient events (Tse, Chapter 10) versus compressed for repeated or irrelevant stimuli (Eagleman, Chapter 11).

Time perception has also been found to be strongly distorted by the execution of saccadic eye movements. Two different types of effects have been observed. Foveating a stimulus can seem to stop time momentarily ('chronostasis'), making the stimulus at the focus of gaze last longer (Yarrow, Chapter 12). On the other hand, events occurring during a saccade become severely temporally compressed (Morrone and Burr, Chapter 13). The neural mechanisms controlling saccades are closely related to those involved in controlling spatial attention, raising the possibility that these temporal distortions have their origin in neural mechanisms related to updating of spatial representations during the shifts of attention that precede saccades (Yarrow, Chapter 12). Indeed similar time compressions are observed for covert shifts of attention as for saccade execution (Morrone and Burr, Chapter 13). Adaptation to fast motion or flickering stimuli can also trigger this type of time compression (Johnston, Chapter 14), and it may be worth exploring whether similar mechanisms underlie the effects of repeated (Eagleman, Chapter 11) or adapted (Johnston, Chapter 14) visual stimuli on time perception. Finally, a compression of time perception has also been shown to occur when a stimulus is perceived to result as a consequence of performing an action ('intentional binding'). Buehner (Chapter 15) considers the roles of intentionality versus causality in determining this effect. It will be interesting for future investigations to explore whether there are common principles of neural function linking action and predicted outcomes that explain time compression after saccades, shifts of attention, and other types of intentional acts.

Section 3 is chunkier, and addresses an aspect of the relationship between attention and time that has not been brought onto a book platform before. It considers how attention can be directed *within* time, to specific moments, in order to optimize performance. The first series of chapters within this section consider how temporal expectations that develop from the inherent temporal structure of task events influence behavioural performance and different types of neural activity. The duration of the interval (or 'foreperiod') between successive stimuli in a task has long been known to influence reaction-time performance ('foreperiod effect'). Furthermore, the effects differ when all foreperiods are fixed across a block of tasks (longer foreperiods lead to longer response times) versus when foreperiods are variable (longer foreperiods lead to shorter response times).

New research using fixed-foreperiod manipulations shows that temporal expectations can be linked to specific expectations about the features of the predicted stimulus (Wagener and Hoffmann, Chapter 16), and that foreperiod effects may involve modulation at perceptual, as well as motor, stages of stimulus processing (Rolke and Ulrich, Chapter 17). Some of the neural mechanisms behind the behavioural foreperiod effects have been revealed at the systems (Burle, Tandonnet, and Hasbroucq, Chapter 18) as well as cellular (Kilavik and Riehle, Chapter 18) levels within the motor system, and are beginning to be explored within other neural systems, such as in brain areas processing reward (Fiorillo, Chapter 19). When variable foreperiods occur within a task, performance can also be influenced by the sequence of intervals intervening between successive events, such that responses to stimuli are shorter after a short preceding interval ('sequential effects'). Current research is aimed at testing the putative roles of automatic associative trace conditioning versus strategic use of temporal conditional probabilities for sequential and variable foreperiod effects (Los, Chapter 21), as well as revealing the neural systems and dynamics involved in their generation (Vallesi, Chapter 22). Prolonged rhythmic sequences of events have also been exploited to investigate the effects of temporal preparation on information processing. Rhythmic stimulation effectively entrains attentional resources, so that perceptual abilities are maximal for stimuli occurring on-beat and fall off gradually and systematically with temporal distance according to the pace of the rhythm (Jones, Chapter 23). Electrophysiological (Praamstra, Chapter 24) and haemodynamic (Schubotz, Chapter 24) imaging methods are being applied to define the neural systems and dynamics involved in generating predictions and optimizing perception based on the temporal regularity between events.

The second series of chapters within this section considers our ability to draw upon predictive temporal information to orient our attention endogenously and voluntarily to the anticipated moment of onset of task-relevant items ('temporal orienting'). This new field of research has benefited from the development of experimental paradigms in which symbolic cues predict or instruct the relevant moments when behavioural target stimuli will occur, building on the tasks initially devised by Posner for investigating spatial orienting of attention. Behavioural investigations have already uncovered many different types of performance benefits conferred by temporal orienting, including improvements in perceptual discriminations, gating subliminal priming, and speeding of motor responses (Correa, Chapter 26). Neuroscientific investigations are beginning to ask how temporal predictions can modulate perceptual and motor processes. But many basic questions still remain to be addressed, such as whether and how temporal predictions can modulate neuronal excitability independently of predictions about other receptive-field properties and the degree of similarity of modulatory mechanisms across different sensory modalities (Nobre, Chapter 27). So far, experiments indicate that temporal orienting can facilitate performance in different sensory modalities, as well as crossmodally, but event-related potentials suggest different patterns of modulation in the auditory as compared to visual modality (Lange and Röder, Chapter 28). Single-unit recordings in visual extrastriate areas are beginning to reveal how temporal orienting may influence the frequency and correlation of neuronal spiking (Anderson and Sheinberg, Chapter 29). Investigations are also being aimed at understanding the neural systems that control temporal orienting, generating the top-down biasing signals. Electrophysiological (Pouthas and Pfeuty, Chapter 30) and haemodynamic (Coull, Chapter 31) brain-imaging methods are being applied to investigate how the neural systems for endogenous temporal orienting relate to those involved in extracting temporal regularities embedded within stimulus sequences and those involved in making explicit timing judgements. Testable theoretical predictions are emerging about the differential roles the cerebral hemispheres may contribute to different types or use of timing functions (Pouthas and Pfeuty, Chapter 30; Coull, Chapter 31).

As will be obvious, the three Sections do not stand in a linear progression. Instead, they take different stances to peer into the multifaceted interplay between attention and time. The view from each of these perspectives contains many unsolved puzzles. There is no prescribed order for travelling through this book. Readers should feel free to sample and jump around according to their interests. We hope that by playing with these unfinished blocks of knowledge, they will get new ideas or forge new connections that will benefit their own research. And that they will also experience some of the enjoyment we got by putting this book together.

Finally, each of the editors would like to thank the other for the many years of support, friendship, and intellectual collaboration. Together, we would like to thank Joachim Hoffmann and Annika Wagener for spurring us onto this project and Martin Baum for his expert guidance through its editorial inception.

Anna C. Nobre
Brain & Cognition Laboratory,
Department of Experimental Psychology,
University of Oxford,
UK

Jennifer T. Coull
Laboratoire de Neurobiologie de la Cognition,
Université de Provence and CNRS,
France

Section 1

Attention is limited in time

Chapter 1

Attending to emerging representations: the importance of task context and time of response

Amelia R. Hunt, Wieske van Zoest, and
Alan Kingstone

What exactly the brain does with sensory input is a fundamental question of cognitive psychology, and the idea that neural processes unfold over time is a cornerstone of techniques used to address this question. In what follows, we focus on human attention, as indexed by the time to respond to stimulus events, and review the use of this behavioural metric. We discuss some of the limitations of using reaction time to make inferences about attention, and describe experiments that extend this approach by examining changes in responses over time and across different response systems.

In the first section we provide a brief history of how reaction-time measures have been used to study attention, highlighting the theoretical framework, the goals, and the limitations of this research approach. But attention may influence reaction time by affecting any one of several different cognitive operations, and the challenge is to tease those cognitive processes apart. In the following three sections, we present three research tactics. One is to look for convergence and divergence in the effect of attention across a range of different responses and tasks. A second approach is to perform a detailed analysis of attentional processing across time while holding the response task itself constant. A third approach is to introduce different responses into the same task and to manipulate when these responses are executed. While no research tactic is perfect, each introduces a level of clarity with regard to the cognitive process that is modulated by attention.

Collectively, our review indicates that much can be gained theoretically, and empirically, by adopting a framework that recognizes a) that the quality of stimulus information changes over time; b) that the cognitive processes available to, or engaged by, stimuli change over time; and c) that different responses may access different types of information because of when that response is executed and/or the type of information required for that response.

A brief history of reaction time

The first explicit proponent of reaction time (RT) as a measure of brain processes was F.C. Donders (1818–1889). He was inspired by his contemporary Helmholtz, who attempted to measure his own nerve conduction speed by stimulating his skin at varying distances from the brain and comparing the time to respond to the stimulation. Donders applied the same logic to demonstrate that when you add basic levels of complexity to a task you can also increase the time the task takes to perform. For example, if pressing a button upon seeing a light takes 300ms, and pressing the left button for a white light or the right button for a red light takes 450ms, the time difference of 150ms would reflect the decision process, cleanly inserted between the process of sensing the light and the process of pressing the button. Although Donders' approach is useful for determining and comparing the time needed to undergo certain transformations, it only goes so far, because it assumes that each stage of the sequence (seeing the light, determining its colour, and pressing the button) is completely independent and can be inserted or removed without affecting the others, which is rarely, if ever, the case.

Sternberg (1968) noted this drawback and refined the method by demonstrating that changes in RT can reveal the underlying mechanisms involved in a task by identifying stages of processing that can be *selectively influenced*. That is, if Factor A influences RT to a similar extent regardless of the presence or absence of Factor B, then the two factors affect independent stages of processing. Alternatively, if manipulation of Factor B changes the influence of Factor A, then the two factors affect the same stage of processing. After this important refinement, the method of using RT to measure mental processes was more widely adopted. A nice example of the utility of Sternberg's logic for studying attention comes from the typical visual search experiment, in which observers must scan an array of some number of items for a pre-specified target. The time to find the target usually increases as distractors are added to the display. This average per-item increase in RT is known as the search slope, and is thought of as an index of how long it takes for attention to search through the items to determine which one is the target. Introducing changes to the search task can alter RT by influencing the processing stages involved in the task. For example, making the target easier to spot among the distractors by giving it some unique, easily identifiable feature decreases the search slope. In other words, changing the relationship between the target and the distractors selectively influences the visual search component of RT. In contrast, changing the number of possible responses selectively influences the process of selecting a response, but would not affect the speed with which the target could be found. In this case, adding possible responses would increase overall RT, but to a similar extent across all possible search array sizes, that is, it would be additive with the distractors' effect. Using this kind of approach, RT can reveal factors that interact with, or are independent from, processes involved in visual selection.

In his 1978 book *Chronometric Explorations of Mind*, Posner laid out the fundamentals of inferring mental processes from RT and changes in performance at various exposure durations. One of the most compelling features of Posner's approach is the way in which chronometric techniques are able to expose changes in the representation of information over time. For instance, in a letter-identification task, responses are faster if the letter is primed by the same letter. When the interval between the prime and the target is short, only physically identical letters produce priming, but when the interval between the prime and the target is longer, the letters can be in different cases or fonts and still produce priming. The change in the effect of different kinds of primes over time suggests the transition of the neural representation of the target letter from a sensory to a more conceptual state. Another classic example is that the time it takes to name an object increases systematically with how many degrees away from upright it is (Shepard and Metzler, 1971). This suggests the representation of the object is mentally rotated in an analogue fashion before the identity can be reported, and further demonstrates that by carefully manipulating stimulus parameters and observing the effect on reaction time, much can be learned about how the mind represents, transforms, and stores information.

Posner's book remains an important description of the rich information about perceptual processes, attention, information accrual, and changes in stimulus representations that can be extracted from chronometric analysis of task performance. Later work has focused more on the processes of attentional selection specifically; however, Posner's 1980 paper with Snyder and Davidson introduced a simple technique for measuring the time required to shift covert visual attention from one location to another, which set the stage for a vast area of research and has been cited over 1000 times as of this writing. They show that when attention is drawn to a location using a spatial cue, RT to detect and/or visually analyse a target appearing there is faster relative to when the target occurs in some other location. Presumably this is because when the target appears at some unattended location, it takes a measurable amount of time for attention to be reallocated appropriately. This simple but elegant demonstration that attention facilitates processing at a spatial location has been used to examine numerous questions, including the effectiveness of various kinds of cues for attracting attention, the dynamics of the attention shift, the processing facilitation attention imbues, and the neural processes supporting spatial selectivity (see also Lupianez, Chapter 2, this volume).

Components of reaction time in attention

While it has been shown time and again that focused attention facilitates reaction time, the underlying mechanism of this facilitation is not singular. The possibilities can be separated into four broad categories, described in the following sections.

Information accrual and quality

The more quickly task-relevant information can be accrued, the more quickly a response can be executed. Attention has been proposed to speed responses by increasing the speed and detail with which information is picked up from the environment. This proposal has found support from a number of studies; for example, Hawkins et al. (1990) found that d′ (a measure of perceptual sensitivity) was heightened at attended locations. Hawkins et al. (1988) showed that attention interacts under-additively with the effect of increasing target luminance, which suggests that increasing luminance and increasing attention have a similar effect on the stimulus. Moreover, early evoked potentials to attended targets are enhanced, suggesting attention acts on early stages of stimulus processing (Van Voorhis and Hillyard, 1977; Mangun and Hillyard, 1987). More recently, Carrasco and others have shown that attention focused on a spatial location influences a range of perceptual processes, including sensitivity to contrast (e.g. Pestilli and Carrasco, 2005), the visual appearance of stimuli (Carrasco, Ling, and Read, 2004; Gobell and Carrasco, 2005), and the speed of visual processing (Carrasco and McElree, 2001).

It is possible to manipulate information accrual by manipulating the duration of the target, and therefore limiting the amount of information that can be accrued. This approach is useful, although it is important to keep in mind that just because a stimulus is no longer physically present does not mean the brain has ceased processing information about it. A weak or incomplete representation can undergo deep, complex, and time-consuming processing by the time a response is actually executed (e.g. Garner, 1970).

Time-consuming shifts

Spatial attention is often likened to a spotlight, illuminating targets inside its focus. Like a spotlight, if attention is directed to the wrong location when the target appears, a measurable amount of time will be needed to disengage from the wrong location, shift across space to the correct location, and engage on the target. Past efforts to measure the time involved in shifting from one location to another have come up with a range of numbers which depend on the kind of cue used and the experimental method used to measure attention, with estimates often ranging from less than 100ms up to 300ms (see Sperling and Weichselgartner, 1995, for an excellent review, or Carlson, Hogendoorn, and Verstraten, 2006, for a recent example).

Whether or not one adopts a spotlight metaphor, there is no escaping the fact that all researchers consider the shifting of attention from its current focus to a new focus to be a time-consuming operation, regardless of whether that shift is spatial in nature, or whether it is between different features of the same or different objects (cf. Duncan, 1984; Serences et al., 2004). Indeed, the idea of disengaging and engaging attention is fundamental to both past (Posner, Cohen, and Rafal, 1982) and present (Corbetta, Patel, and Shulman, 2008) theories of spatial attention, with specific brain regions thought to subserve these operations.

Response priming

It has been shown in a wide range of situations that the location of a stimulus primes responses directed towards its location reflexively, that is, even when the stimulus itself or its spatial position are not relevant to the task at hand. For instance, an irrelevant stimulus suddenly added to a display will attract eye movements (Theeuwes et al., 1998). More generally, responses compatible with the location of a stimulus will be facilitated, even when the location of the stimulus is uninformative in the actual task (known as the Simon effect, e.g. Simon et al., 1970). Debate persists over the exact mechanism behind this response activation (e.g. Bacon and Egeth, 1994; Lu and Proctor, 1994), but it is generally agreed that attention is a mediating factor. In other words, attending to a specific location seems to prime motor responses directed to that location. It is important to note the difference between this phenomenon and what is known as the premotor theory of attention (Rizzolatti et al., 1987); the premotor theory proposes that preparation of a motor response toward a target stimulus is *synonymous* with the allocation of attention to that stimulus. While there is certainly ample evidence for strong links between the attention and motor systems (e.g. Moore and Fallah, 2001, 2004) there is also ample evidence for a functional separation between the two (Klein, 1980; Murthy, Thompson, and Schall, 2001; Hunt and Kingstone 2003a).

Speed–accuracy trade-offs

As described earlier, task-relevant information takes time to accrue, and shifts of attention take time to transpire, but that does not mean that a given subject will always wait until the same moment in the accrual of information and the transpiring of attention shifts to actually execute an overt response. Rather, one can adopt a conservative criterion, and wait until the response will definitely be correct before executing it, at the expense of fast performance. Or one can adopt a more liberal criterion, and sacrifice perfect performance in favour of increased speed. Thus, it is essential when a RT difference is observed also to collect and examine information about performance accuracy, because attention could change RT by changing the threshold for executing a response (e.g. Ivanoff and Klein, 2006).

Using a more liberal criterion would generally produce more errors, though as Pachella (1974) and others have pointed out, having information about response accuracy is not always sufficient to determine whether a speed–accuracy trade-off has occurred. Tasks that are relatively easy to perform will have very low error rate, and for these tasks sacrificing some stimulus information by speeding up responses could have only modest effects on the actual number of erroneous responses executed. Some other tasks might be comparatively more difficult and require relatively more information, and in those tasks, speeding up responses by the same amount could cause a precipitous loss of information and deterioration of performance accuracy. The general lesson here is that while information accrual occurs over time, different tasks may demand different amounts of information for successful performance.

Comparing reaction time effects across responses

A challenge in using RT differences to understand attention has continued to be how to interpret the RT effects of manipulating attention vis-à-vis the multiple components of cognitive processing through which attention could produce a change in RT. Here we outline one approach for investigating what is actually driving the changes in RT produced by manipulations of attention, which is to examine the effect of the same attentional manipulation across multiple types of tasks and response modalities. When multiple tasks and responses converge on the same general pattern of results, it is reasonable to conclude that the process in question is based on a representation or process that is available to all response systems. Sometimes, however, the characteristics of attention change when different responses are used to measure it. Under these circumstances, it suggests that the manipulation has some task-specific or response-related component.

One important example of the utility of this approach comes from the 'inhibition of return' (IOR) literature (see Lupiáñez, Chapter 2, this volume). IOR occurs after attention has been directed to a location by a spatial cue; initially performance is facilitated for targets appearing at the cued location, but after a few hundred milliseconds, the facilitation is replaced by slower responses to a target at the cued location compared to other locations (Posner and Cohen, 1984). The general interpretation is that once the cued location has been attended, there is a bias against directing attention to it a second time. This interpretation is supported by findings that IOR changes perceptual sensitivity at the target location (Handy, Jha, and Mangun, 1999; Prime and Ward, 2006) and interacts with target modality and saliency (Reuter-Lorenz, Jha, and Rosenquist, 1996). However, what might look like attentional costs have been suggested, at least in some circumstances, to reflect a criterion shift instead (e.g. Klein and Taylor, 1994; Ivanoff and Klein, 2006); that is, rather than a change in the rate of information accrual, or a time-consuming shift in the focus of attention, the changes in RT instead result from changes in the threshold for executing a response.

One of the ways in which this question has been pursued is through a comparison of IOR in various task contexts. For example, IOR occurs when attention is drawn reflexively to a location by an abrupt peripheral visual onset, but it does not occur when attention is allocated volitionally based on knowledge of where a target is most likely to appear (Posner and Cohen, 1984). Likewise, IOR is stronger, and begins sooner after the cue onset, when the task is simply to detect the appearance of a target than when the task is to make a discrimination response based on a specific target feature (Lupiáñez et al., 1997; Klein 2000). The very fact that IOR interacts with the task context suggests that there are, at the very least, components of IOR that are not an obligatory, unified consequence of attentional orienting. Taking this further, Hunt and Kingstone (2003b) examined IOR for hand- and eye-movement responses and found a double dissociation; IOR for hand-movement responses interacted with a perceptual luminance manipulation but not a motor manipulation, and IOR for eye-movement responses interacted with a motor manipulation but not a perceptual manipulation. The unique form IOR takes depending on the effector executing the response to the target supports the interpretation that IOR is not a unitary phenomenon influencing some central representation of the stimulus or unitary attentional allocation process, but a collection of task-specific processes that take a similar form (see also Sumner, 2006). Examining IOR across multiple responses can reveal the ways in which these various forms of IOR share common resources and to what degree they are separate.

Another example of response-specificity comes from recent priming literature. Priming is a well-established phenomenon whereby recent experience with a given object facilitates subsequent task performance involving that object. It has generally been assumed that priming occurs because processing the object's features and linking them to a stored representation of the object's identity is more quickly and efficiently performed the second time it occurs. Consistent with this idea, in many brain regions, such as fusiform cortex (which is associated with object identification), there is a reduction in functional magnetic resonance imaging (fMRI) signal strength with repeated presentations (see also Eagleman, Chapter 11, this volume), even as performance improves (e.g. Schacter and Buckner, 1998), suggesting less effort (i.e. neural activity as indexed by blood flow) is required to do the task the second time around. An important detail recently added to this story is that the priming effect is reduced both behaviourally and in the fusiform cortex when the task being performed on the object changes (Dobbins et al., 2004). This result is important because it demonstrates that the facilitation of information processing through repetition is in part specific to a particular task context. This partial specificity suggests that there are actually two components driving the facilitation associated with the prime; one is a general facilitation of perceptual processes that transfers across tasks, and the other is a task-specific component, such as the speed with which a specific response can be executed based on the primed object. Including other responses in priming studies allows for both of these components to be understood separately.

Other examples of the usefulness of converging response systems comes from research probing the putative independence of the dorsal and ventral processing streams (e.g. Aglioti DeSouza, and Goodale, 1995), the performance costs of switching between tasks (Hunt and Klein 2002; Hunt, Ishigami and Klein 2006), and the specificity of oculomotor benefits associated with turning off a fixated light (the gap effect; Saslow, 1967; Ross and Ross, 1980; 1981). These examples illustrate that task and response types can identify the basis for performance effects as central, shared processes or representations, or a more response- and task-specific phenomenon.

Probing responses to the same stimulus over time

A second fruitful approach for carving up the components of attentional effects on RT is to examine how the same response to the same stimulus changes over time. For example, in a study by van Zoest, Donk, and Theeuwes (2004), participants were instructed to saccade to a target (a line segment with a pre-specified orientation) presented in a large array of homogeneously-oriented non-target line segments as well as one additional orientation singleton. The relative salience of the orientation-singleton distractor was varied such that it appeared as less salient, equally salient, or more salient than the target. Task performance was influenced by the salience of the irrelevant distractor only when response latencies were short: eye movements that were executed soon after the presentation of the search display were directed to the most salient element, which meant subjects made very fast and accurate saccades when the target was the most salient item in the display, but incorrect saccades when the target and distractor were equally salient or when the distractor was more salient than the target. As saccadic latency increased, the effect of stimulus-salience decreased; no effect of stimulus-salience was found at the slowest saccadic latencies. On the basis of these results, it was concluded that early visual selection is driven by stimulus features and later selection is driven by goals. In other words, mechanisms of selection change as a function of time.

A reasonable proposal arising from this study was that salience ceased to affect performance at later time-points precisely because voluntary control becomes available, limiting the influence of stimulus-driven control. But further evidence suggests that the role of salience in selection decreases regardless of goal-driven influences (Donk and van Zoest, 2008). When participants were instructed to saccade to the most salient location in a search display, fast saccades were accurate at targeting the most salient feature, but slower saccades (that is, those executed later than 350ms after target onset) were at chance. These results suggest that salience was only transiently represented in the visual system, after which point the representation of saliency was no longer usable for guiding eye movements, even when saliency was the critical feature for accurate performance. If information about target salience had persisted in the visual system, correct selection of the salient location should have been possible across the RT distribution; the fact that performance falters with the passage of time suggests that salience information, which has such a powerful effect on early saccades, degrades over time, even when it is task-relevant.

Therefore, rather than relying on different control mechanisms in selection to explain changes to responses over time, representational change seems to provide a more parsimonious account (see Figure 1.1). The idea here is that salient information dominates the early form of the representation, so when observers respond quickly, salience is prioritized regardless

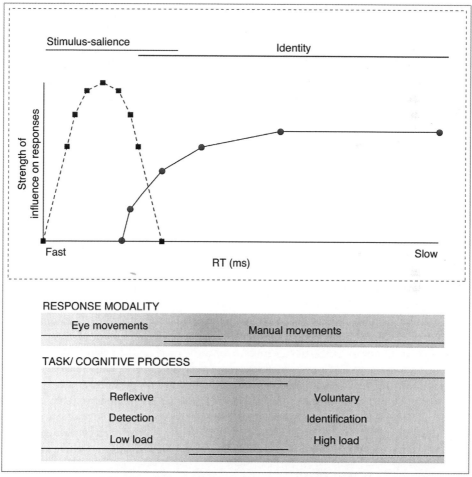

Fig. 1.1 Illustration of changes in the representation of information over time. Early representations are based on stimulus-salience (dotted line), while later representations are based on identity information (solid line). Different response modalities may tap into different representations of information depending on when the response is triggered. Eye movements tend to be executed earlier in time than manual movements, and would therefore be more influenced by stimulus salience. Similarly, different tasks and cognitive processes may have different time courses because they prioritize different components of information.

of its task-relevance. However, as time passes, the representation changes and becomes more sophisticated as other information, such as prior knowledge and observer goals, is integrated. Thus, when observers are slower and more time has been allowed for visual processing, performance is guided by higher-order knowledge. This view contrasts with current models of selection that assume salience to have persistent effects on visual selection unless voluntary goal-driven processes prevent these effects from happening (e.g. Wolfe, Cave, and Franzel, 1989; Treisman and Sato, 1990; Godijn and Theeuwes, 2002). Thus, it may not be so much the mechanism of selection that changes as a function of time, but rather the representation of visual information.

The idea that visual representations become more sophisticated as a function of time is in line with theories of information processing that have emphasized the importance of dynamics in feedforward and recurrent processing (e.g. Li, 1999; Di Lollo, Enns, and Rensink, 2000; Lamme and Roelfsema, 2000; but see Hochstein and Ahissar (2002) for an alternative conceptualization). For example, according to Lamme and Roelfsema (2000), processing that occurs early following the presentation of an image relies on rapid feedforward connections that spread from low-level to high-level areas of the visual cortical hierarchy. During later processing, information from horizontal or feedback connections are incorporated. Whereas initial responses reflect sensory processing by the feedforward sweep, responses at longer latencies correlate with more cognitive or behavioural aspects of sensory processing (and in the context of their argument, with conscious perception of the stimulus). A similar point is made by Di Lollo, Enns, and Rensink (2000), who suggest recurrent signals can reconfigure the initial representation with the consequence that 'the same cells can serve different functions at different stages of processing' (p.501). It is possible that these re-entrant signals from extrastriate visual areas, frontal cortex, and other regions, modulate neural activity to fit the current goals of an observer (Desimone and Duncan, 1995; Kastner and Ungerleider, 2000). In this sense, initial stimulus-driven representations may become goal-driven as more re-entrant signals converge on the representation.

Combining time-course analysis with converging response types

We have discussed the utility of converging tasks and response modalities and the careful analysis of time-course information. Adding these two approaches together can lead to even greater insight into attention. To the extent that different tasks and motor responses depend on different kinds of information, they will be influenced differently by changes in the stimulus representation. The emerging representation of stimuli over time, therefore, can have different effects depending on both the type of response, and the time at which the response is executed. An example comes from a pair of attention-related phenomena known as attentional capture and oculomotor capture. Attentional capture is the more general effect, and is simply the increase in RT to perform a specific task in the presence of an irrelevant distractor. The assumption is that attention is attracted to the irrelevant event and therefore adds to RT the extra time needed to redirect attention appropriately. Oculomotor capture refers to the finding that the eyes can sometimes be directed, in error, to task-irrelevant events (usually a visual transient). So, for example, if the task is to saccade to a single orange circle among an array of red circles, the appearance of an additional red circle will tend to attract eye movements, even though it is not the target. Oculomotor capture was first introduced as a way of studying the movement of attention in the presence of distractors (Theeuwes et al., 1998), but it was later suggested to represent a special case of capture that was different from the more common form of attentional capture (e.g. Ludwig and Gilchrist, 2002; Wu and Remington, 2003). In other words, visual transients may influence eye-movement programming without influencing the manual responses used in typical attentional capture experiments. To reconcile attentional and oculomotor capture, Hunt, von

Mühlenen, and Kingstone (2007) compared manual joystick and eye-movement responses to localize a target in an array. Initially, eye movements and manual responses appeared to be distinct: eye movements were directed towards the sudden onset on about 30% of trials, but manual responses were almost never directed towards the sudden onset. One would be tempted to conclude, based on this result, that oculomotor capture and attentional capture were in fact distinct phenomena. However, manual responses are much slower than eye movements, to the extent that their distributions barely overlap with one another in this context. When RT deadlines were imposed on the responses, in order to bring the RT distributions in line with one another, manual responses began to be directed toward the onset at a similar rate as for eye movements: fast eye and manual responses were directed towards the onset distractor, and slower eye and manual responses were directed towards the target.

The important point to take away about attention here is that the effect of the distractor on target localization was shared across response systems, and there was no evidence of a separation between oculomotor and attentional capture. This suggests that the distractor is influencing a central representation of the visual array that is shared across response systems. We know from the work described earlier (van Zoest et al., 2004; Donk and van Zoest, 2008) that the relative weight of salient information changes over time, such that fast responses are directed towards a salient distractor and later responses are not. Eye movements tend to be executed at a point in time when the effect of the visual distractor is still strong, and manual responses, under normal circumstances, are executed after the power of the distractor has waned (see Figure 1.1). But when the two responses are matched over time, the effect of the distractor begins to look very similar.

A more general question in this respect is what can be learned about attentional processes when both the time course and various response systems are examined in concert. The processing stream can be sampled at different points in time by examining responses across the reaction-time distribution or using reaction-time deadlines, affording the ability to observe changes in the locus of visual attention and the accrual of information over time. Converging evidence across tasks and response types also reveals the degree to which attention is acting on a shared representation or process: if the time course diverges for different responses, there is cause to think the processes involved are task-specific rather than a reflection of some single central process affecting all responses similarly.

Eye movements provide a window into the time course of attentional processes that is much earlier than can normally be obtained using manual responses. Their lower response threshold means they are executed on the basis of less information than hand movements, suggesting they can reveal earlier stages of processing than other kinds of responses. It may be possible to observe the emergence of early attention effects even earlier than the fastest eye movements: recent research suggests that the effects of spatial attention cues can be recorded in the activation of neck muscles as early as 100ms following the cue (Corneil et al., 2008).Other responses, such as long reaches to touch a target, can reveal changes in the trajectory of the reach emerging over more extended periods of time (e.g. Song and Nakayama, 2007). These qualitatively rich measures can reveal subtle or transient influences of attention across time, and by examining a number of different response systems it is possible to separate effects that are response-specific from those influencing central representations or attentional orienting processes.

Conclusions

Attention is a complicated and multifaceted concept that is often studied using a singular number: RT. Multiple stages and aspects of task performance can contribute to RT, and it is not always clear how exactly attention interacts with these various processes to produce faster responses.

We have suggested three approaches for separating the components of RT effects in attentional research: first, measuring effects using multiple response systems to isolate common, central attentional mechanisms from response-specific ones. Second, examining how the same response to the same stimulus changes as a function of time in order to reveal the dynamics of changing representations and the allocation of attention. Finally, combining time-course information with converging responses can reveal the shared and separate time courses of the effects of attention on specific behaviours.

Across all these approaches is the key underlying principle that with the passage of time stimulus representations, and the cognitive processes operating on them, undergo significant modifications. From this perspective one is presented with the novel view that it is absolutely crucial to consider when a response is being executed, because the information available up to the moment of that response, and hence to the attentional processes, will be very different if the response was executed earlier or later in time. As we have discussed in this chapter, appreciation of these dynamics provides the researcher with a number of different ways (we have outlined three) for discovering whether common or distinct attentional processes are being utilized at different moments, with different responses, and different tasks. While we have focused on reaction-time studies, the conceptual framework we have presented here can be applied equally to other domains of measurement where time is of critical importance, such event-related potential (ERP), magnetoencephalography (MEG), and fMRI. We expect that such applications will continue to lead to new and converging insights into human selective attention.

References

Aglioti, S., DeSouza, J.-F. X., and Goodale, M. A. (1995). Size-contrast illusions deceive the eye but not the hand. *Current Biology*, 6, 679–85.

Bacon, W. F. and Egeth, H. E. (1994). Overriding stimulus-driven attentional capture. *Perception & Psychophysics*, 55, 485–96.

Carlson, T. A., Hogendoorn, H., and Verstraten, F. A. J. (2006). The speed of visual attention: What time is it? *Journal of Vision*, 6, 1406–11.

Carrasco, M., Ling, S., and Read, S. (2004). Attention alters appearance. *Nature Neuroscience*, 7, 308–13.
Carrasco, M. and McElree, B. (2001). Covert attention accelerates the rate of visual information processing. *Proceedings of the National Academy of Sciences*, 98, 5363–7.

Corbetta, M., Patel, G., and Shulman, G.L. (2008). The reorienting system of the human brain: from environment to theory of mind. *Neuron*, 58, 306–24.

Corneil, B.D., Muñoz, D.P., Chapman, B.B., Admans, T., and Cushing, S.L. (2008). Neuromuscular consequences of reflexive covert orienting. *Nature Neuroscience*, 11, 13–15.

Desimone, R. and Duncan, J. (1995). Neural mechanisms of selective visual attention. *Annual Reviews of Neuroscience*, 18, 193–222.

Di Lollo, V., Enns, J. T., and Rensink, R. A. (2000). Competition for consciousness among visual events: The psychophysics of reentrant visual processes. *Journal of Experimental Psychology: General*, 129, 481–507.

Dobbins, I.G., Shyner, D.M., Verfaellie, M. and Schacter, D.L. (2004). Cortical activity reductions during repetition priming can result from rapid response learning. *Nature*, 428, 315–19.

Donders, F. C. (1869). On the speed of mental processes. [Translated and reprinted in *Acta Psychologica* (1969), 30, 412–31.]

Donk, M. and van Zoest, W. (2008). Effects of salience are short-lived. *Psychological Science*, 19, 733–9.

Duncan, J. (1984). Selective attention and the organization of visual information. *Journal of Experimental Psychology: General*, 114, 501–17.

Garner, W. R. (1970). The stimulus in information processing. *American Psychologist*, 17, 10–28.

Gobell, J. and Carrasco, M. (2005). Attention alters the appearance of spatial frequency and gap size. *Psychological Science*, **16**, 644–51.

Godijn, R. and Theeuwes, J. (2002). Programming of endogenous and exogenous saccades: evidence for a competitive integration model. *Journal of Experimental Psychology: Human Perception and Performance*, **28**, 1039–54.

Goodale M. A. and Milner, A. D. (1992). Separate visual pathways for perception and action. *Trends in Neuroscience*, **15**(1):20–5.

Handy, T. C., Jha, A. P., and Mangun, R. G. (1999). Promoting novelty in vision: Inhibition of return modulates perceptual-level processing. *Psychological Science*, **10**, 157–61.

Hawkins, H. L., Shafto, M. G., and Richardson, K. (1988). Effects of target luminance and cue validity on the latency of visual detection. *Perception & Psychophysics*, **44**, 484–92.

Hawkins, H. L., Hillyard, S. A., Luck, S. J., Mouloua, M., Downing, C. J., and Woodward, D. P. (1990). Visual attention modulates signal detectability. *Journal of Experimental Psychology: Human Perception and Performance*, **16**, 802–11.

Helmholtz, H. (1890). *Helmholtz's treatise on physiological optics*. J. P. C. Southhall (Ed., 1962) Dover: New York.

Hochstein, S. and Ahissar, M. (2002). View from the top: hierarchies and reverse hierarchies in the visual system. *Neuron*, **36**, 791–804.

Hunt, A. R. and Kingstone, A. (2003a). Covert and overt visual orienting: Linked or independent? *Cognitive Brain Research*, **18**, 102–5.

Hunt, A. R. and Kingstone, A. (2003b). Inhibition of return: dissociating attentional and oculomotor components. *Journal of Experimental Psychology: Human Perception and Performance*, **29**, 1068–74.

Hunt, A. R. and Klein, R. M. (2002). Eliminating the costs of task set reconfiguration. *Memory and Cognition*, **30**, 529–39.

Hunt, A.R., Ishigami, Y. and Klein, R.M. (2006). Eye movements, not hypercompatible mappings, are critical for eliminating the cost of task set reconfiguration. *Psychonomic Bulletin and Review*, **13**, 932–93.

Hunt, A. R., von Mühlenen, A., and Kingstone, A. (2007). The time course of attentional and oculomotor capture reveals a common cause. *Journal of Experimental Psychology: Human Perception and Performance*, **33**, 271–84.

Ivanoff, J. and Klein, R. M. (2006). Inhibition of return: sensitivity and criterion as a function of response time. *Journal of Experimental Psychology: Human Perception and Performance*, **32**, 908–19

Kastner, S. and Ungerleider, L. G. (2000). Mechanisms of visual attention in the human cortex. *Annual Review of Neuroscience*, **23**, 315–41.

Klein, R. M. (1980). Does oculomotor readiness mediate cognitive control of visual attention? In R. Nickerson (Ed.) *Attention and Performance VIII* (pp.259–76). Hillsdale, NJ: Lawrence Erlbaum Associates.

Klein, R. M. (2000). Inhibition of return. *Trends in Cognitive Sciences*, **4**, 138–47.

Klein, R. M., & Taylor, T. L. (1994). Categories of cognitive inhibition, with reference to attention. In D. Dagenbach & T. H. Carr (Eds.), *Inhibitory processes in attention, memory, and language* (pp. 113–150). San Diego, CA: Academic Press.

Lamme, V. A. F. and Roelfsema, P. R. (2000). The distinct modes of vision offered by feedforward and recurrent processing. *Trends in Neuroscience*, **23**, 571–9.

Li, Z. (1999). Contextual influences in V1 as a basis for pop out and asymmetry in visual search. *Proceedings of the National Academy of Sciences*, **96**, 10530–5.

Lu, C. H. and Proctor, R. W. (1994). The influence of irrelevant location information on performance: a review of the Simon and spatial Stroop effects. *Psychonomic Bulletin & Review*, **2**, 174–207.

Ludwig, C. J. H. and Gilchrist, I. D. (2002). Stimulus-driven and goal-driven control over visual selection. *Journal of Experimental Psychology: Human Perception and Performance*, **28**, 902–12.

Lupiáñez, J., Milán, E. G., Tornay, F. J., Madrid, E., and Tudela, P. (1997). Does IOR occur in discrimination tasks? Yes, it does, but later. *Perception & Psychophysics*, **59**, 1241–54.

Mangun, G. R. and Hillyard, S. A. (1987). The spatial allocation of visual attention as indexed by event-related brain potential. *Human Factors*, **29**, 195–211.

Moore, T. and Fallah, M. (2001). Control of eye movements and spatial attention. *Proceedings of the National Academy of Sciences*, **98**, 1273–6.

Moore, T. and Fallah, M. (2004). Microstimulation of the frontal eye fields and its effects on covert spatial attention. *Journal of Neurophysiology*, **91**, 152–62.

Murthy, A., Thompson, K.G., and Schall, J.D. (2001). Dynamic dissociation of visual selection from saccade programming in frontal eye field. *Journal of Neurophysiology*, **86**, 2634–7.

Pachella, R. G. (1974). The interpretation of reaction time in information-processing research. In B. H. Kantowitz (Ed.) *Human information processing: Tutorials in performance and cognition*, pp.41–82. Hillsdale, NJ: Lawrence Erlbaum Associates.

Pestilli, F. and Carrasco, M. (2005). Attention enhances contrast sensitivity at cued and impairs it at uncued locations. *Vision Research*, **45**, 1867–75.

Posner, M. I. (1978). *Chronometric Explorations of Mind*. Hillsdale, NJ: Lawrence Erlbaum Associates.

Posner, M. I. and Cohen, Y. (1984). Component of visual orienting. In H. Bouma and D. Bonwhuis (Eds.) *Attention and Performance X*, pp.551–6. Hillsdale, NJ: Erlbaum.

Posner, M. I., Cohen, A. and Rafal, R. D. (1982). Neural systems control of spatial orienting. *Proceedings of the Royal Society of London, B*, **298**, 187–98.

Posner, M. I., Snyder, C. R., and Davidson, B. J. (1980). Attention and the detection of signals. *Journal of Experimental Psychology: Human Perception and Performance*, **109**, 160–74.

Prime, D. J. and Ward, L. M. (2006). Cortical expressions of inhibition of return. *Brain Research*, **1072**, 161–74.

Reuter-Lorenz, P.A., Jha, A.P., and Rosenquist, J.N. (1996). What is inhibited in inhibition of return? *Journal of Experimental Psychology: Human Perception and Performance*, **22**, 367–78.

Rizzolatti, G., Riggio, L., Dascola, I., and Umilta, C. (1987). Reorienting attention across the horizontal and vertical meridians: evidence in favor of a premotor theory of attention. *Neuropsychologia*, **25**, 31–40.

Ross L. E. and Ross, S. M. (1980). Saccade latency and warning signals: stimulus onset, offset, and change as warning events. *Perception & Psychophysics*, **27**, 251–7.

Ross, S. M. and Ross, L. E. (1981). Saccade latency and warning signals: effects of auditory and visual stimulus onset and offset. *Perception & Psychophysics*, **29**, 429–37.

Saslow, M. G. (1967). Effects of components of displacement-step stimuli upon latency of saccadic eye movements. *Journal of the Optical Society of America*, **57**, 1024–9.

Schacter, D. and Buckner, R. (1998). Priming and the brain. *Neuron* **20**, 185–95.

Serences, J. T., Schwarzbach, J., Courtney, S. M., Golay, X., and Yantis, S. (2004). Control of object-based attention in human cortex. *Cerebral Cortex*, **14**, 1346–57.

Shepard, R. N. and Metzler, J. (1971). Mental rotation of three-dimensional objects. *Science*, **171**, 701–3.

Simon, J. R., Small, A. M., Jr., Ziglar, R. A., and Craft, J. L. (1970). Response interference in an information processing task: Sensory versus perceptual factors. *Journal of Experimental Psychology*, **85**, 311–14.

Song, J. H. and Nakayama, K. (2007). Automatic adjustment of visuomotor readiness. *Journal of Vision*, **7**, 1–9.

Sternberg, S. (1969). Memory-scanning: Mental processes revealed by reaction-time experiments. *American Scientist*, **57**, 421–57.

Sumner, P. (2006). Inhibition vs. attentional momentum in cortical and collicular mechanisms of IOR. *Cognitive Neuropsychology*, **23**, 1035–48.

Sperling, G. and Weichselgartner, E. (1995). Episodic theory of the dynamics of spatial attention. *Psychological Review*, **102**, 503–32.

Taylor, T. L. and Klein, R. M. (1998). On the causes and effects of inhibition of return. *Psychonomic Bulletin and Review*, **5**, 625–43.

Theeuwes, J., Kramer, A. F., Hahn, S., and Irwin, D. E. (1998). The eyes do not always go where we want them to go: Capture of the eyes by new objects. *Psychological Science*, **9**, 379–85.

Treisman, A. M. and Sato, S. (1990). Conjunction search revisited. *Journal of Experimental Psychology: Human Perception and Performance*, **16**, 451–78.

Van Voorhis, S. and Hillyard, S. A. (1977). Visual evoked potentials and selective attention to points in space. *Perception & Psychophysics*, **22**, 54–62.

van Zoest, W. and Donk, M. (2005). The effects of salience on saccadic target selection. *Visual Cognition*, **2**, 353– 75.

van Zoest, W., Donk, M., and Theeuwes, J. (2004). The role of stimulus-driven control in saccadic visual selection. *Journal of Experimental Psychology: Human Perception and Performance*, **30**, 746–59.

Wolfe, J.M., Cave, K.R., and Franzel, S.L. (1989). Guided search: An alternative to the feature integration model for visual search. *Journal of Experimental Psychology: Human Perception and Performance*, **15**, 419–33.

Wu, S. and Remington, R.W. (2003). Characteristics of covert and overt visual orienting: Evidence from attentional and oculomotor capture. *Journal of Experimental Psychology: Human Perception & Performance*, **29**, 1050–67.

Yeshurun, Y. and Carrasco, M. (1998). Attention improves or impairs visual performance by enhancing spatial resolution. *Nature*, **396**, 72–5.

Zhaoping, L. and Guyader, N. (2007). Interference with bottom-up feature detection by higher-level object recognition. *Current Biology*, 17, 26–31.

Chapter 2

Inhibition of return

Juan Lupiáñez

Orienting of attention selectively to the most important location and/or object is crucial for an appropriate interaction with our environment, especially under time pressure. We have therefore developed different attentional mechanisms to accomplish this goal, some of them relying on top-down expectancies (endogenous attention), and others relying on salient characteristics of the environment, which automatically capture attention (exogenous attention) (see Ruz and Lupiáñez, 2002a,b, for reviews). The cost and benefit paradigm, developed by Posner and colleagues (Posner, 1980), has been widely used to study these two mechanisms for the covert orienting of spatial attention. Typically, participants respond to a target presented on a computer screen that is preceded by a spatial cue, which indicates in advance one of the potential target locations (see Figure 2.1). A peripheral onset in one of the potential target locations is used in paradigms aimed at studying exogenous orienting, whereas a centrally presented symbolic cue (e.g. an arrow, a letter, a number, or any other arbitrary symbol) indicating one of the peripheral target locations is normally used in endogenous orienting paradigms. The target can be presented at the same location as the cue, or at a different location. The first case is called the *valid* or *cued-location* condition, whereas the latter is called the *invalid* or *uncued-location* condition. The valid–invalid terminology is typically used with endogenous orienting of attention, as cues are predictive of target location (i.e. they indicate the potential target location with an above-chance probability; e.g. 80% of trials are valid for only 20% invalid), whereas the cued–uncued location terminology is more commonly used with exogenous attention, in which cues usually are not predictive of target location (i.e. 50% of cued and uncued trials).

Importantly, orienting attention in space takes time, which is studied by manipulating the temporal interval, or stimulus onset asynchrony (SOA), between the spatial cue and the target. In fact, exogenous and endogenous orienting have been shown to differ in a variety of ways, perhaps the most important being their time course. Endogenous orienting of attention takes some time to develop so that its facilitatory effects (faster and/or more precise responses at the valid as compared to the invalid location) do not reach asymptote until after 300ms (Müller and Rabbitt, 1989) but, once attention is oriented, facilitation is present for quite long SOAs (at least up to one second). The effects of exogenous orienting have a completely different time course; whereas the facilitatory effect develops much more quickly (it reaches the asymptote by 150ms SOA; Müller and Rabbitt, 1989), the effect reverses after a few hundred milliseconds, so that responses at longer SOAs are slower at the exogenously cued location, as compared to the uncued locations. This effect was first reported by Posner and Cohen (1984), and subsequently named *inhibition of return* (IOR) by Posner et al. (1985), who considered it to reflect an inhibitory bias against returning attention to previously attended locations (see Klein, 2000; and Lupiáñez et al., 2006, for recent reviews).

The IOR mechanism has been shown to operate at environmental rather than retinotopic coordinates (Posner and Cohen, 1984; Maylor and Hockey, 1985), and on both location- and

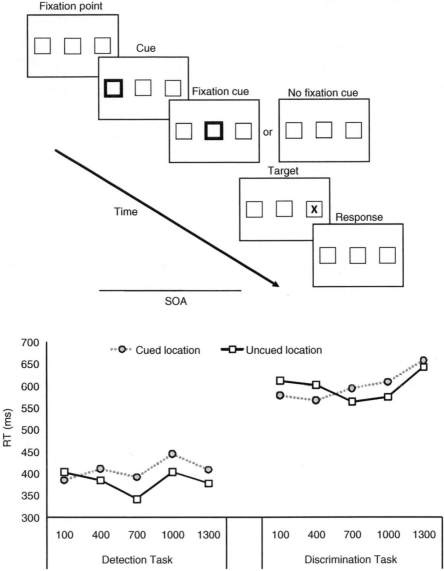

Fig. 2.1 An outline of the standard procedure used to investigate exogenous cueing effects is represented in the top panel. The target can be presented in one of two lateral boxes, while participants are fixating the central box (sometimes this central box is substituted by a dot or a cross, which serves as fixation point). At a variable interval before the target is presented a cue is presented in one of the two peripheral boxes (usually an increment in luminance in the box outline). The target can appear either in the cued or the uncued box, and participants are required to hit a key as soon as it appears (detection task), or one of different keys depending on one target feature (i.e. colour, shape, etc.; discrimination tasks). As shown in the bottom panel (data used with permission from Lupiáñez et al., 1997), the cueing effect shifts from facilitation, observed at short SOAs, to the inhibition of return (IOR) observed at longer stimulus onset asynchronies (SOAs). The point in time at which this transition occurs depends on different factors, mainly on task set: IOR occurs only at longer SOAs in discrimination as compared to detection tasks. Some studies have

Fig. 2.1 (*continued*) incorporated a cue at fixation between the peripheral cue and the target, as in the seminal paper by Posner and Cohen (1984). This fixation cue seems to have no effect on detection tasks, whereas it anticipates the appearance of IOR in discrimination tasks (Prime et al., 2006). Although most researchers have attributed to the fixation cue an important role in disengaging attention from the cued location, it might rather have an important role in how the cue and target representations are treated as the same versus different events (see text for details).

object-based representations (Tipper et al., 1991; Weaver et al., 1998). Thus, responses are slower to targets appearing at the location where a cue was previously presented even when the eyes are moved during the cue–target interval (so that cue and target fall in different positions on the retina), and to targets appearing in cued objects even when the object changes location between cue and target presentation. This has been critical for propounding the IOR as a foraging facilitator, subserving visual search (Klein, 1988; Klein and MacInnes, 1999) (but see Hooge et al., 2005).

This robust IOR effect was first considered to depend upon a hard-wired mechanism, developed to help foraging and search of relevant targets by favouring the inspection of new locations at the detriment of recently explored ones (Posner et al., 1985). However, later research has shown that only under specific conditions is IOR a robust and inflexible effect; mainly when simple detection tasks are used to measure it. In fact, IOR is much stronger in simple detection tasks, and its time course is highly dependent on the task at hand (Lupiáñez et al., 1997). Basically, the time taken for the IOR to appear increases according to the perceptual demands and the sensory-motor complexity of the task (Lupiáñez et al., 2001a; Khatoon et al., 2002). Thus, IOR is now considered to be a rather flexible mechanism with a variable time course depending on different factors.

In any case, the view of IOR as the inhibition of the return of attention to previously attended locations has been maintained until now, and is surely accepted by most researchers in the field, despite mounting contradictory evidence (Berlucchi et al., 2000; Lupiáñez et al., 2004; Rafal et al., 2006) or recent claims for a better name and a different mechanism to explain the effect (Berlucchi, 2006). The aim of the present chapter is to advance our knowledge about the mechanisms underlying IOR. Particular emphasis will be given to the relationship between IOR and the function of disengaging attention, and the effects of task-set on the time course of IOR.

Is inhibition of return due to the inhibition of the return of attention?

Giving such a theoretically suggestive name to the IOR effect has contributed enormously to the confusion between the behavioural *effect* that is measured (i.e. slower responses to targets appearing at previously cued versus uncued locations), and the *mechanism* that is responsible for the effect. The problem is that not much research has been dedicated to understanding the mechanism that produces the IOR effect, as the mechanism suggested by the name of the effect (i.e. the inhibition of the return of attention to previously attended locations) has simply been taken for granted.

Hence, after discovering that the effect in perceptually difficult discrimination tasks only appeared at longer SOAs (Lupiáñez et al., 1997), it was assumed that, for whatever reason, attention might be disengaged from the cued location later in discrimination than in detection tasks (Klein, 2000; Lupiáñez et al., 2001a). Similarly, when IOR was induced to appear at shorter cue-target SOAs (Danziger and Kingstone, 1999; Dodd and Pratt, 2007) its early appearance was interpreted as a consequence of rapid disengagement from the cued location.

Perhaps another reason for accepting the inhibition-of-the-return-of-attention mechanism, is that exogenous and endogenous orienting have traditionally been considered as two ways of orienting a single attentional mechanism (i.e. two ways of 'transporting' the attentional mechanism; Klein and Shore, 2000), rather than as two independent attentional mechanisms. By making this assumption, we would not expect IOR to be observed until attention has been disengaged from the cued location, as attention could not both be oriented towards, and inhibited from returning to, exactly the same location. In other words, the disengagement of attention has been considered a necessary and sufficient condition for IOR to be observed. Therefore, for example, in order to explain the aforementioned discrepancy in IOR effect during detection versus discrimination tasks, it was proposed that task set must affect the speed with which attention is disengaged from the cued location, viz. faster for detection than for discrimination tasks (Klein, 2000).

However, Lupiáñez and Chica (submitted), among others, have recently shown that disengaging attention might be neither necessary nor sufficient for the IOR effect to be observed. On the one hand, IOR can be observed at the location to where endogenous attention is oriented, showing that disengaging attention is not necessary. On the other hand, in some situations, IOR is not observed even after disengaging attention from the cued location (i.e. disengaging attention is not sufficient). Puzzling as they might appear, these kinds of results have been known for a long time in the field, although they have only recently drawn interest from researchers.

Is disengagement of attention necessary for IOR?

The first time I encountered data regarding the independence of IOR from attentional orienting was in a book chapter by Rafal and Henik (1994). Although this paper was not specifically on IOR, one section reported some unpublished data by Berger. She used a paradigm in which a predictive central cue was crossed with a peripheral non-predictive cue, in order to independently manipulate endogenous and exogenous attention, respectively. The target was preceded by a central arrow at fixation predicting one of the two possible target locations (i.e. two boxes, one at each side of fixation), followed by a non-predictive peripheral cue. In this way, it was possible to investigate both the effects of exogenous attention (i.e. facilitation and IOR) and endogenous attention (i.e. costs and benefits), as both predictive and neutral cues were used.

Importantly, it was also possible to test whether exogenous and endogenous attention were independent or, instead, interacted with one another. The pattern of results could not be clearer. The usual costs and benefits of endogenous attention were observed (i.e. slower reaction time [RT] for invalid than neutral trials, and faster RT for valid than neutral trials), suggesting that attention was oriented to the location predicted by the central cue. In parallel, non-predictive peripheral cues led to significant facilitation at short SOAs and IOR at long SOAs. More importantly, the effects of the central predictive and the peripheral non-predictive cues were completely independent from one another. Crucially, significant IOR was observed on endogenously valid trials, i.e. when the target appeared at the location to which attention was oriented and maintained (Figure 2.2; BHR-JEPG-Exp1). In other words, IOR was observed at a location from which attention was not disengaged. I can imagine the authors were as perplexed by this result as I was when I first read their book chapter. This might explain why the results were not published until 10 years later (Berger et al., 2005; note that the results reported in the book chapter correspond to the first experiment of this paper).

Later, Berlucchi and colleagues (Berlucchi et al., 2000) reported an experiment in which they asked participants, in different conditions, either to attend endogenously to one of four locations at which the target could appear, or to divide attention equally across all four locations.

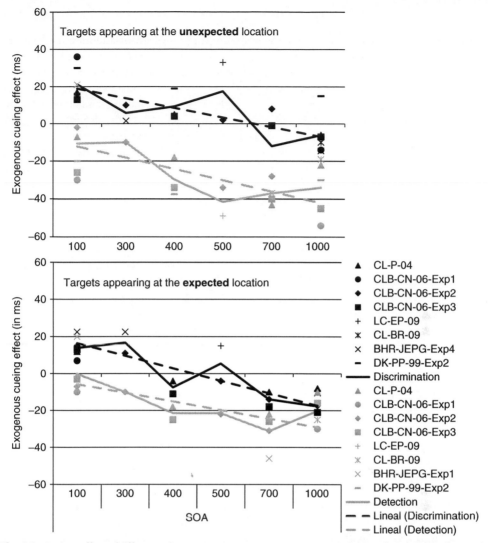

Fig. 2.2 Cueing effects (difference between responses to targets appearing at the peripherally cued versus uncued locations), observed in different experiments, plotted as a function of task, stimulus onset asynchrony (SOA), and spatial orienting of attention. The reported cueing effects reported in the top panel are for targets appearing at the unexpected location. Those reported in the bottom panel are for targets appearing at the expected location, i.e. to where attention has been supposedly disengaged and to where it must return. Note that similar time-courses are observed for each task, independently of attentional orienting. Nevertheless, the cueing effect is more negative (less positive) for detection than for discrimination tasks. Also, differences between detection and discrimination are larger at the unexpected location. Finally, note that at long SOAs (mainly with detection tasks) inhibition of return (IOR) is observed at the expected location, to which attention is supposed to be oriented before the target appears, and therefore to where attention does not have to reorient or return (i.e. disengaging of attention seems to be unnecessary); in contrast, facilitation rather than IOR can be observed in discrimination tasks at the unexpected location, therefore at the location from where attention has been disengaged (i.e. disengaging of attention seems not to be sufficient). Note: CL-P-04: Chica and Lupiáñez (2004); CLB-CN-06: Chica et al. (2006); LC-EP-08: Lupiáñez and Chica (2009); CL-BR-09: Chica and Lupiáñez (2009); BHR-JEPG: Berger et al. (2005); DK-PP-99: Danziger and Kingstone (1999).

Importantly, in one condition, participants were instructed to pay attention exactly to the location at which a non-predictive peripheral cue was presented. Therefore, it was expected that participants would not disengage attention from this location. The results were again clear-cut. First, participants were much faster when the target was presented at the location to which they were attending. Second, and more importantly, IOR was observed equally in all conditions, including the condition where the target was presented at the location to which participants were attending, and therefore from where they had not disengaged attention.

From a historical point of view, it is worth noting that Posner and colleagues (Posner et al., 1982) had already reported an experiment with similar data. They used a paradigm in which the cue predicted the target to appear either at the same or the opposite location as the cue. The authors emphasized the fact that the appearance of the cue produced an early facilitatory effect even though the cue predicted target appearance at the opposite location. However, another important aspect of the data was neglected: IOR was also present when the target appeared at the position to which the participants were attending (i.e. the one predicted by the cue).

Recently, my colleagues and I (Lupiáñez et al., 2004) have used a similar experimental paradigm in order to investigate whether exogenous cueing effects (i.e. facilitation at short SOAs and IOR at long SOAs) are different at endogenously attended and unattended locations. In our study, participants performed three different blocks of trials. In one of the blocks the cue predicted that the target would appear at the cued location on 80% of trials. Therefore, the location of the target could, in this case, be either exogenously cued and endogenously expected, or exogenously uncued and endogenously unexpected. In another block, the cue predicted that the target would appear at the opposite uncued location on 80% of trials (uncued). Thus, this counter-predictive block was composed of trials with uncued but expected location, and trials with cued but unexpected location. Finally, in a third block of trials, the cue was not predictive (i.e. 50% cued and 50% uncued trials). Across the two blocks with predictive cues, the experiment has a factorial design with two factors: Expectancy, which indexed endogenous orienting of attention (i.e. expected versus unexpected location), and Spatial Cueing, which indexed exogenous attention effects (i.e. cued versus uncued location).

The pattern of results, one more time, could not be clearer. In the block with non-predictive cues, the usual transition from facilitation at short SOAs to IOR at long SOAs was observed. Exactly the same pattern of data (i.e. facilitation and IOR) was observed for targets appearing in blocks with predictive cues, at both expected and unexpected locations (see Riggio and Kirsner, 1997, for similar results for facilitation effects with exogenous cues and short SOA). Therefore, of direct relevance to the issues addressed in this chapter, IOR was observed at the location to which participants were attending, and therefore from where they should not have disengaged attention. Similar results have been observed with this paradigm more recently (Chica et al., 2006; 2007).

The same pattern was also observed by Chica and Lupiáñez (2004), when instead of using separate blocks of trials with predictive and counter-predictive cues, the two conditions were manipulated within the same block. In this experiment, the fixation point could take one of two shapes, '−' or '+', indicating that the target would appear either in the same location as the cue ('+') or at the opposite location ('−'). The same pattern of results was observed, i.e. significant IOR was measured at the location to which attention was endogenously oriented (Figure 2.2; CL-P-04 in both detection and discrimination). A similar result has also been observed by Theeuwes and colleagues, who observed slower saccadic eye-movement responses to cued versus uncued locations (IOR) for locations that were actively maintained in spatial working memory (Theeuwes et al., 2006). Thus it seems clear that it is not necessary to disengage attention from the peripherally cued location (or take it out of working memory) for IOR to develop at that location.

Is disengagement of attention sufficient for IOR?

It might be argued, that though not necessary, disengaging of attention could be sufficient for IOR to be observed. In other words, it might be that IOR can be observed even if attention is not disengaged from the cued location, but whenever it is disengaged from the cued location an IOR effect is observed. As first reported by Posner and Cohen (1984), even in detection tasks, it is usual to observe early facilitation at short SOAs with a fast transition to IOR at longer SOAs (Samuel and Kat, 2003). However, in many occasions, IOR has been observed without any hint of facilitation at shorter SOAs (Tassinari et al., 1994; Mele et al., 2008). In fact, contrary to what one might think, it is not very common to observe facilitation at short SOAs in detection tasks; instead, specific conditions are needed for it to be observed. For instance, it has been argued that facilitation is only observed with spatially non-overlapping cues (McAuliffe and Pratt, 2005) and temporally overlapping cues, i.e. when the cue duration is longer than the cue-target SOA (Collie et al., 2000). This may not apply to all situations, as significant facilitation has been reported without temporally overlapping cues (Lupiáñez et al., 1997), and no facilitation was observed in other paradigms that used temporally overlapping cues (Tassinari et al., 1994). Other factors might influence the facilitatory effect, such as: practice (Lupiáñez et al., 2001b), cue saliency (Mele et al., 2008), and presence of catch trials (Okamoto-Barth and Kawai, 2006). Based on these studies and other unpublished data from our lab, the optimal conditions for obtaining facilitation at short SOAs in spatial cueing detection tasks appear to involve: a paradigm with a short enough SOA (around 100ms), in which the cue and target are spatially easy to discriminate, target onset is easy to discriminate, participants are not practised, and the experiment is as short as possible.

The importance of these considerations is twofold. On the one hand, the fact that IOR can occur in the absence of facilitation at short SOAs argues once more against the idea that IOR is due to the inhibition of attention returning to the previously 'visited' location. Furthermore, by understanding why facilitation is not easily observed in detection tasks, we can learn about the nature of the processes underlying facilitation and IOR effects. However, as stated earlier, rather than testing the relationship between facilitation and inhibition, most researchers assume a sequence of orienting and disengaging attention from one location. Explanations centre mainly on the speed with which these stages occur (this transition occurs). For example, it is argued that attention might be disengaged from the cued location earlier in detection than in discrimination tasks (Klein, 2000; Lupiáñez et al., 2001a), or that participants are more motivated to disengage attention from the cued location when catch trials are included—Okamoto-Barth and Kawai (2006) note that most paradigms with detection task include catch trials. In the same vein, one could argue that longer-lasting, temporally overlapping cues might lead participants to maintain attention at the cued location for a longer time (until target appearance), or that participants learn to disengage attention more quickly with practice.

Danziger and Kingstone (1999) went further and directly tested the hypothesis that IOR can be observed at shorter intervals (as short as 50ms) provided that attention is quickly disengaged from the cued location. In their first experiment they used a paradigm with four target locations, suitable for observing facilitation in detection tasks (e.g. temporally overlapping cues were used). They manipulated three experimental conditions. In one of them the cue was non-predictive, whereas in another one the cue predicted the target to appear at the cued location. Facilitation was observed at the short SOA (50ms), independently of whether the cue was predictive or not. However, they tested a third interesting condition where the cue predicted that the target would appear at the location one position clockwise from the cued location. Of course, RT was faster if the target appeared at the predicted location, as compared to a different, uncued location.

This finding confirmed that attention had been oriented to the predicted location, and was therefore disengaged from the cued location. The striking result was that IOR was now observed at the cued location at this short SOA. The authors concluded that the rapid disengagement of attention from the cued location unmasked the IOR effect at an SOA as short as 50ms. Accordingly, since its publication, this paper has been highly cited as a key result supporting the idea that attentional disengagement is sufficient for IOR to be observed.

However, this interpretation is inconsistent with the results of the second experiment reported in Danziger and Kingstone's (1999) paper. They tried to replicate the pattern of results with a different task, which exactly reproduced the critical conditions of the first experiment. In this case, the target was either an upright or inverted uppercase letter 'T', whose orientation participants had to discriminate. With the detection task the same pattern of results was replicated: IOR was observed at the SOA of 50ms provided that attention was disengaged from the cued location (Figure 2.2; DK-PP-99 detection). However, with the discrimination task, significant facilitation was observed at the cued location independently of whether attention had already moved to the expected, adjacent location (Figure 2.2; DK-PP-99 discrimination).

Thus, if we take into account the whole pattern of data, we must conclude that it is not IOR that is unmasked by the disengagement of attention but the cueing effect, which can be either facilitation or IOR, depending on whether a detection or discrimination task is used to measure it. We must also conclude that disengaging attention from the cued location is not sufficient for IOR to be observed. Similar results have been observed by different authors using different paradigms (Riggio and Kirsner, 1997; Chica and Lupiáñez, 2004; Berger et al., 2005; Chica et al., 2006; Lupiáñez and Chica, submitted).

Disengagement of attention and the time course of IOR

Figure 2.2 illustrates the exogenous cueing effect reported in different papers in which the effect of peripheral cues has been measured at different SOAs. Results are plotted separately for detection and discrimination tasks, and for targets appearing at the expected location (where attention is engaged) and unexpected location (from where attention is disengaged).

Several conclusions can be extracted from this figure. It illustrates that disengagement of attention is neither necessary nor sufficient for IOR to be observed. The first part of this statement can be clearly confirmed by looking at data from the expected-location condition. IOR is consistently observed (mainly in detection tasks). The second part of the statement is supported by examining the data from the unexpected-location condition. Facilitation is observed, instead of IOR, in the 100–500ms SOA range in the discrimination task (all points are on the positive side of the scale).

However, the most important conclusion to be extracted from Figure 2.2 concerns the time course of IOR. First, there seems to be a biphasic effect of cueing, with a clear transition from facilitation to IOR, which is independent of the endogenous orienting of attention. A similar time course is observed for targets appearing at expected and unexpected locations. Second the cueing effect is more negative (less positive) when it is measured with a detection task, than when it is measured with a discrimination task. Importantly, task differences in the cueing effect cannot be account for by differences in the speed with which attention is oriented to, or disengaged from, the cued location, since attentional orienting was controlled in all experiments represented in Figure 2.2.

In my opinion, understanding the features of the peripheral cueing effects that are represented in this figure, both facilitation and IOR, is crucial for disentangling the cognitive mechanisms that underlie attentional capture and IOR. However, in order to be able to understand these mechanisms it seems critical not to conflate the behavioural effects that are measured and the mechanisms that produce the effects.

IOR and exogenous versus endogenous attention

Given the aforementioned evidence, we can conclude that both facilitation and IOR at peripherally cued locations can be observed independently of the endogenous orienting of attention. Decidedly, this pattern of results cannot be explained if we assume a) that exogenous and endogenous attention are simply two ways of orienting the spatial attention mechanism, as suggested by the spotlight metaphor (Cave and Bichot, 1999), or b) that the IOR effect results from inhibiting attention from returning to a previously visited location. Therefore, either exogenous and endogenous attention involve independent mechanisms, or IOR is not due to the inhibition of the return of attention.

A variety of different attentional paradigms have shown that exogenous and endogenous attention can be clearly dissociated (Klein and Shore, 2000; Klein, 2004; for reviews, see Funes et al., 2007). For example, Briand and Klein (Briand and Klein, 1987; Briand, 1998) found that peripheral (exogenous) cues conferred larger facilitation during visual search for conjunctions than for features, whereas central (endogenous) cues led to similar effects for conjunction and feature search. In addition, exogenous, but not endogenous, orienting has been shown to induce some perceptual illusions (e.g. the Illusory Line Motion) (Christie and Klein, 2005; Chica et al., 2008), as well as prior-entry effects in temporal order judgements (Shore et al., 2001; Spence, Chapter 7, this volume). Perhaps the clearest results were observed by Funes and colleagues (Funes et al., 2007), who reported a double dissociation between exogenous and endogenous orienting in the context of a spatial Stroop task. Whereas exogenous orienting by non-predictive peripheral cues reduced the spatial Stroop effect, especially at short SOAs, endogenous orienting by predictive central cues increased it, especially at longer SOAs. This pattern of results has been interpreted as evidence that separate attentional systems are triggered by exogenous and endogenous cues, rather than the same system being oriented at different speeds.

Supporting this dissociation, although endogenous disengagement seems to be unrelated to IOR, Prime et al. (2006) have shown that *exogenous* disengagement might lead to IOR. They showed that, in a discrimination task, interposing a cue at fixation between the peripheral cue and the target led to the appearance of IOR, which was not observed if no fixation cue was presented (the fixation cue had no effect on detection and localization tasks, however). We also observed facilitation if no fixation cue was presented, but IOR if it was presented, in a shape discrimination task (Lupiáñez and Chica, submitted). Most researchers in the field will agree that the role of the fixation cue in revealing IOR is consistent with 'its putative role in re-orienting attention away from the cued location' (Prime et al., 2006, p.1310). Several other studies, using both discrimination and detection tasks and in special populations, have shown that IOR is more robust or appears earlier when a cue is presented at fixation, which is interpreted as a central reorienting event, or as a 'cue back' condition (Faust and Balota, 1997; Sapir et al., 2001; Pratt and Fischer, 2002; MacPherson et al., 2003). Similarly, after a peripheral gaze cue (i.e. a face presented at fixation looking left or right), IOR is only observed when attention is exogenously disengaged by the presentation of a fixation cue, not by a change in the direction of the gaze (Frischen et al., 2007, Frischen and Tipper, 2004).

Given that fixation cues are interpreted to disengage attention exogenously, and considering that endogenous disengagement is not sufficient for IOR to be observed (see earlier discussion), it could be argued that only after attention is exogenously disengaged, can IOR be observed, as attention would be exogenously inhibited to return to the cued location even if it was endogenously oriented there. However, this argument would not explain why endogenous disengagement is sufficient in detection tasks, as fixation cues have typically no effect on the IOR effect in the normal population when the effect is measured with detection tasks. Therefore, a different approach should be taken to understand IOR and the role of fixation cues in 'disengaging attention'.

A new framework for understanding peripheral cueing effects

Some authors have used dual-process approaches to explain IOR. Thus, Tipper and colleagues (1997) and Khatoon, et al. (2002; see also Klein, 2000), considered cueing effects to be the addition of two cueing components: decreasing facilitation and increasing inhibition across SOA. According to these authors, different mechanisms increase (facilitation) or decrease (inhibition) the activation of the cue location/object representation over time. When the target appears, the cueing effect that is measured (facilitation or IOR) would depend on whether the net activation is positive or negative.

However, this approach does not explain why even after controlling for any factor related to the processing of the cue and subsequent orient–reorienting processes triggered by it, either facilitation or IOR can be measured depending on task requirements, as we have recently shown (Lupiáñez et al., 2007). In our study, the target could be, for example, an 'X' which was presented in 75% of the trials, and participants were to press a single key when they detected its appearance. We expected participants to adopt an attentional set to detect these targets. In the remaining 25% of the trials, however, either an 'O' or a 'U' could be presented, and participants were to discriminate them by pressing one of two keys. Importantly, the type of target was manipulated within the same block of trials in order to control for any process occurring before target appearance (i.e. attentional capture by the cue and subsequent orienting–reorienting of attention). However, opposite cueing effects were observed for each type of target: whereas significant IOR was observed for the to-be-detected target, significant facilitation was observed for the to-be-discriminated targets. In order to explain this pattern of results a different approach must be taken, in which the same activation of a given location/object representation that is triggered by the cue is detrimental for some detection processes but beneficial for other discrimination processes.

In my opinion, attention is poorly captured by an abrupt onset when it appears at a location or object at which attention was previously captured. The mechanism hindering attentional capture might take place independently of whether attention is endogenously oriented to this location or not, as suggested by all of the experiments reviewed earlier. However, peripheral cueing must also lead to other effects, different from orienting–reorienting of attention and hindering of attentional capture. Figure 2.3 represents three hypothetical effects produced by peripheral cueing, which we have called *detection cost*, *spatial selection* benefit, and *spatial orienting* benefit (Lupiáñez et al., 2007; Lupiáñez and Chica, submitted). The effect ultimately measured in the RT would be the result of the net contribution of each of these effects to performance. Depending on task set and the nature of the target, some of these effects would contribute to performance more than others, leading to different time courses and sizes of the cueing effect (solid versus dashed black lines in Figure 2.3).

Peripheral cues trigger exogenous spatial orienting of attention, thus improving target perception and/or responses to it. However, this effect is short-lived. This '*spatial orienting*' process is the only one usually considered for explaining cuing effects. Therefore inhibitory processes (i.e. an inhibitory rebound or the inhibition of the reorienting of attention) are needed to explain the observed inhibitory after-effects (IOR). However, a peripheral cue is an event occupying a specific location, which can lead to other effects on the processing of subsequent stimuli appearing at the

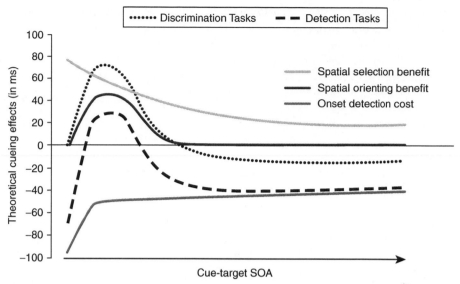

Fig. 2.3 (See also Plate 3) Theoretical cueing effects (in black) usually observed for detection and discrimination tasks as a function of cue-target stimulus onset asynchrony. The greyscale lines represent different cue-triggered processes underlying the cueing effects: spatial orienting of attention (dark grey), onset detection cost (mid grey), and spatial selection benefit (light grey). The different cueing effects for the two tasks are computed as differential contributions of each process to detection and discrimination tasks. Basically, whereas onset detection processes contribute mostly to detection tasks, spatial selection processes are tapped mainly by discrimination tasks.

same location. Targets appearing in close spatiotemporal proximity might be integrated within the same object file (Kahneman et al., 1992), thus being more easily selected for further analysis. Hence, the cue–target integration processes would facilitate processing by helping to select the target location in advance, an effect that is represented in Figure 2.3 as the '*spatial selection*' benefit.

Following the object-file view, if cue and target do not share any task-relevant features, cue–target integration should not interfere with the discrimination of target features, in the same way that the opening of an object file during the perception of a dot in the sky does not interfere with the final discrimination of the dot as a bird (or an airplane) once the object file is updated with subsequent information. However, in case of feature overlap, integration can lead to positive effects, when cue and target are the same object, or negative effects, when cue and target are different objects, as reported in different IOR experiments (Pratt and Abrams, 1999; Milliken et al., 2000; Taylor and Donnelly, 2002). Similar effects have been reported in the priming literature. Hommel and colleagues have consistently observed that when the same stimulus repeats, with exactly the same features and the same response associated to it, responses are faster than when no repetition occurs (complete match benefits). However, when some relevant features repeat but not others, responses are slower (partial match costs; see Hommel, 2004, for a review).

However, the integration of the target within the cue representation, as part of the same event, would produce a cost in detecting the onset of the target, which is represented in Figure 2.3 as the '*onset detection cost*'. To the extent that integration increases as the similarity between cue and target increases, this account would predict that greater costs should occur for detecting targets that were similar to cues (Lupiáñez and Weaver, 1998). Therefore, the explanation is in line with observations that IOR increases the closer to the cue the target is presented, in both space (Bennett and Pratt, 2001) and time (Tassinari et al., 1994, observed greater IOR with simultaneous presentation). The net facilitation or inhibition of responses to peripherally cued targets would result from the sum of spatial orienting, spatial selection benefits, and detection costs. Spatial selection benefits would be more pronounced in discrimination tasks whereas the detection costs would be more pronounced in detection tasks.

These different mechanisms triggered by peripheral cueing may be mediated differentially by different parts of the brain. In this context I find the recent dissociation between ventral and dorsal frontoparietal attentional networks proposed by Corbetta and Shulman to be particularly interesting (Corbetta and Shulman, 2002; Corbetta et al., 2008). In the more recent of these two proposals, they consider the dorsal network, formed by dorsal parietal regions, mainly the intraparietal sulcus (IPS) and superior parietal lobule (SPL), and dorsal frontal cortex regions around the frontal eye field (FEF), responsible for spatial orienting and maintenance of attention. Importantly, they consider this network to be responsible for both stimulus driven (i.e. exogenous) attention and endogenous attention. Perhaps these two ways of orienting attention might underlie the benefits represented in Figure 2.3. Spatial orienting benefits might reflect the spatial orienting of attention, which could be generated either on the basis of endogenous spatial expectations or saliency of external stimuli. Whether this spatial orienting of attention is maintained over time or not will depend on the informative value of the orienting cues. However, it is important to note that, independently of attentional orienting, spatial selection can also be autonomously triggered by stimulus–stimulus interaction processes. Cue–target integration processes (spatial selection benefits in Figure 2.3) might underlie stimulus-driven selection through interactive competition in perceptual areas (Desimone and Duncan, 1995). These two mechanisms might facilitate target selection in parallel by providing an initial advantage in the competition (stimulus driven cue–target integration processes), and by biasing the competition (attentional orienting), thus explaining additive effects in exogenous and endogenous orienting facilitation effects (Riggio and Kirsner, 1997).

Note, however, that if we only had a very good selective attention system (the dorsal attention network), we would be very good at processing only those objects or events that are of a priori interest to us. However, having only this system would be very inefficient, as we would be not able to confront unexpected stimuli, which might be relevant or dangerous, as they would be perfectly filtered out. In this case we need another system that automatically breaks the attentional circuit and prioritizes processing of new potentially relevant objects whenever they come into play. This alternative system is the ventral frontoparietal attentional network proposed by Corbetta and colleagues (Corbetta et al., 2008). This network includes the temporoparietal junction (TPJ) and regions of the ventral frontal cortex (VFC), and is considered to be important for detecting and reorienting to relevant events for which processing should be prioritized. What is called attentional capture in the attention literature (Ruz and Lupiáñez, 2002a,b) might be the triggering of the ventral frontoparietal network by salient relevant events. Of course, targets are especially relevant and this is why the frontoparietal network is especially activated by invalidly cued (i.e. unexpected) targets. However, peripheral abrupt onset cues might also be treated as potentially relevant by the system, especially in the context of a target detection task. Note that the same feature that defines a target in a detection task also defines a cue (i.e. its onset). Thus, I assume that peripheral onsets might somehow trigger the ventral frontoparietal attentional network, even if too transiently to be observed with low temporal resolution neuroimaging techniques, unless cues are predictive and attention is maintained there. Note however, that in this case, the network that would be activated would be the dorsal one, which is responsible for maintaining attention once it is captured (Kincade et al., 2005). In spite of its transient nature, this triggering of the ventral frontoparietal network by peripheral cues might be enough for it to habituate, so that when the target later appears at the same location it would not capture attention any more effectively than if it had appeared in a brand new location. This habituation of the ventral frontoparietal network after having just been triggered by a previous event (i.e. the cue in a cue-target IOR procedure; or the previous target, in a target–target IOR procedure) might underlie what I have called detection cost. The habituation of the detection system might be a consequence of reduced sensorial activity, as indexed by a reduced P1 component for valid targets in IOR experiments. In a recent study we have observed this effect (i.e. reduced P1) for targets appearing at peripherally cued locations, independently of whether they appeared at the expected or unexpected location (Chica and Lupiáñez, 2009).

At first glance, the detection cost proposal seems related to the framework outlined by Dukewich (2009), according to which IOR is due to habituation of the orienting response. Evidence favouring this account comes from studies in which one or more cues are consecutively presented in the same location, and IOR is greater the more cues are presented (Dukewich and Boehnke, 2008). In my opinion, if this approach considers that what is being habituated is the reorienting of attention to the cued location, it seems inconsistent with all the evidence described earlier in which IOR is completely dissociated from the spatial orienting of attention. However, it could be consistent if we consider that what is being habituated is not the orienting of attention in spatial terms, but rather more central orienting and detection, i.e. the prioritization of the target for ongoing behaviour. Following this logic, it could be predicted that less habituation would occur for highly relevant targets, so that no IOR would be observed with them. We have recently reported evidence supporting this prediction, as participants with high anxiety traits did not show IOR for emotionally negative words, whereas significant IOR was observed for neutral and positive words (Pérez-Dueñas et al., 2009). In a different study, no IOR was shown for fearful face targets, independently of anxiety state and trait, whereas significant IOR was observed for neutral and positive faces (Pérez-Dueñas et al., submitted).

In any case, as stated previously, this habituation process or detection cost would be only partially responsible for the effects of peripheral cues on target processing, as spatial orienting and spatial selection benefits would also contribute to performance. Furthermore, these processes might have different time courses, as shown in Figure 2.3. Whereas orienting of attention needs time to develop, both spatial selection and detection cost might be greater the closer in time the target is to the cue. Later on, the effects of these two processes would decay, although benefits due to spatial selection might decay to a greater extent and more quickly than the onset detection cost. The time course of spatial orienting can be easily manipulated by providing spatial information with the cue (attention would be disengaged earlier or later depending on whether the cue is predictive or counter-predictive). Note in Figure 2.2 that the cueing effect is more positive, and the differences between detection and discrimination are larger at the unexpected location, suggesting a more prominent role for spatial selection benefits and detection costs in this case.

The time course of detection cost and spatial selection processes might also be differentially modulated. It is important to note that the time course of IOR is barely modulated in detection tasks (only at very short intervals), whereas large modulations have been reported with discrimination tasks. IOR has been shown to emerge earlier when the target appears at the expected moment in time in discrimination tasks (Milliken et al., 2003), but independent measures of temporal orienting (see Correa, Chapter 26, this volume) and IOR have been observed in detection tasks (Los, 2004; Gabay and Henik, 2008). Similarly, the perceptual difficulty of the task and the presence of distractors (Lupiáñez et al., 2001a) greatly modulates the time course of cueing effects. In detection tasks the system seems to be strongly tuned to base performance almost exclusively on detection processes, so that the effect of peripheral cues is almost invariably negative. By contrast, in tasks in which further target processing is needed, the effect of the peripheral cue will be more or less positive or negative depending on the contribution of the mechanism responsible for spatial selection benefits. Variables traditionally considered to affect attentional maintenance or disengagement, such as cue–target temporal overlap (Collie et al., 2000) or fixation cues (Lupiáñez and Chica, submitted), might modulate this spatial selection process by, respectively, either helping or stopping cue target integration processes.

Finally, a distinctive feature of the proposal forwarded in this paper is that it is *activation* rather than inhibition that leads to the negative cueing effect, i.e. a cost in detecting the target. In other words, according to this view, responses to peripherally cued targets are not slower because attention is inhibited to return to them, but because attention is less effectively captured by them, as they are less new than uncued targets (Milliken, 2002; see also Eagleman, Chapter 11, this volume). And it is due to the lingering activation of the cue that cued location targets are considered less novel by the system. Dorris, et al. (2002) reported evidence supporting this interpretation. Monkeys performed a saccadic IOR task in which they had to foveate a peripheral target, which was preceded by a peripheral cue, while the activity of single neurons in the superior colliculus was recorded. Neurons of the superficial and intermediate layers of the superior colliculus, which showed IOR in their response to visual targets, were not inhibited at the time of target onset. Instead they showed above-baseline increases in activity. This above-baseline activation was enough to hinder the detection of the target as a new event. We have observed a similar result in a reaching task in which participants had to reach a previously cued versus uncued location. The basal electromyographic activation of the muscle responsible for the reaching action was recorded at the moment the target was presented, together with the time in which it was fully activated (reaction time), as well as the time that the reach was completed (contact time). Although reaction and contact time were slower at the cued location (i.e. IOR was observed), the arm ipsilateral to the cue showed increased, not reduced, activity as compared to the contralateral arm, at the moment the target was presented (Huertas et al., submitted).

Conclusions

By equating the name of the effect and the mechanism responsible for it, IOR (i.e. slower responses to targets presented at peripherally cued than uncued locations) has been considered to be the result of the inhibition of attention returning to a previously attended (cued) location. However, disengaging of attention from the cued location (and therefore the return to it) has been proven to be neither necessary nor sufficient for the IOR effect to be observed. A new framework for understanding exogenous cueing effects in general, and IOR in particular, is presented in this chapter. The onset of peripheral cues might trigger not only automatic orienting of attention, but also the activation of an object- or event-representation that is used to process the target (i.e. cue–target integration processes). This activation will benefit target discrimination processes (spatial selection benefit) but hinder onset-detection processes (detection cost). These processes have different time courses and are differently tapped by different tasks. Therefore, the cueing effect that is measured (facilitation or IOR) will depend on the cue-target SOA as well as on the task to be performed with the target.

References

Bennett, P. J. and Pratt, J. (2001). The spatial distribution of inhibition of return. *Psychological Science*, **12**, 76–80.

Berger, A., Henik, A., and Rafal, R. (2005). Competition between endogenous and exogenous orienting of visual attention. *Journal of Experimental Psychology: General*, **134**, 207–21.

Berlucchi, G. (2006). Inhibition of return: A phenomenon in search of a mechanism and a better name. *Cognitive Neuropsychology*, **23**, 1065–74.

Berlucchi, G., Chelazzi, L. and Tassinari, G. (2000). Volitional covert orienting to a peripheral cue does not suppress cue-induced inhibition of return. *Journal of Cognitive Neuroscience, 12*, 648–63.

Briand, K. A. (1998). Feature integration and spatial attention: More evidence of a dissociation between endogenous and exogenous orienting. *Journal of Experimental Psychology: Human Perception and Performance, 24*, 1243–56.

Briand, K. A. and Klein, R. M. (1987). Is Posner's "beam" the same as Treisman's "glue"?: on the relation between visual orienting and feature integration theory. *Journal of Experimental Psychology: Human Perception and Performance, 13*, 228–41.

Cave, K. R. and Bichot, N. P. (1999). Visuospatial attention: beyond a spotlight model. *Psychonomic Bulletin & Review, 6*, 204–23.

Chica, A. B. and Lupiáñez, J. (2004). Inhibition of return without return of attention. *Psicothema, 16*, 248–54.

Chica, A. B. and Lupiáñez, J. (2009). Effects of endogenous and exogenous attention on visual processing: An Inhibition of Return study. *Brain Research 1278*, 75–85.

Chica, A. B., Charras, P., and Lupiáñez, J. (2008). Endogenous attention and illusory line motion depend on task set. *Vision Research, 48*, 2251–9.

Chica, A. B., Lupiáñez, J., and Bartolomeo, P. (2006). Dissociating inhibition of return from endogenous orienting of spatial attention: Evidence from detection and discrimination tasks. *Cognitive Neuropsychology, 23*, 1015–34.

Chica, A. B., Sanabria, D., Lupiáñez, J. and Spence, C. (2007). Comparing intramodal and crossmodal cuing in the endogenous orienting of spatial attention. *Experimental Brain Research, 179*, 353–64.

Christie, J. and Klein, R. M. (2005). Does attention cause illusory line motion? *Percept Psychophys, 67*, 1032–43.

Collie, A., Maruff, P., Yucel, M., Danckert, J., and Currie, J. (2000). Spatiotemporal distribution of facilitation and inhibition of return arising from the reflexive orienting of covert attention. *Journal of Experimental Psychology: Human Perception and Performance 26*, 1733–45.

Corbetta, M. and Shulman, G. L. (2002). Control of goal-directed and stimulus-driven attention in the brain. *Nature Reviews Neuroscience, 3*, 201–15.

Corbetta, M., Patel, G., and Shulman, G. L. (2008). The reorienting system of the human brain: from environment to theory of mind. *Neuron, 58*, 306–24.

Danziger, S. and Kingstone, A. (1999). Unmasking the inhibition of return phenomenon. *Perception & Psychophysics, 61*, 1024–37.

Desimone, R. and Duncan, J. (1995). Neural mechanisms of selective visual attention. *Annual Review in Neurosciences, 18*, 193–222.

Dodd, M. D. and Pratt, J. (2007). Rapid onset and long-term inhibition of return in the multiple cuing paradigm. *Psychological Research, 71*, 576–82.

Dorris, M. C., Klein, R. M., Everling, S., and Munoz, D. P. (2002). Contribution of the primate superior colliculus to inhibition of return. *Journal of Cognitive Neuroscience, 14*, 1256–63.

Dukewich, K. R. (2009). Reconceptualizing inhibition of return as habituation of the orienting response. *Psychonomic Bulletin & Review, 16*, 238–51.

Dukewich, K. R. and Boehnke, S. E. (2008). Cue repetition increases inhibition of return. *Neuroscience Letters, 448*, 231–5.

Faust, M. E. and Balota, D. A. (1997). Inhibition of return and visuospatial attention in healthy older adults and individuals with dementia of the Alzheimer type. *Neuropsychology, 11*, 13–29.

Frischen, A. and Tipper, S. P. (2004). Orienting attention via observed gaze shift evokes longer term inhibitory effects: Implications for social interactions, attention, and memory. *Journal of Experimental Psychology: General, 133*, 516–33.

Frischen, A., Bayliss, A. P., and Tipper, S. P. (2007). Gaze cueing of attention: visual attention, social cognition, and individual differences. *Psychological Bulletin, 133*, 694–724.

Funes, M. J., Lupiáñez, J. and Milliken, B. (2007). Separate mechanisms recruited by exogenous and endogenous spatial cues: evidence from a spatial Stroop paradigm. *Journal of Experimental Psychology: Human Perception and Performance*, **33**, 348–62.

Gabay, S. and Henik, A. (2008). The effects of expectancy on inhibition of return. *Cognition*, **106**, 1478–86.

Hommel, B. (2004). Event files: feature binding in and across perception and action. *Trends in Cognitive Sciences*, **8**, 494–500.

Hooge, I. T., Over, E. A., Van Wezel, R. J., and Frens, M. A. (2005). Inhibition of return is not a foraging facilitator in saccadic search and free viewing. *Vision Research*, **45**, 1901–8.

Huertas, F., Funes, M. J., Castellote, J., and Lupiáñez, J. (submitted). Activation rather than inhibition leads to inhibition of return.

Kahneman, D., Treisman, A., and Gibbs, B. J. (1992). The reviewing of object files: object-specific integration of information. *Cognitive Psychology*, **24**, 175–219.

Khatoon, S., Briand, K. A., and Sereno, A. B. (2002). The role of response in spatial attention: direct versus indirect stimulus-response mappings. *Vision Research*, **42**, 2693–708.

Kincade, J. M., Abrams, R. A., Astafiev, S. V., Shulman, G. L., and Corbetta, M. (2005). An event-related functional magnetic resonance imaging study of voluntary and stimulus-driven orienting of attention. *Journal of Neuroscience*, **25**, 4593–604.

Klein, R. M. (1988). Inhibitory tagging system facilitates visual search. *Nature*, **334**, 430–1.

Klein, R. M. (2000). Inhibition of return. *Trends in Cognitive Sciences*, **4**, 138–47.

Klein, R. M. (2004). On the control of visual orienting. In Posner, M. I. (Ed.) *Cognitive neuroscience of attention*. New York, Guilford Press.

Klein, R. M. and MacInnes, W. J. (1999). Inhibition of return is a foraging facilitator in visual search. *Psychological Science*, **10**, 346–52.

Klein, R. M. and Shore, D. I. (2000). Relations among modes of visual orienting. In Monsell, S. and Driver, J. (Eds.) *Attention & Performance XVIII: Control of Cognitive Processes*. Cambridge: The MIT Press.

Los, S. A. (2004). Inhibition of return and nonspecific preparation: separable inhibitory control mechanisms in space and time. *Perception & Psychophysics*, **66**, 119–30.

Lupiáñez, J. and Chica, A. B. (submitted). Inhibition of return and attentional disengagement.

Lupiáñez, J. and Weaver, B. (1998). On the time course of exogenous cueing effects: a commentary on Tassinari et al. (1994). *Vision Res*, **38**, 1621–8.

Lupiáñez, J., Klein, R. M., and Bartolomeo, P. (2006). Inhibition of return: twenty years after. *Cognitive Neuropsychology*, **23**, 1003–14.

Lupiáñez, J., Milan, E. G., Tornay, F. J., Madrid, E., and Tudela, P. (1997). Does IOR occur in discrimination tasks? Yes, it does, but later. *Perception & Psychophysics*, **59**, 1241–54.

Lupiáñez, J., Milliken, B., Solano, C., Weaver, B., and Tipper, S. P. (2001a). On the strategic modulation of the time course of facilitation and inhibition of return. *Q J Exp Psychol A*, **54**, 753–73.

Lupiáñez, J., Weaver, B., Tipper, S. P., and Madrid, E. (2001b). The effects of practice on cueing in detection and discrimination tasks. *Psicológica*, **22**, 1–23.

Lupiáñez, J., Decaix, C., Sieroff, E., Chokron, S., Milliken, B., and Bartolomeo, P. (2004). Independent effects of endogenous and exogenous spatial cueing: inhibition of return at endogenously attended target locations. *Experimental Brain Research*, **159**, 447–57.

Lupiáñez, J., Ruz, M., Funes, M. J., and Milliken, B. (2007). The manifestation of attentional capture: facilitation or IOR depending on task demands. *Psychology Research*, **71**, 77–91.

MacPherson, A. C., Klein, R. M., and Moore, C. (2003). Inhibition of return in children and adolescents. *Journal of Experimental Child Psychology*, **85**, 337–51.

Maylor, E. A. and Hockey, R. (1985). Inhibitory component of externally controlled covert orienting in visual space. *Journal of Experimental Psychology: Human Perception and Performance*, **11**, 777–87.

McAuliffe, J. and Pratt, J. (2005). The role of temporal and spatial factors in the covert orienting of visual attention tasks. *Psychology Research*, **69**, 285–91.

Mele, S., Savazzi, S., Marzi, C. A., and Berlucchi, G. (2008). Reaction time inhibition from subliminal cues: is it related to inhibition of return? *Neuropsychologia*, **46**, 810–19.

Milliken, B. (2002). Commentary on Ruz and Lupiáñez's "A review of attention capture: On its automaticity and sensitivity to endogenous control". *Psicológica*, **23**, 355–356.

Milliken, B., Tipper, S. P., Houghton, G., and Lupiáñez, J. (2000). Attending, ignoring, and repetition: on the relation between negative priming and inhibition of return. *Perception & Psychophysics*, **62**, 1280–96.

Milliken, B., Lupiáñez, J., Roberts, M., and Stevanovski, B. (2003). Orienting in space and time: Joint contributions to exogenous spatial cuing effects. *Psychonomic Bulletin & Review*, **10**, 877–83.

Müller, H. J. and Rabbitt, P. M. (1989). Reflexive and voluntary orienting of visual attention: time course of activation and resistance to interruption. *Journal of Experimental Psychology: Human Perception and Performance*, **15**, 315–30.

Okamoto-Barth, S. and Kawai, N. (2006). The role of attention in the facilitation effect and another "inhibition of return". *Cognition*, **101**, B42–50.

Pérez-Dueñas, C., Acosta, A., and Lupiáñez, J. (submitted). Attentional capture hypothesis to faces in trait and state anxiety.

Pérez-Dueñas, C., Acosta, A., and Lupiáñez, J. (2009). Attentional capture and trait anxiety: evidence from inhibition of return. *Journal of Anxiety Disorders* **23**, 782–90

Posner, M. I. (1980). Orienting of attention. *The Quarterly Journal of Experimental Psychology*, **32**, 3–25.

Posner, M. I. and Cohen, Y. (1984). Components of visual orienting. In Bouma, H. and Bouwhuis, D. (Eds.) *Attention and Performance X*. London, Lawrence Erlbaum.

Posner, M. I., Cohen, Y., and Rafal, R. D. (1982). Neural systems control of spatial orienting. *Philosophical Transactions of the Royal Society of London B*, **298**, 187–98.

Posner, M. I., Rafal, R. D., Choate, L. S., and Vaughan, J. (1985). Inhibition of return: Neural basis and function. *Cognitive Neuropsychology*, **2**, 211–28.

Pratt, J. and Abrams, R. A. (1999). Inhibition of return in discrimination tasks. *Journal of Experimental Psychology: Human Perception and Performance*, **25**, 229–42.

Pratt, J. and Fischer, M. H. (2002). Examining the role of the fixation cue in inhibition of return. *Canadian Journal of Experimental Psychology: Revue Canadienne De Psychologie Experimentale*, **56**, 294–301.

Prime, D. J., Visser, T. A. W., and Ward, L. M. (2006). Reorienting attention and inhibition of return. *Perception & Psychophysics*, **68**, 1310–23.

Rafal, R. and Henik, A. (1994). The neurology of inhibition: Integrating controlled and automatic processes. In Dagenbach, D. and Carr, T. H. (Eds.) *Inhibitory Processes in Attention, Memory and Language*. San Diego, CA, Academic Press.

Rafal, R., Davies, J., and Lauder, J. (2006). Inhibitory tagging at subsequently fixated locations: Generation of "inhibition of return" without saccade inhibition. *Visual Cognition*, **13**, 308–23.

Riggio, L. and Kirsner, K. (1997). The relationship between central cues and peripheral cues in covert visual orientation. *Perception & Psychophysics*, **59**, 885–99.

Ruz, M. and Lupiáñez, J. (2002a). A review of attentional capture: on its automaticity and sensitivity to endogenous control. *Psicológica*, **23**, 283–309.

Ruz, M. and Lupiáñez, J. (2002b). Attentional capture and its manifestation on performance: New perspectives in the study of the attentional capture phenomena: Reply to comments. *Psicológica*, **23**, 366–9.

Samuel, A. G. and Kat, D. (2003). Inhibition of return: a graphical meta-analysis of its time course and an empirical test of its temporal and spatial properties. *Psychonomic Bulletin & Review*, **10**, 897–906.

Sapir, A., Henik, A., Dobrusin, M., and Hochman, E. Y. (2001). Attentional asymmetry in schizophrenia: disengagement and inhibition of return deficits. *Neuropsychology*, **15**, 361–70.

Shore, D. I., Spence, C., and Klein, R. M. (2001). Visual prior entry. *Psychological Science*, **12**, 205–12.

Tassinari, G., Aglioti, S., Chelazzi, L., Peru, A., and Berlucchi, G. (1994). Do peripheral non-informative cues induce early facilitation of target detection? *Vision Research*, **34**, 179–89.

Taylor, T. L. and Donnelly, M. P. (2002). Inhibition of return for target discriminations: the effect of repeating discriminated and irrelevant stimulus dimensions. *Perception & Psychophysics*, **64**, 292–317.

Theeuwes, J., Van der Stigchel, S., and Olivers, C. N. (2006). Spatial working memory and inhibition of return. *Psychonomic Bulletin & Review*, **13**, 608–13.

Tipper, S. P., Driver, J., and Weaver, B. (1991). Object-centred inhibition of return of visual attention. *Quarterly Journal of Experimental Psychology*, **A**, 289–98.

Tipper, S. P., Rafal, R., Reuterlorenz, P. A., Starrveldt, Y., Ro, T., Egly, R., and Danzinger, S. (1997). Object-based facilitation and inhibition from visual orienting in the human split-brain. *Journal of Experimental Psychology: Human Perception and Performance*, **23**, 1522–32.

Weaver, B., Lupiáñez, J., and Watson, F. L. (1998). The effects of practice on object-based, location-based, and static-display inhibition of return. *Perception & Psychophysics*, **60**, 993–1003.

Acknowledgements

This research was supported by the Spanish Ministerio de Educación y Ciencia (Research Projects SEJ2005-01313PSIC and PSI2008-03595PSIC).

Chapter 3

The attentional blink: temporal constraints on consciousness

Kimron L. Shapiro and Jane E. Raymond

Our subjective conscious experience is something akin to watching a continuous, carefully edited movie. It unfolds before us in what seems like an instantaneous, on-line, accurate representation of the external world. However, numerous examples (e.g. the absence of the perception of motion during a rapid eye movement), show that instead, consciousness is comprised of a series of highly interpreted representations of a few carefully selected objects in the external world. In the last 15 years or so, a large body of empirical data has made it increasingly clear that high-level mechanisms associated with selective attention severely limit the flow of information into the limited capacity of consciousness. In this chapter we address specifically how the temporal limits of selective attention work to constrain consciousness. Selective attention can be thought of as a set of neural mechanisms that facilitate the conscious perception of task-relevant information and inhibit the processing of task-irrelevant information. An important but often neglected aspect of task relevance in the context of selective attention is predictability. If, for example, an experimental task requires participants to identify a red letter, then, after a very few trials they can predict where targets are likely to appear (somewhere on a computer screen), how big the letters might be, the brightness and specific hue of the target, the range of other colours they will see, and so on. Predictability reduces the number of possible objects or events that could be considered to be task relevant and this leads to improved performance on a wide range of measures. Thus, predictability should aid selective attention and, indeed, numerous studies have shown this to be so (e.g. Miniussi et al., 1999). In the latter half of this chapter we explore this issue by reviewing some recent findings concerning the link between temporal predictability and limits of temporal attention.

We focus our discussion on the attentional blink. This behaviourally evident effect, first described by us (with Karen Arnell) in 1992 has produced a wealth of both empirical data and theoretical views that have greatly informed our understanding of the temporal constraints on conscious experience. The attentional blink is a demonstration that selection of information from an ongoing rapid serial visual presentation (RSVP) of images is episodic in nature. It shows that selection of a briefly presented and behaviourally relevant target (T1) usually results in a remarkably reduced ability to select a second behaviourally relevant target (T2), if that target is presented (and masked) within about a half second of the presentation of the (masked) first target (T1) (Raymond, Shapiro, and Arnell, 1992). The transient reduction in the ability to report T2 is called the attentional blink (AB).

There are a number of key features of this effect that have piqued the curiosity of cognitive neuroscientists and continue to raise interesting issues for understanding temporal constraints on consciousness. First, the effect is variable in that the AB does not occur on every trial. Average performance on the T2 task during the critical half-second AB interval rarely hits floor, meaning that on a significant proportion of trials T2 report reflects conscious awareness of the target.

A possible mechanism for this is discussed in the first of six empirical projects we review here. Second, the effect is not explicable by low-level sensory processes. Performance on the T2 task remains high throughout the AB interval if the T1 stimulus is no longer behaviourally relevant, even though it is physically, i.e. perceptually, salient. This points out that the effect is attentional in its basis and that top-down demands of the T1 stimulus play a key role in affecting subsequent processing. In relating this to predictability, we review three different experiments that manipulated aspects of predictability of the T1 stimulus. In addition, we explore a series of manipulations investigating not just predictability of a single element in the RSVP stream but the predictability of both the timing and spatial characteristics of the entire stream. Third, information in T2 is processed at a high level even on trials when it cannot be successfully reported. Unreported T2 items can subsequently prime responses to later items (Shapiro, et al., 1997) and evoke an electrophysiological marker indicative of high level semantic processing (Luck, Vogel, and Shapiro, 1996). These features, as well as other characteristics of the AB, all point to this phenomenon as reflecting a complex set of processes that control the mechanisms that gate the flow of information into consciousness. At the end of the chapter we refer to this by discussing some recent work linking temporal attention with motivation.

For now, though, we begin the chapter with a brief review of the basic AB paradigm and follow that with a summary of the extant formal and informal models of the AB. Then, we review and discuss six different empirical studies that bear on the issue of predictability as it relates to temporal attention.

Attentional blink basics

The AB paradigm (Raymond et al. 1992) requires participants to report the identity, or detect the occurrence, of two targets presented as part of a RSVP sequence of centrally presented stimuli. In previous studies, letters and digits have primarily been used as stimuli, with the rate of presentation varying between 6–20 items per second. (However, other studies have used faces, objects, scenes, false fonts, and words of all types as well as combinations of stimuli from different sense modalities.) In the canonical dual-task paradigm participants are presented with a randomly chosen series of letters, from which they have to identify the only white letter in a series of black letters (first target task; T1) and then report whether a black letter 'X' (second target task; T2) occurred in the subsequent letter stream. T2 is presented on only 50% of trials (enabling a false alarm rate to be calculated) and when presented, occurs with an interval separating the two targets of between 100–800ms. Report of both targets is required after the stimulus stream terminates, typically in the correct order. Performance on the T2 task (percentage correct or d′), conditional on correct T1, is usually plotted (see Figure 3.1) as a function of lag (stimulus onset asynchrony [SOA] between T1 and T2). The signature of the AB is a statistically significant drop in performance for medium lags (between about 100–500ms) relative to longer lags or relative to performance at the same lags in a single-task control condition (wherein T1 is ignored). The canonical AB procedure presents T1 and T2, items appearing immediately after each target (T1-mask and T2-mask), and numerous filler items (appearing before T1, during any interval after the T1 mask and before T2, and also after the T2 mask). A shorter, skeletal version has also been frequently used. It eliminates all the filler items leaving only T1, its mask, T2 and its mask (Duncan, Ward, and Shapiro, 1994).

There have been many hundreds of studies using the AB and related procedures. We refer the reader to two recent reviews of some of this work. (Dux and Marois, in press; Olivers and Meeter, 2008). The AB has been extensively used to probe the complex processes supporting consciousness (e.g. perception, selective attention, and working memory) and the result of this

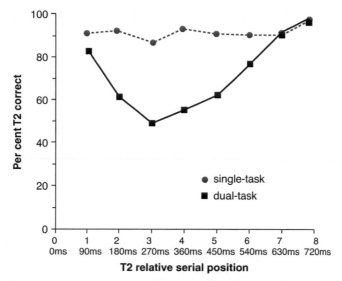

Fig. 3.1 Depicts the group mean percentage of trials in which the second target (T2) was correctly detected, plotted as a function of the relative serial position (lag) and stimulus onset asynchrony (SOA) between T1 and T2. Circle symbols represent data obtained in the single-target (baseline) condition in which subjects were told to ignore T1. Square symbols represent data obtained in the dual-target (experimental) condition in which subjects were told to identify T1.

many facetted body of empirical data is a significant advance in the development of theory concerning how sensory information becomes represented at the level of consciousness.

Theoretical views

Although there are a number of different ideas to explain the AB, all current theories place the mechanism leading to it at a relatively late stage of processing, i.e. after sensory processing and at or after a stage related to selective attention. These theories fall into three main categories, though we hasten to point out that the distinctions between these categories are blurred by neural mechanisms that do not necessarily respect such pigeonholing: 1) filter-based views: the AB reflects the workings of a mechanism designed to filter out non-relevant visual information; 2) consolidation bottleneck: the AB represents a bottleneck in the transfer of highly-processed information into a short-term memory cache that eventually makes information available to consciousness; and 3) retrieval complications: the AB reflects errors in retrieval of information from a short-term memory cache into consciousness. Note: none of these theories explicitly address how predictability of either stimuli or events would affect the AB.

We begin with filter theories because in the first report of the AB (Raymond et al., 1992) a simple version of this idea was advanced. Raymond and colleagues proposed that the AB resulted when the T1 mask item signalled to a central processor that the potential for representational confusion—at high levels, as in binding errors, (Treisman, 1996)—was too high and that any incoming stimuli should be suppressed. The basic notion of a suppression process evoked as a response to distractors subsequently formed the basis of an account put forward by Olivers and Meeter (2008; Olivers, Chapter 4, this volume). They proposed a 'boost and bounce' theory (complete with connectionist formalization) in which each stimulus in the RSVP stream is filtered at a high level for its featural and semantic information. When information matches the target (and thus gains entry into a durable cache accessible by consciousness), a (slightly delayed) temporary 'boost' to subsequent incoming information is given; if such information fails to match the template, a bounce (suppression signal) is directed at incoming stimuli. The size of the bounce is determined by the size of the 'threat', i.e. the bigger the signal, the larger the bounce. The AB is assumed to reflect the temporal dynamics of this system. If the boost from T1 (matching the target template) becomes active at the time of the T1 mask, then the T1 mask's signal gets amplified but because it is not a target, it initiates a big 'bounce' that then gets applied to subsequent stimuli, causing an AB. A different filter theory was proposed by Di Lollo and colleagues (Di Lollo et al., 2005; Kawahara, Enns, and Di Lollo, 2006). They argued that the AB occurs when humans are required to switch from filtering *out* distractors in the pre-target stream to filtering *in* the T1 stimulus when it appears. They propose that the switch in the input filter after T1 has been processed leaves the filter not configured (producing a 'temporary loss of control'), a state that results in weak processing of T2 and leaves it especially susceptible to backward masking (Seiffert and Di Lollo, 1997). As a group these theories emphasize the role of top-down target selection processes and thus link the AB very closely to selective attention as it might operate prior to durable storage of information in a cache, such a visual working memory (WM), accessible by consciousness.

The second category of theories is somewhat similar but places greater emphasis on limited capacity mechanisms needed to transfer current perceptual representations into a durable short-term memory cache. Chun and Potter (1995) suggested a *two-stage* account that argued the AB occurs because report requires information to pass through two stages, an initial, fast-decay, unlimited capacity stage followed by a slow-acting, conceptual consolidation stage with a limited capacity of one. In this view, the second target is unable to be consolidated into a sufficiently durable memory (to support post-stream report) because the necessary stage-two mechanism is engaged with the first target and the representation of T2 decays before it becomes available (or is overwritten by its mask). Jolicoeur and his colleagues (Jolicoeur, 1998, 1999; Jolicoeur and Dell'Acqua, 1998) expanded this account to connect it to the psychological refractory period (PRP) (Pashler, 1994; see also Sigman, Chapter 5; Ruthruff and Pashler, Chapter 9, this volume) phenomenon, which argues for central capacity limitations in humans' ability to process two temporally adjacent stimuli such as occurs in both PRP and the AB.[1]

An early computational model of the AB was built around this notion of a limited capacity second stage of consolidation (Taylor and Rogers, 2002). At the heart of Taylor and Rogers' model sits an inverse model controller (IMC) whose function is to boost stimuli, having arrived via input and object map modules, in order to admit them to a limited capacity working memory. According to this model, the AB occurs when T2 cannot be admitted because the IMC is admitting T1.[2] Formally modelling the Chun and Potter two-stage model, Bowman and Wyble (2007) proposed a 'Simultaneous Type/Serial Token (STST) Model' (recently emerged in an extended version, (Wyble, Bowman, and Nieuwenstein, 2009). At the centre of this theory is the notion that the AB occurs when two targets are unable to be *episodically* distinguished one from the other. The theory posits that, whereas all stimuli in the RSVP sequence can be represented at a conceptual stage (referred to as *type* representation), access for report of these stimuli can only occur when they have been bound to a *token* in WM. This process is enabled by a mechanism

---

[1] It is important to note that the PRP task requires an RT response to both targets and thus introduces a response requirement, which is absent in the traditional AB paradigm.

[2] Note the similarity to Chun and Potters (2005) account, which posits that T2 is not admitted to a limited capacity store because the T1 is still being processed.

called a 'blaster' and allows a target to be episodically distinguished from other stimuli. The AB occurs when the blaster mechanism is suppressed as a result of being engaged in tokenizing the first target.

Recently there have been a series of physiological investigations into neuropharmacological factors that may affect the consolidation process as described earlier. Nieuwenhuis and his colleagues (Nieuwenhuis et al., 2005; see also Olivers, Chapter 4, this volume) suggest the AB occurs as a consequence of the refractory nature of the locus coeruleus (LC), whose involvement in the AB arises as a result of the mediating effects of the noradrenergic system.[3] According to these investigators, it has been proposed that the LC is involved in attentional tasks, releasing norepinephrine to enhance the receptivity of neurons. As the response of the LC is phasic with an approximately 200-ms activity period, the AB occurs when this brainstem nucleus is in its refractory period, lasting about 500ms, which corresponds to the duration of the AB interval. Although Nieuwenhuis failed to find empirical evidence to support this hypothesis (Nieuwenhuis et al., 2007), Dolan's group (De Martino, Strange, and Dolan, 2008) have found behavioural evidence that the adrenergic system has a modulatory influence on selective attention as revealed with the AB paradigm.

A third category of theories places the cause of the AB late in processing at the stage where information is retrieved out of a short-term memory cache and made available to consciousness. This view was expressed in a seminal AB paper (Shapiro, Raymond, and Arnell, 1994) and was developed on the basis of evidence that difficulty manipulations to the first target task had no effect on the magnitude of the 'blink'. These data suggested that retrieval *interference* lay at the basis of the AB phenomenon. The basic idea here is that the two targets and their respective masks compete for retrieval from a short-term memory cache into a report (or consciousness) stage. Higher weighting of the first target prevents consistent retrieval of the second. A modification to this account (Duncan, Ward, and Shapiro, 1994; Ward, Duncan, and Shapiro, 1996) incorporated the *attentional dwell time* hypothesis to suggest that the AB occurs because the two targets compete for limited attentional resources with the loser giving way to extended processing of the winner. A related idea was put forward by Dehaene and his colleagues (Dehaene, Sergent, and Changeux, 2003). They proposed a global workspace model where a stimulus must enter a global neuronal space for it to become consciously accessible. In this global workspace, neuronal assemblies project to multiple distal areas of the brain enabling conscious awareness of the stimulus. According to their model, whereas T1 is able to enter this workspace and ignite the neuronal ensemble, T2 is prevented from doing so until T1 has been fully processed. In this sense this model is similar to a two-stage model but instead places emphasis on consciousness-related processing rather than memory consolidation. The 'Attentional Cascade' model put forward by Shih (2008) is a formal mathematical model that combines the interference models and the two-stage memory model. Two channels are postulated, a *mandatory* pathway and a *bottom-up salience* pathway, both of which potentially provide entry into an *attentional window*. If a stimulus arrives that matches the target template, then an 'enhancement' process occurs that makes the stimulus available to consciousness. The mandatory pathway activates conceptual long-term memory whereas the salience pathway refers to activity driven by more perceptual factors. The AB occurs when the mechanism responsible for consolidating the second target into a durable (i.e. working) memory is unavailable as it is still engaged with the first.

---

[3] Note that this is not an empirical observation but one made on the basis of the known characteristics of the noradrenergic system.

One of the most significant features of the AB is that the effect is present on only about half of trials. The basis for this is not well addressed by any of the extant models because none of them directly address organismic-level factors that may fluctuate from trial to trial. Here we review one study that suggests that this variability results as a consequence of changes in the modulation of communication patterns among different brain areas.

Synchronization and the attention blink

Using a variant of the standard AB paradigm, Gross et al. (2004) required experimental participants, while undergoing magnetoencephalography (MEG) recording, to report any occurrence(s) of the letters 'X' and 'O' in each of a series of RSVP streams containing 15 black letters. Each stream could contain one, two, or none of the targets. Critically, when two targets occurred, they were separated by a short interval (lag 2; 300ms), which placed T2 in the middle of the AB interval, or by a long interval (lag 6; 900ms), which placed T2 outside the AB interval. At the end of each stream, participants reported how many targets occurred and identified them accordingly. As can be seen in Figure 3.2A, the typical AB outcome was manifest, as revealed by a significantly reduced ability to report T2 at the short lag, relative to the long lag, in the dual-target (white squares) condition.[4]

For the analysis of the MEG data, Gross and colleagues examined long-range synchronization among multiple areas of the brain as a means of determining whether such a mechanism could predict when an AB would occur. Synchronization has been proposed as a mechanism for inter-area communication (Varela et al., 2001) and is defined as phase-locked oscillatory activity between two or more cortical areas. Importantly, these cortical areas must be phase-locked to each other, rather than to the external stimulus driving the oscillations. The steps to arrive at this analysis are each detailed and complex and will only be described superficially here.

The first step was to perform a time–frequency analysis in order to determine in *what* frequency range and *when* the oscillations occurred that lay at the basis of the synchronization analysis. They determined that such oscillations had a frequency of about 15Hz, placing it at the boundary of the beta oscillatory band, and occurred at approximately 400ms following the occurrence of accurately reported targets. Functional tomographic maps were created using the method of dynamic imaging of coherent sources (DICS), which uses spatial filters in the frequency domain to localize *where* in the brain a particular frequency of oscillation is occurring. We determined the involvement of eight brain regions, including occipital cortex, as well as bilateral frontal, temporal, and posterior parietal areas, and the cingulum. This analysis then enabled us in Step 3 to determine the degree of synchronization among those regions identified in Step 2 and to distinguish two 'networks', one involved in distractor-only trials and another in trials on which two targets were presented. Although the two identified networks were composed of the set of brain areas identified in Step 2, the specific areas among which the largest modulation of synchronization occurred differed importantly. The 'distractor-related' network principally involved the occipital cortex in synchronization with (left) frontal and (left) temporal areas, whereas the 'target-related' network involved the (right) posterior parietal area in synchronization with (left) temporal and (left) frontal areas. The final step was to examine modulation of this target-related network to the critical elements responsible for yielding the AB, i.e. the two targets and their respective masks. As shown in Figure 3.2B, we divided trials into the four possible types: distractor only, single target, dual target where T2 was correctly identified (i.e. no AB occurred), and

---

4 Negative lags reveal T1 performance and the 'Focused Attention' condition (black circles) shows data for when only one target was presented.

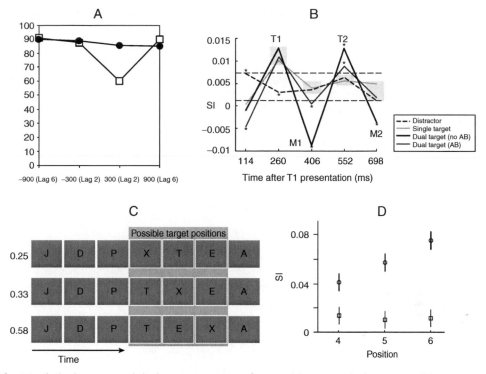

Fig. 3.2 A) Single-target and dual-target responses of 10 participants. In dual target conditions (white squares), negative and positive lags refer to performance for T1 and T2, respectively. In the single-target conditions (black circles), negative and positive lags refer to the lag of the single target as a function of where the other target would have occurred had it been presented. B) Phase synchronization index (SI) reflecting the cortical components of five successive stimuli, comprising a distractor, two targets (T1, T2), and target masks (M1, M2). The x-axis specifies time after presentation of the first target. Each point represents the mean SI in a 60-ms window centred at 260ms after the respective stimulus. Values at 260ms quantify the network synchronization to the first target (T1), and values at 114ms represent the network synchronization corresponding to the distractor preceding the first target. Conditions are: black, no AB; dark grey, AB; light grey, target; dotted line, distractor. The dashed lines mark the extent of SI in trials containing only distractors. Points marked with an asterisk are significantly different from their neighbours at the same position (P <0.05, Kruskall–Wallis test), whereas points within the same shaded area are not significantly different. Negative values arise from the filtering of the SI time courses. C) Schematic representation of the predictability of target occurrence. The figure shows the first seven stimuli of the rapid serial visual stream. A target (in this case 'X') could occur at position 4 (see top row), 5, or 6 with equal probability. If a distractor is presented at position 4 (see middle row) the probability is increased for a target to appear at position 5. Presentation of another distractor at position 5 (see bottom row) further increases the probability for target occurrence at position 6. Numbers to the left of each row represent the conditional probability for target occurrence at position 4 (top), 5 (middle), and 6 (bottom), given that no target was presented up to this position (only behaviourally relevant trials, i.e. trials with target) were considered). D) Modulation of phase synchronization (SI) by stimuli at different temporal positions in the presentation stream. The mean of 11 points surrounding the maximum (~260ms) and minimum (~114ms) temporal window was computed across subjects for all cortical connections of the target-related network for targets (circles) and for distractors (boxes). Lines extending from the mean indicate the standard error. The SI modulation (difference of synchronization and desynchronization) increased with temporal stimulus position for target trials only.

dual target where T2 was not identified correctly (i.e. an AB occurred). The dependent variable, referred to as a synchronization index, could vary from −1 to +1, reflecting synchronization at positive values and *de*-synchronization at negative values. Whereas synchronization is thought to reflect an active communication channel among the neural areas involved, de-synchronization is believed to reflect a lack of communication, colloquially speaking. This final analysis showed an equal amount of synchronization on all trials on which T1 was reported correctly and an equivalent amount on T2 trials when it was reported correctly. Trials on which T2 was not reported correctly, i.e. an AB occurred or no T2 was presented, revealed a significantly lower degree of synchronization. The unexpected finding was that there was a significantly larger degree of *de*-synchronization to both the T1 and T2 masks on trials when no AB occurred. As it has been shown that masks reduce target accuracy and are critical to the production of the AB (Seiffert and Di Lollo, 1997), this outcome was interpreted to reflect that T2 was more likely to survive the AB when those areas processing the mask were unable to communicate with each other, presumably as a result of the decreased synchronization.

These findings can be construed as support for either filter theories or retrieval complication theories. If, according to filter theories, the T1 mask item is not well processed (due to lack of brain synchronization) then it is less likely to effect a suppression (or 'bounce' as proposed by Olivers and Meeter, 2008) and thus less likely to cause an AB. Similarly if the target mask items are not well represented or even entered in WM (due to lack of brain synchronization) then they are less likely to become competitors during retrieval.

Of considerable relevance to the topic of the present book is an AB study examining whether a temporal judgement on T1 produces an AB. The study took as its departure point a finding from Shapiro et al. (1994) where a judgement of the *duration* (short versus long) of a 'gap' between two non-targets as the T1 task produced no AB. Sheppard and colleagues (2002) replicated this outcome but went on to ascertain whether the attenuation of the AB was due to the lack of interference between a non-spatial (i.e. gap) stimulus (T1) and a spatial stimulus (T2) or, alternatively, the requirement to make a duration judgement on T1. In a subsequent condition, Sheppard and colleagues replaced the judgement of the duration of the gap with an identical duration judgement of a letter stimulus, i.e. was the letter displayed for a short or long duration. In this condition, even though a stimulus with spatial information was presented and according to the Interference account (above) should have resulted in an AB, no AB was found. However, when the same stimulus (letter) was required to be judged for its identity (even though selected on the basis of its duration (i.e. longer than the other, non-target, stream elements) an AB resulted. These experiments suggest that judgements of duration do not cause an AB, though whether this is a general case or specific to the (spatial) T2 judgement required, has not yet been determined.

Predictability and temporal selection: empirical findings

A goal of this chapter, in addition to summarizing theoretical views of the AB, is to discuss how the ability to predict aspects of an expected target or other aspects of an RSVP stream might modify access of information to consciousness. In this next section we review five studies that address this issue. The first concerns predicting *when* T1 is about to appear; the second and third address the issue of *what* T1 is likely to be when it appears in an RSVP stream. After this we review a study that examines the effect of predictability of the timing and size of distractors in the RSVP stream. Lastly, we present a study showing that prior experience that causes value predictions (i.e. predictions of reward and punishment) to become associated with stimuli can also alter the AB.

When will T1 occur?

If humans are able to predict when a behaviourally relevant stimulus is likely to appear, are they also able to prepare the machinery for consciousness so as to become especially efficient? And, if so, what neural mechanism might be able to effect this preparation? Using an RSVP stream, Dehaene and his colleagues (Naccache, Blandin, and Dehaene, 2002) showed that when the occurrence of a brief target is temporally predictable versus unpredictable, performance is enhanced. This confirms previous reports that temporal predictability improves the allocation of attention (e.g. Miniussi et al., 1999; see also Correa, Chapter 26; Nobre, Chapter 27, this volume). But what is the neural machinery producing this preparation? Gross and colleagues (2006) reasoned that evidence might be found in the magnitude of long-range synchronization as participants in an AB task prepare for the occurrence of the first target. The AB experiment described earlier (Gross et al., 2004) provided a means to search for this 'anticipatory signature' because the first target could only appear at one of three possible temporal moments after the onset of the RSVP stream. With this sort of predictable temporal sequence, the passing of each possible moment when the target could occur increases the probability of its occurrence at the next possible moment (Figure 3.2C). Accordingly, Gross and colleagues (2006) examined the magnitude of synchronization to targets occurring at each possible moment with the prediction that synchronization magnitude would track the probability of the target's occurrence. Their prediction was correct, as shown in Figure 3.2D: a significant increase in synchronization occurred to targets on dual-target trials (dark vertical lines; circle symbols), relative to distractors (light vertical lines; box symbols) when no targets occurred. Thus, Gross and colleagues (2006) provide evidence that neural preparation can occur and that long-range synchronization may be a viable mechanism for linking top-down (expectation) with bottom-up (perceptual) information processing mechanisms.

What will T1 be?

Can prediction of what T1 is likely to be facilitate processing and, in so doing, reduce the AB effect for subsequent stimuli? The answer to this is probably 'no' (but see Visser, 2007). For example, in a standard AB experiment where the T1 stimulus was always the same (the letter S) thus requiring participants merely to detect *if* a white letter occurred, a conventionally sized AB was found (Shapiro et al., 1994). This indicates that top-down expectation of what a target will be cannot mitigate the AB effect. However, there is other evidence that predictability expressed in a different form can eliminate the AB effect entirely. Raymond (2003) reasoned that a low-level form of predictability is inherent in apparent motion. An illusion of apparent (or long-range) motion can be produced by presenting a series of brief static images of the same object in rapid succession. On successive frames, the object is displaced spatially (leading to the perception of translational motion), seen from a different viewpoint (leading to the perception of object rotation), or slightly transformed, (leading to the perception that the original object is morphing into another object). A widely accepted view of why one consciously perceives only one object instead of multiple objects during such a display is that the initial image in the apparent motion sequence allows the formation of a high-level object representation, with successive images requiring only that the existing representation be updated. Presumably, a combination of re-entrant processing and low-level motion analysis is used to choose between updating an old object representation versus creating a new representation. Such a mechanism would match a perceptual representation with current sensory information to test a prediction of what the next image in a sequence will be. In this sense, prior experience with an object (at least sufficient to create a current object representation) should reduce the need for selective attention (see also Eagleman, Chapter 11, this volume) and mitigate the consequent difficulties in detecting later targets. In other words, would items that are currently represented as objects (i.e. predicted to remain in the scene) still cause an AB when new information about them became available and is task relevant?

To test these ideas, Raymond (2003) presented a standard AB stream (in terms of timing, image size, etc.) but used stimuli that were primarily repeated presentations of the same object (a trident), seen in different viewpoints. In some conditions, another object (an arrowhead) was presented as T1 or T2, or both. The T1 stimulus was defined as the item having a thick central bar; the task was to identify the item (as a trident or arrowhead). The T2 stimulus was the presentation of a small line presented either on the foot of the trident or the nose of the arrowhead; the task was to report whether it was present or absent. In all conditions the filler items, including those presented before T1, were trident images. In two conditions the T1 was also a trident (i.e. able to make use of an already created trident representation) and in two it was an arrowhead (requiring a new object representation). In a fully crossed design, T2 was a trident on two conditions and an arrowhead on two conditions. The results were clear. Whenever T1 was an 'old' object (trident), no AB was observed, even when T1 and T2 were different objects (trident, arrowhead, respectively). However, when T1 was a new object (arrowhead), then an AB was observed, even when T1 and T2 were versions of the same object (both arrowheads). These results make sense if one proposes that when the T1 object was a trident (old), its object representation was fully predictable from preceding filler items (also tridents). This leaves the mechanism needed to create a new object representation fully available for T2. However, when T1 was an arrowhead (new object), this mechanism was engaged so that when T2 was presented it could not be represented sufficiently. These results argue strongly for the notion that the AB results as a temporal limitation of the mechanism needed to create new high-level object representations, or in other words, the mechanisms that deal with the unpredictable occurrence of a new object.

Kellie and Shapiro (2004) explored related ideas in a series of experiments that presented a sequence of highly similar images in an AB task. In their experiments the RSVP stream comprised a set of images made by morphing the image of a pipe to that of a saucepan. In one condition, each successive image was a partial morph between the two objects, presented in the appropriate sequence so that the pipe appeared to smoothly morph itself into a saucepan. The successive updating of each previous image by a just slightly different image promotes object constancy, leading to a morphing effect. In terms of object representations, each successive image in such a display is similar enough to maintain activation of a single object representation. In the other condition, the same partial morph images were presented, but this time in a random sequence. In both cases, T1 and T2 were partial (ambiguous) morph images each overlaid with a different surface texture (circles for T1, squares for T2). The tasks were to identify the size (large or small) of the textural elements. The key finding was that no AB was found for the smooth morph sequence condition but a significant AB for the random sequence. These results, like those of Raymond (2003), support the notion that the AB involves mechanisms used in the creation of new, high-level object representations. In the smooth morph condition, no new object representation was needed to do the T1 (or T2) task, whereas in the random condition, new object representations would have had to be activated whenever the series presented an image that was significantly different from its predecessor.

Temporal and spatial predictability of distractors

In a recent series of experiments, Martin, Enns, and Shapiro (in submission) investigated the effects of predictability of the temporal and spatial components of an AB stream (see also Correa, Chapter 26, this volume). Given that the attentional blink represents a failure of attention to sustain selection over time, in their initial experiment they manipulated the predictability of the temporal characteristics of every non-target element in the RSVP stream, leaving intact the timing of critical items, i.e. T1, T2, and their respective masks, as in the canonical AB paradigm. Although the critical items each had an SOA of 100ms, the SOA between all other items in the stream varied around a mean of 100ms (ranging between 34–221ms). The participants' task was to identify the only two coloured letters in a stream of black letters. As shown in Figure 3.3 (circle symbols), AB magnitude was dramatically reduced by the arrhythmic stream, relative to the canonical (regular) condition (square symbols). They reasoned that perhaps the arousal caused by the unpredictability of the RSVP stream required more attentional resources to be devoted to the task, thus enhancing performance. If this were true, then unpredictability on other aspects of the stimulus stream should have the same effect. So, in a subsequent experiment, they returned the AB to its canonical regular temporal rhythm (100ms SOA between all stimuli) but created unpredictability by varying the size of the letters. The critical items were presented in the same size (18 point) as used in the previous experiment, but all other stream items varied randomly between 14–22 point, in a spatial manipulation that mirrored the temporal manipulation of the previous condition. Surprisingly, instead of attenuating the AB, as was seen with the temporally arrhythmic distractor items, a dramatic and significant *increase* in AB magnitude relative to the canonical AB task was found (Figure 3.3). Clearly, arousal was inadequate to explain this pattern of results because there was no reason to predict more arousal in the temporal unpredictability condition than in the spatial unpredictability condition. Perhaps, whereas unpredictable conditions increase arousal generally, the temporal manipulation calls attention to the variable

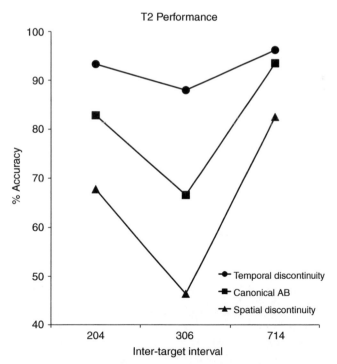

Fig. 3.3 Depicts second target (T2) accuracy (y-axis) as a function of SOA between T1 and T2 for the Temporal Discontinuity condition (circle symbols), the Canonical condition (square symbols), and the Spatial Discontinuity condition (triangle symbols).

timing aspect of the stream and the spatial manipulation calls attention to the *spatial* nature of the stimuli. Given that this particular AB task requires a judgement of the spatial configuration (i.e. identity) of the targets, the latter manipulation may conflict more with the target task than the former. Thus these data indicate that unpredictability in a *task-relevant* domain can hinder performance and are consistent with the view that predictability aids selective attention.

Outcome-value prediction and temporal attention

In a recent series of studies, Raymond and O'Brien (2009) examined how an entirely different form of prediction might influence the temporal limits of attention. Specifically they asked whether previously learned associations with specific stimuli might facilitate target selection from RSVP streams in single- and dual-task conditions. It is well established that via instrumental learning, specific stimuli can acquire value prediction codes that allow the brain to predict the value (the quantity of a reward or punishment) and the likelihood of its occurrence, given a specific action (Padoa-Schioppa and Assad, 2006). To test whether such motivation codes might influence selection, Raymond and O'Brien asked participants to play a simple choice game wherein they learned to associate different faces with a high or low probability of a monetary win or loss, or no outcome. After value learning reached a criterion level, these faces, as well as other novel faces, were used as T2 targets (with scrambled face masks) in an AB procedure that required participants to report whether the T2 face was 'old' (from the learning task) or 'new'. T1 was a non-face abstract image requiring a simple texture judgement. When the lag between T1 and T2 was long (800ms; outside of the AB interval), face recognition was significantly better for faces associated with highly probable wins or losses (no effect of valence), compared to faces associated with a low or no probability of an outcome. This indicates that prediction regarding the probability of an outcome facilitates processing. To determine if attention was driving this effect, T2 recognition when the T1–T2 lag was short (200ms; in the AB interval) and attention was largely unavailable was compared to T2 recognition in the long-lag condition. Interestingly, even during the AB the facilitatory effect of a high outcome-probability association persisted, suggesting that this effect of motivation is independent of attention. Furthermore, faces that were previously associated with wins (high or low probability) fully escaped the AB, showing no decrement in recognition relative to the long-lag condition. However, faces that were previously associated with loss (high or low probability) or no outcome showed a conventional AB effect (significant reduction in recognition performance). This pattern of outcome indicates that whereas outcome-probability codes can facilitate processing independently of attention, codes for predicting the valence (win/loss) of an outcome interact with attention. Specifically, stimuli associated with reward (wins) preferentially gain access to consciousness when attention is limited but stimuli associated with punishment (losses) do not. These results show that predictions of value acquired in another context can persist to affect conscious recognition processes even when the outcomes are irrelevant to the present task.

Conclusions

To summarize, the AB effect and the paradigm used to measure it have proved highly useful for examining the processes that give rise to conscious perception. By revealing the conditions that produce this temporary failure in the perception system, the AB paradigm has shown that the transfer of sensory information to consciousness can be time-consuming and can trigger a set of neural events (such as synchronization) that, in more naturalistic circumstances, probably aid the selection of task relevant information for consciousness. Clearly, other factors related to predictability and continuity in the environment contribute to the processes that lead to consciousness by limiting the set of stimuli that can be considered task-relevant and by involving other systems in the brain, such as motivation. Although not reviewed here, the AB in recent years has been used to address a wide range of questions concerning the constraints on human consciousness. Among them are questions of how perceptual and attentional processes develop through the lifespan; how brain damage and disease alter such processes; how emotional and other content in stimuli affect processing; and how individual differences on a spectrum of variables determines these constraints. Placing the human organism under temporal pressure to process and respond to complex visual information has proved a fruitful and feasible way to probe the mechanism that determines awareness of stimuli and to discover its limitations.

References

Bowman, H. and Wyble, B. (2007). The simultaneous type, serial token model of temporal attention and working memory. *Psychological Review,* **114**(1), 38–70.

Chun, M. M. and Potter, M. C. (1995). A two-stage model for multiple target detection in rapid serial visual presentation. *Journal of Experimental Psychology Human Perception and Performance,* **21**(1), 109–27.

De Martino, B., Strange, B. A., and Dolan, R. J. (2008). Noradrenergic neuromodulation of human attention for emotional and neutral stimuli. *Psychopharmacology (Berl),* **197**(1), 127–36.

Dehaene, S., Sergent, C., and Changeux, J. P. (2003). A neuronal network model linking subjective reports and objective physiological data during conscious perception. *Proceedings of the National Academy of Sciences of the United States of America,* **100**(14), 8520–5.

Di Lollo, V., Kawahara, J., Shahab Ghorashi, S. M., and Enns, J. T. (2005). The attentional blink: resource depletion or temporary loss of control? *Psychological Research,* **69**(3), 191–200.

Duncan, J., Ward, R., and Shapiro, K. L. (1994). Direct measurement of attentional dwell time in human vision. *Nature,* **369**(6478), 313–15.

Dux, P. and Marois, R. (in press). On how humans search for targets through time: A review of the attentional blink. *Attention, Perception, & Psychophysics.*

Gross, J., Schmitz, F., Schnitzler, I., Kessler, K., Shapiro, K., Hommel, B., et al. (2004). Modulation of long-range neural synchrony reflects temporal limitations of visual attention in humans. *Proceedings of the National Academy of Sciences of the United States of America,* **101**(35), 13050–5.

Gross, J., Schmitz, F., Schnitzler, I., Kessler, K., Shapiro, K., Hommel, B., et al. (2006). Anticipatory control of long-range phase synchronization. *European Journal of Neuroscience,* **24**(7), 2057–60.

Jolicoeur, P. (1998). Modulation of the attentional blink by on-line response selection: Evidence from speeded and unspeeded Task-sub-1 decisions. *Memory & Cognition,* **26**(5), 1014–32.

Jolicoeur, P. (1999). Concurrent response-selection demands modulate the attentional blink. *Journal of Experimental Psychology: Human Perception & Performance,* **25**(4), 1097–113.

Jolicoeur, P. and Dell'Acqua, R. (1998). The demonstration of short-term consolidation. *Cognitive Psychology,* **36**(2), 138–202.

Kawahara, J., Enns, J. T., and Di Lollo, V. (2006). The attentional blink is not a unitary phenomenon. *Psychological Research,* **70**(6), 405–13.

Kellie, F. J. and Shapiro, K. L. (2004). Object file continuity predicts attentional blink magnitude. *Perception & Psychophysics,* **66**(4), 692–712.

Luck, S. J., Vogel, E. K., and Shapiro, K. L. (1996). Word meanings can be accessed but not reported during the attentional blink. Nature, **383**(6601), 616–18.

Miniussi, C., Wilding, E. L., Coull, J. T., and Nobre, A. C. (1999). Orienting attention in time. Modulation of brain potentials. *Brain,* **122**(Pt 8), 1507–18.

Naccache, L., Blandin, E., and Dehaene, S. (2002). Unconscious masked priming depends on temporal attention. *Psychological Science,* **13**(5), 416–24.

Nieuwenhuis, S., Gilzenrat, M. S., Holmes, B. D., and Cohen, J. D. (2005). The role of the locus coeruleus in mediating the attentional blink: a neurocomputational theory. *Journal of Experimental Psychology: General,* **134**(3), 291–307.

Nieuwenhuis, S., van Nieuwpoort, I. C., Veltman, D. J., and Drent, M. L. (2007). Effects of the noradrenergic agonist clonidine on temporal and spatial attention. *Psychopharmacology (Berl),* **193**(2), 261–9.

Olivers, C. N. and Meeter, M. (2008). A boost and bounce theory of temporal attention. *Psychologial Review,* **115**(4), 836–63.

Padoa-Schioppa, C. and Assad, J. A. (2006). Neurons in orbitofrontal cortex encode economic value. *Nature,* **441**, 223–6.

Pashler, H. (1994). Dual-task interference in simple tasks: Data and theory. *Psychological Bulletin,* **116**(2), 220–44.

Raymond, J. E. (2003). New objects, not new features, trigger the attentional blink, *Psychological Science,* **14**, 54–9.

Raymond, J. E. and O'Brien, J. (2009) Selective visual attention and motivation: The consequences of value learning in an attentional blink task. Psychological Science, **20**(8):981–8.

Raymond, J. E., Shapiro, K. L., and Arnell, K. M. (1992). Temporary suppression of visual processing in an RSVP task: An attentional blink? *Journal of Experimental Psychology Human Perception and Performance,* **18**(3), 849–60.

Seiffert, A. E. and Di Lollo, V. (1997). Low-level masking in the attentional blink. *Journal of Experimental Psychology: Human Perception and Performance,* **23**(4), 1061–73.

Shapiro, K. L., Raymond, J. E., and Arnell, K. M. (1994). Attention to visual pattern information produces the attentional blink in rapid serial visual presentation. *Journal of Experimental Psychology Human Perception and Performance,* **20**(2), 357–71.

Shapiro, K., Driver, J., Ward, R., and Sorensen, R. E. (1997). Priming from the attentional blink: A failure to extract visual tokens but not visual types. *Psychological Science,* **8**(2), 95–100.

Sheppard, D. M., Duncan, J., Shapiro, K. L., and Hillstrom, A. P. (2002). Objects and events in the attentional blink. *Psychological Science,* **13**(5), 410–15.

Shih, S. I. (2008). The attention cascade model and attentional blink. *Cognitive Psychology,* **56**(3), 210–36.

Taylor, J. G. and Rogers, M. (2002). A control model of the movement of attention. *Neural Networks,* **15**(3), 309–26.

Treisman, A. (1996). The binding problem. *Current Opinion in Neurobiology,* **2**, 171–8.

Varela, F., Lachaux, J. P., Rodriguez, E., and Martinerie, J. (2001). The brainweb: phase synchronization and large-scale integration. *Nature Reviews Neuroscience,* **2**(4), 229–39.

Visser, T. A. (2007). Masking T1 difficulty: processing time and the attentional blink. *Journal of Experimental Psychology Human Perception and Performance,* **33**(2), 285–97.

Ward, R., Duncan, J., and Shapiro, K. (1996). The slow time-course of visual attention. *Cognitive Psychology,* **30**(1), 79–109.

Wyble, B., Bowman, H., and Nieuwenstein, M. (2009). The attentional blink provides episodic distinctiveness: Sparing at a cost. *Journal of Experimental Psychology: Human Perception and Performance* **35**, 787–807.

Chapter 4

The attentional boost and the attentional blink

Christian N. L. Olivers

Selective visual attention is the ability to prioritize relevant over irrelevant visual information. Over the past century or so, researchers have addressed many fundamental questions with regard to selective attention, ranging from why it is there (e.g. limited capacity resources, binding of features, enabling awareness and action, or noise reduction), *what* it selects (e.g. locations, features, or objects), which way it is driven (bottom-up, by salient stimulus properties; or top-down, by behavioural goals), and how it is implemented (e.g. through enhancement of relevant, or suppression of irrelevant representations). One aspect of selective attention that remains elusive is its time course (Box 4.1). When does what happen? The purpose of this chapter is to point out some consistency in the findings from a subset of classic attention tasks, ranging from cueing to the attentional blink. The consistency suggests a common underlying attentional dynamic, which I will refer to as the *attentional boost*.

The attentional boost

In a classic study, Folk and colleagues (1992) found evidence for a rapid, automatic, but at the same time goal-driven, attentional response. When observers performed a visual search task in

---

Box 4.1 Early versus late selection

An age-old debate in attention research has been whether selection occurs 'early' or 'late' (Deutsch and Deutsch, 1963; Treisman, 1969; Lavie and Tsal, 1994; Vogel et al., 2005). Although the terms suggest a particular time course, 'early' and 'late' refer more to the level or locus than to the moment of selection. Early selection is the filtering on the basis of relatively low-level properties such as colour and orientation. Late selection refers to filtering on the basis of higher level, semantic, or response-related representations. Although in the classic textbook information-processing chain (sensation → perception → response selection) this ordering of representations indeed correlates with early and late moments in time, there is now ample research indicating that information does not just flow linearly, in a feedforward fashion, through the cognitive system. Cortical areas are activated within 50–100ms from each other, including presumably higher-order areas (Nowak and Bullier, 1997; Schroeder et al., 2001; Foxe and Simpson, 2002). Moreover, activity in a particular area, and presumably the representation it carries, can change over time as a function of recurrent processes. Attention onset latencies show that higher areas like IT and V4 are modulated before lower areas such as V2 and V1a (see Schroeder et al., 2001, for a review). This would be expected if attention is subject to, or expresses itself as, extensive feedback processing.

which they had to identify a red target among white distractors, response times (RTs) were affected by a red cue preceding the search display, even though this cue had no predictive value concerning the target position or identity. Search RTs were not affected by at least equally salient cues defined by abrupt onset, indicating that the cueing effect was goal-driven. Consistent with this, the converse pattern was found when the search target was defined by onset: now onset cues affected RTs, but colour cues did not. Folk and colleagues argued that the automatic deployment of attention is contingent upon task settings.

For the present purpose, there are two important aspects of this finding. First, even though goal-driven mechanisms are involved, the deployment of attention is automatic and rapid. Folk et al. (1992) showed that cueing effects already occurred for cue-target SOAs of 50ms, and appeared to reach asymptote at 100–150ms (see also Folk et al., 2002; and Leblanc and Jolicoeur, 2005). Second, when attention is triggered by a feature (e.g. red), it does not only affect that feature, but automatically boosts other aspects of the cued object such as its location and identity. After all, if it did not, invalid red cues would not lead to costs (as their redness would equally prime the target), and valid cues would not lead to benefits in discrimination tasks (as the response is decoupled from the selection cue). This latter point may sound trivial, but it at least suggests that once activity in the relevant population of neurons (e.g. those coding for redness) is triggered, this activity rapidly feeds back to the source of the triggering signal (i.e. its location), and from there the modulation may spread to other properties, such as shape and identity. This rapid surge of recurrent activity, enhancing the entire object and its location within 100–150ms, is what I will refer to as the attentional boost.

Spatial cueing

Evidence for a rapid attentional boost also comes from classic peripheral cueing tasks (Posner, 1980; Jonides, 1981). In these tasks, it is found that attention to a peripheral visual target is facilitated when the target's location is indicated by a cue that appears at the same position. In one of the few studies that explored cue-target timing in detail, Cheal and Lyon (1991) found that benefits from peripheral cues peaked at 100ms. In a different paradigm, Carlson and colleagues (2006) presented an array of multiple running clocks, one of which could be cued. Participants were asked to tell the time on this clock at the time it was cued. With peripheral cues, the participants were consistently late by about 140ms. Such rapid orienting is usually interpreted as evidence for pure stimulus-driven attention, especially because in many tasks the cue has no predictive value concerning the target position. However, I would like to argue here that although peripheral cueing results are consistent with an automatic process, this process is unlikely to be purely stimulus-driven: if the cues were not directly task-relevant (as they were in the previously mentioned studies), then they were at least indirectly task-relevant, as they resembled the target in terms of both abruptness and potential location of appearance, consistent with contingent automatic capture (Ansorge and Heumann, 2003).

Object substitution

The object-substitution masking paradigm (Enns and Di Lollo, 1997) may provide further evidence for a 100–150-ms attentional boost. In the typical version of the task, participants are asked to identify a briefly presented target object among a number of distractor objects. The target is defined by a simultaneously appearing surrounding cue that is quite dissimilar to the target (e.g. four dots where the target is a ring). Importantly, the cue also serves as a mask, as it may remain visible after the target has already disappeared. When it does, performance deteriorates. Enns and Di Lollo argued that the mask replaces the target in awareness. Of most interest for the present purpose, the time course of substitution masking is remarkably similar to that of cueing, as the effect of the common onset mask reaches maximum between 80–160ms from onset (Di Lollo et al., 2000). I would like to argue here that this is no coincidence, and that object-substitution masking is in part attentional in nature (see Bachmann, 2005; and Woodman and Luck, 2003, for related arguments). The target-defining signal triggers a localized attentional boost, which needs 100–150ms to accrue. By the time it reaches its peak, the target signal is gone, while the mask is still there. This enhanced mask then pushes the weaker target out of competition. A prediction then is that substitution masking is reduced when attention is allowed to peak earlier. Indeed, the effect disappears when the target is pre-cued by 90–135ms (Di Lollo et al., 2000).

Transient attention

Further explorations of the time course of attention suggest that cueing effects do not remain constant across time. This was first noticed by Posner and Cohen (1984), who found that after about 300ms, responses to targets at cued locations were slowed, rather than speeded, as compared to uncued locations. The phenomenon has become known as *inhibition of return* (IOR), and is thought to facilitate orienting towards previously unexplored locations (Lupiáñez, Chapter 2, this volume). IOR also occurs following feature-based cueing (Gibson and Amelio, 2000). In IOR studies, the cue is typically only 50% valid, and observers are often cued back to the centre of the screen. It therefore makes sense to orient away from the cued location. However, peripheral cues lose a considerable part of their facilitative effect even when they are 100% valid and observers are not drawn away from the cued location. In a classic study, Nakayama and Mackeben (1989) asked observers to identify a target in a cluttered display, followed by a mask. A preceding cue indicated the target position with 100% validity. As expected, performance increased with increasing SOA between cue and target display, up to about 100ms. Beyond this peak, however, increasing SOAs resulted in gradually decreasing benefits. This suggests that the initial attentional boost is temporary in nature. Nakayama and Mackeben referred to this temporary enhancement in performance as *transient attention*, and argued that it is largely automatic, but not necessarily low-level. Note that the cue was always relevant in their paradigm, so effects may not have been entirely stimulus-driven. Similar transient attentional functions have been found or hypothesized by others using various different paradigms (Weichselgartner and Sperling, 1987; Müller and Rabbitt, 1989; Cheal and Lyon, 1991; Hikosaka et al., 1993; Mackeben and Nakayama, 1993; Suzuki and Cavanagh, 1997; Kristjánsson et al., 2001; Nothdurft, 2002; Bachmann and Oja, 2003; Scharlau et al., 2006; Shimozaki et al., 2007). Box 4.2 considers whether IOR and transient attention should be regarded as the same mechanism.

Box 4.2 Are inhibition of return and transient attention one and the same thing?

Could transient attention contribute to IOR, or vice versa? Might they be one and the same process? These are questions that scientists have not even begun to answer. Although Nakayama and Mackeben (1989) used the term *decay* to refer to the declining part of the transient attention function, there is no reason why this might not be caused by some form of inhibition. Unfortunately, any debate on whether there is inhibition involved in each case is troubled by the fact that a suitable baseline has been lacking—if one could be found at all (Jonides and Mack, 1984). In transient-attention studies, the cue is always valid, and there

---

Box 4.2 Are inhibition of return and transient attention one and the same thing? *(continued)*

is typically no baseline condition. In IOR studies, the usual condition for comparison is when the target appears at the uncued location (i.e. the invalid cue condition), which would probably not classify as a neutral baseline.

There appear to be a few dissociations between the two effects. For one, in IOR studies, the cue is typically 50% valid, and the effect is strongest when attention is first cued towards and then drawn away again from the target location before the target appears (by cueing observers back to the centre of the screen). In transient attention studies, effects occur without such explicit withdrawals of attention. The cue is usually 100% valid, and thus observers have every incentive to keep on focusing on the cued location. Second, transient attention effects have typically been found in target-discrimination tasks, whereas IOR is difficult, though not impossible, to find with such tasks (see Klein, 2000, for a review). Finally, transient attention paradigms have made use of accuracy measures, whereas IOR is usually measured through RTs. Effects on these different types of measures may have different origins (Prinzmetal et al., 2005). For example, IOR appears to be, for at least a large part, motor-based (Klein and Taylor, 1994), whereas the accuracy effects of transient attention appear to have a more perceptual origin. Systematic studies are needed to determine whether these differences are insurmountable.

Important for the remainder of this chapter is the finding that the rapid attentional boost is not limited to basic properties such as colour or abrupt onset. Recently, Wyble et al. (2009) found an at least equally fast attentional response when cues were defined by alphanumeric category (i.e. look for the digit among letters), resulting in enhanced processing of a subsequent target within about 110ms and the advantage largely gone by 220ms. This opens up the possibility that the attentional boost also plays an important role in yet another paradigm: the attentional blink.

The attentional blink

As explained in the preceding chapter (Shapiro and Raymond, Chapter 3), the attentional blink is the marked drop in performance that occurs for the second of two targets (T1 and T2) when it occurs within 500ms from the first (Raymond et al., 1992). This has led researchers to conclude that attention has a rather slow 'dwell time' of hundreds of milliseconds (Duncan et al., 1994). Apparently, attention is occupied by the need to process T1, a period during which it is unavailable for, or slow to respond to, T2. The prevalent theories of the past 15 years have all been based on this general idea of a T1-induced depletion of limited capacity resources or bottleneck blockage (Shapiro et al., 1997).

Escaping the blink

Although researchers have tended to focus on the 500-ms dip in performance, there are indications that the 100–150-ms mark is crucial in explaining the attentional blink. This becomes clear when we look at conditions in which T2 appears to escape from the blink. One such condition is when T2 immediately follows T1, at lag 1, which is typically at about 100ms. In fact, at this time T2 is often identified even better than T1. This *lag-1 sparing* has been a puzzle for limited-capacity or bottleneck theories, and to account for it, they have assumed a variety of additional hypotheses, often involving the creation of some form of combined episodic, token, or event-type representation of T1 and T2 (Bowman and Wyble, 2007; Chun, 1997; Jolicoeur et al., 2002; Hommel and

Akyürek, 2005; Kessler et al., 2005). But a simpler explanation may be to assume that, like other relevant visual events, T1 triggers a rapid attentional boost. This boost reaches its peak within about 100ms, which is the time at which T2 appears. Hence T2 is spared (see also Raymond et al., 1992; Chua et al., 2001).

It has been suggested that lag-1 sparing and the attentional blink are independent phenomena (Visser et al., 1999). However, against this goes the finding that, when it is a *distractor*, the lag-1 item appears to play an important part in explaining the attentional blink: when the lag-1 distractor intervening the two targets is replaced with a blank, the attentional blink is strongly reduced (Raymond et al., 1992; Chun and Potter, 1995; Grandison et al., 1997; Seiffert and Di Lollo, 1997; Breitmeyer et al., 1999). Perhaps even more remarkable is that the attentional blink disappears when the distractors between the two targets are replaced with even more targets. For example, compare two conditions in a study by Olivers et al. (2007; see also Di Lollo et al., 2005). In the *TDT* condition, the two targets were separated by a distractor. As expected, an attentional blink was found: performance for the last target was considerably worse than for the first. In the *TTT* condition, the first and last targets were separated by another target. Despite the fact that it was still in the same temporal position as in the *TDT* condition, and despite the fact that it now had to be reported along with two other targets instead of only one, this last target was identified considerably more often than in the two-target case (up to the level of the first target). In other words, sparing spread to lag 2.[1] Thus, whether the final target is reported or not does not so much depend on T1, but on whether the intervening item is a distractor. Note that this goes directly against a T1-induced resource-depletion explanation of the attentional blink. Note further that with the stream rates used by Olivers et al. (100–135ms/item), the intermediate distractor in the *TDT* sequence must have exerted its effect on the final target quite rapidly, within about 100–150ms.

Another case found by Olivers and colleagues (2007), in which a target was relatively immune to the attentional blink, also points towards a strong role for distractors, and a rapid attentional response. In the *TDTT* condition, the second target was preceded by a distractor, and an attentional blink was found for this target. However, the third target, which was preceded by a target, turned out to be almost completely spared, especially compared to a *TDDT* condition in which it was preceded by a distractor. In other words, even once induced, the attentional blink could be reversed within a single SOA of roughly 100ms.

Boost and bounce theory

The previously discussed results suggest that rather than reflecting an attentional inertia of several hundreds of milliseconds, the attentional blink is the result of more dynamic attentional processes that respond within roughly 100ms to important changes in the stream. Recently, Olivers and Meeter (2008; see Raymond et al., 1992, for an important theoretical predecessor) proposed a theory of how this may work. The theory has been implemented in a computational model. It assumes that a task-relevant visual event (such as a target in a rapid stream of distractors, or a cue in a cueing task) automatically triggers goal-driven attentional feedback that amplifies its location. This boost is rapid (in the model, it reaches its peak at 90ms after target detection), and transient (it decays within the next 300ms or so). A further assumption is that a distractor generates exactly the opposite response, a transient inhibitory *bounce* with the same time course as the boost function. One way to envisage this is that the inhibition is responsive to the initial activation

---

[1] This result depended little on whether or not the first and/or intermediate targets were perceived correctly.

of an item. The stronger the distractor activity, the stronger is the inhibitory response. As the distractor activity dissipates, so does the need to suppress it.

Figure 4.1A shows how the theory accounts for the attentional blink pattern, as simulated in Figure 4.1B. The top panel shows the initial bottom-up activation for each item. Prior to T1, only distractors are encountered, and, as shown in the middle panel, each of these triggers some inhibitory feedback sufficiently strong to keep them out of working memory (see Olivers and Watson, 2006, for evidence for such a pre-T1 inhibitory state). Then, T1 appears and triggers the attentional boost. At the usual presentation rates of 100ms/item, T1 benefits somewhat (sufficient for its detection), but the bulk of the boost actually arrives *after* T1, at the post-T1 item. The attentional blink occurs when this post-T1 item is a distractor. The distractor accidentally receives the maximal enhancement intended for T1, resulting in a very strong distractor signal. This strong signal then automatically results in a bounce—a proportionally strong transient inhibitory response, which, in effect, temporarily closes off working memory from the RSVP stream. Just like the boost reaches its maximum after T1, the bounce reaches its maximum after the post-T1 distractor. If this next item turns out to be a target, an attentional blink will arise, as the now

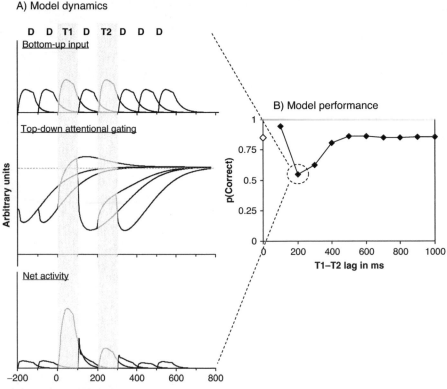

Fig. 4.1 Simulation of the basic attentional blink paradigm. A) The model's dynamics for a T2 at lag 2 is shown in detail, with 1) the bottom-up sensory signal; 2) the transient attentional response (as a combination of both excitatory and inhibitory feedback); 3) the net activity, which is the combined (i.e. multiplied) bottom-up and top-down activity. B) The model's performance is shown for T1 (the open marker on the Y axis), and for T2 as a function of T1-T2 lag. Reproduced from Olivers, C. N. L. and Meeter, M. (2008). A boost and bounce theory of temporal attention. *Psychological Review*, **115**, 836–63 (adapted with permission from APA Journals).

strong inhibition prevents it from mustering sufficient activity to make it into working memory (the bottom panel shows the net activity of T1 and T2, as a function of bottom-up activity and attentional feedback). Nevertheless, this inhibited target will still generate some attentional enhancement of its own, and if there were to be yet another, immediately following target, this third target would often escape from the blink.

According to boost and bounce theory, the attentional blink is completely determined by the temporal dynamics of excitatory and inhibitory selection mechanisms following T1 and its trailing distractors. The important deviation from existing theories is that the blink is not caused by T1 occupying a vital bottleneck or limited capacity processing stage. Instead, boost and bounce theory assumes rather run-of-the-mill attentional selection or 'gating' mechanisms: enhance the input when a target is encountered, suppress the input when it is a distractor. As shown in Olivers and Meeter (2008), the model explains a number of other temporal attention findings, including transient attention (Weichselgartner and Sperling, 1987; Nakayama and Mackeben, 1989), the effect of blanks on the attentional blink (Chun and Potter, 1995), and the effects of varying the stream speed (Bowman and Wyble, 2007). The general theory can also account for why the attentional blink is sometimes reduced when observers are distracted (Olivers and Nieuwenhuis, 2005): A weaker attentional response to T1 will also lead to a weaker inhibitory response to the subsequent distractor.

In an important deviation from limited-capacity theory, 'boost and bounce' theory assumes that the attentional blink is time-locked not to T1, but to the post-T1 distractor instead. The prediction then is that the attentional blink can be postponed if somehow the post-T1 items are no longer treated as a distractor. Olivers and Meeter (2008) tested this prediction as follows (see Figure 4.2a): participants were asked to report the red letters in a stream of black digits. Thus, we assumed that observers would treat redness as an important cue for targets, and blackness as an important cue for distractors. The crucial manipulation was the color of the post-T1 distractor: In the *standard* condition, this distractor was black, and we expected a normal attentional blink to occur. In the *T1+1red* condition, this distractor was red and thus more target-like than a typical distractor. The model predicts that the inhibition triggered by such a distractor will be at most weak, and thus the attentional blink will be postponed until the first 'real' (in this case black) distractor is encountered. Similarly, the attentional blink should be postponed even further when two post-T1 distractors are made red, as was the case in the *T1+2red* condition. Figure 4.2b shows the model's predictions, and Figure 4.2c shows the empirical evidence that the attentional blink is indeed shifted in time.

Transient attention in other models

There are now a number of models of temporal attention that postulate a central role for a rapid, transient attentional response (Bowman and Wyble, 2007, Nieuwenhuis et al., 2005, Fragopanagos et al., 2005). However, unlike boost and bounce theory, all these models still reserve an important role for limited capacity resources. For example, in Bowman and Wyble's (2007) simultaneous type serial token (ST²) model, an attentional *blaster* is necessary to temporarily enhance target representations so that an episodic representation or 'token' (required for report) can be created. T1 triggers this blaster, but the process of tokenization is limited to a single target at a time and thus seeks to temporarily suppress the blaster. Being denied the blaster, T2 will often fail to reach the episodic stage, resulting in an attentional blink (see Wyble et al., 2009, for recent adjustments that bring the ST2 and boost and bounce models closer together).

The locus coeruleus norepinephrine (LC-NE) model of Nieuwenhuis and colleagues (2005) proposes that the attentional blink is the consequence of the dynamics of the locus coeruleus, the

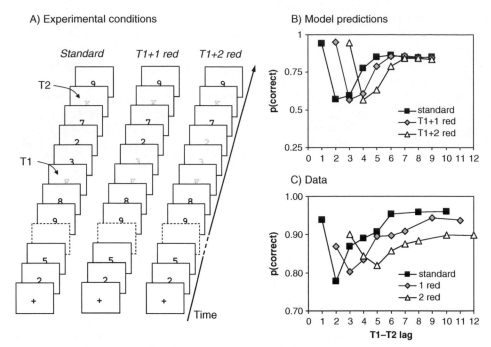

Fig. 4.2 Postponing the attentional blink. A) In the *Standard* condition, targets were red (here drawn in grey) letters among black digit distractors. In the *T1+1 red* condition the distractor immediately following T1 was also red. In the *T1+2* red condition, the two distractors following T1 were red. B) The boost and bounce model's predictions: The attentional blink is postponed. C) Average accuracy data from 18 participants for T2 as a function of T1–T2 lag. Reproduced from Olivers, C. N. L. and Meeter, M. (2008). A boost and bounce theory of temporal attention. *Psychological Review*, **115**, 836–63 (adapted with permission from APA Journals).

brain-stem nucleus responsible for the release of norepinephrine in the neocortex. The norepinephrine release is believed to have a transient attention-enhancing effect, and, according to Nieuwenhuis et al., is a necessary condition for target awareness. Interestingly, activity in the locus coeruleus peaks around 100ms after target onset but is then followed by a refractory period of between 200–400ms (Usher et al., 1999). According to Nieuwenhuis et al., lag-1 sparing corresponds directly to the peak, whereas the attentional blink corresponds directly to the refractory period. Although there are many similarities, again, the LC-NE model differs from the boost and bounce model in that the former is in essence a limited-capacity resource model: T1 uses up a vital resource which it requires for detection (namely locus coeruleus firing, and norepinephrine release). This resource is then temporarily unavailable to subsequent targets (due to the refractory period). The LC-NE model therefore has difficulty explaining sparing and escaping from the blink.

Neurophysiological evidence for the boost in the brain

One of the major advantages of the LC-NE model is that it provides a clear neurophysiological correlate of transient attention: The phasic burst of activity in the locus coeruleus, followed by a transient norepinephrine release in the cortex. The locus coeruleus itself certainly responds rapidly enough to account for fast transient attention effects, although little is known on whether the cortical release of norepinephrine follows a similar time course. Others have placed transient attention effects in more specific cortical areas: the adjusted CODAM model by Fragopanagos et al. (2005; see also Bowman and Wyble, 2007) proposes superior parietal cortex and the temporo-parietal junction as potential generators of what they call the 'attention control signal'. For the time being, boost and bounce theory also assumes that the transient attentional feedback is generated cortically, when those areas that code for task-relevant properties are being triggered by matching incoming stimuli. One promising area in this respect may be LIP (regarded as the monkey homologue of human intra-parietal sulcus). Many LIP neurons feature a rapidly on-setting but transient activation function, and most importantly, they appear to flexibly code for task-relevant stimuli, allowing them to perform a gating function (e.g. Bisley and Goldberg, 2003; Freedman and Assad, 2006).

It is possible that norepinephrine-release further enhances this gating of sensory input, thus aggravating the attentional blink. Other subcortical contenders for phasic attention effects are the thalamus (Bachmann, 1984) and the basal ganglia (Frank et al., 2001). The latter could operate through phasic disinhibition of the thalamus, and/or through the cortical release of dopamine, a neurotransmitter thought to play a role in working-memory functioning. There is some indirect evidence for a role for dopamine in the attentional blink (Olivers and Nieuwenhuis, 2006; Colzato et al., 2008,)

Besides these originally model-based hypotheses, is there more direct neurophysiological evidence for a rapidly and transiently responding attention function? A popular method for measuring the time course of cognitive functioning in humans is electroencephalography (EEG). It has revealed attentional modulations of several event-related potentials (ERPs) in the electrical signal measured from the scalp (see Luck, 2006, for a review). Spatial attention appears effective as early as 70–100ms after target onset, as expressed in the modulation of the P1 component. ERP modulations appear to occur considerably later when spatial attention cannot be directed in advance. For example, when selection is based on a non-spatial feature, then the earliest modulation appears to arise in the P2 and N2 components, starting around 150ms after stimulus onset, peaking even later, and lasting for 100–300ms (though see Hillyard and Anllo-Vento, 1998; Hopf et al., 2004; Schoenfeld et al., 2007, for earlier feature-based effects). This effect is referred to as the *selection negativity*. Consistent with the idea of an attentional boost, this feature-based modulation then appears to culminate in the focusing on the spatial source of the feature, as indexed by the spatially sensitive N2pc component, which peaks around 200–250ms after stimulus onset (e.g. Lien et al., 2008), although others have argued that the N2pc may also reflect distractor suppression (Luck and Hillyard, 1994; Hickey et al., 2009).

At first sight, the difference between the relatively early spatial cueing effects and the relatively late feature-based selection effects on ERP argue against a common underlying mechanism such as the attentional boost proposed here. Moreover, the late feature-based effects by themselves may appear inconsistent with a rapid (100–150ms) transient attentional response as found in the behavioural data. However, a direct comparison of these findings is very difficult. The early P1 modulations in spatial attention studies are measured in response to the *target* stimulus, and only occur when attention has been directed to a location well in advance (either by a cue or by sustained attention to one particular location). Thus, what is measured is the dynamics of target processing under a certain attentional state, not the dynamics of attention itself (that is, how the attentional response develops and changes over time). Moreover, whereas ERP data typically provide an *absolute* time estimate of a certain cognitive event (including, for example, the time for the visual signal to reach the cortex), behavioural experiments typically only focus on the time course of the process of interest by making use of the relative time difference between two stimuli (the typical SOA manipulation). It would therefore be more informative to look at ERPs in response to the *cue*, or in response to the target but as a function of *cue-target SOA*. The few studies that have looked at the direct response to the cue so far have only used central, symbolic cues (e.g. Eimer et al., 2002; Green and McDonald, 2008), which makes these studies less relevant for the rapid automatic response discussed here. Interestingly, the few studies that have looked at peripheral cueing as a function of SOA have indeed found that modulations of the P1 (among other components) are reduced or reversed with increasing SOA, consistent with transient attention and IOR (Hopfinger and Mangun, 1998; McDonald et al., 1999; Prime and Ward, 2004).

Finally, other neurophysiological evidence consistent with a fast, transient attentional response comes from studies using transcranial magnetic stimulation. These have reported maximum disruption of performance when the pulse is applied around 100ms post stimulus onset, in spatial as well as feature-based selection tasks (Ashbridge et al., 1997; Chambers et al., 2004). The one method that is lacking here is functional magnetic resonance imaging (fMRI), which, due to its low temporal resolution, has proven to be less useful in determining the exact timing of attention.

Conclusions

It is clear that a lot is still unknown about the dynamics of attention. What I have argued here is that a variety of paradigms, ranging from spatial cueing to the attentional blink, reveal a common underlying time course. There is ample behavioural evidence that attention acts rapidly and often transiently in response to the detection of a relevant stimulus. A number of important questions remain outstanding. For one, the previous section suggests that important progress can be made in the neurophysiological domain. Furthermore, I have restricted treatment to the type of attention that is automatically triggered given a certain task set. This begs the question as to how the time course of such contingent attention relates to the time course of pure stimulus-driven processes on the one hand, and pure voluntarily-driven attention on the other. Another question concerns the special role of space. Most researchers will agree that the location of a stimulus is more rapidly detected than its exact features. But does the fact that a spatially-defined target leads to earlier attentional modulation than a feature-defined target reflect just that—quicker detection and hence the quicker triggering of attention? Or is the attentional modulation itself, including its time course, inherently different when invoked by spatial information as compared to features? Time will tell, is the apt pun here.

References

Ansorge, U. and Heumann, M. (2003). Top-down contingencies in peripheral cuing: The roles of color and location. *Journal of Experimental Psychology: Human Perception and Performance, 29*, 937–48.

Ashbridge, E., Walsh, V., and Cowey, A. (1997). Temporal aspects of visual search studied by transcranial magnetic stimulation. *Neuropsychologia, 35*, 1121–31.

Bachmann, T. (1984). The process of perceptual retouch: Nonspecific afferent activation dynamics in explaining visual masking. *Perception & Psychophysics, 35*, 69–84.

Bachmann, T. (2005). Object substitution and its relation to other forms of visual masking: reply to James Enns. *Vision Research, 45*, 381–5.

Bachmann, T. and Oja, A. (2003). Flash-lag without change in feature space is alive and well at late intervals after stream onset. *Perception, S32*, 126–7.

Bisley, J. W. and Goldberg, M. E. (2003). Neuronal activity in the lateral intraparietal area and spatial attention. *Science, 299*, 81–6.

Bowman, H. and Wyble, B. P. (2007). The simultaneous type, serial token model of temporal attention and working memory. *Psychological Review, 114*, 38–70.

Breitmeyer, B., Ehrenstein, A., Pritchard, K., Hiscock, M., and Crisan, J. (1999). The roles of location specificity and masking mechanisms in the attentional blink. *Perception & Psychophysics*, **61**, 798–809.

Carlson, T. A., Hogendoorn, H., and Verstraten, F. A. J. (2006). The speed of visual attention: What time is it? *Journal of Vision*, **6**, 1406–11.

Chambers, C. D., Payne, J. M., Stokes, M. G., and Mattingley, J. B. (2004). Fast and slow parietal pathways mediate spatial attention. *Nature Neuroscience*, **7**, 217–18.

Cheal, M. L. and Lyon, D. R. (1991). Central and peripheral precuing of forced-choice discrimination. *Quarterly Journal of Experimental Psychology*, **43A**, 859–80.

Chua, F. K., Goh, J., and Hon, N. (2001). Nature of codes extracted during the attentional blink. *Journal of Experimental Psychology: Human Perception and Performance*, **27**, 1229–42.

Chun, M. M. (1997). Types and tokens in visual processing: A double dissociation between the attentional blink and repetition blindness. *Journal of Experimental Psychology: Human Perception and Performance*, **23**, 738–55.

Chun, M. M. and Potter, M. C. (1995). A two-stage model for multiple detection in RSVP. *Journal of Experimental Psychology: Human Perception and Performance*, **21**, 109–27.

Colzato, L. S., Slagter, H. A., Spapé, M., and Hommel, B. (2008). Blinks of the eye predict blinks of the mind. *Neuropsychologia* **46**:3179–83.

Deutsch, J. A. and Deutsch, D. (1963). Attention: Some theoretical considerations. *Psychological Review*, **70**, 80–90.

Di Lollo, V., Enns, J. T., and Rensink, R. A. (2000). Competition for consciousness among visual events: The psychophysics of reentrant processes. *Journal of Experimental Psychology: General*, **129**, 481–507.

Di Lollo, V., Kawahara, J., Ghorashi, S. M. S., and Enns, J. T. (2005). The attentional blink: resource depletion or temporary loss of control? *Psychological Research*, **69**, 191–200.

Duncan, J., Ward, R. and Shapiro, K. (1994). Direct measurement of attentional dwell time in human vision. *Nature*, **369**, 313–15.

Eimer, M., Van Velzen, J., and Driver, J. (2002). Cross-modal interactions between audition, touch, and vision in endogenous spatial attention: ERP evidence on preparatory states and sensory modulations. *Journal of Cognitive Neuroscience*, **14**, 254–71.

Enns, J. T. and Di Lollo, V. (1997). Object substitution: A new form of masking in unattended visual locations. *Psychological Science*, **8**, 135–9.

Folk, C., Remington, R. W. and Johnston, J. C. (1992). Involuntary covert orienting is contingent on attentional control settings. *Journal of Experimental Psychology: Human Perception and Performance*, **18**, 1030–44.

Folk, C. L., Leber, A. B., and Egeth, H. E. (2002). Made you blink! Contingent attentional capture produces a spatial blink. *Perception & Psychophysics*, **64**, 741–53.

Foxe, J. J. and Simpson, G. V. (2002). Flow of activation from V1 to frontal cortex in humans: a framework for defining "early" visual processing. *Experimental Brain Research*, **142**, 139–50.

Fragopanagos, N., Kockelkoren, S., and Taylor, J. G. (2005). A neurodynamic model of the attentional blink *Cognitive Brain Research*, **24**, 568–86.

Frank, M. J., Loughry, B., and O'Reilly, R. (2001). Interactions between frontal cortex and basal ganglia in working memory: a computational model. *Cognitive, Affective & Behavioral Neuroscience*, **1**, 137–60.

Freedman, D. J. and Assad, J. A. (2006). Experience-dependent representation of visual categories in parietal cortex. *Nature*, **443**, 85–8.

Gibson, B. S. and Amelio, J. (2000). Inhibition of return and attentional control settings. *Perception & Psychophysics*, **62**, 496–504.

Grandison, T. D., Ghirardelli, T. G., and Egeth, H. E. (1997). Beyond similarity: Masking of the target is sufficient to cause the attentional blink. *Perception & Psychophysics*, **59**, 266–74.

Green, J. J. and McDonald, J. J. (2008). Electrical neuroimaging reveals timing of attentional control activity in human brain. *Plos Biology*, **6**, 730–8.

Hickey, C., Di Lollo, V., and McDonald, J. J. (2009). Electrophysiological indices of target and distractor processing in visual search. *Journal of Cognitive Neuroscience*, **21**, 760–75.

Hikosaka, O., Miyauchi, S., and Shimojo, S. (1993). Focal visual attention produces illusory temporal order and motion sensation. *Vision Research*, **33**, 1219–40.

Hillyard, S. A. and Anllo-Vento, L. (1998). Event-related brain potentials in the study of visual selective attention. *Proceedings of the National Academy of Sciences USA*, **95**, 781–7.

Hommel, B. and Akyürek, E. G. (2005). Lag-1 sparing in the attentional blink: Benefits and costs of integrating two events into a single episode. *The Quarterly Journal of Experimental Psychology*, **58**, 1415–33.

Hopf, J.-M., Boelmans, K., Schoenfeld, M. A., Luck, S. J., and Heinze, H. J. (2004). Attention to features precedes attention to locations in visual search: Evidence from electromagnetic brain responses in humans *Journal of Neuroscience*, **24**, 1822–32.

Hopfinger, J. B. and Mangun, G. R. (1998). Reflexive attention modulates processing of visual stimuli in human extrastriate cortex. *Psycholigical Science*, **9**, 441–7.

Jolicoeur, P., Tombu, M., Oriet, C., and Stevanovski (2002). From perception to action: Making the connection. In Prinz, W. and Hommel, B. (Eds.) *Attention and Performance, Vol XIX: Common mechanisms in perception and action*. Oxford: Oxford University Press.

Jonides, J. (1981). Voluntary versus Automatic Control over the Mind's Eye's Movement. In Long, J. and Baddeley, A. (Eds.) *Attention and Performance IX*. Hillsdare, NJ: Lawrence Erlbaum.

Jonides, J. and Mack, R. (1984). On the cost and benefit of cost and benefit. *Psychological Bulletin*, **96**, 29–44.

Kessler, K., Schmitz, F., Gross, J., Hommel, B., Shapiro, K., and Schnitzler, A. (2005). Cortical mechanisms of attention in time: Neural correlates of the lag-1 sparing phenomenon. *European Journal of Neuroscience*, **21**, 2563–74.

Klein, R. M. (2000). Inhibition of return. *Trends in Cognitive Sciences*, **4**, 138–47.

Klein, R. M. and Taylor, T. L. (1994). Categories of cognitive inhibition with reference to attention. In Dagenbach, D. and Carr, T. H. (Eds.). *Inhibitory Processes in Attention, Memory, and Language*. San Diego, CA: Academic Press.

Kristjánsson, Á., Mackeben, M., and Nakayama, K. (2001). Rapid, object-based learning in the deployment of transient attention. *Perception*, **30**, 1375–87.

Lavie, N. and Tsal, Y. (1994). Perceptual load as a major determinant of the locus of selection in visual attention. *Perception & Psychophysics*, **56**, 183–97.

Leblanc, E. and Jolicoeur, P. (2005). The time course of the contingent spatial blink. *Canadian Journal of Experimental Psychology*, **59**, 124–31.

Lien, M.-C., Ruthruff, E., Goodin, Z., and Remington, R. W. (2008). Contingent attentional capture by top-down control settings: converging evidence from event-related potentials. *Journal of Experimental Psychology: Human Perception and Performance*, **34**, 509–30.

Luck, S. J. (2006). The operation of attention – millisecond by millisecond – over the first half second. In Ögmen, H. and Breitmeyer, B. G. (Eds.) *The first half second: The microgenesis and temporal dynamics of unconscious and conscious visual processing*. Cambridge, MA: MIT Press.

Luck, S. J. and Hillyard, S. A. (1994). Electrophysiological correlates of feature analysis during visual search. *Psychophysiology*, **31**, 291–308.

Mackeben, M. and Nakayama, K. (1993). Express attentional shifts. *Vision Research*, 33, 85–90.

McDonald, J. J., Ward, L. M., and Kiehl, K. A. (1999). An event-related brain potential study of inhibition of return. *Perception & Psychophysics*, **61**, 1411–23.

Müller, H. J. and Rabbitt, P. M. A. (1989). Reflexive and voluntary orienting of visual attention: time course of activation and resistance to interruption. *Journal of Experimental Psychology: Human Perception and Performance*, **15**, 315–30.

Nakayama, K. and Mackeben, M. (1989). Sustained and transient components of focal visual attention. *Vision Research*, **29**, 1631–47.

Nieuwenhuis, S., Gilzenrat, M. S., Holmes, B. D., and Cohen, J. D. (2005). The role of the locus coeruleus in mediating the attentional blink: A neurocomputational theory. *Journal of Experimental Psychology: General,* **134**, 291–307.

Nothdurft, H.-C. (2002). Attention shifts to salient targets. *Vision Research,* **42**, 1287–306.

Nowak, L. G. and Bullier, J. (1997). The timing of information transfer in the visual system. In Rockland, K. S., Kaas, J. H., and Peters, A. (Eds.) *Cerebral Cortex, Vol. 12: Extrastriate Cortex in Primates.* New York:Plenum Press.

Olivers, C. N. L. and Meeter, M. (2008). A boost and bounce theory of temporal attention. *Psychological Review,* **115**, 836–63.

Olivers, C. N. L. and Nieuwenhuis, S. (2005). The beneficial effect of concurrent task-irrelevant mental activity on temporal attention. *Psychological Science,* **16**, 265–9.

Olivers, C. N. L. and Nieuwenhuis, S. (2006). The beneficial effects of additional task load, positive affect, and instruction on the attentional blink. *Journal of Experimental Psychology: Human Perception and Performance,* **32**, 364–79.

Olivers, C. N. L. and Watson, D. G. (2006). Input control processes in rapid serial visual presentation: Target selection and distractor inhibition. *Journal of Experimental Psychology: Human Perception and Performance,* **32**, 1083–92.

Olivers, C. N. L., Van der Stigchel, S., and Hulleman, J. (2007). Spreading the sparing: Against a limited-capacity account of the attentional blink. *Psychological Research,* **71**, 126–39.

Posner, M. I. (1980). Orienting of Attention, The VIIth Sir Frederic Bartlett Lecture. *Quarterly Journal of Experimental Psychology,* **32**, 3–25.

Posner, M. I. and Cohen, Y. (1984). Components of visual orienting. In Bouma, H. and Bouwhuis, D. G. (Eds.) *Attention and Performance X: Control of Language Processes.* Hillsdale, NJ, Lawrence Erlbaum.

Prime, D. J. and Ward, L. M. (2004). Inhibition of return from stimulus to response. *Psycholigical Science,* **15**, 272–6.

Prinzmetal, W., McCool, C., and Park, S. (2005). Attention: Reaction time and accuracy reveal different mechanisms. *Journal of Experimental Psychology: General,* **134**, 73–92.

Raymond, J. E., Shapiro, K. L., and Arnell, K. M. (1992). Temporary suppression of visual processing in an RSVP task: An attentional blink? *Journal of Experimental Psychology: Human Perception and Performance,* **18**, 849–60.

Scharlau, I., Ansorge, U., and Horstmann, G. (2006). Latency facilitation in temporal-order judgments: Time course of facilitation as a function of judgment. *Acta Psychologica,* **122**, 129–59.

Schoenfeld, M. A., Hopf, J.-M., Martinez, A., Mai, H. M., Sattler, C., Gasde, A., et al. (2007). Spatio-temporal analysis of feature-based attention. *Cerebral Cortex,* **17**, 2468–77.

Schroeder, C. E., Mehta, A. D., and Foxe, J. J. (2001). Determinants and mechanisms of attentional modulation of neural processing. *Frontiers in Bioscience,* **6**, 672–84.

Seiffert, A. E. and Di Lollo, V. (1997). Low-level masking in the attentional blink. *Journal of Experimental Psychology: Human Perception and Performance,* **23**, 1061–73.

Shapiro, K. L., Arnell, K. M., and Raymond, J. E. (1997). The attentional blink. *Trends in Cognitive Sciences,* **1**, 291–6.

Shimozaki, S. S., Chen, K. Y., Abbey, C. K., and Eckstein, M. P. (2007). The temporal dynamics of selective attention of the periphery as measured by classification images. *Journal of Vision,* **7**, 1–20.

Suzuki, S. and Cavanagh, P. (1997). Focused attention distorts visual space: An attentional repulsion effect. *Journal of Experimental Psychology: Human Perception and Performance,* **23**, 443–63.

Treisman, A. (1969). Strategies and models of selective attention. *Psychological Review,* **76**, 282–99.

Usher, M., Cohen, J. D., Servan-Schreiber, D., Rajkowski, J., and Aston-Jones, G. (1999). The role of locus coeruleus in the regulation of cognitive performance. *Science,* **283**, 549–54.

Visser, T. A. W., Zuvic, S. M., Bischof, W. F., and Di Lollo, V. (1999). The attentional blink with targets in different spatial locations. *Psychonomic Bulletin & Review,* **6**, 432–6.

Vogel, E. K., Woodman, G. F., and Luck, S. J. (2005). Pushing around the locus of selection: Evidence for the flexible-selection hypothesis *Journal of Cognitive Neuroscience,* **17**, 1907–22.

Weichselgartner, E. and Sperling, G. (1987). Dynamics of automatic and controlled visual attention. *Science,* **238**, 778–80.

Woodman, G. F. and Luck, S. J. (2003). Dissociations among attention, perception and awareness during object-substitution masking. *Psychological Science,* **14**, 605–11.

Wyble, B., Bowman, H., and Nieuwenstein, M. R. (2009). The attentional blink provides episodic distinctiveness: sparing at a cost. *Journal of Experimental Psychology: Human Perception and Performance* **35**, 787–807.

Wyble, B., Bowman, H., and Potter, M. C. (2009). Categorically defined targets trigger spatiotemporal visual attention. *Journal of Experimental Pscyhology: Human Perception and Performance,* **35**, 324–37.

Acknowledgement

This work was supported by NWO Vidi grant 452-06-007 from the Netherlands Organization for Scientific Research.

Chapter 5

A stream of thought: temporal organization of mental operations

Mariano Sigman

A ubiquitous aspect of brain function is its quasi-modular and massively parallel organization, with a large number of processors (neurons, columns, or entire areas) operating simultaneously (Hubel and Wiesel, 1959). For example, in the visual modality, a yet undefined number of visual areas perform different feature analyses, and within each area a parallel ensemble of cortical columns simultaneously sample the visual scene (Felleman and Van Essen, 1991) allowing rapid coverage of a wide field of view. This vast parallel machine can perform, with seemingly no effort and extreme rapidity, tasks that, until recently, were judged virtually impossible for contemporary artificial machines, such as invariant object recognition.

The paradox, however, is that this extraordinary parallel machine is incapable of doing various mental calculations in parallel or even to perform a single large arithmetic calculation that requires multiple steps. How come it is so easy to recognize moving objects, but so difficult to multiply 357 times 289? And why, if we can simultaneously coordinate walking, group contours, segment surfaces, talk, and listen to noisy speech, can we only make one decision at a time?

Many studies on decision-making have described, both at the psychological and neurophysiological level, a temporal stream of operations including stimulus encoding, accumulation of evidence, response selection, and response triggering (Romo et al., 2002). In a typical decision task, the entire sequence of operations happens in a fraction of a second. In contrast, when the task architecture involves a number of interconnected operations, as in simple arithmetic (where the result of a partial operation needs to be piped to the subsequent step), response times can last many seconds and are associated with highly demanding mental effort. Multi-step human cognition has been modelled by applying the computer-science notion of 'production system' as a general framework (the 'Adaptive Control of Thought – Rational' theory; see Anderson et al., 2004). It consists of a general mechanism for selecting production rules fuelled by sensory, motor, goal, and memory modules. These models, as well as other similar enterprises (see Meyer and Kieras, 1997) emphasize the chained nature of cognition: at any moment in the execution of a task, information placed in buffers of specialized modules acts as data for the central production system, which in turn outputs new information to the buffers.

This general framework has been very productive in understanding scheduling and information flow in multi-step cognition (Anderson et al., 2004). However, this is done at a cost. Each task is modelled with a specific program, which requires an enormous number of parameters to be assigned to it. A comparably simpler approach, which resulted in a rich goldmine for understanding the dynamics of information processing, involved dual-task interference paradigms, such as the psychological refractory period (PRP) and the attentional blink (AB). The logic of these experiments resembles the classic scattering methodology in physics in which the internal structure of an element (particle, molecule, here a cognitive task) is understood by colliding it with an experimental probe.

In this chapter I review behavioural and physiological PRP experiments, which provide evidence for the dynamic organization of two qualitatively different operations involved in a task: 1) dedicated circuits (analogous to compiled routines in software design) that can very rapidly and in parallel execute stereotyped programs typically related to encoding, memory retrieval, or execution of learned motor programs; and 2) a slow and serial, large-scale system, broadly related to attention, conscious processing and effortful mental operations, capable of pooling and routing information in a flexible manner.

Parsing a cognitive task into serial and parallel processing states

When two tasks are presented simultaneously (or within a short interval), a delay in the execution of the second task is systematically observed (Telford, 1931; Smith, 1967; Kahneman, 1973; Pashler and Johnston, 1989; Ruthruff and Pashler, Chapter 9, this volume). A natural interpretation of this effect is that subjects are unable to carry out certain processing steps involving the second stimulus until they have finished with the first. When the effect was first observed, it was considered analogous to the refractory period of neurons (even if these two effects involve completely different time scales) and thus the effect received the somehow misleading term 'psychological refractory period' (PRP) (Pashler and Johnston, 1998). The PRP has been related to the broad notion of attention since it occurs even when the two tasks do not share any sensory or motor representation and arises exclusively from the superposition of both tasks (Pashler and Johnston, 1998).

Different mechanisms by which attentional limitations may result in the PRP have been reviewed by Pashler and Johnston and can broadly be divided into three categories (Pashler and Johnston, 1998): 1) single-channel or bottleneck models, according to which certain critical mental operations are carried out sequentially; 2) a capacity-sharing model, which argues that processing for different tasks proceeds in parallel, with processing efficiency being modulated by the resources allocated to the task; 3) a cross-talk model, which suggests that even with existing machinery to carry out different tasks at once, processing streams are actively kept separate to avoid dual-task interference. While a lot of research has been devoted to argue in favour of one of these theories, they are not necessarily incompatible: First, the bottleneck model is a limited case of the capacity-sharing model. When resources to the less-attended task progressively decrease, the capacity-sharing model becomes equivalent to a bottleneck model when these resources reach zero. Second, active inhibition for preventing cross-talk may lead, de facto, to single-channel architecture. Finally, different stages within a task may be subject to partially shared resources or to full seriality. In this chapter I will show that while the purely sequential model suffices to explain a broad number of observations in most PRP experiments, some departures have to be considered in order to explain all the data.

The PRP-bottleneck model considers that tasks involve three stages of processing (Figure 5.1A): a perceptual P-component, a central C-component, and a motor M-component, where only the C-component results in a bottleneck (Sternberg, 1969; Schweickert, 1980; Pashler and Johnston, 1989; Pashler, 1994; Ruthruff et al., 2001). This model can be seen as a simple extension of the Chun and Potter two-stage model, developed to explain attentional limitations in rapid serial visual presentations (Chun and Potter, 1995; see also Shapiro and Raymond, Chapter 3, this volume). PRP experiments have mainly associated the central C-component to 'response selection', the mapping between sensory information and motor action (Pashler and Johnston, 1998), which is consistent with the idea that seriality emerges for flexible routing of information. The P-component involves an initial stage of encoding and should probably be referred to as the

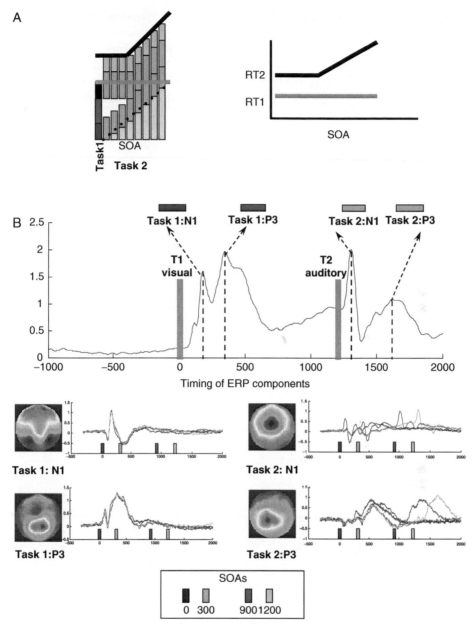

Fig. 5.1 (See also Plate 1) A) Left panel: scheme of the main PRP effect. The vertical axis labels response time. The leftmost column indicates the first task (Task 1), the remaining columns the second task (Task 2), and each box within the columns represents a different stage of processing: from bottom to top *Perceptual (P)*, *Central (C)* and *Motor (M)* components. The pale grey boxes for task 2 indicate stimulus onset asynchrony (SOA). Right panel: the expected dependence of the bottleneck model for RT2 and RT1 as a function of increasing SOA. B) Identifying the response components (N1 and P3), for each task when performed at the longest SOA (1200ms) outside of the interference regime. B) Time-course of the components: components of Task 1 (left panels) are utterly unaffected by SOA. The N1 component of Task 2 (top right panel) tightly follows the stimulus presentation, as would be expected by a P-component. The P3 component of Task 2 (bottom right) reflects a bottleneck for short SOAs as would be expected by a C-component.

S-component (for sensory) to avoid the misunderstanding that this process by itself may lead to conscious perception. The late M-component is thought of as the implementation of the motor response by a dedicated circuit. The central stage is the only one that provides a bottleneck, in the sense that the central C-component of multiple tasks cannot be carried out simultaneously. The PRP bottleneck model leads to a large number of parameter-free predictions (Sigman and Dehaene, 2005). Here, I summarize some relevant ones. I use the term short or long SOA (stimulus onset asynchrony) depending on whether the second stimulus (i.e. Task 2) is presented before or after completion of Task 1.[1]

1) SOA does not affect RT1 (RT for Task 1), which reflects the first-come, first-served aspect of the model. RT2 (RT for Task 2) decreases with a slope of -1 for short SOA durations. This is because the onset of the central component of Task 2 is not locked to Task 2 stimulus presentation, but rather to the completion of the central component of Task 1. For long SOAs, the two tasks are independent and thus RT2 is independent of SOA. Due to RT1 and RT2 variability, the transition between these two regimes is smooth. In this chapter I will follow the convention by which RT2 is measured from the onset of the trial. This is not the most usual convention but it has a great advantage for the analysis of human physiology data, as will become evident later. Under this convention, the prediction of the model is that RT2 does not change for short SOAs (this emphasizes that the completion of Task 2 is locked to the onset of Task 1) but for long SOAs, when the two tasks are independent, increasing SOA will increase RT2 proportionally (see Figure 5.1A).

2) All factors affecting Task 1 should increase RT1. If these manipulations affect P and C-components then this effect should propagate to RT2. This effect is only observed at short SOAs, since for long SOAs the two tasks are independent. Manipulations affecting the M-component of Task 1 do not propagate to Task 2 since it is a post-bottleneck manipulation.

3) Factors affecting the C- and M-components of Task 2 should increase RT2 independently of SOA. In contrast, factors affecting the P-component of Task 2 should increase RT2 only for large SOA values. This is one of the critical predictions of the model, since it implies that certain computations required for Task 2 completion can be performed during Task 1 queuing and thus argues for coexistence of serial and parallel processing within the same task.

We have extensively studied a PRP paradigm in which the main experimental task (Task 1) is a number-comparison task, which involves deciding whether a digit presented on the screen is larger or smaller than a fixed reference, performed simultaneously or quasi-simultaneously with a probe task (Task 2) (tone discrimination) at varying SOAs. Different manipulations of the number task can render it more difficult including: *notation* (target number presented in Arabic digits or as a spelt word); *distance* (numerical distance between the target number and the reference); and *response complexity* (whether subjects were asked to tap once or twice to indicate their choice). These manipulations change the difficulty of the task: mean response time slows down when numerical distance decreases and when numbers are presented as spelt words (Moyer and Landauer, 1967; Dehaene, 1996; Sigman and Dehaene, 2005). These effects are additive – that is, the mean increase due to the distance factor is independent of the effect of notation (Dehaene, 1996), thus establishing the first indication that they involve independent processing stages and can be factored separately from the task (Sternberg, 1969; 2004).

---

[1] SOAs are defined as short when $SOA+P2 < P1 + C1$, i.e. whenever sensory processing of Task 2 has completed before the bottleneck is free.

A surprising observation resulted from an analysis of the effects of these factors on RT variability. Although the precise dependence of the mean and variance of an RT distribution may vary (Wagenmakers and Brown, 2007), a simultaneous increase in the mean and dispersion of RTs is expected from any stochastic (noisy) process. Indeed, the distance manipulation, as expected, resulted in a significant increase in dispersion, which paralleled an increase in the mean. Strikingly however, the notation and response complexity factors, while inflicting a substantial change in the mean, did not affect the dispersion of the RT distribution.

By exploring the number task within a PRP paradigm, we showed that the three experimental factors mapped onto distinct stages of the PRP model: notation, numerical distance, and response gesture mapped on to the P-, C-, and M-components respectively. Thus, the numerical distance manipulation was the only one that affected the variance of the response and a serial processing stage. We postulated that the accumulation of evidence over time to reach a decision constitutes the only central process in a simple cognitive task, while all other stages can proceed in parallel with stages of another task (Sigman and Dehaene, 2005).

The PRP-bottleneck model argues that the timing of each processing stage is affected by interference. All other characteristics (duration, precision, variability…) are unaffected according to the model. Beyond purely chronometric measures, this hypothesis establishes a critical prediction for simple decision tasks; If the processing stages involved in a cognitive task are merely rescheduled during dual-task performance, the quality of the decision should be unaffected by a concurrent task.

In the previously described task, the number is presented as a symbol (digit or word). Thus, as in most previous studies, error rates are very low. To study whether the quality of the decision changes during the PRP, we performed a number task in which numbers were presented as a set of dots in a brief visual display. In this situation, subjects have only approximate information regarding numerosity, mimicking a more realistic decision-making situation that would rely upon noisy evidence for making a choice. Confirming the prediction of the bottleneck model, we showed that while response times replicated the main effects of interference observed in prior dual-task studies, the distribution of errors as a function of the numerical distance (which in single-task performance decreases according to the Weber fraction) were utterly unaffected by interference (Kamienkowski and Sigman, 2008).

Serial and parallel processing in the human brain: network dynamics and architecture

Methodological developments

What is the neurophysiological basis for the postulated stream of processing stages, and particularly for the central decision stage? The PRP-bottleneck model predicts that task interference results exclusively from a change in the dynamics of the processing stages within each task, without additional engagement of other brain areas. This constitutes a challenge for neurophysiology since it implies that during dual-task interference there are shifts in time without any corresponding change in the total amount of activity. This challenge explains why most previous studies have relied on the fine-grained temporal resolution of the event-related potential (ERPs) methodology. These experiments have systematically shown delayed (and occasionally also reduced) components, such as the N2PC, P3, and lateralized readiness potentials during PRP tasks (Osman and Moore, 1993; Luck, 1998; Arnell and Duncan, 2002; Dell'Acqua et al., 2005; Brisson and Jolicoeur, 2007). Using time-resolved functional magnetic resonance imaging (fMRI) (Menon et al., 1998; Formisano and Goebel, 2003), Dux and collaborators showed delayed activity in prefrontal cortex during a PRP paradigm (Dux et al., 2006), suggesting that a frontal network was one of the fundamental nodes responsible for the central bottleneck of information processing. None of those studies, however, provided a complete analysis of the neurocognitive task architecture at the whole-brain level.

We sought to achieve such a full decomposition. This ambitious goal required some methodological advances: to estimate changes in onset latency and response duration (Bellgowan et al., 2003), and to cluster the timing information into distinct stages based on a precise model of the stages in the task. We first demonstrated that fMRI could be used to recover the timing of all the stages in a complex composite task, reconstructing the controlled stream of brain activations in a sequence of cognitive operations (sensory, motor, verbal) (Sigman et al., 2007). Our Fourier-based methodology (described thoroughly in Sigman et al., 2007) showed that single-event fMRI can reveal changes in activation timing with a precision of 100–200ms. We then used this methodology in a simplified version of the PRP experiment described in the previous section. Only four SOA values (two short and two long) were used, the number task was presented second, numbers were presented only in Arabic digits, and a single response modality was required. We performed independent identical experiments with both time-resolved fMRI and with high-density ERP recordings (Sigman and Dehaene, 2008).

Factorizing a physiological stream into processing stages and investigating their temporal superposition

To understand the dynamics of different brain processes involved in the dual-task condition, we first decomposed the ERP data using scalp templates identified from the ERP recorded at the largest SOA, during which the execution of both tasks does not overlap in time. We simply identified the main topographies at each local maximum of the total voltage power recorded over all electrodes (Figure 5.1B, top panel), which could easily be identified as the N1 and P3 components corresponding to each task. Our aim was to understand the dynamics and architecture of these basic response components within the interference regime.

To do so, we decomposed the ERP at each time point for each SOA condition into a linear combination of the four scalp templates—simply referred as the 'time course of the ERP components'. The time course of the N1 and P3 components of Task 1 was utterly unaffected by changes in SOA values (Figure 5.1B, bottom left panels) indicating that, as predicted by the sequential model, the processing stages of Task 1 unfolded strictly identically both within and outside the interference regime. This observation also testifies to the efficiency of the decomposition procedure, which was able to identify the visual components of Task 1 even when they were superimposed with simultaneously occurring auditory components.

The time course of the Task-2 components showed a very different pattern (Figure 5.1B, bottom right panels). The N1 component was strictly time locked to Task 2 onset, as would be expected for a perceptual component of Task 2, peaking at a fixed latency after Task-2 onset. The time course of the P3 component, on the other hand, showed little effect of SOA for the short SOAs but a shift proportional to the change in SOA for the long SOAs, as would be expected for a central C-component of Task 2. The data suggest that Task-2 presentation immediately engages a sensory processing stage that unfolds over a period of about 300ms after Task-2 onset, followed by a central component which starts about 250ms after Task-2 onset and peaks at 380ms, but is systematically delayed by the simultaneous presence of a comparable component of a concurrent task.

While the sequential model was capable of explaining the bulk of the observations, some details of the ERP analysis did suggest significant departures: a modulation of the amplitude of the N1 component, reflecting sensory attenuation during concurrent task processing; ramping of the N1 component, revealing Task-2 sensory expectation after Task-1 completion, and the emergence of the Task-2 P3 component before stimulus presentation. These important departures will be discussed in the next section.

Serial and parallel processing in the human brain

ERPs provide high temporal resolution, but they are notoriously imprecise for spatial localization. Here, we took advantage of the fact that the PRP phenomenon induces delays of several hundred milliseconds which, as discussed previously, are measurable with fMRI. For the context of this chapter, it is important to know that the analysis is based on the *phase* of the response, which provides an estimate of the 'temporal centre of mass' and thus: 1) for a change in the onset of neural activation, only the phase of the haemodynamic response should vary, not the amplitude. The change in the phase should be identical to the change in delay; 2) for a change in the duration of activation, both phase and amplitude should increase, with the slope of the phase change reflecting half of the actual change in the duration of neuronal activation (Sigman et al., 2007).

We therefore recorded whole-brain fMRI images at a sampling time (TR) of 1.5 seconds, and computed the phase and amplitude of the haemodynamic response. A large network of brain areas (Figure 5.2A) exhibited phases consistently falling within the expected response latency for a task-induced activation. As expected for a complex dual-task experiment with visual and auditory stimuli, active regions included bilateral visual occipitotemporal cortices, bilateral auditory cortices, motor, premotor, and cerebellar cortices, and a large-scale bilateral parieto-frontal network. How is this large network organized in time during dual-task performance? As with the ERPs, we relied on the sequential model to determine our analytical strategy. Our method allowed us to parse the responsive brain areas into five different networks based on their temporal profile. The functional neuroanatomy of these networks was, for the most part, in tight accordance with the theoretical predictions.

For the brain network involved exclusively in Task 1, timing of the activation, and hence the phase of the fMRI response, should not change with SOA. This Task-1 network (Figure 5.2B, lower left, blue) comprised regions in extra-striate visual cortex, left motor cortex, and the most medial part of the posterior parietal cortex as well as an extended subcortical network. This network is that which would be expected for a visual number-comparison task requiring a right-hand response. For the brain network involved in the perceptual P-component of Task 2, the phase of the fMRI response should increase in direct proportion to SOA. This second cluster (Figure 5.2B, bottom, yellow) comprised bilateral auditory cortex, including Heschl's Gyrus – a plausible network for sensory processing of the second task (auditory tone discrimination). For the networks involved the central C- and motor M- components of Task 2, activations should be unchanged for short SOAs—due to queuing—and thus a delay should only be observed at long SOAs. FMRI voxels with this non-linear temporal profile (Figure 5.2B, lower right, red) were found in the right motor cortex, right supplementary motor area (SMA) (Task 2 responses were given with the left hand), and bilateral intraparietal sulcus. Interestingly this cluster also included the most medial parts of the visual cortex.

Estimating these networks assumes that the distinct dynamic processes of the two tasks always engage distinct brain regions. We therefore investigated one of the most interesting theoretical predictions: that the serial bottleneck may result from a broad network shared between both tasks, even though sensory and response modalities of the two tasks were distinct. Since the phase estimates the centre-of-mass of the response, regions involved in both tasks should show an increase in phase corresponding roughly to one-half of the increase in SOA. This profile corresponded to a large cluster, including bilateral posterior parietal cortex, premotor cortex, SMA,

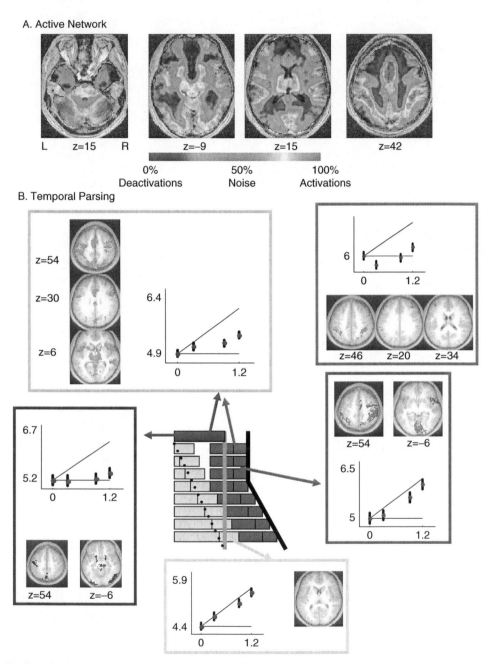

Fig. 5.2 (See also Plate 2) A) Networks activated (red) and deactivated (blue) during dual-task performance as identified by a phase coherence analysis. B) Parsing the brain network into distinct dynamic processing stages, according to their phase profile.

anterior part of the insula, and the cerebellum (Figure 5.2B, top left, cyan). For all these regions, if the effect of SOA is simply to alter the onset time of distinct processes, the amplitude of the fMRI activation should remain constant. This was indeed a very consistent experimental observation, in striking contrast with the broad repertoire of phase profiles. This indicates that all of the above changes corresponded to purely dynamic reorganization of task components, without any change in activation strength.

In summary, we measured the phase of the fMRI response in the whole brain at high temporal resolution, in order to parse the brain network involved in dual-task performance into distinct processing stages. We found regions whose timing was not affected by SOA, suggesting that they are involved exclusively in Task 1. Regarding Task 2 activations, sensory areas tracked the objective time of stimulus presentation, while a bilateral parieto-prefrontal network correlated with the dual-task sequential delay. Without performing the same experiment in the reverse task order, we cannot distinguish between C and M-components of this network, since both show the same temporal profile (see the scheme in Figure 5.2). An extended bilateral network was shared by both tasks during the extent of dual-task performance.

Beyond the simple sequential model: a hierarchical scheme for decision-making and executive control

I have previously shown that a simple sequential model of task architecture successfully accounts for most behavioural and neurophysiological observations of a simple PRP experiment. However, in each instance, we observed small but consistent and reproducible departures, which suggested that the model is necessarily incomplete. The first marked departure came from behavioural observations. Responses to Task 1 in the PRP paradigm, while independent of SOA, were found to be slower than when performing the task in isolation (Jiang et al., 2004; Sigman and Dehaene, 2005). We reasoned that this could be related to an executive control stage that is engaged before performance of the first task. We hypothesized that in situations in which task order is unknown, this executive time should increase, reflecting a hierarchical decision processes: first, which task to respond to, and second, the specific decision involved in each task. This hypothesis was verified in a new series of experiments in which we concluded that in this situation of task uncertainty, executive components (engaging and disengaging in a task) had to be incorporated into our original model, in order to account for these critical behavioural observations (Sigman and Dehaene, 2006).

Evidence for the involvement of such executive components could also be derived from the human physiology data. In the ERP analysis we observed that, while the timing of the peak of the N1 component of Task 2 was in strict accordance with the predictions of the bottleneck model, several other observations deviated from this model. First, the amplitude of the sensory N1 component decreased during the interference regime. Second, the temporal course of the N1 component ramped prior to stimulus presentation, probably reflecting task expectation and preparation. Finally, an auditory P3 component emerged at long SOAs, even before any auditory stimulus was presented. This anticipatory component peaked around 500ms, thus coinciding nicely with the end of the visual P3 evoked by Task 1. This ERP sequence is compatible with the hypothesis that, as soon as they completed Task 1, subjects re-oriented their attention to prepare for Task 2, reflecting an executive component of task engagement (De Jong, 1993; Logan and Meiran et al., 2000; Gordon, 2001; Ruthruff et al., 2001; Sigman and Dehaene, 2006). In addition it suggests that the absence of attentional top-down control may explain the amplitude attenuations observed during interference (Gilbert and Sigman, 2007).

The involvement of executive mechanisms in the PRP was also suggested by a cluster of voxels in the fMRI experiment that would not have been predicted by the purely sequential model. These voxels showed a purely non-linear pattern, with an increase in phase at the shortest SOA (Figure 5.2B, top right, green), and comprised a bilateral fronto-parietal network previously shown to be responsible for processing bottlenecks in dual-task performance (Marois et al., 2000; Marois and Ivanoff, 2005; Dux et al., 2006) and to be engaged in effortful but not automatic tasks (Ashbridge et al., 1997).

The extended network of areas affected by the PRP suggests that a broad array of processes cause the delay. Although this large set of areas might implement just one single cognitive stage of response selection, it seems more likely to correspond to the deployment of multiple hierarchically organized executive operations (Koechlin and Jubault, 2006; Koechlin et al., 2003). We thus proposed a model in which decisions could occur serially at any of several possible levels of the cognitive architecture. This model allows for simple task decisions (which key should I press for this stimulus?), but also higher-level executive decisions (which of these two stimuli should I process first? Am I finished with the first stimulus? Can I orient attention to the second?). Our evidence so far suggests that all of these decisions involve overlapping parieto-prefrontal networks and are serially arranged in time—such that the need for a higher-level decision pushes all other lower-level decisions further back in time.

Pause for thought: evidence from introspection and metacognition

Our approach for understanding cognitive architecture involved a variety of methodologies. An aspect common to most of them was the combination of chronometry (through additive factor analysis; see Hunt, van Zoest, and Kingstone, Chapter 1, this volume) with other experimental tools such as electroencephalography (EEG) and time-resolved fMRI. Recently, we have also investigated whether chronometric techniques could be used to address, in a precise quantitative manner, the introspective knowledge of one's own mental content (Wundt, 1897/1999; Jack and Roepstorff, 2003; Overgaard, 2006).

To explore which processing stages were accessible to introspection during the PRP, we explored the number-comparison task with the new twist that participants could also indicate their introspective estimation of response time by clicking with the mouse on a continuous graded scale, spanning from 0–1200ms and labelled every 300ms. The results we obtained were extremely clear-cut. Introspective RT turned out to be an extremely reliable and sensitive measure, tightly correlated with objective RT in a single-task context, and sensitive to factors (e.g. notation) that affect response time by as little as 50ms. In a PRP task, however, the objective processing delay was totally absent from introspective estimates. During the interference regime, the participants were totally unaware that their responses to the second task had been slowed by as much as 300ms. Thus, awareness and accessibility to introspection seemed to be tightly linked to the availability of the central decision system. When this system was available, all stages of a cognitive task contributed to introspective RT, but when it was occupied by another task, participants were no longer aware of the duration of the perceptual and queuing stages of the PRP task (Corallo et al., 2008).

These results suggest that a mental clock continues to operate throughout the performance of a PRP task (RT to Task 1 is well estimated introspectively). The salient events of the trial are stored with 'time stamps' derived from this clock, which are retrievable later (presumably with some noise added due to forgetting or storage failures). During the PRP interference regime the time stamp applied to stimulus 2 is the time by which the central (bottleneck-dependent) parts of Task 1 have been completed.

Discussion: cognitive architecture of the never-halting machine

Several cognitive theories have shared the hypothesis that while most mental and neural operations are modular, certain specific controlled processes require a distinct functional architecture that can establish flexible links amongst existing processors. This process has been called the central executive (Baddeley, 1986), the supervisory attentional system (Shallice, 1988), the anterior attention system (Posner, 1994), the capacity limited stage (Chun and Potter, 1995), or the global workspace (Baars, 1989; Dehaene and Naccache, 2001). Yet in all of these different versions, four critical aspects are shared: 1) binding of information from many different modules; 2) uniqueness of its contents; 3) sustained activity for a few hundred milliseconds and 4) its relation to attentional control and mental effort. These aspects are also characteristic of consciousness and thus it has been proposed that engagement of the central system may be a requirement for conscious processing (Baars, 1989; Dehaene and Naccache, 2001). Chun and Potter's two-stage model (2005) proposes that an early stage permits the rapid, initial evaluation of the visual world. Only during a second, capacity-limited stage, does information become conscious when the neural population that represents it is mobilized into a state of coherent activity at the level of the whole brain (Baars, 1989; Chun and Potter, 1995; Dehaene and Naccache, 2001).

Combining models, psychophysics, and human physiology, we can disentangle the unfolding of processing stages during a compound cognitive task. The data have converged to a model that proposes:

+ Initial perceptual processing of incoming stimuli, which is performed in a modular (parallel) fashion and, as indexed by the N1 latency of the ERP, is extremely reliable in time

+ Followed by a central process, indexed by the P3 component of the ERP, involved in the flexible coordination of information according to specific task requirements, which is intrinsically serial and involves noisy accumulation of evidence to reach a decision.

Our findings of Task-2 dynamics in the PRP fit well with ERP data from other interference experiments, such as the AB (Sergent et al., 2005). In these experiments, it was found that the first approximately 270ms, indexed by P1 and N1 components, were independent of conscious access, and this was followed by a centrally distributed P3 component, involving a prefrontal and parietal network, which was engaged only in trials in which the stimulus accessed conscious processing.

These results have led to the proposal that the P3 component of the EEG may index access to a global coherent workspace associated with flexible coordination of information, which in turn may mediate conscious reportability (Sergent et al., 2005). According to this theory, this state provides a global 'broadcasting' system enabling communication between arbitrary and otherwise not directly connected brain processors (Baars, 1989; Dehaene and Naccache, 2001). In most psychological tasks, the relation between stimuli and responses is entirely arbitrary and thus requires temporary mapping between otherwise independent processors. Supporting this interpretation, interference is drastically reduced for highly practised or non-arbitrary tasks (Lien and Proctor, 2002; Greenwald, 2003). More evidence for the existence of a common processing bottleneck involved in conscious access and in the flexible routing of information results from hybrid behavioural experiments which combine the PRP and the AB (Jolicoeur, 1999; Wong, 2002; Marois and Ivanoff, 2005).

A basic sketch of the postulated brain dynamics during the AB and the PRP illustrates this idea (Figure 5.3). In both experimental designs, certain aspects of T2[2] processing—indexed by the

---

[2] T2 refers to the second task in the PRP. In the AB responses are not speeded and thus subjects are not asked to respond to the presence of the second stimuli (S2). Here I refer to T2 in the AB as the conscious perception of the second stimulus (S2).

N1 and mediated by a transient activation of sensory cortex—can proceed while T1 engages a broad and coherent state of processing that occupies the central workspace. While the nature of this T2 sensory memory is not fully understood and requires theoretical and experimental investigation (Sperling, 1960; Gegenfurtner and Sperling, 1993) it appears to constitute a labile form of memory (Graziano and Sigman, 2008; 2009; Zylberberg et al., 2009) which can be overriden by the presence of a mask, consistent with current theories and experimental evidence of masking by object substitution (Di Lollo et al., 2000). The presence of a mask after T2 can thus lead to the AB phenomenon, whereby participants fail to detect the presence of a second stimulus despite a strong initial perceptual activation. In the absence of masking, T2 can access the workspace and is therefore processed after the delay known as the PRP. AB and PRP are therefore envisaged as two very similar phenomena, arising from the constraints with which operations can be carried out in parallel versus those which require serial processing.

While there are no direct correlates of these findings in single-cell neurophysiology (there is currently no demonstration of the PRP in non-human primates), some chronometric aspects can be related to the dynamics of neuronal activation in single tasks. The neurophysiological bases of perceptual decision making have been studied in tactile (Romo et al., 2002) and visual discrimination tasks (Shadlen and Newsome, 1996; Thompson et al., 1996). These studies have revealed direct physiological correlates of the accumulation process postulated in formal response-time models. Some neurons appear to code for the current perceptual state. For instance, neurons in area MT appear to encode the amount of evidence for motion in a certain direction (Shadlen and Newsome, 1996). Other neurons, distributed in multiple areas, including posterior parietal cortex, dorsolateral prefrontal cortex, and frontal eye fields, appear to integrate this sensory information and thus show stochastically increasing firing rates in the course of decision-making (Shadlen and Newsome, 1996). In agreement with the accumulation model of decision-making, the rate of increase varies with the quality of sensory evidence, and the response is emitted when the firing exceeds a threshold (Shadlen and Newsome, 1996). Furthermore, accumulation of information about the upcoming response appears in the firing train after a latency of about 200ms (Roitman and Shadlen, 2002), which is relatively fixed for a given task and might thus index the duration of the initial perceptual stage.

Further evidence of such a dynamic arrangement comes from recordings from the primary visual cortex of awake monkeys, which have shown that a visual stimulus first evokes a transient response, followed by a sustained wave of activity (Lamme and Roelfsema, 2000; Li et al., 2006) at a latency of about 200ms, nicely coincident with the latency of integration in parietal and prefrontal areas and of the engagement of the P3 process. These two responses have very different functional dependencies: the first transient response is largely determined by stimulus properties and can be explained by classical bottom-up receptive field properties In contrast, the second response can be modulated by different cognitive, attentive, and contextual factors. For instance, it is amplified if the local stimulus is salient and attended (as in figure-ground experiments) and it can virtually disappear if the stimulus is masked (which presumably precludes its access to awareness) or by anaesthetics. This specificity suggests an engagement of the central workspace system in the second wave of activity and implies that the same neuron may be involved in distinct processing stages within the same task. Further experiments are required to determine whether this second wave of activity shows a dual-task delay characteristic of the serial processing bottleneck.

Conclusions

Altogether, neurophysiological and brain-imaging studies suggest that, beyond an initial and relatively reliable perceptual delay of about 200ms, a decision stage begins which involves a

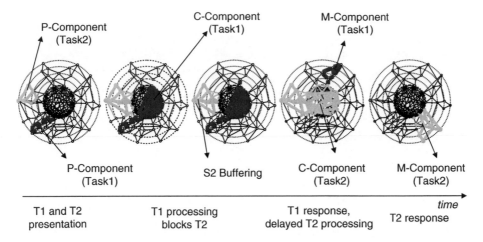

P-Component
(Task2)

C-Component
(Task1)

M-Component
(Task1)

P-Component
(Task1)

S2 Buffering

C-Component
(Task2)

M-Component
(Task2)

time

T1 and T2
presentation

T1 processing
blocks T2

T1 response,
delayed T2 processing

T2 response

PSYCHOLOGICAL REFRACTORY PERIOD

- T2 is sustained and thus can access the workspace after a delay.
- This delay is inaccessible to introspection.

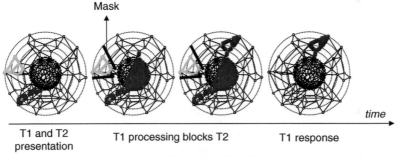

Mask

time

T1 and T2
presentation

T1 processing blocks T2

T1 response

ATTENTIONAL BLINK

- S2 is masked and does not access consciousness.

Fig. 5.3 A simple sketch of the dynamics of modular (P- and M-components) and central (C-component) processing during the PRP and the attentional blink. Each network constitutes a symbolic representation of the hierarchy of connections between brain processors symbolized by concentric circles (after Dehaene, Kerszberg, and Changeux, 1998). Higher levels of this hierarchy are assumed to be widely interconnected by long-distance interconnections. The activation of this system brings together several peripheral processors in a coherent brain-scale activation pattern (black circles) and has been suggested to be a requirement for conscious access (Dehaene, Kerszberg, and Changeux, 1998). Peripheral levels represent modules which can work in parallel, including P- and C- components of the PRP. Here we suggest that the activation of this system establishes a processing bottleneck which may be responsible for the PRP (top row) and the AB (bottom row). In each row the highlighted segments schematically represent the activation related to Stimulus 1 (light grey) and Stimulus 2 (dark grey). In the top row, the second stimulus (S2) can be held in a local memory. It can access the central stage when it becomes available, thus resulting in a delay (PRP). In the bottom row, the second stimulus' processing stream is masked before accessing the central processing stage and thus remains unconscious (the blink). T = Task.

process of noisy accumulation of evidence and the joint activation of a distributed network of areas, with partially changing topography as a function of the nature of the task, but with frequent if not systematic coactivation of parietal and premotor regions. The activation of this distributed network seems to be required for combining information flexibly in different sensory, mnemonic, and motor modalities according to specific task-requirements. Our results show that the engagement of this network provides a major contribution to response time variability and is responsible for establishing the PRP bottleneck. Thus, while certain neural computations, probably mediated by hard-wired circuits confined to small portions of sensory space, can be very fast, precise, and parallel, linking such information together in a coherent workspace is a slow, variable, and intrinsically sequential computation.

The challenge for the next few years will be to understand which precise biophysical mechanisms are involved in this coherent workspace and why they result in such distinctive dynamic and architectonic properties. At present, our results simply suggest that this bottleneck might occur because the cerebral accumulation system is broadly distributed and largely shared across tasks, and thus must be entirely 'mobilized', at any given moment, by whichever task is currently performed. Considerable research has examined the neurophysiology of a single cognitive operation, but much less is known on how we chain these basic operations into complex tasks. The results described here constitute a first step towards a progressive understanding of the chaining of simple computations into complex compound tasks.

References

Allport, D. et al. (1994). Shifting intentional set: exploring the dynamic control of tasks. In C. Umilta, and M. Moscovitch (Eds.) *Attention and Performance XV*, pp.421–52. Cambridge, MA: MIT Press.

Anderson, J. R. et al. (2004). An integrated theory of the mind. *Psychol Rev,* **111**, 1036–60.

Arnell, K. M. and Duncan, J. (2002). Separate and shared sources of dual-task cost in stimulus identification and response selection. *Cognit Psychol,* **44**, 105–47.

Ashbridge, E. et al. (1997). Temporal aspects of visual search studied by transcranial magnetic stimulation. *Neuropsychologia,* **35**, 1121–31.

Baars, B. J. (1989). *A Cognitive Theory of Consciousness.* Cambridge: Cambridge Univesity Press.

Baddeley, A. D. (1986). *Working Memory.* Oxford: Clarendon Press.

Bellgowan, P. S. et al. (2003). Understanding neural system dynamics through task modulation and measurement of functional MRI amplitude, latency, and width. *Proc Natl Acad Sci U S A,* **100**, 1415–19.

Brisson, B. and Jolicoeur, P. (2007). A psychological refractory period in access to visual short-term memory and the deployment of visual-spatial attention: multitasking processing deficits revealed by event-related potentials. *Psychophysiology,* **44**, 323–33.

Chun, M. M. and Potter, M. C. (1995). A two-stage model for multiple target detection in rapid serial visual presentation. *J Exp Psychol Hum Percept Perform,* **21**, 109–27.

Corallo, G., Sackur, J., Dehaene, S., and Sigman, M. (2008). Limits on introspection: distorted subjective time during the dual-task bottleneck. *Psychol Sci.* **19**(11):1110–17.

De Jong, R. (1993). Multiple bottlenecks in overlapping task performance. *J Exp Psychol Hum Percept Perform* **19**, 965–80.

Dehaene, S. (1996). The organization of brain activation in number comparison: event-related potential and the additive-factor methods. *J Cogn Neurosci,* **8**, 47–68.

Dehaene, S. and Naccache, L. (2001). Towards a cognitive neuroscience of consciousness: basic evidence and a workspace framework. *Cognition,* **79**, 1–37.

Dell'Acqua, R. et al. (2005). Central processing overlap modulates P3 latency. *Exp Brain Res,* **165**, 54–68.

Di Lollo, V. et al. (2000). Competition for consciousness among visual events: the psychophysics of reentrant visual processes. *J Exp Psychol Gen,* **129**, 481–507.

Duncan, J. and Owen, A. M. (2000). Common regions of the human frontal lobe recruited by diverse cognitive demands. *Trends Neurosci,* **23**, 475–83.

Dux, P. E. et al. (2006). Isolation of a central bottleneck of information processing with time-resolved fMRI. *Neuron,* **52**, 1109–20.

Felleman, D. J. and Van Essen, D. C. (1991). Distributed hierarchical processing in the primate cerebral cortex. *Cereb Cortex,* **1**, 1–47.

Formisano, E. and Goebel, R. (2003). Tracking cognitive processes with functional MRI mental chronometry. *Curr Opin Neurobiol,* **13**, 174–81.

Gegenfurtner, K. R. and Sperling, G. (1993). Information transfer in iconic memory experiments. *J Exp Psychol Hum Percept Perform,* **19**, 845–66.

Gilbert, C. D. and Sigman, M. (2007). Brain states: top-down influences in sensory processing. *Neuron,* **54**, 677–96.

Graziano, M. and Sigman, M. (2008). The dynamics of sensory buffers: geometric, spatial, and experience-dependent shaping of iconic memory. *J Vis,* **8**, 9.1–13.

Graziano, M. and Sigman, M. (2009). The spatial and temporal construction of confidence in the visual scene. *PLoS One,* **4**, e4909.

Greenwald, A. G. (2003). On doing two things at once: III. Confirmation of perfect timesharing when simultaneous tasks are ideomotor compatible. *J Exp Psychol Hum Percept Perform,* **29**, 859–68.

Hubel, D. H. and Wiesel, T. N. (1959). Receptive fields of single neurones in the cat's striate cortex. *J Physiol,* **148**, 574–91.

Jack, A. I. and Roepstorff, A. (2003). Trusting the subject I. *J Conscious Stud,* **9**, 9–10.

Jiang, Y. et al. (2004). Functional magnetic resonance imaging provides new constraints on theories of the psychological refractory period. *Psychol Sci,* **15**, 390–6.

Jolicoeur, P. (1999). Concurrent response-selection demands modulate the attentional blink. *J Exp Psychol Hum Percept Perform,* **25**, 1097–113.

Kahneman, D. (1973). *Attention and Effort.* Englewood Cliffs, NJ: Prentice-Hall.

Kamienkowski, J. E. and Sigman, M. (2008). Delays without mistakes: response time and error distributions in dual-task. *PLoS One,* **3**, e3196.

Koechlin, E. and Jubault, T. (2006). Broca's area and the hierarchical organization of human behavior. *Neuron,* **50**, 963–74.

Koechlin, E. et al. (2003). The architecture of cognitive control in the human prefrontal cortex. *Science,* **302**, 1181–5.

Lamme, V. A. and Roelfsema, P. R. (2000). The distinct modes of vision offered by feedforward and recurrent processing. *Trends Neurosci,* **23**, 571–9.

Li, W. et al. (2006). Contour saliency in primary visual cortex. *Neuron,* **50**, 951–62.

Lien, M. C. and Proctor, R. W. (2002). Stimulus-response compatibility and psychological refractory period effects: implications for response selection. *Psychon Bull Rev,* **9**, 212–38.

Logan, G. D. and Gordon, R. (2001). Executive control of visual attention in dual tasks. *Psychol Rev,* **108**, 393–434.

Luck, S. J. (1998). Sources of dual-task interference: evidence from human electrophysiology. *Psychol Sci,* **9**, 223–7.

Marois, R. et al. (2000). Neural correlates of the attentional blink. *Neuron,* **28**, 299–308.

Marois, R. and Ivanoff, J. (2005). Capacity limits of information processing in the brain. *Trends Cogn Sci,* **9**, 296–305.

Meiran, N. et al. (2000). Component processes in task switching. *Cognit Psychol,* **41**, 211–53.

Menon, R. S. et al. (1998). Mental chronometry using latency-resolved functional MRI. *Proc Natl Acad Sci U S A,* **95**, 10902–7.

Meyer, D.E. and Kieras, D. E. (1997). A computational theory of executive cognitive processes and multiple-task performance: Part 1. Basic mechanisms. *Psychol Rev,* **104**, 3–65.

Moyer, R. S. and Landauer, T. K. (1967). Time required for judgements of numerical inequalities. *Nature*, **215**, 1519–20.

Osman, A. and Moore, C. M. (1993). The locus of dual-task interference: psychological refractory effects on movement-related brain potentials. *J Exp Psychol Hum Percept Perform*, **19**, 1292–312.

Overgaard, M. (2006). Introspection in science. *Conscious Cogn*, **15**, 629–33.

Pashler, H. (1994). Dual-task interference in simple tasks: data and theory. *Psychol Bull*, **116**, 220–44.

Pashler, H. and Johnston, J. C. (1989). Chronometric evidence for central postponement in temporally overlapping tasks. *QJEP*, **41A**, 19–45.

Pashler, H. and Johnston, J. C. (1998). Attentional limitations in dual-task performance. In H. Pashler (Ed.) *Attention*, pp.55–89. Hove: Psychology Press/Erlbaum.

Posner, M. I. (1994). Attention: the mechanisms of consciousness. *Proc Natl Acad Sci U S A*, **91**, 7398–403.

Roitman, J. D. and Shadlen, M.N. (2002). Response of neurons in the lateral intraparietal area during a combined visual discrimination reaction time task. *J Neurosci*, **22**, 9475–89.

Romo, R. et al. (2002). From sensation to action. *Behav Brain Res*, **135**, 105–18.

Ruthruff, E. et al. (2001). Processing bottlenecks in dual-task performance: structural limitation or strategic postponement? *Psychon Bull Rev*, **8**, 73–80.

Schweickert, R. (1980). Critical-path scheduling of mental processes in a dual task. *Science*, **209**, 704–6.

Sergent, C. et al. (2005). Timing of the brain events underlying access to consciousness during the attentional blink. *Nat Neurosci*, **8**, 1391–400.

Shadlen, M. N. and Newsome, W. T. (1996). Motion perception: seeing and deciding. *Proc Natl Acad Sci U S A*, **93**, 628–33.

Shallice, T. (1988). *From neuropsychology to mental structure*. Cambridge: Cambridge University Press.

Sigman, M. and Dehaene, S. (2005). Parsing a cognitive task: a characterization of the mind's bottleneck. *PLoS Biol*, **3**, e37.

Sigman, M. and Dehaene, S. (2006). Dynamics of the central bottleneck: dual-task and task uncertainty. *PLoS Biol*, **4**, e220.

Sigman, M. and Dehaene, S. (2008). Brain mechanisms of serial and parallel processing during dual-task performance. *J Neurosci*, **28**, 7585–98.

Sigman, M. et al. (2007). Parsing a sequence of brain activations at psychological times using fMRI. *Neuroimage*, **35**, 655–68.

Smith, M. C. (1967). Theories of the psychological refractory period. *Psych Bull*, **67**, 202–13.

Sperling, G. (1960). *The information available in brief visual presentations*. Washington, DC: APA.

Sternberg, S. (1969). The discovery of processing stages: Extension of Donders' method. In W. G. Koster (Ed.) *Attention and performance II*, pp.276–315. Amsterdam.

Sternberg, S. (2004). Separate modifiability and the search for processing modules. In N. Kanwisher & J. Duncan (Eds.), *Attention and Performance XX*. Oxford: Oxford University Press.

Telford, C.W. (1931). The refractory phase of voluntary and associative responses. *J Exp Psych*, **14**, 1–36.

Thompson, K. G. et al. (1996). Perceptual and motor processing stages identified in the activity of macaque frontal eye field neurons during visual search. *J Neurophysiol*, **76**, 4040–55.

Wagenmakers, E. J. and Brown, S. (2007). On the linear relation between the mean and the standard deviation of a response time distribution. *Psychol Rev*, **114**(3), 830–41.

Wong, K. F. E. (2002). The relationship between attentional blink and psychological refractory period. *J Exp Psychol Hum Percept Perform*, **28**, 54–71.

Wundt, W. M. (1897/1999). *Outlines of Psychology*. London: Thoemmes Press.

Zylberberg, A. et al. (2009). Neurophysiological bases of exponential sensory decay and top-down memory retrieval: a model. *Front Comput Neurosci*, **3**, 4.

Chapter 6

Vigilant attention

Ian H. Robertson and Redmond O'Connell

Human beings find it surprisingly difficult to attend to unchanging or unchallenging repetitive stimuli and responses. We have little difficulty concentrating when navigating a complex traffic junction or playing a fast and difficult computer game, yet when all that is required of us is to sit in a lecture hall for an hour and take in what a single person is saying, we struggle. Why do civil engineers build curves into highways across flat land where there is no geographical or geological need to do so? They do so because our brains cannot reliably focus attention for even quite modest periods without requiring the small attentional and psychomotor challenge that the bends induce. This chapter discusses vigilant attention, an attention system of the brain that has evolved with certain limitations—to the extent that engineers throughout the world have to spend billions of euros every year to try to compensate for its failings. Vigilant attention is also extremely sensitive to disorders and damage to the brain, and can be a major source of difficulty in everyday life in conditions such as traumatic brain injury (Robertson et al., 1997), attention deficit hyperactivity disorder (Bellgrove et al., 2005), and tau-opathy related neurodegeneration (O'Keeffe et al., 2007).

One reason why the vigilant attention system may have evolved imperfectly is because there are survival advantages associated with periodic disengagement from the current focus of attention—in other words 'lapses'. While under certain circumstances continually directing attention to the burrow where the prey might emerge is adaptive, such prolonged attention if overly focused may lead to lack of detection of danger and consequently becoming the prey oneself. Vigilant attention and drifting attention may therefore both have separate costs and benefits. Today, however, we live in a constantly changing world where the fast pace of techno-logical advances has presented us with challenges and dangers that the human race has never faced before. It is only in very recent history that a simple lapse of attention by a single individual could result in the death or injury of hundreds of people, as in the cases of air and rail travel. Similarly, our system of education has transformed such that a heavy premium is now placed on one's ability to maintain focus over long periods of time. The purpose of this chapter is to eluci-date the nature of this often-ignored and poorly understood type of attention. Attention research has long been plagued by terminological confusion. Before elaborating on the components we believe are important in vigilant attention, the following are our working definitions of some of the relevant terms in this area.

Vigilant attention

We define vigilant attention as: 'the ability to self-sustain mindful, conscious processing of stimuli whose repetitive, non-arousing qualities, would otherwise lead to habituation and distraction by other stimuli' (Robertson et al., 1997). As we will discuss later on, vigilant attention is closely linked to a predominantly right hemispheric fronto-parietal system and acts in close linkage with the midbrain noradrenergic system to maintain optimal levels of responding during fluctuating levels of arousal.

Vigilance

Following the seminal work of Mackworth in the late 1940s, vigilance is a term to describe the slow increase in error rate that occurs over periods of between 30 minutes and 1 hour in the context of perceptual detection tasks involving the detection of very rare targets amongst large numbers of monotonous and homogeneous stimuli (Mackworth, 1957). As we will outline in later sections, recent work has demonstrated that vigilant attention can fluctuate over periods of less than a minute. We do not, therefore, use the term vigilance because it has come to imply the time-on-task decline in performance apparent only over long periods.

Arousal

While acknowledging there are many different neurotransmitters associated with arousal, for the purposes of this chapter we define arousal as the tonic and phasic levels of locus coeruleus (LC)-mediated noradrenergic activation, whose action both enhances signal-to-noise ratio of neural signals underpinning perceptual and cognitive representations and increases error rate, particularly at high levels of noradrenaline (NA) activation. Arousal varies with circadian rhythms and shows an inverted-U function such that performance is impaired when NA levels are both below and above optimal levels (Aston-Jones and Cohen, 2005). The term 'alerting', used by Posner and Petersen in their seminal article on the attention systems of the brain (Posner and Petersen, 1990), is approximately co-terminous with the above working definition of arousal, albeit that 'alerting' has connotations of the behavioural (e.g. reaction-time shortening contingent on phasic 'alerting' stimuli), as well as on the phenomenological ('feeling alert') aspects of the more biologically defined concept of 'arousal'.

Sustained attention

Sustained attention is the capacity to maintain accurate responding over time across tasks which can be effortful and demanding, or monotonous and undemanding. Sustained attention tasks may not show the same time-on-task declines that monotonous, Mackworth-type tasks show, if they are perceptually, motorically, or cognitive challenging, as the external challenge drives the arousal system and does not place demands on the vigilant attention system, which has a specific role in maintaining accurate responding in situations where such externally-mediated modulation of arousal is not present.

The neural basis of vigilant attention

Attention can be defined as the capacity to allocate processing resources selectively to particular stimuli or classes of stimuli. There are many different ways in which the brain does this, and these can be broadly arranged into a continuum according to which the allocation is driven by bottom-up, externally driven factors at one end, versus top-down, internally driven factors at the other. If a truck horn blares in my ear as I am about to step off the road, all my processing resources will be allocated to the relevant stimuli in an almost entirely bottom-up way. If I am proofreading this chapter for minor typographical errors, on the other hand, the attention required for this tedious task is almost entirely top-down.

Imaging studies have indicated that vigilant attention is controlled by a right lateralized cortical network that includes the anterior cingulate gyrus, the right dorsolateral prefrontal cortex, and the inferior parietal lobule (Sturm and Willmes 2001). This network monitors and modulates activity in subcortical regions governing arousal to match current task demands (Critchley et al. 2003, Foucher et al. 2005). Posner and Peterson (1990) identified the midbrain LC as the critical arousal hub supporting the alert state by increasing perceptual signal-to-noise ratios via the neurotransmitter NA. The LC is the principal midbrain source of NA and has inputs from prefrontal cortex and the anterior cingulate cortex. It projects particularly strongly to inferior parietal cortex and somatosensory cortex, but also throughout frontal pole and the temporal parietal junction (Berridge and Waterhouse, 2003).

LC activity increases when animals are observed as being behaviourally alert (Aston-Jones, Chiang, and Alexinsky, 1991), and the appearance of a low-probability target stimulus among foils leads to increased LC activity and widespread noradrenergic release (Berridge and Waterhouse, 2003). The influence of the LC system in humans was demonstrated by Smith and Nutt (1996) who reported that suppressing the release of NA through clonidine administration resulted in the sorts of attentional lapses that are characteristic of diminished vigilant attention. Pharmacological studies by Coull and her colleagues have found similarly close links between noradrenergic function and vigilant attention (Coull et al., 1995). More recently, our group has demonstrated a specific linkage in humans between NA activity and performance on a vigilant attention task in healthy adults who differ in a genotype that codes for an enzyme (dopamine β-hydroxylase) that controls the availability of NA in the brain. Individuals whose genotype was associated with relatively low noradrenergic availability showed significantly increased errors of commission (Greene et al., 2009). Our group has also reported similar results in children diagnosed with attention deficit/hyperactivity disorder (Bellgrove et al., 2006).

Vigilant attention versus arousal

In 1908, Yerkes and Dodson studied the effects of different degrees of arousal (by varying the degree of shock) on the ability of mice to learn discriminations between the luminance of two compartments (Yerkes and Dodson, 1908). They found that where lightness levels were easily discriminated, the mice performed better at high levels of arousal, whereas difficult light discriminations were best learned at low levels of arousal. On the basis of these experiments, they formulated the Yerkes–Dodson law. This law proposed that any task will have an optimal level of arousal below and beyond which performance will decline; they hypothesized this optimal level is lower in challenging tasks than in routine tasks. Similarly, Broadbent (1971) showed that while stress can improve performance on routine, non-demanding tasks, the same levels of stress can impair performance on more complex and demanding tasks. These classic psychological studies, suggesting an interaction between arousal levels, optimal performance, and degree of challenge in a task, mesh well with the notion of exogenous modulation of arousal as previously discussed. They also suggest, however, that the relationship between the system for vigilant attention and that of arousal may not be a simple one of mutual facilitation, and a number of other more recent studies support such a view.

As mentioned earlier, vigilant attention can be impaired through administration of drugs—for instance, clonidine—that inhibit NA release. One study by Smith and Nutt (1996), for example, confirmed that NA suppression in humans led to lapses of vigilant attention but they also showed that this effect was much attenuated when the participants were exposed to loud white noise while performing the task. This suggests that external stimuli can induce 'bottom-up' or exogenous modulation of the cortical systems for vigilant attention. Coull and her colleagues confirmed that this is indeed the case (Coull et al., 1995), showing that clonidine-induced noradrenergic suppression impaired vigilant attention performance much more when the task was familiar than when it was unfamiliar—and thus more challenging. Furthermore, research by Arnsten and Contant (1992) showed that clonidine affected delayed response performance during a delay period *less* when a distractor was interpolated into the delay period than when the period was free of distractors. This apparently paradoxical effect, where the deleterious effect of a drug is reduced by making the task more *difficult*, is a key finding in understanding how the vigilant attention system might function. More recently, a functional magnetic resonance imaging (fMRI) study by Coull and colleagues (2004) explored the functional anatomical correlates of exogenous modulators of attention in a group of participants who were sedated by an alpha-2 adrenergic receptor agonist. The improvement in performance following phasic white noise stimulation was associated with a selective increase in activation of the left medial pulvinar nucleus of the thalamus. What these findings suggest is that this system can be engaged by both endogenous and exogenous means; furthermore, where exogenous activation takes place, we argue, this considerably reduces the demands on the endogenous components of the system.

Progress has been made in identifying the neurophysiological basis for this attention-arousal coupling. For example, LC activity has been shown to correlate closely with behavioural performance where monkeys have to detect relatively rare (20% probability) visual targets among foils, but optimal performance was achieved not at maximum levels of LC activity, but rather at intermediate levels (Usher et al., 1999). Increased tonic LC noradrenergic activity was linked to decreased responsivity of LC neurons to target stimuli, as well as to poor behavioural performance. These authors proposed that high tonic LC activity offers a mechanism for sampling new stimuli and behaviours by decreasing attentional selectivity and increasing the behavioural responsiveness to unexpected or novel stimuli. Intermediate levels of tonic LC activity, on the other hand, allow the optimizing of performance in a stable environment. In a comprehensive review of catecholamine modulation of prefrontal cognitive function, Arnsten showed that many studies have confirmed the findings of Usher and colleagues in showing a Yerkes–Dodson type inverted-U relationship between levels of NA release on the one hand, and behavioural performance on the other (Arnsten, 1998). She also concludes that different neuropsychiatric conditions may reveal impairment in executive control of complex behaviours for reasons of either deficient or excessive levels of NA respectively.

In a study by Paus and colleagues (1997), volunteers were asked to perform a simple continuous performance task, a measure of vigilant attention, for around 60 minutes. Every 10 minutes, regional cerebral blood flow (via positron emission tomography [PET]) and an electroencephalogram (EEG) were measured. Over the 60 minutes, they saw reductions in blood flow in subcortical structures including the thalamus, substantia innominate, and putamen, and in right hemisphere cortical areas, including frontal and parietal cortex. Increases in low theta activity, associated with reduction in arousal, were also observed on the EEG as the task progressed. Importantly, however, the changes in the subcortical (arousal) network were not correlated over time with the changes in the right fronto-parietal (attentional) network. In other words, even though both arousal and vigilant attention declined, they declined independently. Furthermore, despite the reduction in blood flow in the right hemisphere 'attentional' network and the subcortical 'arousal' network, the number of successful target detections did not significantly decline over the hour of the task. Paus and his colleagues argued that this was because detection of targets in the vigilance task became more automatic and hence less dependent on vigilant attention, whose capacity waned over the course of the task.

It is this type of result that leads to the use of the term *vigilant* attention rather than *sustained* attention. Sustained attention may include situations that require sustained *performance* but which may actually make limited demands on vigilant attention. This distinction is perhaps best captured by consideration that 'maintaining' responsivity to an arbitrary but overlearned stimulus such as one's own name does not require an active maintenance of attention at all (Cherry, 1953)

Such a conclusion would be supported by Coull et al. (Coull, Fackowiak, and Frith, 1998) who also found decreases in thalamic and right fronto-parietal perfusion over an 18-minute task period in which participants had to respond to any stimulus appearing intermittently (within a range of 1–30 seconds) on the screen. In contrast, when the task was made relatively more difficult by requiring participants to respond selectively to red Bs interspersed among red and blue Bs and Gs, no significant decline in the right frontal and parietal cortices was observed. This is in line with the earlier arguments concerning the effects of exogenous demand on vigilant attention, and suggests that this right fronto-parietal system for vigilant attention is, at least in part, a system that is needed to maintain alert and reasonably accurate responding in the absence of strong external demands or stimuli that otherwise promote alert responding.

Assuming this to be the case, then a major role of the right fronto-parietal system is to modulate arousal, particularly where that arousal is not externally generated by task demand or stimulus. Taken together, the studies outlined here underline the functional and anatomical distinction between arousal, which is mediated by subcortical networks, and vigilant attention, which is mediated by a primarily cortical network.

The time course of vigilant attention

In the laboratory, vigilant attention has typically been examined using variants of the continuous performance task during which participants monitor a stream of stimuli over an extended period of time for the occurrence of a rare target stimulus to which they must make a response. These tasks have been designed to mimic 'real world' situations in which low signal probability places us at risk of a critical lapses of attention (e.g. the train driver who passes a red light or the airport security officer who fails to notice a weapon on the luggage x-ray). Performing such tasks is tedious and undemanding, leading to a gradual decrement in performance over time. This phenomenon is known as the 'vigilance decrement' and it, rather than overall accuracy, has been used as the key metric of vigilant attention in numerous studies (Parasuraman, Nestor, and Greenwood, 1989; Swanson et al., 2004). In other words, it has been argued that vigilant attention only comes into play when it is needed to offset the reductions in arousal that occur with increasing time-on-task. But in everyday life we are also susceptible to momentary fluctuations in goal-directed attention in the context of much shorter periods of time-on-task (e.g. putting coffee on your cornflakes instead of in your cup). Accuracy over relatively short periods of time (seconds to minutes) may be equally informative by providing a more sensitive measure of the moment-to-moment efficiency of top-down mechanisms. Functional imaging and electrophysiological studies have supported these observations by demonstrating that activity in the vigilant attention network can vary over shorter periods of less than a minute (Makeig and Jung, 1996; Paus et al., 1997; Weissman, Roberts, and Visscher, 2006).

While we know that arousal levels shift over periods of several minutes, comparatively little is known about the typical time course of fluctuations in the cortical vigilant attention network. A few studies have begun to shed some light on this question. An fMRI study by Weissman and colleagues (2006) investigated the consequences of fluctuations in activity in frontal control regions prior to the onset of a critical stimulus during a global/local selective attention task. The results indicated that slower RTs were correlated with reduced activity in key frontal control regions including the right inferior frontal gyrus and anterior cingulate cortex. A clear impression of the timing of these fluctuations was not possible due to the lag between an event and the subsequent haemodynamic response but the effect was estimated to have emerged 1–2 seconds prior to target onset.

Another fMRI study that may be informative in this regard was recently conducted by Eichele and colleagues (2008). In this study, which did not explicitly measure vigilant attention, participants performed a speeded visual flanker task but again the goal was to explore the extent to which performance lapses were foreshadowed by changes in neural activity. In this case the authors used independent components analysis to isolate a number of predictive activation patterns in frontal control regions that began to emerge as early as 30 seconds before an error was made. These data are highly suggestive of a gradually diminishing attentional engagement that eventually increases the risk of making an error.

Following on from this work, we exploited the higher temporal resolution of EEG to uncover the neural signature of lapsing vigilant attention. In this study participants performed a new paradigm that demands the continuous deployment of vigilant attention (O'Connell et al., 2009). The Continuous Temporal Expectancy Task requires a continuous stream of patterned stimuli to be monitored for the occurrence of a target pattern, which is identified by its markedly longer duration (see Figure 6.1). Standard and target stimuli are perceptually identical aside from the difference in

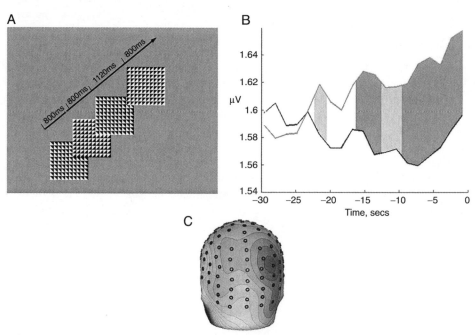

Fig. 6.1 (See also Plate 4) A) Continuous Temporal Expectancy Task (CTET). During this test of vigilant attention, participants were asked to monitor a continuous stream of checker stimuli centrally presented and flickering at a rate of 25Hz. Standard stimuli were presented for 800ms and participants were required to monitor for the occurrence of target stimuli defined by their longer duration (1120ms) relative to other stimuli. Target detection was indicated by a speeded button press. B) Alpha amplitude calculated for the 30 seconds preceding a target onset and averaged separately for correctly (hit, dark grey) and incorrectly (miss, pale grey) detected targets. Significant alpha-band divergences emerged up to 20 seconds before a lapse of attention. C) Scalp topography showing that the increase in alpha-power prior to a miss was most prominent over right inferior parietal scalp sites.

their duration. The advantages of this design are twofold: first, matching the physical features of target and standard stimuli bypasses the sometimes problematic issue of target salience automatically engaging attention and obviating the top-down processes under investigation, and second, a continuous demand is imposed on top-down attention because stimulus classification cannot be completed until the stimulus has disappeared. By tracking changes in a range of well-known attention-sensitive markers in the EEG while participants performed the temporal expectancy task, we were able to chart the elements of compromised brain activity across multiple timescales and hierarchical processing levels prior to lapses of attention. Our data revealed specific maladaptive trends with slow endogenous increases in alpha-band power beginning approximately 20 seconds before a momentary lapse followed by short-term (3–4 seconds pre-error) disruption of task-related monitoring mechanisms that was indexed by two event-related components; the P300 and contingent negative variation. The gradual increase in alpha amplitude (see Figure 6.1) appears consistent with the emergence of cortical idling or a resting state as controlled monitoring processes go off-line (Pfurtscheller and Lopes da Silva, 1999; Mantini et al., 2007).

These studies highlight the fact that although vigilant attention is subject to gradual decrements with time-on-task, equal consideration must be given to sub-minute fluctuations in attentional engagement. This underlines a major flaw of the typical continuous performance/vigilance-decrement paradigms that have been used in the field. Since there are large gaps between the responses made by the participant during continuous performance tasks, it is not actually possible to measure moment-to-moment changes in engagement. Extensive work in our lab has demonstrated that vigilant attention can be better isolated by adopting task paradigms that require continuous routine action, and analysis strategies, such as Fourier transform of reaction time data, pre-error EEG time series, that can elucidate the temporal characteristics of the underlying neural networks (Manly et al., 2003; Dockree et al., 2005; Johnson et al., 2007; O'Connell et al., 2009).

Another paradigm that has proved particularly useful in our studies of vigilant attention has been the Sustained Attention to Response Test (Robertson et al., 1997). In this task, a predictable series of single digits (1–9) is presented in sequence and subjects are required to press a response key to each number except the number 3, which occurs every ninth digit. Thus unlike traditional CPTs, the SART requires participants to *respond* to non-target stimuli while *withholding* their response on the appearance of the target stimulus. The simplicity of the SART tends to encourage a routine response set, placing heavy demands on the individual's ability to endogenously sustain attention to the overall goal of withholding to the No-Go target during the inter-target intervals. In addition, the regular occurrence of target stimuli means that the task can be sensitive to relatively brief lapses of attention. In this manner the SART is thought to provide a better analogue of the kinds of real-life situations in which failures of attention occur. Importantly, PET and fMRI studies have confirmed that performance of the SART activates the same aforementioned right lateralized vigilant attention network (Manly et al. 2003; Fassbender et al. 2004; O'Connor et al. 2004) and it has been demonstrated that the SART is better able to discriminate between patients with prefrontal brain injury than traditional CPTs (Robertson et al., 1997; Manly et al., 2003; O'Keeffe, Dockree, and Robertson, 2004).

Improving vigilant attention

A better understanding of the neuroanatomy and time course of vigilant attention can feed directly into the development of rehabilitative strategies. We have shown, for example, that the interaction between cortical vigilant attention networks and subcortical arousal systems can be exploited to alleviate deficits in patients with traumatic brain injury. We found that performance could be significantly improved, at least temporarily, by increasing arousal through exogenous mechanisms, such as random sounds played unpredictably during a test of vigilant attention (Manly et al., 2004).

More recently, we have also shown that people with impaired executive functions can be trained to self-regulate their levels of arousal and hence improve attention and reduce error. In a study that was designed to capitalize on our understanding of the vigilant attention system we developed a training protocol in which participants learn to modulate their own arousal levels consciously, known as Self-Alert Training. During Self-Alert Training participants view their own arousal levels, as indexed by skin-conductance levels that are measured with the galvanic skin response. First, the experimenter generates a loud exogenous stimulus, clapping or rapping on the table, so that the participant can see the immediate increase in arousal that this engenders. Then, using a strategy previously validated by Robertson and colleagues (Robertson et al. 1995), the exogenous stimulus is gradually phased out and internalized to the point that the participant is able to self-alert at will. Participants were then asked to self-alert periodically while performing the Sustained Attention to Response Task. Comparing this technique to a control condition involving practising a video game, we found significant short-term improvements in both performance accuracy and reaction-time variability. This training protocol was a brief pilot version designed to investigate, in a preliminary fashion, whether repeated volitional modulation of autonomic arousal would trigger increased top-down control of sustained attention. The training procedure lasted between 30–40 minutes in each case and therefore would therefore be of limited utility as a rehabilitative strategy in its current form. The next challenge is to use this knowledge in the development of more complete rehabilitative strategies that can produce improvements in everyday living for people who suffer from attention deficits.

Conclusions

When you have driven your train a hundred times through a light that was always green, it is all too easy for the brain to miss the yellow light that appears on the 101st journey—and to let the train-driving motor programme run on, unsupervised—occasionally to catastrophe. If that yellow light is detected, the accelerator handle released, and the train slowed down in preparation to stop at the next light, it is thanks to the right hemisphere of the brain, and in particular the right dorsolateral prefrontal and inferior parietal cortices, working in concert with subcortical thalamic and mesencephalic circuits. Repeated, unchallenging stimuli in the context of highly practised actions diminish arousal, dull sensory responsiveness, and blunt vigilant oversight of one's actions and environment. The reciprocal actions of a right hemisphere cortical network on the one hand, and a subcortical arousal network on the other, have evolved to protect against such a potentially dangerous diminution of awareness and monitoring. Because so much of what we do is practised and automatic, this system is needed throughout our waking day. The next time you walk into a room, scratch your head and wonder—'now why did I come in here?'—you are witnessing a minor inefficiency of this system.

We further conceive of the right parietal-prefrontal network and its interactions with the subcortical arousal systems as the circuitry by which vigilant attention is maintained. Although we can conceive of this system as somewhat independent and autonomous, in order to be responsive to changing task demands, changing performance levels, or changing physiological resources such as might be depleted by fatigue, monitoring processes must be tightly coupled with, or intrinsic to, its functioning. Therefore, the circuitry can be 'boosted' either exogenously by sensory stimuli or endogenously, by the right fronto-parietal vigilant elements of the system. Within this system, we believe that the prefrontal cortex plays a central role in maintaining and monitoring optimal arousal levels to match current task demands. This system also works in the service of current task goals and close interaction between it and goal representations are to be expected. Consequently, the type of attentional control that has been the focus of this chapter need not be isolated from the other aspects of attention linked to selection, working memory, and switching that were mentioned at the beginning of this chapter.

References

Arnsten, A. F. T. (1998). Catecholamine modulation of prefrontal cortical cognitive function. *Trends in Cognitive Sciences*, 2, 436–47.

Arnsten, A. F. T. and Contant, T. A. (1992). Alpha-2 adrenergic agonists decrease distractibility in aged monkeys performing the delayed response task. *Psychopharmacology*, 108, 159–69.

Aston-Jones, G. and Cohen, J. D. (2005). An integrative theory of locus coeruleus-norepinephrine function: adaptive gain and optimal performance. *Annual Review of Neuroscience*, 28, 403–50.

Aston-Jones, G., Chiang, C., and Alexinsky, T. (1991). Discharge of noradrenergic locus coeruleus neurons in behaving rats and monkeys suggests a role in vigilance. In C. D. Barnes and O. Pompeiano (Eds.), *Progress in Brain Research*, 88, 501–20.

Bellgrove, M. A., Gill, M., Hawi, Z., Kirley, A., and Robertson, I. H. (2005). Dissecting the attention deficit hyperactivity disorder (ADHD) phenotype: sustained attention and spatial attention asymmetries in relation to dopamine transporter (DAT1) transporter. *Neuropsychologia*, 43, 1847–57.

Bellgrove, M. A., Hawi, Z., Gill, M., and Robertson, I. H. (2006). The cognitive genetics of attention deficit hyperactivity disorder (ADHD): sustained attention as a candidate phenotype. *Cortex*, 42(6), 838–45.

Berridge, C. W. and Waterhouse, B. D. (2003). The locus-coeruleus-noradrenergic system: modulation of behavioral state and state-dependent cognitive processes. *Brain Research Reviews*, 42, 33–84.

Broadbent, D. E. (1971). *Decision and stress*. London: Academic Press.

Cherry, E. C. (1953). Some experiments on the recognition of speech, with one and with two ears. *Journal of Acoustical Society of America*, 25, 975–9.

Coull, J. T., Middleton, H. C., Robbins, T. W., and Sahakian, B. J. (1995). Clonidine and diazepam have differential effects on tests of attention and learning. *Psychopharmacology*, 120, 322–32.

Coull, J. T., Fackowiak, R., and Frith, C. D. (1998). Monitoring for target objects: activation of right frontal and parietal cortices with increasing time on task. *Neuropsychologia*, 36, 1325–34.

Coull, J.T., Jones, M.E., Egan, T.D., Frith, C.D., and Maze, M. (2004). Attentional effects of noradrenaline vary with arousal level: selective activation of thalamic pulvinar in humans. *Neuroimage*, 22(1):315–22.

Critchley, H. D., Mathias, C. J., Josephs, O., O'Doherty, J., Zanini, S., Dewar, B. K., et al. (2003). Human cingulate cortex and autonomic control: converging neuroimaging and clinical evidence. *Brain*. 126(Pt 10):2139–52.

Dockree, P.M., Kelly, S.P., Robertson, I.H., Reilly, R.B., Foxe, J.J. (2005). Neurophysiological markers of alert responding during goal-directed behavior: a high-density electrical mapping study. *Neuroimage*, 27(3):587–601.

Eichele, T., Debener, S., Calhoun, V.D., Specht, K., Engel, A.K., Hugdahl, K., et al. (2008). Prediction of human errors by maladaptive changes in event-related brain networks. *Proc Natl Acad Sci U S A*. 105(16):6173–78.

Fassbender, C., Murphy, K., Foxe, J.J., Wylie, G.R., Javitt, D.C., Robertson, I.H., et al. (2004). A topography of executive functions and their interactions revealed by functional magnetic resonance imaging. *Brain Res Cogn Brain Res*. 20(2):132–43.

Foucher, J.R., Otzenberger, H., and Gounot, D. (2004). Where arousal meets attention: a simultaneous fMRI and EEG recording study. *NeuroImage*, 22:688–97.

Greene, C., Bellgrove, M. A., Gill, M., and Robertson, I. H. (2009). Noradrenergic genotype predicts lapses in sustained attention. *Neuropsychologia*, 47, 591–4.

Johnson, K.A., Kelly, S.P., Bellgrove, M.A., Barry, E., Cox, M., Gill, M., Robertson, I.H. (2007). Response variability in attention deficit hyperactivity disorder: evidence for neuropsychological heterogeneity. *Neuropsychologia*. 45(4):630–38.

Mackworth, N. W. (1957). Some factors affecting vigilance. *Advancement of Science*, 53, 389–93.

Makeig, S. and Jung, T.-P. (1996). Tonic, phasic, and transient EEG correlates of auditory awareness in drowsiness. *Cognitive Brain Research,* **4**(1), 15–25.

Manly, T., Owen, A. M., Datta, A., Lewis, G., Scott, S., Rorden, C., et al. (2003). Enhancing the sensitivity of a sustained attention task to frontal damage. Convergent clinical and functional imaging evidence. *Neurocase,* **9**, 340–9.

Manly, T., Heutink, J., Davison, B., Gaynord, B., Greenfield, E., Parr, A., et al. (2004). An electronic knot in the handkerchief: 'Content free cueing' and the maintenance of attentive control. *Neuropsychological Rehabilitation,* **14**, 89–116.

Mantini, D., Perrucci, M. G., Del Gratta, C., Romani, G. L., and Corbetta, M. (2007). Electrophysiological signatures of resting state networks in the human brain. *Proceedings of the National Academy of Sciences,* **104**(32), 13170–5.

O'Connell, R. G., Dockree, P. M., Robertson, I. H., Bellgrove, M. A., Foxe, J. F., and Kelly, S. P. (2009). Uncovering the neural signature of lapsing attention – electrophysiological changes predict errors up to 30 seconds before they occur. *Journal of Neuroscience,* **29**(26), 8604–611.

O'Connor, C., Manly, T., Robertson, I.H., Hevenor, S.J., and Levine, B. (2004). An fMRI of sustained attention with endogenous and exogenous engagement. *Brain Cogn.* **54**(2):133–35.

O'Keeffe, F. M., Dockree, P. M., and Robertson, I. H. (2004). Poor insight in traumatic brain injury mediated by impaired error processing? Evidence from electrodermal activity. *Cognitive Brain Research,* **22**, 101–12.

O'Keeffe, F. M., Murray, B., Coen, R. F., Dockree, P. M., Bellgrove, M. A., Garavan, H., et al. (2007). Loss of insight in frontotemporal dementia, corticobasal degeneration and progressive supranuclear palsy. *Brain,* **130**, 753–64.

Parasuraman, R., Nestor, P., and Greenwood, P. (1989). Sustained-attention capacity in young and older adults. *Psychology and Aging,* **4**, 339–45.

Paus, T., Zatorre, R. J., Hofle, N., Caramanos, Z., Gotman, J., Petrides, M., et al. (1997). Time-related changes in neural systems underlying attention and arousal during the performance of an auditory vigilance task. *Journal of Cognitive Neuroscience,* **9**, 392–408.

Pfurtscheller, G. and Lopes da Silva, F. H. (1999). Event-related EEG/MEG synchronization and desynchronization: basic principles. *Clinical Neurophysiology,* **110**(11), 1842–57.

Posner, M. I. and Petersen, S. E. (1990). The attention system of the human brain. *Annual Review of Neuroscience,* **13**, 25–42.

Robertson, I. H., Tegner, R., Tham, K., Lo, A., and Nimmo-Smith, I. (1995). Sustained attention training for unilateral neglect: theoretical and rehabilitation implications. *Journal of Clinical and Experimental Neuropsychology,* **17**, 416–30.

Robertson, I. H., Manly, T., Andrade, J., Baddeley, B. T., and Yiend, J. (1997). Oops!: performance correlates of everyday attentional failures in traumatic brain injured and normal subjects: The Sustained Attention to Response Task (SART). *Neuropsychologia,* **35**, 747–58.

Smith, A. and Nutt, D. (1996). Noradrenaline and attention lapses. *Nature,* **380**, 291.

Sturm, W. and Willmes, K. (2001). On the functional neuroanatomy of intrinsic and phasic alertness. *Neuroimage,* **14**(1 Pt 2):S76–84.

Swanson, J. M., Casey, B. J., Nigg, J. T., Castellanos, F. X., Volkow, N. D., and Taylor, E. (2004). Clinical and cognitive definitions of attention deficits in children with attention-deficit/hyperactivity disorder. In M. Posner (Ed.), *Cognitive Neuroscience of Attention* pp.430–47. New York: Guilford.

Usher, M., Cohen, J. D., Servan-Schreiber, D., Rajkowski, J., and Aston-Jones, G. (1999). The role of locus cueruleus in the regulation of cognitive performance. *Science,* **283**, 549–53.

Weissman, D. H., Roberts, K. C., and Visscher, K. M. (2006). The neural bases of momentary lapses in attention. *Nat Neurosci,* **9**, 971–8.

Yerkes, R. M. and Dodson, J. D. (1908). The relation of strength of stimulus to rapidity of habit-formation. *Journal of Comparative and Neurological Psychology,* **18**, 459–82.

Chapter 7

Prior entry: attention and temporal perception

Charles Spence

Does attention speed-up perceptual processing? Or, in other words, does attending to (or expecting) a particular stimulus mean that it will be perceived earlier in time than if attention had been directed elsewhere? This seemingly simple question is in fact one of the oldest in the field of experimental psychology (see Mollon and Perkins, 1996; Spence et al., 2001). However, while researchers have been investigating the topic of temporal perception for more than two centuries now, it has only been in the last decade or so that convincing psychophysical evidence in support of the existence of 'prior entry' (as the phenomenon is known; see Titchener, 1908) has finally been obtained (Pashler, 1998; Shore and Spence, 2005). Exciting progress has recently come from research utilizing cognitive neuroscience techniques such as event-related potentials (ERPs) in order to investigate just how early in human information processing the effects of prior entry can be observed (McDonald et al., 2005; Vibell et al., 2007; submitted). This chapter provides a brief review of the empirical literature investigating the effects of attention on multisensory temporal perception in humans.

The problem with measuring the perception of temporal order

The problem when investigating the effects of attention on temporal perception is that (unlike in the spatial domain) it is impossible for a person to index (at a fine temporal scale) when exactly a given stimulus or event was perceived as occurring. Instead, researchers have to rely on a person's judgements of the *relative* timing of an event of interest with respect to another (comparison or marker) stimulus. The techniques that have been used most frequently to study the effects of attention on temporal perception in humans are the temporal order judgement (TOJ) task and the simultaneity-judgement (SJ) task. For both tasks, the stimulus onset asynchrony (SOA) between the two to-be-judged stimuli on each trial is normally varied using the method of constant stimuli (e.g. Spence et al., 2001), or else some form of adaptive staircase procedure (e.g. Sternberg et al., 1971; Stelmach and Herdman, 1991; Zampini et al., 2005a). In a prototypical TOJ study, participants have to report which stimulus was presented first (or, on occasion, second; see Frey, 1990; Parise and Spence, 2009; Shore et al., 2001), while in the SJ task, participants report whether the two stimuli were presented simultaneously or not. Occasionally, these two tasks are combined into a so-called ternary response task (S. A. Stone, 1926; Stelmach and Herdman, 1991; Jaśkowski, 1993; Zampini et al., 2007), where participants either report which stimulus was

Box 7.1 Psychometric data fitting

By fitting psychometric functions to the data from TOJ studies, researchers can extract two key performance indicators: 1) participants' sensitivity to the temporal order in which the two stimuli were presented, known as the just noticeable difference (JND); and 2) the amount of time by which one stimulus has to precede the other in order for the two stimuli to be perceived as simultaneous, known as the point of subjective simultaneity (PSS; note that this value actually reflects the SOA at which participants make each response equiprobably). The JND is conventionally defined as half the temporal interval between the 75% and 25% points on the psychometric function. Researchers typically fit a Gaussian function to SJ data, with the width (or standard deviation) of the distribution providing a measure of a participant's sensitivity to asynchrony (i.e. in some sense equivalent to the JND), and the peak of the distribution taken to indicate the PSS. It is, however, unclear whether SJs and TOJs actually measure the same thing or not: the fact that various experimental manipulations have been shown to have different effects on SJs and TOJs (see Guerrini et al., 2003; Shore et al., 2005; Vatakis et al., 2008b), has led some researchers to argue that they measure somewhat different things, and even that they may reflect different underlying mechanisms (e.g. Mitrani et al., 1986; Jaśkowski, 1991; Stelmach and Herdman, 1991).

It is important to note that the TOJ, SJ, and ternary response tasks are all subject to potential response biases. Consequently, which task is more appropriate depends on the specific experimental question that is being addressed (and, in particular, on the specific kinds of response bias that one is trying to avoid). So, for example, SJs appear to be more appropriate than TOJs for assessing the effects of attention on the perceived time of arrival of an event (i.e. when trying to measure the effects of prior entry; see Schneider and Bavelier, 2003; Zampini et al., 2005b), whereas TOJs are more appropriate than SJs for answering questions about multisensory temporal perception related to the 'unity assumption' (Vatakis et al., 2008a; Vatakis and Spence, 2007, 2008; Parise and Spence, 2009).

presented first, or else that the two stimuli appeared to have been presented simultaneously (see Box 7.1).[1]

While participants are normally encouraged to make unspeeded perceptual judgements (though see Prinzmetal et al., 2005; Santangelo and Spence, 2009), analysis of the distribution of reaction times (RTs) from TOJ studies can also be informative (Heath, 1984): So, for example, if a wide enough range of SOAs are tested, one often finds that RTs in the TOJ task are more-or-less normally distributed around the point of subjective simultaneity (PSS; see Box 7.1), thus highlighting the fact that participants respond most slowly when they are least certain with regard to the temporal order in which two stimuli were presented (Shore et al., 2001).

---

[1] While the latter approach might, at first, seem preferable in terms of providing a more nuanced measure of people's perceptual experience, it should be noted that the ternary task suffers from the problem that participants vary markedly in how frequently they choose the simultaneous response option when they are given three (rather than just two) response alternatives (e.g. compare the results reported by Jaśkowski, 1993, and Stelmach and Herdman, 1991; see also Schneider and Bavelier, 2003).

Prior attention: attention and the perception of temporal order

There are at least two different effects that attention might be expected to have on temporal perception: First, it might lead to the *prior entry* (or earlier arrival) of the attended stimulus relative to the same stimulus when attention happens to have been directed elsewhere (i.e. an effect on the perceived temporal order of the stimuli). In addition, however, attention might also be expected to improve the resolution of temporal perception for the attended stimulus (i.e. an effect on the sensitivity of participants' temporal judgements) (Brown, Chapter 8; Ruthruff and Pashler, Chapter 9; Tse, Chapter 10; Eagleman, Chapter 11, this volume). The focus in this chapter will be on the prior entry effect. Initially, prior entry research was designed to evaluate one of the putative causes leading to the '*personal equation*' (see Box 7.2). One influential early suggestion was that the personal equation simply reflected individual differences in how observers chose to allocate their attention to the auditory and/or visual modalities. The idea being that an observer who directed their attention to the sound of the clock would perceive the transit at a different point in time as compared to another observer whose visual attention had been focused on the movement of the star instead (Bessel, 1822).

The first studies of prior entry focused on assessing the effects of voluntarily (i.e. endogenously) attending to a particular sensory modality on the perception of stimuli presented in that

Box 7.2 The eye and ear method

Scientists first became interested in the topic of temporal perception when they realized that there were individual differences in observers' measurements of the time of stellar transits (i.e. measuring the time at which a star crossed the hairline of the telescope's eyepiece; Bessel, 1822). Traditionally, stellar transits were measured by 'the eye and ear method'; That is, an observer would judge the time of the visual event (the transit) with respect to the sound of the second hand of the clock ticking in the background (Cairney, 1975b). In fact, it was just such measurement differences between the Astronomer Royal, Nevil Maskelyne, and his assistant David Kinnebrook (of around 800ms) in 1796 at the Greenwich Observatory that led both to Kinnebrook being fired (see Mollon and Perkins, 1996), and to German scientists, such as Fechner and Wundt, launching the fields of psychophysics and experimental psychology. Practically speaking, the problem of these reliable inter-observer differences in the measurement of stellar transits was solved by the introduction of the '*personal equation*': defined as the amount of time to be added to or taken away from one observer's measurements in order to bring them into alignment with those of other observers (Bessel, 1822; Cairney, 1976b).

The notion that the existence of the personal equation might reflect individual differences in which sensory modality people preferentially attended to emerged from the observation that if one observer shouted when the star crossed the hairline while another observer judged the time of the shout relative to sound of clock, their errors were greatly reduced (presumably because each observer only had to attend to a single sensory modality under such conditions; see Spence et al., 2001). While, at first, researchers attempted to investigate the factors modulating multisensory temporal perception using variants of the complication situation, problems of interpretation (associated with participants' eye movements to the moving stimulus etc.; Cairney, 1975b) soon led to the development of the TOJ task, and thence to studies of prior entry (e.g. Hamlin, 1895; Drew, 1896; Stone, 1926).

modality relative to stimuli presented at around the same time in another sensory modality (Hamlin, 1895; Drew, 1896; Stone, 1926). More recently, however, the focus of research has shifted to investigating the effects of *spatial* attention on the perception of temporal order, i.e. to investigate whether stimuli that happen to be presented at an attended location will be perceived earlier in time than stimuli presented at around the same time from another ('relatively unattended') location (Stelmach and Herdman, 1991). It is important to note here that attention researchers have made a distinction between the endogenous and exogenous orienting of spatial attention (e.g. Spence and Driver, 1994; Klein and Shore, 2000; Corbetta and Shulman, 2002; Prinzmetal et al., 2005; 2009). Psychophysical research has now shown that both forms of attentional allocation can give rise to significant prior entry effects (e.g. Shore et al., 2001; Yates and Nicholls, 2009; though see also Schneider and Bavelier, 2003).

Prior entry and attention to a sensory modality

Several early studies demonstrated that endogenously attending to a particular sensory modality resulted in the prior entry (or relatively earlier arrival into awareness) of stimuli subsequently presented in that modality (Stone, 1926; Sternberg et al., 1971; Wilberg and Frey, 1977; 1990; Frey, 1990). In particular, Stone observed a 46-ms prior entry effect (see Sternberg and Knoll, 1973) when attention was directed to either the auditory or tactile modality (note that this pair of modalities was chosen in order to avoid any concerns relating to eye movements that had confounded earlier studies involving the 'complication' situation; see Cairney, 1975b). Sternberg and his colleagues, in an unpublished conference presentation given at a meeting of the Psychonomics Society in 1971, reported a 55-ms prior entry effect when attention was directed to either audition or touch, and a 30-ms prior entry effect when attention was directed to audition or vision instead.[2] Importantly, however, many other studies failed to show any such prior entry effect (see Hamlin, 1895; Drew, 1896; Vanderhaeghan and Bertelson, 1974; Cairney, 1975a; Frey and Wilberg, 1975). Such an inconsistent pattern of results led Pashler (1998, p.260) to argue that '*At present, the empirical evidence for prior entry is unconvincing*'. Spence and his colleagues (2001) were, however, able to highlight a number of methodological and interpretational problems with *all* previous studies—both the significant prior entry effects reported by certain researchers and the null effects reported by others.

Spence and his colleagues (2001; see also Cairney, 1975a) pointed out that the apparent prior entry effects reported in early studies might simply have reflected some form of response bias, given that participants' attention was manipulated along the same dimension that they had to respond to: that is, participants might simply have given as their response the stimulus that they had been instructed to attend to when uncertain of the correct response. This form of *decisional* bias is distinct from the *perceptual* change that Titchener (1908) clearly had in mind when he first

---

[2] One important confound with these early studies is that while the researchers involved argued that they were studying the effects of attending to a sensory modality on prior entry they may actually have been studying the effects of spatial attention instead, since the stimuli in the different sensory modalities were always presented from different spatial locations (e.g. sounds presented over headphones while visual stimuli were presented from a tachistoscope screen or from LEDs, and tactile stimuli were delivered to the participant's fingertip positioned elsewhere). Hence, any instruction to attend to a particular sensory modality was also, in effect, an instruction for the participant to focus their attention on a particular spatial location (see Spence et al., 2001, on this point).

outlined the concept of prior entry (see also Jaśkowski, 1993).[3] On the other hand, the null results reported in other studies (Hamlin, 1895; Drew, 1896; Vanderhaeghen and Bertelson, 1974; Cairney, 1975a; Frey and Wilberg, 1975) could equally have reflected the failure by the experimenters concerned to manipulate their participants' attention successfully. This concern is a particularly plausible one for studies in this area, given the taxing nature of the TOJ task that participants had to perform (again, see Spence et al., 2001, for a fuller discussion of these confounds).

Spence and colleagues (2001) introduced the *orthogonal-responding TOJ task* in order to reduce the likelihood that response bias would affect participants' TOJ performance. Specifically, attention was manipulated in one dimension (i.e. 'attend vision' or 'attend touch') while the participants had to judge the temporal order of the stimuli along another (orthogonal) dimension (e.g. 'Was the first stimulus presented on the left or right?'). The visual and tactile stimuli in Spence et al.'s studies were always presented from the same set of spatial locations on either side of fixation. This feature of the design ensured that the experimenter's instruction to direct attention to a particular sensory modality provided no information to the participants with regard to where the stimuli were likely to be presented (thus ruling out spatial attention as the cause of any prior entry effects that they obtained). Furthermore, in order to ensure that their participants' attention was indeed endogenously focused in the desired manner (i.e. on either the visual or tactile modality), Spence et al. manipulated the probability of stimuli being presented in each modality. In particular, they varied the relative proportions of unimodal tactile and unimodal visual TOJ trials in the different blocks of experimental trials. So, for example, the majority of stimuli (75%) in the 'attend touch' blocks were tactile (as compared to just 25% visual stimuli), while these stimulus probabilities were reversed in the 'attend vision' blocks (see Figure 7.1).

Spence et al.'s (2001) results revealed that the visual stimulus had to be presented further in advance of the tactile stimulus in order for the stimuli to be judged as simultaneous (or rather, for the PSS to be achieved) when participants' attention had been endogenously directed toward the tactile modality than when attention had been directed toward the visual modality instead (see Figure 7.1). In other words, when attending to the tactile modality, a tactile stimulus was perceived as occurring at the same time as a visual stimulus that had actually been presented much earlier. In effect, the perception of the tactile stimulus had been shifted forward in time relative to the visual stimulus with which it was being compared. Using a very similar methodology, Zampini and his colleagues subsequently demonstrated significant prior entry effects when attention was directed to either the auditory or visual modality (see Zampini et al., 2005b), or when participants were expecting painful laser heat stimuli versus visual stimuli (Zampini et al., 2007). The painful stimulus in the latter study had to be presented 29ms further in advance of the visual stimulus (the illumination of an LED) in order for participants to perceive the stimuli as having been presented simultaneously when participants were expecting vision than when they were expecting a painful stimulus instead.

It is worth noting that the magnitude of the prior entry effects reported in these (and other) published studies has varied quite substantially—so, for example, while Spence et al. (2001) reported a 126-ms effect when attention was directed to vision versus touch (see Figure 7.1),

---

[3] Once again, it is important to note that the majority of these studies have utilized a non-orthogonal TOJ design (e.g. Kanai et al., 2007). Orthogonal-responding TOJ paradigms (e.g. Yates and Nicholls, 2009), and SJ tasks (see Schneider and Bavelier, 2003) are, however, now being used more frequently. Note that Jaśkowski (1993) found that the visual prior entry effects observed in a non-orthogonal TOJ design disappeared when a ternary response task was used (though see Stelach and Herdman, 1991, for contradictory evidence).

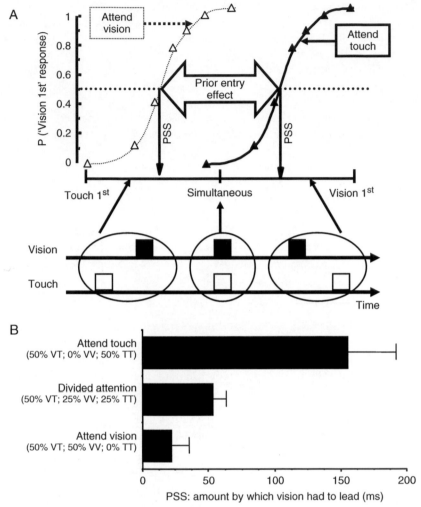

Fig. 7.1 A) Beneath the graph are three stimulus pairs (touch first, simultaneous, and vision first) of the sort typically presented in studies of the effect of attention on temporal perception. The graph above shows two schematic psychometric functions, one for data collected when a participant's attention was directed toward the visual modality and the other (on the right) for when attention had been directed to the tactile modality instead. The PSS for each function is calculated as the 50% point on the psychometric function. The prior entry effect (shown) is calculated as the difference in the PSS between these two attention conditions. B) Graph highlighting the prior entry effect reported by Spence et al. (2001; experiment 2) in their prior entry study of the effects of endogenously attending to a sensory modality. The mean PSS is presented for the various attention conditions: Attend touch, divided attention, and attend vision. The proportions of different trial types presented in the various blocks of trials are shown below each condition: VT = crossmodal visual-tactile TOJ trial; VV = unimodal visual TOJ trial; TT = unimodal tactile TOJ trial. Note the shift in the PSS as a function of participants' attention being endogenously focused on either the tactile or visual modality (or else divided between the two modalities). Error bars indicate the between-participant standard error of the means. Panel B adapted and redrawn from Spence, C., Shore, D. I., and Klein, R. M. (2001). Multisensory prior entry. *Journal of Experimental Psychology: General*, **130**, 799–832.

a prior entry effect of just 14ms was observed in Zampini et al.'s (2005b) audiovisual prior entry study. One generalization that can be drawn here is that the largest prior entry effects are reported in those studies where a non-orthogonal TOJ design is used (i.e. under conditions that are most open to potential response bias confounds; see Spence et al., 2001). Smaller prior entry effects have typically been reported in those studies where an orthogonal TOJ design is used, and the smallest prior entry effects of all are observed in those studies where a simulteneity-judgement task is used (see Stelmach and Herdman, 1991; Schneider and Bavelier, 2003; Wada, 2003; Zampini et al., 2005b). This pattern of results has led certain researchers to argue that while response bias can certainly be reduced by the use of an orthogonal-responding TOJ design, it can only be ruled out completely by the use of an SJ task (see Schneider and Bavelier, 2003; Zampini et al., 2005b).

Prior entry and spatial attention

In recent years, the focus of prior entry research has shifted away from studying the effects of attending to a sensory modality to assessing the effects of attending to a particular location (either endogenously or exogenously; see Klein and Shore, 2000; Corbetta and Shulman, 2002; Prinzmetal et al., 2005) on the perception of temporal order. Many studies have now shown that stimuli presented at the attended location will be perceived earlier in time (relative to other stimuli). While the majority of this research has focused on the effects of visual spatial attention (e.g. Stelmach and Herdman, 1991; Hikosaka et al., 1993a; Jaśkowski, 1993; Neumann et al., 1993; Shore et al., 2001; Schneider and Bavelier, 2003) similar results have also been reported in unimodal auditory (Kanai et al., 2007) and unimodal tactile studies (Yates and Nicholls, 2009).

Shore and his colleagues (2001) attempted to eliminate residual response-bias effects from their study of the effects of exogenous and endogenous visual spatial orienting on prior entry by averaging the performance of their participants on 'Which came first?' and 'Which came second?' orthogonal TOJ tasks. The participants judged the order of presentation of two visual stimuli (a horizontal and a vertical line segment presented from either the same or opposite sides, to the left or right of fixation). Attention was directed to one or other side by means of the presentation of a peripheral (exogenous) or central arrow (endogenous) precue at the start of each trial. Shore and his colleagues argued that any response bias should have had an equal and opposite effect on performance in these two tasks, and hence would be cancelled out, leaving just the perceptual prior entry effect. Their results showed that exogenous visual orienting led to a significantly larger prior entry effect than did endogenous orienting (mean prior entry effects of 61ms and 17ms, respectively; see also Stelmach and Herdman, 1991; Jaśkowski, 1993; Schneider and Bavelier, 2003; though see Prinzmetal et al., 2005). Yates and Nicholls (2009) have recently reported a similar pattern of results in the tactile modality. Interestingly, the residual effect of response bias in Shore et al.'s orthogonal TOJ design was estimated at 13ms (this value was calculated by dividing the difference between the prior entry effects in the 'Which first?' and 'Which second?' TOJ tasks by two). This value compares favourably with the 60-ms response bias effect observed in previous non-orthogonal TOJ designs (see Frey, 1990; Shore et al., 2001).

Psychophysicists have recently demonstrated that prior entry effects can also result from the crossmodal spatial cuing of exogenous spatial attention (Shimojo et al., 1997; Spence and Lupiáñez, 1998; Lupiáñez et al., 1999; Wada, 2003; Hongoh et al., 2008; Santangelo and Spence, 2009). The participants in an experiment reported by Lupiáñez and his colleagues (1999) were presented with a spatially-non-predictive visual cue on either the left or right side at the start of each trial. Participants then had to make unspeeded TOJs concerning which of two tones, one high and the other low in pitch (one presented on either side of fixation at SOAs of 15–250ms, varied using the method of constant stimuli) had been presented first. The onset of the first tone occurred 150ms after the onset of the visual cue. A small but significant prior entry effect was observed. Hongoh et al. (2008) have recently documented similar crossmodal spatial cuing effects on unimodal TOJs. In their study, a spatially-non-predictive auditory cue was presented on either the left or right 100ms prior to participants making a red vs. green visual orthogonal TOJ (see also Shimojo et al., 1997; Santangelo and Spence, 2009).

Spence and colleagues (Spence and Lupiáñez, 1998; Lupiáñez et al., 1999) conducted a further study in which a spatially non-predictive auditory cue (a brief white-noise burst) was presented prior to a pair of visual and tactile stimuli, again one presented on either side of fixation (see Figure 7.2A). Participants made orthogonal TOJs regarding which modality stimulus had been presented first, regardless of the side on which the first stimulus happened to be presented. Even though the participants were instructed to ignore the spatially-uninformative sound as much as possible, the results nevertheless demonstrated that the stimulus subsequently presented on the side of the task-irrelevant sound was speeded-up relative to the stimulus that happened to

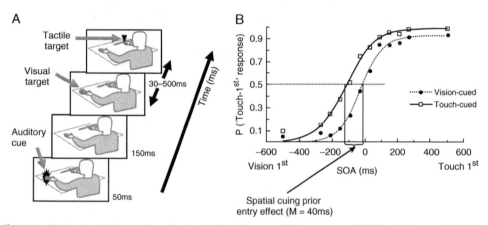

Fig. 7.2 A) Schematic illustration of a typical trial in one of the crossmodal TOJ studies conducted by Lupiáñez, Baddeley, and Spence (1999). At the start of each trial, an auditory cue was briefly and unpredictably presented from a loudspeaker cone placed by the participant's left or right hand. This was followed by the presentation of a pair of visual and tactile stimuli, one presented to either side of central fixation. These TOJ stimuli were separated by an SOA of 30–500 ms (varied using the method of constant stimuli). Participants made an unspeeded discrimination response regarding which modality (vision or touch) appeared to have been presented first (each modality was presented first on 50% of the trials), while trying to ignore the auditory cue which was spatially-non-predictive with regard to the side where the first TOJ stimulus was presented. B). Mean proportion of touch-first responses as a function of the stimulus onset asynchrony (SOA) between the visual and tactile stimuli. Trials on which the visual stimulus was presented on the side of the auditory cue are shown by the dotted line, while trials on which the tactile stimulus was presented on the auditorily-cued side are shown by the solid line. The visual stimulus had to lead by a greater interval for the PSS to be achieved when the side of the tactile stimulus was cued than when the side of the visual stimulus was cued instead. Adapted and redrawn from Spence, C., McDonald, J., and Driver, J. (2004). Exogenous spatial cuing studies of human crossmodal attention and multisensory integration. In C. Spence and J. Driver (Eds.), *Crossmodal space and crossmodal attention*, pp.277–320. Oxford: Oxford University Press.

be presented on the other side (see Figure 7.2B). Taken together, these results suggest that prior entry can be elicited by the exogenous orienting of spatial attention that follows the peripheral presentation of spatially non-predictive visual, auditory, and tactile cues. Interestingly, Hongoh et al.'s (2008) results suggested that the more eccentrically the cue is presented, the larger the prior entry effect that may be observed.

The cognitive neuroscience of prior entry

So much for the behavioural manifestation of prior entry; what about the neural substrates (or consequences) of the effect? Neuroscience evidence demonstrating the modulation of early responses in sensory brain areas would provide strong support for the genuinely perceptual nature of the prior entry effect. However, the first study to look explicitly at the attentional modulation of TOJs using event-related brain potentials actually failed to demonstrate any such effect of spatial attention on the timing of the earliest event-related potentials (ERPs) to visual stimuli in visual cortex (McDonald et al., 2005). The participants in McDonald et al.'s study had to judge which of two differently-coloured lateralized visual stimuli (one presented from either side of fixation) had been presented first. Attention was exogenously directed to one side or the other by means of a brief non-predictive auditory tone presented 100–300ms before onset of the first visual stimulus (just as in Hongoh et al.'s, 2008, study).

Although a robust prior entry effect (M = 69ms) was observed behaviourally, this did not appear to lead to any observable temporal shift in the latency of the early brain potentials associated with the presentation of the visual stimulus on the side of the auditory cue. That is, the contralateral N1 and P1 components (these early ERPs, which originate from extrastriate cortex, are assumed to represent the initial volley of neural input into these cortical areas) were observed at the same latency (as the ipsilateral components), no matter whether the visual stimulus was presented on the side of the auditory cue or not. No latency effects were observed for the N1 or N2 either. A small (5-ms) P2 latency effect was observed over contralateral cortex. However, it was difficult to interpret the latter effect unambiguously in terms of prior entry given the possibility of stimulus-related artefacts. By contrast, McDonald and colleagues observed a significant modulation of signal strength for posterior ERPs in the 80–140-ms time-range. That is, neural activation in visual cortex associated with the processing of the exogenously attended visual signal was amplified, as has been observed in many previous ERP studies of spatial attention.

McDonald et al. (2005) concluded that the psychophysical shifts in the PSS that they observed were not caused by perceptual prior entry (i.e. from a change in the latency of early perceptual processing), but rather that they arose from modulations of signal strength (i.e. gain-modulation) in early visual-cortical pathways. However, before accepting this conclusion, it is worth remembering that researchers have argued that different kinds of attention (in particular, exogenous and endogenous) can have qualitatively different effects on human perception and performance (see Spence and Driver, 1994; Klein and Shore, 2000; Corbetta and Shulman, 2002; Prinzmetal et al., 2005; 2009; Lupiáñez, Chapter 2, this volume), and that McDonald et al. only looked at the effects of crossmodal exogenous spatial orienting.

More recently, Vibell et al. (2007) reported a study in which attention was directed to a sensory modality (rather than to a particular spatial location as in McDonald et al.'s, 2005, study), and which came to a dramatically different conclusion. Using an orthogonal crossmodal TOJ paradigm, attention was endogenously directed to either vision or touch. The participants had to respond which side the first stimulus had been presented on. A 38-ms prior entry effect was observed behaviourally. Importantly, latency shifts of the early visual evoked potentials were also observed.[4] In particular, the latencies of the early visual P1, N1, N2, all peaked slightly (but significantly) earlier in time over contralateral (than over ipsilateral) cortex when the visual stimulus was attended as compared to when attention was directed to the tactile modality instead (see Figure 7.3A). Specifically, P1 and N1 were temporally shifted by 3–4ms. A 14-ms latency shift of the late P300 potential was also observed. Interestingly, the mean amplitude of the P1 and N1

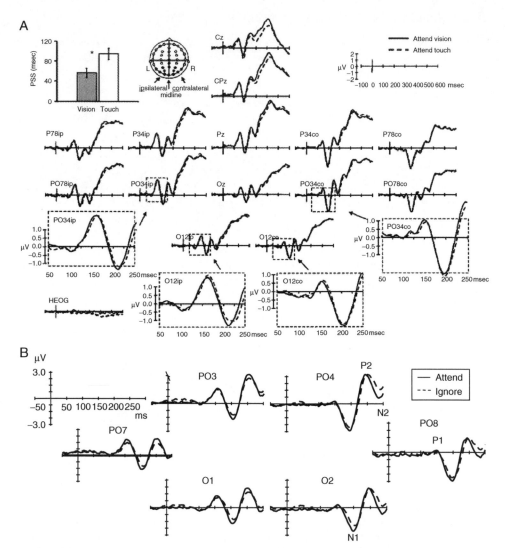

Fig. 7.3 A) The bar graph in the upper left corner of this figure shows the PSS in the attend-vision and attend-touch conditions, and the significant behavioral prior entry effect reported by Vibell et al. (2007) in their prior entry study. Grand-averaged ERP waveforms for visual stimuli in the attend-vision (solid lines) and the attend-touch (dashed lines) conditions show both latency and

---

4   Note that due to concerns relating to the possibility of neural interactions taking place between the two stimuli presented in the TOJ task, only ERPs elicited by the visual stimuli on the majority of trials where they were presented first were analysed.

Fig. 7.3 (*continued*) amplitude modulation of the evoked potentials as a function of the attention condition. A bird's-eye view of the electrode montage used in the experiment is shown above. Waveforms are shown for the electrodes used to analyze the visual and P300 potentials, and these are shaded black on the montage schematic. Blow-ups of the early portion of the waveforms at PO3/4 and O1/2 electrodes, where the early prior-entry effects and amplitude modulations were largest, are shown. Positive voltage is plotted upward. Reproduced with permission from Vibell, J., Klinge, C., Zampini, M., Spence, C., and Nobre, A. C. (2007). Temporal order is coded temporally in the brain: early ERP latency shifts underlying prior entry in a crossmodal temporal order judgment task. *Journal of Cognitive Neuroscience*, **19**, 109–20. B) Early ERP amplitude and latency modulations highlighted by Vibell et al.'s (submitted) study of the effects of endogenous spatial attention on the prior entry effect. Grand-averaged ERP waveforms for visual stimuli presented on the attended (solid lines) and (relatively) unattended sides (dashed lines). The graphs highlight the modulation of both the latency and amplitude of the evoked potentials as a function of the attention condition. Significant amplitude effects were observed for the P1, while the N1, P2, and N2 showed significant attention effects on both the amplitude and latency measures. Note that the latency shift recorded for N1 (c. 3-4 ms) was only marginally-significant in this study. Positive voltage is plotted upward. Adapted from with permission from Vibell, J., Klinge, C., Zampini, M., Spence, C., and Nobre, A. C. (submitted). ERP study of the spatial prior-entry effect.

components for the attended visual stimuli were also enhanced over selected scalp locations (just as in McDonald et al.'s study), hence suggesting that the subjective perception of temporal order may result from some (as yet) unknown combination of neural latency and amplitude modulation effects.

There are a number of possible reasons why these two ERP studies (McDonald et al., 2005; Vibell et al., 2007) may have arrived at such different conclusions regarding the neural consequences (or correlates) of the prior entry effect. Theoretically interesting suggestions here include the possibility that: 1) there may actually be differences between the mechanisms of attention to sensory modalities and attention to spatial locations (cf. Spence et al., 2001; Macaluso et al., 2002); and/or 2) there are differences between the mechanisms underlying the exogenous and endogenous orienting of attention (see Klein and Shore, 2000; Corbetta and Shulman, 2002; Schneider and Bavelier, 2003; Prinzmetal et al., 2005). Alternatively, however, one less-interesting methodological explanation for the null result is simply that McDonald et al. used a lower sampling rate (the ERP signals were digitized at 250Hz as compared to a sampling rate of 500Hz in Vibell et al.'s study) and thus may have missed the small early effects (c. 3–4ms) reported in the latter study.

In order to test the hypothesis that the effects of attention to a sensory modality may be somehow qualitatively different from the effects of attending to a particular spatial location, Vibell et al. (submitted) recently investigated whether directing attention to a particular spatial location would result in a similar latency shifts of the early visual evoked potentials as when attention was endogenously directed to a particular sensory modality. The experiment was essentially identical to that reported by Vibell et al. (2007) but now participants' (N = 15) attention was directed to either the left or right side of space (i.e. rather than to the visual or tactile modality), and participants reported which sensory modality (vision or touch) had been presented first. A significant prior entry effect was, once again, observed behaviourally (M = 28ms), with the stimulus presented at the attended location being perceived relatively earlier in time than when attention was directed to the other side. Importantly, however, while the subsequent analysis of the ERP data revealed some significant modulations in the speed of perceptual analysis (note, once again, that only the ERPs associated with the presentation of the visual stimuli were analysed), they started later than in Vibell et al.'s (2007) study (see Figure 7.3B).

When taken together, the results of Vibell et al.'s (2007; submitted) two ERP studies therefore suggest that different mechanisms may underlie the effects of endogenously attending to a sensory modality versus endogenously attending to a specific spatial location (cf. Spence et al., 2001; Macaluso et al., 2002). The results suggest that attending endogenously to a location modulates peak latencies slightly later in information processing than does endogenously attending to a sensory modality. It will be an interesting question for future research to determine whether prior entry effects associated with the endogenous versus exogenous orienting of spatial attention are also underpinned by somewhat different neural mechanisms.

Conclusions

The last few years have seen a rapid growth of interest in the effects of attention on temporal perception in humans. Researchers have now managed to eliminate the many methodological confounds that have bedevilled the interpretation of so much of the early research in this area. By eliminating these confounds, psychologists have now started to provide convincing empirical evidence in support of the existence of the prior entry effect. The results of a number of studies now show that attention does indeed speed the relative latency of perceptual processing no matter the dimension or channel (e.g. modality or location) along which attention is oriented, and no matter whether attention is directed in an endogenous or exogenous manner (Shore et al., 2001; though see also Schneider and Bavelier, 2003). The available research has also highlighted the fact that decisional-level effects (e.g. response biases) have contributed (to a varying degree) to the results reported in the *majority* of prior entry studies that have been published to date. In fact, it appears that only studies incorporating an SJ (Schneider and Bavelier, 2003; Zampini et al., 2005b) or ternary response task (Zampini et al., 2007) can be considered to be completely immune from the potential influence of response bias on measures of the prior entry effect.

Although researchers have made great progress in furthering our understanding of the phenomenon of prior entry in recent years, there are still a number of important questions awaiting future research:

1) The latest ERP research (discussed earlier) has demonstrated just how early in human information processing the effects of prior entry can occur (at least when attention is directed endogenously to a particular sensory modality). What is more, the evidence reported by Vibell et al. (2007) has shown that temporal information (at least at the fine timescales measured in prior entry studies) is (at least to a certain extent) represented temporally in the brain. Future research will hopefully speak to the question of whether there is, as has often been proposed, a 'simultaneity centre' in the human brain for making conscious temporal comparisons (e.g. Efron, 1963; Corwin and Boynton, 1968; Noesselt et al., submitted). Furthermore, given that other species (such as chinchillas) can also direct their attention to a particular sensory modality (as a function of the task that currently happens to be relevant; see Delano et al., 2007), it would be interesting to determine whether they also experience prior entry effects, and if so, to conduct neurophysiological studies of the phenomenon at the cellular level (cf. Liang et al., 2002; Wada et al. 2005). The rapid development of intracranial recording techniques in awake humans could also prove useful here (cf. Thesen et al., 2008; Walter and Crow, 1961).

2) Over the last few years, the focus of much of the multisensory research has started to move away from the study of pairs of simplistic and essentially (semantically) meaningless stimuli (e.g. beeps, flashes, and brief taps on the fingertip; see Spence et al., 2001, for a review),

stimuli that have no relation to one another (cf. Spence, 2007). Instead, researchers are increasingly studying the temporal constraints on the perception of simultaneity/temporal order for more realistic (and typically complex) stimuli (e.g. Vatakis and Spence, 2007; 2008; Vatakis et al., 2008). Interestingly, it has now been shown that when realistic, meaningfully related, audiovisual stimuli are presented asynchronously, participants are sometimes more likely to bind them (than when unrelated, or incongruent, audiovisual stimuli are presented), due presumably to the 'unity assumption' (Vatakis and Spence, 2007, 2008; Vatakis et al., 2008a; see Parise and Spence, 2009).

It remains an intriguing question for future research as to whether prior entry effects may be reduced, or even eliminated, under conditions where the two to-be-judged sensory stimuli are meaningfully (or at least plausibly) related to one another (cf. Kanai et al., 2007). One hypothesis here is that prior entry might only affect the relative time of arrival of unrelated sensory stimuli (that is, for pairs of stimuli about which the participant has no assumption of unity (Spence, 2007; Vatakis and Spence, 2007; Parise and Spence, 2009) or no reason to infer common cause. It may be that when pairs of sensory stimuli are presented at about the same time, attention can either prioritize the processing of one of the stimuli if they happen to be unrelated to one another (i.e. if they are attributed by the brain to different objects or events), or else help to bind them (across time and space) if they are perceived to be meaningfully related to one another (see Neisser, 1976; Spence et al. 2003; Buehner, Chapter 15, this volume). The latter idea links to the notion—made popular by research on feature integration theory—that attention serves to bind stimuli that refer to the same object or event intramodally (e.g. Treisman and Gelade, 1980; Treisman, 1996).

3) Finally, it is somewhat ironic that while individual differences in the timing of auditory and visual stimuli is what prompted researchers to start investigating temporal perception in humans more than two centuries ago, we still have no clear understanding of what exactly underlies these individual differences (that are still reported; e.g. Stone et al., 2001). One possibility here is that they might reflect fundamental differences in the distribution of a person's attention between different sensory modalities. Alternatively, however, they might simply reflect some form of strategic shift in attentional set in response to the particular experimental situation under investigation. Resolving this long-standing issue still represents an important issue for future study.

References

Bessel, F. W. (1822). *Astronomische Beobachtungen auf der Königlichen Universitäts-Sternwarte in Königsberg* [Astronomical observations at the Royal University Observatory in Koennigsberg]. Konigsberg.

Cairney, P. T. (1975a). Bisensory order judgement and the prior entry hypothesis. *Acta Psychologica*, 39, 329–40.

Cairney, P. T. (1975b). The complication experiment uncomplicated. *Perception*, 4, 255–65.

Corbetta, M. and Shulman, G. L. (2002). Control of goal-directed and stimulus-driven attention in the brain. *Nature Reviews Neuroscience*, 3, 201–15.

Corwin, T. R. and Boynton, R. M. (1968). Transitivity of visual judgments of simultaneity. *Journal of Experimental Psychology*, 78, 560–8.

Delano, P. H., Elgueda, D., Hamame, C. M., and Robles, L. (2007). Selective attention to visual stimuli reduces cochlear sensitivity in chinchillas. *Journal of Neuroscience*, 27, 4146–53.

Drew, F. (1896). Attention: Experimental and critical. *American Journal of Psychology*, 7, 533–73.

Efron, R. (1963). The effect of handedness on the perception of simultaneity and temporal order. *Brain*, 86, 261–84.

Frey, R. D. (1990). Selective attention, event perception and the criterion of acceptability principle: Evidence supporting and rejecting the doctrine of prior entry. *Human Movement Science*, **9**, 481–530.

Frey, R. D. and Wilberg, R. B. (1975). Selective attention and the judgment of temporal order. In J. Salmela (Ed.), *Mouvement 7*, pp.63–5. Quebec: Canadian Society for Psychomotor Learning and Sport Psychology.

Guerrini, C., Berlucchi, G., Bricolo, E., and Aglioti, S. M. (2003). Temporal modulation of spatial tactile extinction in right-brain-damaged patients. *Journal of Cognitive Neuroscience*, **15**, 523–36.

Hamlin, A. J. (1895). On the least observable interval between stimuli addressed to disparate senses and to different organs of the same sense. *American Journal of Psychology*, **6**, 564–75.

Heath, R. A. (1984). Response time and temporal order judgement in vision. *Australian Journal of Psychology*, **36**, 21–34.

Hikosaka, O., Miyauchi, S., and Shimojo, S. (1993a). Focal visual attention produces illusory temporal order and motion sensation. *Vision Research*, **33**, 1219–40.

Hikosaka, O., Miyauchi, S., and Shimojo, S. (1993b). Voluntary and stimulus-induced attention detected as motion sensation. *Perception*, **22**, 517–26.

Hongoh, Y., Kita, S., and Soeta, Y. (2008). Separation between sound and light enhances audio-visual prior entry effect. *IEICE Transactions on Information and Systems*, **E91-D**, 1641–8.

Jaśkowski, P. (1991). Two-stage model for order discrimination. *Perception & Psychophysics*, **50**, 76-82.

Jaśkowski, P. (1993). Selective attention and temporal-order judgement. *Perception*, **22**, 681–9.

Kanai, K., Ikeda, K., and Tayama, T. (2007). The effect of exogenous spatial attention on auditory information processing. *Psychological Research*, **71**, 418–26.

Klein, R. M. and Shore, D. I. (2000). Relationships among modes of visual orienting. In S. Monsell and J. Driver (Eds.) *Control of cognitive processes: Attention and performance XVIII*, pp.195–208. Cambridge, MA: MIT Press.

Liang, H., Bressler, S. L., Ding, M., Truccolo, W. A., and Nakamura, R. (2002). Synchronized activity in prefrontal cortex during anticipation of visuomotor processing. *Neuroreport*, **13**, 2011–15.

Lupiáñez, J., Baddeley, R., and Spence, C. (1999). 'Crossmodal links in exogenous spatial attention revealed by the orthogonal temporal order judgment task.' Paper presented at the 1st International Multisensory Research Conference: Crossmodal Attention and Multisensory Integration. Oxford 1st – 2nd October. http://www.wfubmc.edu/nba/IMRF/99abstracts.html

Macaluso, E., Frith, C. D., and Driver, J. (2002). Directing attention to locations and to sensory modalities: multiple levels of selective processing revealed with PET. *Cerebral Cortex*, **12**, 357–68.

McDonald, J. J., Teder-Sälejärvi, W. A., Di Russo, F., and Hillyard, S. A. (2005). Neural basis of auditory-induced shifts in visual time-order perception. *Nature Neuroscience*, **8**, 1197–202.

Mitrani, L., Shekerdjiiski, S., and Yakimoff, N. (1986). Mechanisms and asymmetries in visual perception of simultaneity and temporal order. *Biological Cybernetics*, **54**, 159–65.

Mollon, J. D. and Perkins, A. J. (1996). Errors of judgement at Greenwich in 1796. *Nature*, **380**, 101–2.

Neisser, U. (1976). *Cognition and reality: Principles and implications of cognitive psychology*. San Francisco: Freeman.

Neumann, O., Esselmann, U., and Klotz, W. (1993). Differential effects of visual-spatial attention on response latency and temporal-order judgment. *Psychological Research*, **56**, 26–34.

Noesselt, T., Bergmann, D., Heinze, H.-J., Münte, T., and Spence, C. (submitted). Spatial coding of multisensory temporal relations in human superior temporal sulcus.

Parise, C. and Spence, C. (2009). 'When birds of a feather flock together': Synesthetic correspondences modulate audiovisual integration in non-synesthetes. *PLoS ONE* **4**, e5664

Pashler, H. E. (1998). *The psychology of attention*. Cambridge, MA: MIT Press.

Prinzmetal, W., Zvinyatskovskiy, A., Gutierrez, P., and Dilem, L. (2009). Voluntary and involuntary attention have different consequences: The effect of perceptual difficulty. *Quarterly Journal of Expeirmental Psychology*, **62**, 352–69.

Prinzmetal, W., McCool, C., and Park, S. (2005). Attention: Reaction time and accuracy reveal different mechanisms. *Journal of Experimental Psychology: General*, **134**, 73–92.

Santangelo, V. and Spence, C. (2009). Crossmodal exogenous orienting improves the accuracy of temporal order judgments. *Experimental Brain Research* **194**, 577–86.

Schneider, K. A. and Bavelier, D. (2003). Components of visual prior entry. *Cognitive Psychology*, **47**, 333–66.

Shimojo, S., Miyauchi, S., and Hikosaka, O. (1997). Visual motion sensation yielded by non-visually driven attention. *Vision Research*, **12**, 1575–80.

Shore, D. I. and Spence, C. (2005). Prior entry. In L. Itti, G. Rees, and J. Tsotsos (Eds.), *Neurobiology of attention*, pp.89–95. North Holland: Elsevier.

Shore, D. I., Spence, C., and Klein, R. M. (2001). Visual prior entry. *Psychological Science*, **12**, 205–12.

Shore, D. I., Gray, K., Spry, E., and Spence, C. (2005). Spatial modulation of tactile temporal-order judgments. *Perception*, **34**, 1251–62.

Spence, C. (2007). Audiovisual multisensory integration. *Acoustical Science and Technology*, **28**, 61–70.

Spence, C. and Driver, J. (1994). Covert spatial orienting in audition: Exogenous and endogenous mechanisms facilitate sound localization. *Journal of Experimental Psychology: Human Perception and Performance*, **20**, 555–74.

Spence, C. and Lupiáñez, J. (1998). *Crossmodal links in attention revealed by the orthogonal temporal order judgment task*. Paper presented at II Congreso de la Sociedad Espanyola de Psicologia Experimental (SEPEX 98). Granada, Spain, 17th December.

Spence, C., Shore, D. I., and Klein, R. M. (2001). Multisensory prior entry. *Journal of Experimental Psychology: General*, **130**, 799–832.

Spence, C., Baddeley, R., Zampini, M., James, R., and Shore, D. I. (2003). Crossmodal temporal order judgments: When two locations are better than one. *Perception & Psychophysics*, **65**, 318–28.

Spence, C., McDonald, J., and Driver, J. (2004). Exogenous spatial cuing studies of human crossmodal attention and multisensory integration. In C. Spence and J. Driver (Eds.), *Crossmodal Space and Crossmodal Attention*, pp.277–320. Oxford: Oxford University Press.

Stelmach, L. B. and Herdman, C. M. (1991). Directed attention and perception of temporal order. *Journal of Experimental Psychology: Human Perception and Performance*, **17**, 539–50.

Sternberg, S. and Knoll, R. L. (1973). The perception of temporal order: Fundamental issues and a general model. In S. Kornblum (Ed.) *Attention and Performance IV*, pp.629–85. London: Academic Press.

Sternberg, S., Knoll, R. L., and Gates, B. A. (1971, November). *Prior entry reexamined: Effect of attentional bias on order perception*. Paper presented at the meeting of the Psychonomic Society, St. Louis, Missouri, USA.

Stone, J. V., Hunkin, N. M., Porrill, J., Wood, R., Keeler, V., Beanland, M., Port, M., and Porter, N. R. (2001). When is now? Perception of simultaneity. *Proceedings of the Royal Society B*, **268**, 31–8.

Stone, S. A. (1926). Prior entry in the auditory-tactual complication. *American Journal of Psychology*, **37**, 284–7.

Thesen, T., Blumberg, M. A., Spence, C., Carlson, C. E., Cash, S. S., Doyle, W. K., et al. (2008). 'The effects of task and attention on visual-tactile processing: Human intracranial data.' Paper presented at the 9th IMRF meeting, Hamburg, Germany, 16–19th July, 2008.

Titchener, E. B. (1908). *Lectures on the elementary psychology of feeling and attention*. New York: Macmillan.

Treisman, A. (1996). The binding problem. *Current Opinion in Neurobiology*, **6**, 171–8.

Treisman, A. M. and Gelade, G. (1980). A feature-integration theory of attention. *Cognitive Psychology*, **12**, 97–136.

Vanderhaeghen, C. and Bertelson, P. (1974). The limits of prior entry: nonsensitivity of temporal order judgments to selective preparation affecting choice reaction time. *Bulletin of the Psychonomic Society*, **4**, 569–72.

Vatakis, A. and Spence, C. (2007). Crossmodal binding: evaluating the "unity assumption" using audiovisual speech stimuli. *Perception & Psychophysics*, **69**, 744–56.

Vatakis, A. and Spence, C. (2008). Evaluating the influence of the 'unity assumption' on the temporal perception of realistic audiovisual stimuli. *Acta Psychologica*, **127**, 12–23.

Vatakis, A., Ghazanfar, A., and Spence, C. (2008a). Facilitation of multisensory integration by the 'unity assumption': is speech special? *Journal of Vision*, **8**(14), 1–11.

Vatakis, A., Navarra, J., Soto-Faraco, S., and Spence, C. (2008b). Audiovisual temporal adaptation of speech: temporal order versus simultaneity judgments. *Experimental Brain Research*, **185**, 521–9.

Vibell, J., Klinge, C., Zampini, M., Spence, C., and Nobre, A. C. (2007). Temporal order is coded temporally in the brain: Early ERP latency shifts underlying prior entry in a crossmodal temporal order judgment task. *Journal of Cognitive Neuroscience*, **19**, 109–20.

Vibell, J., Klinge, C., Zampini, M., Spence, C., and Nobre, A. C. (submitted). ERP study of the spatial prior-entry effect.

Wada, Y. (2003). Crossmodal attention between vision and touch in temporal order judgment task. *Shinrigaku Kenkyu*, **74**, 420–7.

Wada, M., Moizumi, S., and Kitazawa, S. (2005). Temporal order judgment in mice. *Behavioural Brain Research*, **157**, 167–75.

Walter, W. G. and Crow, H. (1961). Depth recording from human brain. *Excerpta Medica International Congress Series*, **37**, 64–5.

Wilberg, R. B. and Frey, R. D. (1977). The prior entry phenomenon: In search of determinants of the effect. In B. Kerr (Ed.) *Human performance and behaviour*, pp.237–40. Banff: Canadian Society for Psychomotor Learning and Sport Psychology.

Wilberg, R. B. and Frey, R. D. (1990). Prior entry: Information processing requirements and the judgment of temporal order. In Geissler, H.-G., Müller, M. H., and Prinz, W. (Eds.) *Psychophysical explorations of mental structures*, pp.253–67. Goettingen, Germany: Hogrefe and Huber Publishers.

Yates, M. J. and Nicholls, M. E. R. (2009). Somatosensory prior entry. *Attention, Perception & Psychophysics* **71**, 847–59.

Zampini, M., Bird, K. S., Bentley, D. E., Watson, A., Barrett, G., Jones, A. K., et al. (2007). 'Prior entry' for pain: Attention speeds the perceptual processing of painful stimuli. *Neuroscience Letters*, **414**, 75–9.

Zampini, M., Guest, S., Shore, D. I., and Spence, C. (2005a). Audio-visual simultaneity judgments. *Perception & Psychophysics*, **67**, 531–44.

Zampini, M., Shore, D. I., and Spence, C. (2005b). Audiovisual prior entry. *Neuroscience Letters*, **381**, 217–22.

Time perception is modulated by attention, perception, and action

Chapter 8

Timing, resources, and interference: attentional modulation of time perception

Scott W. Brown

The research described here is part of a larger theoretical framework of time perception. Many models posit the existence of an internal clock mechanism that underlies our experience of time (e.g. Treisman, 1963; Allan, 1992). This mechanism includes a pacemaker that emits a series of neural pulses and a counter/accumulator that records the pulses and establishes an internal representation or temporal record of the interval. Attention influences the content of the temporal record by affecting the pulse count. According to the attentional gate model (Block and Zakay, 1996; Zakay and Block, 1996), a gating component is situated between the pacemaker and the accumulator. Attention directed towards time causes the gate to become wider, allowing more pulses to enter the accumulator. The result is that perceived time is lengthened. When attention is directed away from time, the gate narrows, fewer pulses are counted, and perceived time is shortened.

Prospective and retrospective timing

The distinction between the prospective and retrospective paradigms has important implications for the study of attention and time perception. In the prospective paradigm, subjects are told in advance that they will be required to estimate the duration of an impending interval, and so are fully aware that the task is about time. They consciously attend to any available temporal cues and may even engage in timekeeping strategies such as counting or rhythmically tapping if conditions permit. The vast majority of timing studies are prospective. In the retrospective paradigm, however, subjects are unaware that the task is about time and, instead, are given a surprise duration estimation task once the interval has already elapsed. These subjects are more attentive to the non-temporal features of the stimulus environment, and their temporal awareness is relatively low. Retrospective timing studies are less common, mainly because subjects can provide only one time judgement. After that initial judgement, subjects will begin attending to time, which makes any subsequent judgements prospective rather than retrospective.

Paradigm comparison studies

The ideal situation is to compare directly the two paradigms in the same experiment. Unfortunately, only a relatively small number of these studies exist (see Block and Zakay, 1997 for a review). Practical considerations in the form of the extra time, effort, and expense in testing larger numbers of subjects than usual serve to limit research in this area. In an early paper (Brown, 1985), I compared prospective and retrospective time judgements of subjects who performed various attentional distractor tasks. The subjects in Experiment 1 judged the time they spent performing a perceptual-motor task configured to represent different degrees of difficulty. The task involved a star pattern printed on a sheet of paper. Depending on instructions, subjects simply concentrated on the figure (control condition), traced around the narrow border of the figure with a pencil (easy condition), or traced around the figure using a mirror-drawing apparatus (difficult condition). The main results showed that (a) prospective judgements were longer and more accurate than retrospective judgements, and (b) both prospective and retrospective judgements became shorter and/or more inaccurate with increases in distractor task difficulty (this interference effect is discussed more fully in the section that follows). In Experiment 2, subjects were tested under three auditory conditions: control (listen to speech-like noise over headphones); easy (attend to one channel of a dichotic tape consisting of two lists of words); and difficult (attend to both channels of the dichotic tape). As before, prospective judgements tended to be longer and more accurate than retrospective judgements, and both types of judgements became increasingly inaccurate as the distractor task become more difficult. The findings reveal differences in the accuracy of prospective and retrospective timing, but also point to an essential similarity, as time judgements under both paradigms were affected in the same way by distractor task demands.

The problem of one retrospective time judgement per subject

The restriction of one time judgement per subject presents a practical problem for researchers studying retrospective timing. Brown and Stubbs (1988) devised a procedure to circumvent this limitation. This method entails psychophysical scaling, which involves the relation between changes in stimulus intensity and corresponding changes in perceived intensity. In this instance, we compared prospective and retrospective time judgements of varying stimulus durations. Subjects in each paradigm listened to a series of four musical selections, each of a different duration, and then estimated the duration of the four selections. This procedure produces four separate time judgements from each subject. In line with standard psychophysical methodology, power functions were created by plotting the log of the time judgements against the log of the stimulus durations. The main interest centres on the slope of the power function. The slope reflects the correspondence between changes in physical and perceived time. Figure 8.1 depicts power functions based on the averaged data of four prospective groups and eight retrospective groups. The figure shows that the slopes were flatter and responses more variable for the retrospective judgements compared with the prospective judgements. Note that none of the slopes are flat, which would be the case if all intervals were perceived to be the same. The fact that even retrospective judgements show some correspondence with changes in duration indicates that although these subjects were not consciously attending to time, they were processing temporal information in an incidental or implicit fashion outside conscious awareness. Despite a lack of accuracy, these subjects had at least some idea about how much time had passed.

This same methodology was used to explore the effects of concurrent distractor tasks on prospective and retrospective timing. Brown and Stubbs (1992) presented four musical selections of different durations to prospective and retrospective groups, who then judged the durations of the selections. In addition, half the subjects in each paradigm performed a proofreading task as they listened to the music; the remaining subjects were assigned to a control condition without any proofreading requirement. There were three main findings. First, psychophysical slopes relating perceived and physical time were steeper for the prospective subjects and flatter for the retrospective subjects, a finding that replicates the previous research. Second, there was a trade-off between temporal and distractor task performance. The prospective subjects were more accurate at judging time but worse at proofreading, whereas the retrospective subjects worse at

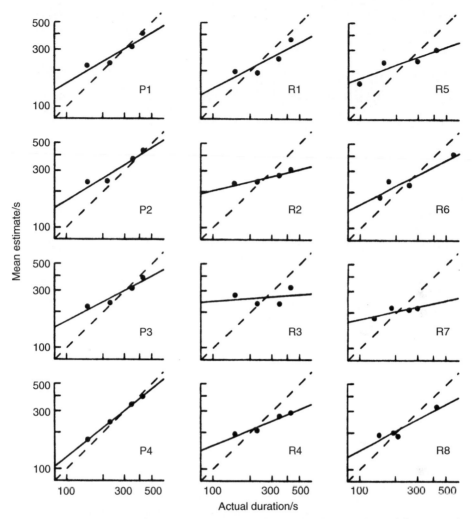

Fig. 8.1 Power functions (best-fitting linear regression plots on log–log coordinates) for mean time judgements as a function of actual duration of musical selections for different groups. Dashed lines represent a perfect correspondence between time judgements and stimulus duration. Groups P1–P4 were tested under the prospective paradigm and groups R1–R8 were tested under the retrospective paradigm. Reprinted with permission from Brown, S. W. and Stubbs, D. A. (1988). The psychophysics of retrospective and prospective timing. *Perception,* **17**, 297–310.

timing but better at proofreading. This same trade-off also was obtained in a recent scaling study in which prospective and retrospective subjects listened to four auditory prose passages under control and target-detection conditions (Brown and Rowden-Tibbetts, 2007). This pattern can be explained in terms of task priorities. Time was the important feature for the prospective subjects and proofreading (or target detection) was important for the retrospective subjects, and so these tasks received the most attention. The third finding was that the proofreading task interfered with both retrospective and prospective judgements. This result indicates that even though retrospective conditions involve only implicit timing, this incidental processing depends on attentional resources. The proofreading task requires attention, and it altered the allocation of resources sufficiently to disrupt temporal processing in both paradigms.

Do the two paradigms involve similar or different timing processes?

The experience of time is undoubtedly different under the two paradigms. Prospective timing involves heightened temporal awareness and conscious attention to the passage of time, whereas retrospective timing involves incidental temporal processing and a greater reliance on memory and reconstructive processes to gauge the duration of events. Does this mean that the underlying timing processes are different for the two paradigms? The argument that they are different is bolstered by research showing that subjects in the two paradigms respond differently to certain experimental manipulations (e.g. Block, 1992; Zakay and Block, 2004). On the other hand is research showing that subjects in prospective and retrospective conditions respond similarly to various distractor tasks, which supports the position that any differences that occur are differences in degree, not in kind (e.g. Brown, 1985; Brown and Stubbs, 1988, 1992). In the largest paradigm comparison study to date involving some 510 subjects, Kurtz and Strube (2003) employed the same star tracing task used in Brown (1985, Exp. 1). They found that time judgements for all subjects, both prospective and retrospective, decreased from the easy to difficult star tracing conditions, a result that parallels the original study. At this point, further investigations are needed to resolve the conflicting results seen in the retrospective data.

One way to view the prospective/retrospective distinction is in terms of a continuum spanning different degrees of attentiveness to time (Brown and Stubbs, 1992). The prospective paradigm, along with conditions of expectancy and anticipation, are instances of high-resolution timing, which is characterized by enhanced temporal alertness and attentiveness to temporal cues. The retrospective paradigm, absorbing situations, and conditions involving heavy processing demands all fall at the low-resolution timing end of the scale. Temporal awareness under these circumstances is minimal, with temporal information processing being conducted in a subconscious, incidental fashion. In this perspective, prospective and retrospective timing are closely related, and any differences that occur can be traced to different degrees of attentiveness to time.

Dual-task processing and interference

It is obvious from everyday life that attentiveness to the flow of time has an enormous influence in shaping our temporal experience. The adage 'time flies when you're having fun' captures the idea that when attention is distracted away from time by having fun or, more generally, by engaging in some absorbing activity (Brown, 2008b), less time seems to have passed by. Attentiveness to non-temporal information diminishes our temporal awareness. This basic observation serves as the basis for dual-task experiments in which attention is divided between concurrent temporal and distractor tasks (see also Sigman, Chapter 5; Ruthruff and Pashler, Chapter 9, this volume).

The interference effect and attentional resources

In two reviews (Brown, 1997, 2008b), I examined a large number of experimental studies showing an interference effect on prospective time judgement performance when subjects are also required to perform a simultaneous distractor task. Compared with single-task, timing-only conditions, time judgements become shorter, more variable, and/or more inaccurate under dual-task conditions. Of some 77 experiments reviewed, 91% showed the interference effect. It is the most robust, well-replicated finding in the time perception literature. There are two especially notable findings about this effect. First, timing performance is extremely sensitive to processing demands. Although many studies show that increases in task demands generally lead to greater disruption in timing performance, even weak demands will produce a substantial impairment in time judgement performance (Brown, 2008b). Second, virtually any type of distractor task will produce the interference effect. One might imagine that verbal tasks would cause interference by disrupting counting processes, but the effect also extends to tasks such as visual search, pattern detection, and manual tracking, tasks with little (or no) verbal component at all. Rather, the effect represents a basic attentional phenomenon in which the diversion of resources to any distractor task is sufficient to disrupt normal temporal processing.

A resource theory of attention (e.g. Navon and Gopher, 1979; Navon, 1984) readily accounts for the interference effect. Resource theorists conceive of attention as a limited pool of energy that is responsible for all cognitive processing. These limited resources are allocated to various task demands on a priority basis. If a person performs concurrent tasks, then resources must be distributed between them, with the result that each task may receive a less-than-optimal supply of attention. This reduction in processing capacity typically produces a decrement in task performance, as many dual-task experiments have shown. Similarly, performing concurrent temporal and distractor tasks leads to a division of resources. Fewer resources devoted to timing disrupt time judgement performance (Hicks et al. 1977; Zakay, 1989; Brown, 1997). This description of the interference effect is predicated on the idea that timing itself is an attentional demanding task (cf. Ruthruff and Pashler, Chapter 9, this volume). Michon (1972, 1985; Michon and Jackson, 1984) is a strong advocate for this position, arguing that timekeeping requires attentional resources. In this view, time judgements are no different from any other perceptual judgements in that all these tasks are supported by limited-capacity attention.

Interference and multiple timing

These ideas were tested in the context of a multiple timing paradigm devised by Brown and West (1990). The rationale is that if timing requires processing capacity, then performing two or more simultaneous timing tasks should result in an interference effect similar to that observed in the standard temporal/distractor dual-task situation. In one experiment (Exp. 1), subjects viewed a computer screen in which the letters A, B, C, and D each appeared in one of the four quadrants. The letters appeared in a random order, had asynchronous onsets and offsets, and each lasted for different amounts of time. In the control condition, subjects monitored the duration of the letter A and ignored the other letters; once all letters had disappeared from the screen, the subjects reproduced the duration of A. In the experimental conditions, subjects were instructed to time one letter (A), two letters (A and B), three letters (A, B, and C), or all four letters. Following stimulus presentation, one of the target letters was selected randomly for temporal reproduction. The results, expressed in terms of absolute error, are shown in Figure 8.2. Time judgement error increased linearly from less than 10% to more than 30% as subjects divided their attention between increasing numbers of temporal targets. Different variations on the multiple timing task involving different time judgement methods, experimental designs, and subject populations have yielded similar results (Brown and West, 1990, Exp. 2; Brown et al. 1992; Ambro and Czigler, 1998; Vanneste and Pouthas, 1999). These findings demonstrate that keeping track of time is a resource-demanding process.

Interference and event structure

Brown and Boltz (2002) sought to integrate research on the interference effect and event structure. Event structure involves the organization of the stimulus environment, which can

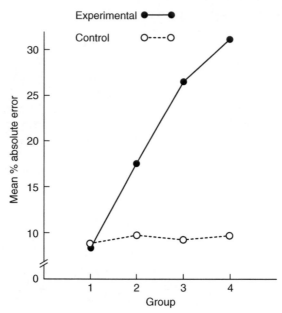

Fig. 8.2 Mean percentage absolute error of time judgements in control and experimental conditions for four groups. In the experimental condition, Groups 1, 2, 3, and 4 attended to 1, 2, 3, or 4 temporal targets, respectively. In the control condition, the groups attended to one temporal target. Reprinted from Brown, S. W. and West, A. N. (1990). Multiple timing and the allocation of attention. *Acta Psychologica*, **75**, 103–21, with permission from Elsevier.

range from coherent (highly organized, predictable, easily attended to and remembered events) to incoherent (disorganized, unpredictable events that are difficult to track and remember). Coherent events are associated with more accurate time judgements (e.g. Jones and Boltz, 1989; Boltz, 1992, 1998). In the Brown and Boltz (2002) paper, we combined distractor task demands (target detection) with musical sequences (Exp. 1) and narrative prose (Exp. 2) that varied in structural coherence. Both experiments showed that task demands and event structure affected timing performance. Time judgements were less accurate under the interference and incoherent structure conditions. The two factors also worked in combination by exerting a greater decrement in timing performance than either one alone. Overall, the distractor task imposed a stronger effect; structure exerted its main influence when task demands were greatest. These findings show that different aspects of attention can influence perceived time.

Interference and individual differences

Virtually everyone has trouble trying to monitor the passage of time while simultaneously performing another task. However, there are reliable individual differences in the degree to which timing is disrupted. Brown et al. (1995) developed a temporal signal-detection task to identify individual differences in timing performance. Signal detection involves the ability to distinguish a target stimulus from background sensory noise. Subjects were tested in a duration discrimination procedure in which they judged whether a visual stimulus was presented for certain target duration or for a slightly longer duration. Performance data were used to calculate measures of

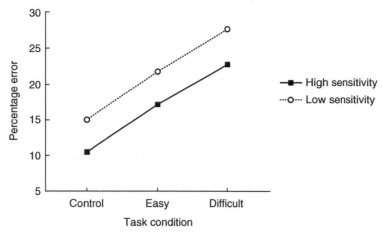

Fig. 8.3 Mean percentage absolute error in time judgements for subjects with high and low temporal sensitivity as a function of task condition. Subjects in the control, easy, and difficult conditions rehearsed 0, 3, or 7 two-digit numbers, respectively, throughout the stimulus interval. Reprinted with permission from Brown, S. W. (1998), Influence of individual differences in temporal sensitivity on timing performance. *Perception, 27*, 609–25.

perceptual sensitivity, which allowed subjects to be classified into high and low temporal sensitivity groups. Brown et al. (1995) demonstrated that performance on the temporal signal-detection task was related to performance on other timing tasks and situations. In a later study (Brown, 1998b), this methodology was used to investigate whether high and low temporal sensitivity groups would respond similarly to distractor task demands. After completing the temporal signal-detection procedure, subjects were tested on a time judgement task in which they reproduced the duration of a series of numerical displays. During each display interval, subjects monitored the passing time and also rehearsed 0, 3, or 7 two-digit numbers for a subsequent recall test. The absolute error of the temporal reproductions for the high and low sensitivity groups is depicted in Figure 8.3. The figure shows two main results. First, replicating the earlier findings, the high-sensitivity subjects were more accurate at judging time than were the low-sensitivity subjects. Secondly, although error increased linearly as a function of rehearsal task difficulty for both groups, the low-sensitivity subjects averaged approximately 4.5–5.0% more error in each task condition compared with the high-sensitivity subjects. This pattern suggests that the interference effect is a fundamental phenomenon in time perception, but that individual differences in timekeeping ability can moderate the extent to which a distracting task disrupts timing.

Practice and automaticity

Practice is an important element in the successful performance of most tasks. With practice, the task becomes predictable, routine, easier to execute, and performance improves (Laberge and Samuels, 1974; Logan, 1988, 1989). According to resource theorists, one experiences these benefits because of the development of automaticity. Automaticity refers to a reduction in the resources required to perform a skilled task (Moors and De Houwer, 2006). Due to practice, various resource-demanding components of task performance drop out of conscious awareness and are performed automatically, requiring far less capacity than otherwise. This lessened demand on resources has important implications for cognitive functioning. For example, automaticity training has been used as a means of improving dual-task performance (Ahissar et al. 2001; Ruthruff et al. 2001). The standard procedure is to practise one task sufficiently to achieve some degree of automatization; then the automatized task is performed concurrently with another task in a dual-task arrangement. Because the automatized task uses fewer resources than usual, resource competition with the other task is minimized and interference is reduced.

Automaticity offers a unique approach for investigating attentional allocation and the interference effect in timing. If practice on a task reduces its resource demand, then pairing that task with a concurrent timing task should diminish the interference effect. More resources would be available for timekeeping, which in turn would improve time judgement performance. Such an outcome would provide a converging operation for establishing timing as an attentional process.

The attenuation effect

In the initial research based on this idea (Brown, 1998a, Exp. 1), subjects were tested in a pre-test/practice/post-test paradigm. The task was pursuit-rotor tracking. Both the pre-test and post-test consisted of a timing-only single-task condition and a timing + tracking dual-task condition. Between the pre-test and post-test was a series of practice sessions on the tracking task alone, which was designed to at least partially automatize tracking performance. The results showed the expected interference effect in timing performance from the single-task to dual-task conditions on the pre-test. On the post-test, however, the dual-task condition exhibited a sharp reduction in interference. This reduction in interference because of practice on the distractor task is known as the attenuation effect. In follow-up research (Brown and Bennett, 2002), the same pattern of results was obtained with another tracking task (Exp. 1) and a mirror-reversed reading task (Exp. 2). In each case, the interference effect was not eliminated, but it was reduced substantially as a result of practice on the task. In related research, Sawyer (1999) had subjects judge time while they performed a concurrent mirror-tracing task. Practice on the tracing task improved timing accuracy, particularly for those performing a more difficult version of the task. All these findings demonstrate that the changing dynamics of attentional allocation can have a profound effect on perceived time.

Attenuation from the other direction

If practice on a distractor task minimizes the interference effect by making more resources available for the concurrent timing task, then what about providing practice on the timing task? Would practise at judging time automatize timekeeping skills, thus lowering the degree of resource competition between temporal and distractor tasks and reducing dual-task interference? This hypothesis was tested in attenuation experiments in which subjects received practice at judging time (Brown, 2008a). In Experiment 1, subjects were tested on a series of practice trials in which they judged time under training (feedback) or control (no feedback) conditions. As expected, the training group exhibited less time judgement error compared with the control group. Subsequently, all subjects participated in dual-task test trials involving concurrent timing and digit memory tasks. The digit memory task was designed to impose different degrees of attentional demand by varying the memory load between 0, 3, and 6 three-digit numbers to rehearse during the interval. The main results showed that increases in memory load lead to an increase in time judgement error for both the training and control groups. However, the training group maintained a constant reduction in error of approximately 4 percentage points across the three memory load conditions, compared with the control group. That is, time-judgement skill training attenuated the interference effect.

Experiment 2 followed the same basic design of the first experiment, except that the practice trials involved concurrent timing and memory load conditions. Otherwise, the procedure was the same as before, with subjects in the practice trials assigned to control and training groups. When tested later on the test trials, the control group showed a steady increase in time judgement error from approximately 9% to 19% across the three memory load conditions. In contrast, the training group maintained a constant degree of timing error (averaging less than 9%) across the memory load conditions. Time judgement practice with feedback under dual-task conditions had not just attenuated the interference effect, but had actually eliminated the effect altogether. A key factor contributing to the effectiveness of the procedure is that the make-up of the practice trials closely corresponded to the make-up of the test trials. Automaticity research suggests that practice is most beneficial when training conditions match testing conditions (e.g. Schneider, 1985; T. L. Brown and Carr, 1989). These attenuation studies show that practice on either the distractor task or the timing task is effective in minimizing the interference effect.

Bidirectional interference and resource specialization

A resource view of timing emphasizes the capacity demands of attending to time and the division of resources that occurs when one also performs a concurrent distractor task. The allocation of resources to multiple tasks implies that each task must necessarily receive less attention than normal. In this instance, one may predict that performance on both tasks would be compromised because of resource scarcity. In other words, one would expect a pattern of bidirectional (mutual) interference, in which performance on each task suffers. Although dual-task studies on the interference effect typically report a substantial adverse impact on timing performance, there is less information about performance on the concurrent distractor task. Because most investigators are concerned with timing processes, distractor task performance is usually ignored. In a review of the interference literature (Brown, 2006), I found only 33 studies that measured performance on both the temporal and distractor tasks, and that also included conditions in which subjects performed each task separately as well as concurrently. About half the studies showed bidirectional interference, and half showed interference with the timing task only. Why do some studies show the expected result and some do not? Is there something about the nature of the distractor tasks that makes a difference, and can this tell us anything about the cognitive processes that support timing functions? The answers to these questions lead to a reconsideration of the resource theory of attention.

Resource theory, revisited

Based on interference patterns obtained with the dual-task paradigm, some theorists conceive of an attentional system consisting of multiple pools of independent, special-purpose resources (e.g. Navon and Gopher, 1979, 1980; Wickens, 1980, 1991). These specialized resource pools are geared to handle specific types of processing demands. For example, separate resource pools may be dedicated to such functions as executive control, verbal/phonological processing, visuospatial processing, etc. (Wickens, 1991; Baddeley, 1992, 1993). This theoretical framework helps account for why it is that some concurrent tasks interfere with one another, whereas others do not. Tasks that interfere depend on the same resource pool, thus limiting the amount of attention each task receives; tasks that do not interfere depend on separate resource pools and so are able to proceed independently. In tasks that produce partial interference, as in the case of one task showing interference and the other task being unaffected, shared resources may be more important for one task than for the other (Navon and Gopher, 1980; Tsang et al. 1995).

How does a multiple resource theory apply to timing and the interference effect? As noted earlier, a survey of dual-task timing studies found that only some of the studies demonstrated bidirectional interference (Brown, 2006). Broadly speaking, the experiments showing evidence of bidirectional interference tended to involve what may be characterized as executive tasks, such as comprehension, mental arithmetic, and attentional control. Executive functions are those cognitive processes that direct actions, supervise behaviour, and are responsible for planning, judgement, and reasoning (Miyake et al., 2000). Bidirectional interference patterns suggest that time perception is closely related to the resources that support these executive functions.

Executive resources and timing

My initial research on bidirectional interference (Brown, 1997) illustrates the issue. Interference patterns between concurrent timing tasks and three different distractor tasks were examined. The distractor tasks were manual tracking (Exp. 1), visual search (Exp. 2), and mental arithmetic (Exp. 3). In each case, the distractor task interfered with temporal judgements. As for distractor task performance, however, concurrent timing disrupted only mental arithmetic. Mutual interference between the timing and arithmetic tasks suggests that they rely on common resources. Given that mental arithmetic is associated with executive resources, the implication is that timing is dependent on those same resources.

Other research has involved distractor tasks chosen specifically because of their association with executive functioning. Brown and Frieh (2000) examined interference patterns between concurrent timing and memory updating tasks. The updating task involved the presentation of a series of random digits. The digit sequence stopped at unpredictable times, at which point the task was to report the three or five most recently presented items. This task, requiring continual monitoring of the flow of information, is regarded as a traditional executive task (Towse and Valentine, 1997; Baddeley et al. 1998). The results provided partial support for the executive resource hypothesis. Timing and updating produced mutual interference in the easy version of the updating task (report the three most recently presented digits). The difficult version of the task (report the five most recent digits) was equally poor with or without concurrent timing. In another study (Brown, 2006), timing was combined with one of the most well-studied executive tasks, random generation. Random generation requires that the subject produce a continual series of items (usually verbalizing numbers or letters) in a random order. Randomization is an appropriate task to test an executive resource model of timing, as many empirical studies have shown that randomization interferes with other established executive tasks (e.g. Robbins et al. 1996; Baddeley et al., 1998). Furthermore, task performance may be assessed with an array of sensitive statistical measures designed to measure randomness. The procedure involved having subjects perform timing and digit randomization tasks separately and in combination. The results showed that, compared with single-task conditions, dual-task conditions disrupted both timing performance and randomization performance. This pattern of bidirectional interference implies strongly that timing and randomization processes rely on the same set of attentional resources.

Research with executive tasks continues in my laboratory. A project involving tasks representing three main executive functions was recently completed (Brown et al. 2009). The executive functions are shifting, updating, and inhibition (Miyake et al. 2000). The experiments used the attentional sharing procedure, in which subjects were instructed to divide attention in specified proportions between temporal and distractor tasks (e.g. 25% of attention to one task and 75% to the other). The results showed that: (1) temporal judgements became increasingly disrupted as attention was directed less to time and more to the executive task, and (2) executive task performance was progressively impaired as attention was directed away from that task and more towards time. This even trade-off in performance between the temporal and executive tasks is characteristic of tasks that rely on the same cognitive resources and mechanisms.

Executive functioning may also account for one particular aspect of the interference effect. Why are time judgements so sensitive to the presence of distractor task demands, even for tasks that do not depend on executive resources? In several papers (Brown, 1997, 2006, 2008b), I have argued for a coordination hypothesis as an explanation of the classic interference effect. One critical executive function involves managing dual-task situations. Multitasking requires coordinating cognitive operations, organizing inputs, integrating information, and scheduling responses. Interference studies have shown that executive resources are required to implement these coordination functions (Bourke et al. 1996; Logie et al. 2004). In a dual-task situation involving concurrent temporal and distractor tasks, the coordination functions place a demand on executive resources, which are also required for the timing task. Given that timing is very sensitive to attentional allocation, the diversion of resources to coordinative functions acts to disrupt timing performance. These ideas are supported by a series of dual-task timing studies by Dutke (2005). Dutke found that coordinative demands impaired timing performance, whereas non-coordinative demands left performance unimpaired.

Sequencing and timing

The idea of resource specialization in timing also has led to a line of research on the relation between sequencing and timing. This research stems from the notion that sequencing and timing both involve temporal information processing. Both tasks involve the perception and processing of a succession of events, and so both may share common attentional resources or cognitive mechanisms. Moreover, there is conceptual basis for linking these processes together. Sequencing is an essential feature of the executive functions of coordination, integration, and planning (Baddeley, 1992). This connection between sequencing, timing, and executive resources points to a basic underlying similarity between these processes.

Research reported by Brown and Smith-Petersen (2002) was designed to compare judgements of time and judgements of order. Subjects viewed a series of wordlists presented on a screen. Prior to each list, subjects were instructed to attend to the list duration, the temporal order of the words, or both duration and temporal order. The results showed strong evidence of bidirectional interference. Compared with single-task conditions, attention to order interfered with time judgements and attending to time interfered with order judgements. Further, we found that a concurrent mental subtraction task interfered equally with both time judgements and temporal order judgements by causing both types of judgements to become less accurate.

Brown and Merchant (2007) obtained patterns of bidirectional interference with a different set of sequencing tasks. In Experiment 1, subjects verified a series of reasoning statements that described the ordering of a pair of letters. In Experiment 2, subjects monitored an alphabetic sequence of letters and responded with a key press whenever they detected an omission in the sequence. These tasks were done singly and in conjunction with a concurrent timing task. Although the sequencing tasks are very different, they produced similar results. In both experiments, concurrent sequencing interfered with temporal judgements. Likewise, the concurrent timing task interfered with sequencing performance. These performance trade-offs between timing and sequencing indicate that common mechanisms support these tasks.

A different approach to studying the relation between timing and sequencing is to manipulate the degree to which executive tasks emphasize sequencing. The rationale is that a timing task should interfere more with a task requiring a greater involvement of sequencing resources compared with one requiring a lesser involvement. Brown and Usher (2005) had subjects perform executive tasks involving either sequence or similarity judgements. These tasks were performed alone and with a concurrent timing task. A screen displayed a series of pairs of statements describing familiar actions. In the sequencing condition, subjects judged whether the two actions were presented in the correct or incorrect temporal order. In the similarity condition, subjects judged whether the two actions were related or unrelated. The data showed that both tasks interfered with timing, and that concurrent timing also interfered with both the sequencing and similarity tasks. However, concurrent timing exerted a stronger impact on the sequencing task. The results make two basic points. First, they show that these tasks, dependent on the executive functions of reasoning and judgement, both rely on the same resources used by timing. Secondly, the differential degree of interference suggests that there is a greater overlap of resources between timing and sequencing judgements than between timing and similarity judgements.

Conclusions

The research has involved various techniques for modifying attention to time, including manipulations of temporal awareness via the prospective and retrospective paradigms, temporal/distractor dual-task processing, practice and automaticity, and variations in the nature of the distractor tasks. All these different approaches have produced a consistent set of findings. Like most tasks, interval timing requires attentional resources, and time judgement performance is influenced strongly by the allocation of those resources. This is not to say that timing is entirely a conscious process. Timing is also an implicit process, as evidenced by retrospective experiments. Timing probably falls into the domain of 'partially automatic' processes, those processes that have both intentional and incidental components (Hampson, 1989). Partially automatic processes are susceptible to attentional allocation and dual-task interference, as in the case of retrospective timing.

The research points to several different directions for future investigations. More research on the interference effect involving tasks that tap into different cognitive functions may provide a more detailed picture specifying the resources important for timing. There is also need of a finer-grained analysis of temporal/distractor dual-task performance, which may lead to a better description of the dynamics of timekeeping under interfering conditions. Finally, research on brain function holds great promise, because this area brings together empirical work on timing, attention, and executive processes. Studies in neuroimaging (Coull et al. 2004), brain injury (Harrington et al. 1998), and cognitive aging (Block et al. 1998), in conjunction with performance-based research, will expand our knowledge of the connection between attention and time.

References

Ahissar, M., Laiwand, R., and Hotchstein, S. (2001). Attentional demands following perceptual skill training. *Psychological Science,* **12**, 56–62.

Allan, L. G. (1992). The internal clock revisited. In F. Macar, V. Pouthas, and W. J. Friedman (Eds.) *Time, Action, and Cognition: Towards Bridging the Gap*, pp.191–202. Dordrecht: Kluwer Academic Publishers.

Ambro, A. and Czigler, I. (1998). Parallel estimation of short durations in humans. In V. DeKeyser, G. d'Ydewalle, and A. Vandierendonck (Eds.) *Time and the Dynamic Control of Behavior*, pp.143–56. Seattle, WA: Hogrefe and Huber.

Baddeley, A. D. (1992). Is working memory working? The fifteenth Bartlett lecture. *Quarterly Journal of Experimental Psychology,* **44A**, 1–31.

Baddeley, A. D. (1993). Working memory or working attention? In A. D. Baddeley and L. Weiskrantz (Eds.) *Attention: Selection, Awareness, and Control*, pp.152–70. New York: Oxford University Press.

Baddeley, A. D., Emslie, H., Kolodny, J., and Duncan, J. (1998). Random generation and the executive control of working memory. *Quarterly Journal of Experimental Psychology,* **51A**, 819–52.

Block, R. A. (1992). Prospective and retrospective duration judgment: The role of information processing and memory. In F. Macar, V. Pouthas, and W. J. Friedman (Eds.) *Time, Action, and Cognition: Towards Bridging the Gap,* pp.141–52. Dordrecht: Kluwer Academic Publishers.

Block, R. A. and Zakay, D. (1996). Models of psychological time revisited. In H. Helfrich (Ed.) *Time and Mind,* pp.171–95. Seattle, WA: Hogrefe and Huber.

Block, R. A. and Zakay, D. (1997). Prospective and retrospective duration judgments: A meta-analytic review. *Psychonomic Bulletin and Review,* **4**, 184–97.

Block, R. A., Zakay, D., and Hancock, P. A. (1998). Human aging and duration judgments: A meta-analytic review. *Psychology and Aging,* **13**, 584–96.

Boltz, M. G. (1992). The incidental learning and remembering of event durations. In F. Macar, V. Pouthas, and W. J. Friedman (Eds.) *Time, Action, and Cognition: Towards Bridging the Gap,* pp.153–63. Dordrecht: Kluwer Academic Publishers.

Boltz, M. G. (1998). The processing of temporal and nontemporal information in the remembering of event durations and musical structure. *Journal of Experimental Psychology: Human Perception and Performance,* **24**, 1087–104.

Bourke, P. A., Duncan, J., and Nimmo-Smith, I. (1996). A general factor involved in dual-task performance decrement. *Quarterly Journal of Experimental Psychology,* **49A**, 525–45.

Brown, S. W. (1985). Time perception and attention: the effects of prospective versus retrospective paradigms and task demands on perceived duration. *Perception and Psychophysics,* **38**, 115–24.

Brown, S. W. (1997). Attentional resources in timing: interference effects in concurrent temporal and nontemporal working memory tasks. *Perception and Psychophysics,* **59**, 1118–40.

Brown, S. W. (1998a). Automaticity versus timesharing in timing and tracking dual-task performance. *Psychological Research,* **61**, 71–81.

Brown, S. W. (1998b). Influence of individual differences in temporal sensitivity on timing performance. *Perception,* **27**, 609–25.

Brown, S. W. (2006). Timing and executive function: bidirectional interference between concurrent temporal production and randomization tasks. *Memory and Cognition,* **34**, 1464–71.

Brown, S. W. (2008a). The attenuation effect in timing: Counteracting dual-task interference with time judgment skill training. *Perception,* **37**, 712–24.

Brown, S. W. (2008b). Time and attention: Review of the literature. In S. Grondin (Ed.) *Time Perception,* pp.111–38. Bingley: Emerald.

Brown, S. W. and Bennett, E. D. (2002). The role of practice and automaticity in temporal and nontemporal dual-task performance. *Psychological Research,* **66**, 80–9.

Brown, S. W. and Boltz, M. G. (2002). Attentional processes in time perception: Effects of mental workload and event structure. *Journal of Experimental Psychology: Human Perception and Performance,* **28**, 600–15.

Brown, S. W. and Frieh, C. T. (2000). Information processing in the central executive: Effects of concurrent temporal production and memory updating tasks. In P. Desain and L. Windsor (Eds.) *Rhythm Perception and Production,* pp.193–6. Lisse: Swets and Zeitlinger.

Brown, S. W. and Merchant, S. M. (2007). Processing resources in timing and sequencing tasks. *Perception and Psychophysics,* **69**, 439–49.

Brown, S. W. and Rowden-Tibbetts, D. K. (2007). 'Effects of attentional demands and event structure on the psychophysical scaling of prospective and retrospective time judgments.' Paper presented at the New England Sequencing and Timing (NEST) 17th annual meeting, Haskins Laboratories, New Haven, CT. March, 2007.

Brown, S. W. and Smith-Petersen, G. A. (2002). 'Time and attention: Interference effects in duration judgment and temporal order memory tasks.' Paper presented at the New England Sequencing and Timing (NEST) 12th annual meeting, Yale University, New Haven, CT. March, 2002.

Brown, S. W. and Stubbs, D. A. (1988). The psychophysics of retrospective and prospective timing. *Perception,* **17**, 297–310.

Brown, S. W. and Stubbs, D. A. (1992). Attention and interference in prospective and retrospective timing. *Perception,* **21**, 545–57.

Brown, S. W. and Usher, S. R. (2005). *Effects of concurrent timing on sequence versus similarity judgments.* Paper presented at the New England Sequencing and Timing (NEST) 15th annual meeting, Yale University, New Haven, CT. March, 2005.

Brown, S. W. and West, A. N. (1990). Multiple timing and the allocation of attention. *Acta Psychologica,* **75**, 103–21.

Brown, S. W., Collier, S. A., and Night, J. C. (2009). 'Timing and executive resources: Dual-task interference patterns between temporal production and switching, updating, and inhibition tasks.' Paper presented at the New England Sequencing and Timing (NEST) 19th annual meeting, Haskins Laboratories, New Haven, CT. March, 2009.

Brown, S. W., Stubbs, D. A., and West, A. N. (1992). Attention, multiple timing, and psychophysical scaling of temporal judgments. In F. Macar, V. Pouthas, and W. J. Friedman (Ed) *Time, Action, and Cognition: Towards Bridging the Gap,* pp.129–40. Dordrecht: Kluwer Academic Publishers.

Brown, T. L. and Carr, T. H. (1989). Automaticity in skill acquisition: Mechanisms for reducing interference in concurrent performance. *Journal of Experimental Psychology: Human Perception and Performance,* **15**, 686–700.

Coull, J. T., Vidal, F., Nazarian, B., and Macar, F. (2004). Functional anatomy of the attentional modulation of time estimation. *Science,* **303**, 1506–8.

Dutke, S. (2005). Remembered duration: working memory and the reproduction of intervals. *Perception and Psychophysics,* **67**, 1404–13.

Hampson, P. J. (1989). Aspects of attention and cognitive science. *Irish Journal of Psychology,* **10**, 261–75.

Harrington, D. L., Haaland, K. Y., and Knight, R. T. (1998). Cortical networks underlying mechanisms of time perception. *Journal of Neuroscience,* **18**, 1085–95.

Hicks, R. E., Miller, G. W., Gaes, G., and Bierman, K. (1977). Concurrent processing demands and the experience of time-in-passing. *American Journal of Psychology,* **90**, 431–46.

Jones, M. R. and Boltz, M. (1989). Dynamic attending and responses to time. *Psychological Review,* **96**, 459–91.

Kurtz, R. M. and Strube, M. J. (2003). Hypnosis, attention, and time cognition. *International Journal of Clinical and Experimental Hypnosis,* **51**, 400–13.

Laberge, D. and Samuels, S. J. (1974). Toward a theory of automatic information processing in reading. *Cognitive Psychology,* **6**, 293–323.

Logan, G. D. (1988). Automaticity, resources, and memory: Theoretical controversies and practical implications. *Human Factors,* **30**, 583–98.

Logan, G. D. (1989). Automaticity and cognitive control. In J. S. Uleman and J. A. Bargh (Eds.) *Unintended Thought,* pp.52–74. New York: Guilford.

Logie, R. H., Cocchini, G., Della Sala, S., and Baddeley, A. D. (2004). Is there a specific executive capacity for dual task coordination? Evidence from Alzheimer's disease. *Neuropsychology,* **18**, 504–13.

Michon, J. A. (1972) Processing of temporal information and the cognitive theory of time experience. In J. T. Frasier, F. C. Haber, and G. H. Muller (Eds.) *The Study of Time,* pp.242–58. New York: Springer-Verlag.

Michon, J. A. (1985) The compleat time experiencer. In J. A. Michon and J. L. Jackson (Ed), *Time, Mind, and Behavior,* pp.20–52. New York: Springer-Verlag.

Michon, J. A. and Jackson, J. L. (1984) Attentional effort and cognitive strategies in the processing of temporal information. In J. Gibbon and L. Allan (Eds.) Timing and Time Perception. *Annals of the New York Academy of Sciences,* **423**, 298–321. New York: New York Academy of Sciences.

Miyake, A., Friedman, N. P., Emerson, M. J., Witzki, A. H., Howerter, A., and Wager, T. D. (2000). The unity and diversity of executive functions and their contributions to complex "frontal lobe" tasks: a latent variable analysis. *Cognitive Psychology,* **41**, 49–100.

Moors, A. and De Houwer, J. (2006). Automaticity: a theoretical and conceptual analysis. *Psychological Bulletin,* **132**, 297–326.

Navon, D. (1984). Resources—a theoretical soup stone? *Psychological Review,* **91**, 216–34.

Navon, D. and Gopher, D. (1979). On the economy of the human-processing system. *Psychological Review,* **86**, 214–53.

Navon, D. and Gopher, D. (1980). Task difficulty, resources, and dual-task performance. In R. S. Nickerson (Ed), *Attention and Performance VIII*, pp.297–315. Hillsdale, NJ: Erlbaum.

Robbins, T. W., Anderson, E. J., Barker, D. R., Bradley, A. C., Fernyhough, C., Henson, R., et al. (1996). Working memory in chess. *Memory and Cognition,* **24**, 83–93

Ruthruff, E., Johnston, J. C., and Van Selst, M. (2001). Why practice reduces dual-task interference. *Journal of Experimental Psychology: Human Perception and Performance,* **27**, 3–21.

Sawyer, T. F. (1999). Allocation of attention and practice in the production of time intervals. *Perceptual and Motor Skills,* **89**, 1047–51.

Schneider, W. (1985). Training high-performance skills: fallacies and guidelines. *Human Factors,* **27**, 285–300.

Towse, J. N. and Valentine, J. D. (1997). Random generation of numbers: a search for underlying processes. *European Journal of Cognitive Psychology,* **9**, 381–400.

Treisman, M. (1963). Temporal discrimination and the indifference interval: implications for a model of the "internal clock". *Psychological Monographs,* **77**, 1–31.

Tsang, P. S., Shaner, T. L., and Vidulich, M. A. (1995). Resource scarcity and outcome conflict in time-sharing performance. *Perception and Psychophysics,* **57**, 365–78.

Vanneste, S. and Pouthas, V. (1999). Timing in aging: the role of attention. *Experimental Aging Research,* **25**, 49–67.

Wickens, C. D. (1980). The structure of attentional resources. In R. S. Nickerson (Ed), *Attention and Performance VIII*, pp. 239–57. Hillsdale, NJ: Lawrence Erlbaum.

Wickens, C. D. (1991). Processing resources and attention. In D. L. Damos (Ed), *Multiple-task Performance*, pp.3–34. London: Taylor and Francis.

Zakay, D. (1989). Subjective time and attentional resource allocation: an integrated model of time estimation. In I. Levin and D. Zakay (Eds), *Time and Human Cognition: A Life-span Perspective*, pp.365–97. Amsterdam: Elsevier.

Zakay, D. and Block, R. A. (1996). The role of attention in time estimation processes. In M. A. Pastor and J. Artieda (Eds), *Time, Internal Clocks and Movement*, pp.143–64. Amsterdam: Elsevier.

Zakay, D. and Block, R. A. (2004). Prospective and retrospective duration judgments: an executive-control perspective. *Acta Neurobiologiae Experimentalis,* **64**, 319–28.

Chapter 9

Mental timing and the central attentional bottleneck

Eric Ruthruff and Harold Pashler

Time estimations are important in everyday life. When the stoplight ahead turns yellow, for example, one needs to estimate whether there is sufficient time to enter and exit the intersection. As noted elsewhere in this book, however, the ability to estimate time is impaired under conditions of divided attention (e.g. Hicks, Miller, and Kinsbourne, 1976; Brown, 1985, 1997; Mattes and Ulrich, 1998; Brown, Chapter 8, this volume). In many cases, authors have interpreted these results as reflecting a diversion of processing resources from the timing task to another task, so that both tasks receive a partial share of the available resources. The purpose of the present chapter is to evaluate the specific alternative hypothesis that timing might be subject to a discrete central processing bottleneck (Pashler, 1984; Welford, 1952), so that timing cannot take place until central operations have finished. To begin, we briefly review the evidence for a central bottleneck, and then relate this research to studies of timing under divided attention.

Central bottleneck model

Traditional dual-task studies (with non-temporal tasks) often reveal dramatic interference between tasks that require planning and production of responses (for reviews, see Pashler and Johnston, 1998; Lien and Proctor, 2002). There are many different dual-task paradigms, but perhaps the most widely used approach is to present two different stimuli, each requiring production of its own speeded motor response. By varying the time between these stimuli—known as the stimulus onset asynchrony (SOA)—we can vary the degree to which the tasks need to be performed concurrently. Typically, the task presented first (Task 1) is performed quickly at all SOAs. But response times to the task presented second (Task 2) are usually elevated by several hundred milliseconds at short SOAs (e.g. 50ms) relative to long SOAs (e.g. 1000ms). This dual-task interference effect has been termed the psychological refractory period (PRP) effect (see also Sigman, Chapter 5, this volume). The term 'refractory period' came from the hypothesis that the interference stems from a temporary cognitive sluggishness immediately following an act of cognition (analogous to the neuronal refractory period); although that hypothesis has long since been discarded, the name for the phenomenon stuck.

The robustness of PRP interference across a wide range of tasks, input modalities, and output modalities led Welford (1952) to propose the central bottleneck model. The key assumption, shown in Figure 9.1A, is that while central operations of one task are underway, central operations of all other tasks must wait. The term 'central operation' is rather vague, but is usually taken to refer to the decision-making processes that take place after perception but before response execution.

Note that the central bottleneck model implies a discrete view of dual-task interference, postulating a complete inability to carry out more than one central operation at a time.

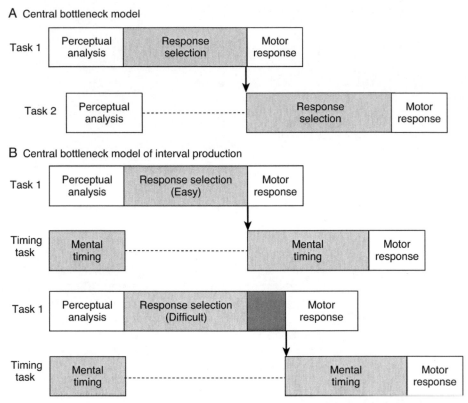

Fig. 9.1 A) The central bottleneck model, as applied to a traditional dual-task experiment. At short stimulus onset asynchronies (SOAs), like the one shown in the figure, the central stage of Task 2 (e.g. response selection) must wait for the central stage of Task 1 to finish. B) The central bottleneck model as applied to a mental timing task (interval production). The key assumption is that mental timing cannot take place while central operations are underway for any other task.

Dual-task interference thus is assumed to result primarily from processing delays (represented by the dotted line in Figure 9.1A), not from a slowing of mental processes that run concurrently (e.g. Kahneman, 1973). There is considerable evidence to favour this discrete view (e.g. Pashler, 1984, 1994; McCann and Johnston, 1992; Ruthruff, Pashler, and Hazeltine, 2003; Sigman and Dehaene, 2005), although there continues to be controversy about whether graded sharing of capacity among central processes can be ruled out (Navon and Miller, 2002; Tombu and Jolicoeur, 2002, 2003; Miller, Ulrich, and Rolke, 2009).

One major goal of research on this topic has been to determine the precise processing locus of the 'central' bottleneck. Studies have demonstrated convincingly that response selection is subject to the central processing bottleneck (e.g. Pashler, 1984, 1994; Pashler and Johnston, 1989; McCann and Johnston, 1992), at least relatively early in practice (see Hazeltine, Teague, and Ivry, 2001; Schumacher et al., 2001; Ruthruff et al., 2006; Maquestiaux et al., 2008). Subsequent studies have associated the bottleneck with a wide range of additional mental processes, including mental rotation (Ruthruff, Miller, and Lachmann, 1995), encoding into short-term memory (Jolicoeur, 1999; Ruthruff and Pashler, 2001), long-term memory retrieval (Carrier and Pashler, 1995; Byrne and Anderson, 2001), complex stimulus categorizations (Johnston and McCann, 2006), and even the discrimination of facial expressions (Tomasik et al., 2009). The diversity of mental processes subject to the processing bottleneck suggests the existence of a single very general-purpose processing mechanism, perhaps analogous to the CPU (central processing unit) of a computer (although not necessarily anatomically localized). We refer to this putative mechanism or resource as the *central mechanism.*

Of course, not all mental processes require the central mechanism. If tasks were performed entirely sequentially, with no temporal overlap in any mental processes, then the time to complete two tasks in dual-task conditions would be equal to the *sum* of the times to complete the tasks in single-task conditions. Dual-task interference is rarely ever this severe, however, suggesting that some mental processes can overlap in time. Research indicates that perceptual processes often do not require the central mechanism; specific examples include letter identification (Pashler and Johnston, 1989; Luck, 1998; Johnston and McCann, 2006), word identification (at least for skilled readers; Ruthruff et al., 2008), and retrieval of images from long-term memory (Green, Johnston, and Ruthruff, 2007).

It appears that response-execution processes are also not subject to the bottleneck, under many circumstances. To study this issue, Osman and Moore (1993) used one task that required either a left-hand or right-hand response (Task 1, presented first) and another task that required a left-foot or right-foot responses (Task 2, presented second). With such tasks, one can determine when subjects begin preparing a response by measuring lateralized readiness potentials—the difference in brain potentials between the motor cortices of the left and right hemispheres. Osman and Moore found that preparation of the manual response to Task 2 began before the foot response to Task 1 had been completed (i.e. response executions overlapped). Lien et al. (2007) found similar results with a vocal task followed by a manual task. Behavioural studies have yielded similar conclusions. If motoric processes are sequential then, at short SOAs in the PRP paradigm, any manipulation that prolongs Task-1 response execution should also delay the Task-2 response. Contrary to this prediction, Pashler and Christian (1994) found that increasing the complexity of Task-1 response execution (e.g. saying 'one' versus saying 'one two three four five') increased response times to Task 1 but had relatively little effect on response times to Task 2 (see also Bratzke et al., 2008). Thus Task-2 response execution does not generally need to wait until Task-1 response execution has finished. Ulrich et al. (2006), however, found that increases in the complexity of the manual response to Task 1 (short versus long movements of a lever) increased response time to Task 1 and also caused a similar increase in response times to Task 2, which also required a manual response. A tentative conclusion from these studies is that response execution is not wholly subject to the central bottleneck, at least when the tasks use distinct response modalities (e.g. vocal versus manual).

In sum, results from recent dual-task studies are generally consistent with the original claim that the bottleneck generally encompasses central processes (loosely defined as deciding how to respond to the stimulus), but not necessarily perceptual processes or response execution. However, the precise boundary between bottleneck and non-bottleneck processes is still being mapped out.

Mental timing under divided attention

Most studies examining attentional limitations in mental timing have asked subjects to estimate time while performing some fairly continuous distracting task (Brown, Chapter 8, this volume). The mental activities required in these tasks have been quite diverse, ranging from perceptuo-motor coordination (e.g. mirror drawing) to fine perceptual discriminations (e.g. loudness or brightness) to demanding cognitive operations (e.g. problem-solving). Typically, the subject reports either a numerical estimate of the duration of some event (*time estimation*), pushes a button after a specified time interval has elapsed (*interval production*), or reproduces the duration of some recently experienced event (*interval reproduction*). Sometimes, subjects are asked to judge durations after the fact (*retrospective timing*), although the present article concerns only cases where subjects know in advance that they are to record the duration of some interval (*prospective timing*).

Overwhelmingly, these studies show that concurrent tasks interfere with prospective timing (Hicks, Miller, and Kinsbourne, 1976; Zakay, Nitzan, and Glicksohn, 1983; Brown, 1985, 1997; Fortin and Rousseau, 1998; Zakay and Block, 1996, 1997; Mattes and Ulrich, 1998; Zakay, 1998; Rammsayer and Ulrich, 2005). Specifically, performing a concurrent task usually leads to a foreshortening of perceived time and an increase in the variability of time estimates. These interference effects typically become more severe as the difficulty of the concurrent task increases (e.g. Zakay, Nitzan, and Glicksohn, 1983; Brown, 1985, 1997).

As an example, Brown (1985, Experiment 1; Brown, Chapter 8, this volume) asked subjects to perform one of three tasks on a 6-pointed star: (1) attend the star (no response required); (2) trace the outline of the star; or (3) trace the star using a mirror. After either 16 or 32 seconds of performing these tasks, the experimenter then asked the subject to verbally report how much time had elapsed. Half were tested under prospective conditions (they knew in advance they would be asked to make time judgements) and half under retrospective conditions. Of primary interest here is the observation that the mean prospective time estimates decreased (by about 27%) as the difficulty of the concurrent task increased.

Previous findings clearly indicate that time perception benefits from 'attention', in the most global sense of that term (and, conversely, suffers from a lack of attention). However, they do not tell us whether mental timing is subject to the central bottleneck (see Figure 9.1B). Indeed, the link between these literatures has rarely been discussed. One limitation of most previous timing studies—with respect to evaluating a central bottleneck account—is the use of continuous concurrent tasks, which require central mechanisms only intermittently. If subjects switch back and forth between the timing task and the concurrent task, at times of their choosing, the central bottleneck hypothesis makes no clear predictions regarding the amount of interference. Another limitation is that researchers typically compare timing performance in dual-task versus single-task blocks, which differ not only in the availability of central mechanisms, but also in overall mental load. Even in studies that compared multiple dual-task conditions differing in difficulty (e.g. the different curve tracing conditions of Brown, 1985, Experiment 1), the different conditions are completed in separate blocks of trials or even using different groups of subjects. So load is still confounded with competition for central mechanisms. The problem is that, as mental task load increases, the quality of advance preparation for any particular task decreases, and task performance suffers (Gottsdanker, 1979; Rogers and Monsell, 1995). Even if mental timing is not subject to the central bottleneck, timing accuracy might degrade in dual-task blocks due to poorer preparation for timing. As a simple analogy, it would take longer to launder two heavy blankets together (compared to laundering only one) because the heavier load would prolong drying time. This load effect reflects a kind of capacity limitation, but it is clearly not the case that the dryer somehow deals with each blanket one at a time. Furthermore, this confound between load and task difficulty makes it nearly impossible to generate precise predictions from the central bottleneck model. Indeed, the success of the PRP paradigm (which varies SOA, the time between stimuli, rather than the number of tasks) stems largely from the fact that it reduces the impact of task load. A further concern is that, in some previous studies, the concurrent task was initiated prior to the onset of the stimulus whose duration is to be timed. Consequently, it is possible that the interference reflects not a difficulty in timekeeping per se, but rather a failure to detect the onset of the interval to be timed (see Lejeune, 1998).

Time production

We have investigated the attentional demands of time perception using a new type of procedure (Ruthruff and Pashler, 2008). Our specific goal was to determine whether mental timing must be postponed while central mechanisms select a speeded response to a concurrent task (see Figure 9.1B). Because the concurrent task requires subjects to rapidly decide which of several responses is appropriate for a given stimulus (decision-making), it should engage central attentional mechanisms.

As a starting point, we examined the ability to produce a fixed time interval in parallel with a concurrent task requiring a comparison of the brightness of two filled squares. As shown in Figure 9.2A, subjects were required to make their brightness response in less than 1 second and then press a key when 1.5 seconds had elapsed since stimulus onset (time production). Because the stimulus used for the brightness task was also used for the timing task, there was no danger that divided attention would cause subjects to fail to notice the onset of the interval to be timed. We assumed that the brightness task would receive priority in dual-task blocks because of the requirement to respond quickly. Consistent with this assumption, brightness discriminations were just as fast in dual-task blocks as in single-task blocks.

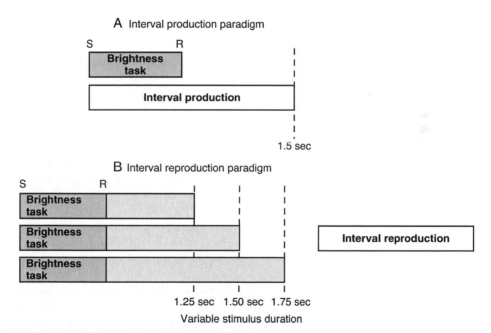

Fig. 9.2 A) Dual-task condition with interval production. Upon stimulus onset, subjects were to perform the brightness discrimination and to begin producing a 1.5-second interval. B) Dual-task condition with interval reproduction. Upon stimulus onset, subjects were to perform the brightness discrimination and also to estimate the stimulus duration (the actual duration was 1.25, 1.5, or 1.75 seconds). They could reproduce this duration any time after stimulus offset.

The key manipulation was the difficulty of the brightness judgement. In the easy condition the brightness difference was large, whereas in the difficult condition the brightness difference was much more subtle. These conditions were randomly intermixed within dual-task blocks, so that difficulty would not be confounded with load (i.e. the number of pending tasks to be prepared was the same). In single-task blocks, decreasing the difference in brightness increased the time to complete the brightness discrimination by nearly 100ms. The critical question was how this manipulation would influence time production in dual-task blocks. If subjects can keep track of time while performing the speeded brightness discrimination, without interference, then their timing performance should not depend much on the difficulty of the brightness discrimination. They should simply produce intervals of about 1.5 seconds (± error) in both the easy and difficult conditions. But if timing requires central attentional mechanisms, attempts to produce a 1.5-second interval should be strongly biased by the difficulty of the intervening brightness discrimination. The reason is that subjects would not be able start their mental timer until *after* completing the brightness discrimination (see Figure 9.1B). Consequently, they should fail to record the extra time taken while performing the difficult version of the concurrent task. It follows that their time productions should be much longer with a difficult brightness discrimination than with an easy discrimination. We refer to this phenomenon as *carryover*. In the extreme, the carryover onto the timing task (i.e. the lengthening of time productions) should be just as large as the effect on the brightness discrimination itself (100% carryover).

The mean produced time interval across single and dual-task blocks was 1481ms (SD = 192ms), which is very close to the target value (1500ms). Subjects received feedback after each time production, which presumably helped them to hone in on the target value. More importantly, carryover was nearly 100%. In dual-task blocks, the brightness manipulation slowed performance on the brightness discrimination by 82ms, and increased time productions by 80ms. The most straightforward explanation is that, as depicted in Fig 9.1B, subjects did not actually begin keeping track of time until after the brightness discrimination was finished (or, at least, until after the stage(s) influenced by our difficulty manipulation). In other words, the data suggest that timing requires the same central attentional mechanisms that are needed to select a response to Task 1.

This conclusion is supported by the timing variability data. In dual-task blocks, brightness discriminations took about 500ms and had a standard deviation (SD) of 97ms. By comparison, the average SD of the (1500ms) time productions in single-task blocks was 214ms. Assuming that timing variance is proportional to the duration being timed, the SD for a 500-ms interval would be about 124ms. Thus, timing estimates appear to be more variable than brightness discriminations. Hence, if subjects do not keep track of time during the brightness discrimination, time productions will inherit the variability of the approximately 500-ms brightness discrimination, rather than the variability of 500ms of mental timing. This leads to the surprising prediction that timing variability should actually *decrease* in dual-task blocks. Indeed, the SD of time productions was significantly smaller in dual-task blocks (SD = 171ms) than in single-task blocks (SD = 214ms).

One might propose that a failure to keep track of time during the brightness discrimination should lead, overall, to production of an interval much longer than the target interval (e.g. because no counts are made while the brightness discrimination is underway). However, this did not happen: mean time productions were 21ms shorter (marginally significant) in the dual-task condition (1471ms) than in the single-task condition (1492ms) and quite close to the target interval (1.5 sec). However, because subjects were given trial-by-trial feedback on the accuracy of their produced time intervals, they presumably learned to compensate for the missed time. In other words, we propose that subjects first performed the brightness judgement (taking about 500ms), then timed out an interval of about 1000ms to produce a total interval of about 1500ms.

In principle, subjects could have learned two different compensations—one for the easy brightness judgement and one for the difficult one—eliminating the carryover onto time productions. Clearly, this did not happen. It seems that people learn to make a single, overall compensation (which can be prepared in advance of each trial), but do not make different compensations for specific conditions (which are mixed together unpredictably and thus cannot be anticipated).

Time reproduction

When the task required time production, the nearly 100% carryover suggests that subjects could not keep track of time while simultaneously performing a speeded brightness discrimination. These findings, however, fall short of demonstrating that mental timing wholly usurps central attentional mechanisms, in general. Subjects might have information about the elapsed time that cannot be used in time production, but can be used when making other types of timing judgements. Moreover, one might suggest that subjects begin timing after completing the brightness discrimination not because they are compelled to do so by basic cognitive architecture, but rather because this strategy simplifies the timing task. Instead of timing out the full 1.5-second interval, they need only time out the period remaining after completing the brightness discrimination (roughly 1 second). As noted earlier, brightness-task response time was relatively consistent from trial to trial, so the amount of error introduced by not timing during that task would probably be less than the error associated with mental timing of the same interval.

To address this issue, we conducted a series of follow-up experiments with a different kind of timing response. Instead of producing a time interval during the brightness discrimination (interval production), we asked subjects to keep track of the stimulus duration and subsequently reproduce this interval (known as interval reproduction). Thus, as shown in Figure 9.2B, subjects first classified the brightness of a stimulus, and then attempted to reproduce the duration of that stimulus. To make the task challenging, we used a variable stimulus duration of 1.25, 1.5, or 1.75 seconds. The bottleneck model predictions parallel those of the previous experiment with time production, but with an important twist. If subjects can time only after completing the brightness discrimination, then they should perceive a shorter stimulus duration in trials with a difficult brightness discrimination than with an easy discrimination. However, the effect of this estimation bias on time reproductions should be opposite in sign to the effect observed on time productions. Specifically, time reproductions should be *reduced* following the more difficult brightness discrimination, by the same amount that the brightness response is increased (100% carryover).

We found that the mean reproduced time interval was significantly shorter in the difficult condition (1415ms, SD = 209ms) than in the easy condition (1448ms, SD = 200ms). Although this 33-ms carryover effect went in the predicted direction, it was only 22% of the 147-ms lengthening of the brightness judgement itself with difficult discriminations (see Figure 9.3). These results—in contrast to those we obtained with time production—suggest that mental timing is far from being completely subject to a central bottleneck.

One caveat is that, as the stimulus duration increased by 500ms (from 1.25 to 1.75 seconds), interval productions increased by only 194ms. Thus, only 38.8% of the change in stimulus duration was reflected in time productions. Given that the perceived estimate of the stimulus duration on any given trial is noisy, subjects might combine this noisy estimate with a relatively stable estimate of the mean stimulus duration. The result would be regression-to-the-mean in stimulus reproductions. Critically, this regression might also limit the carryover of difficulty effects onto the timing task. Nevertheless, the 22% carryover of difficulty effects is significantly less than the 38.8% of variation in stimulus duration that is reflected in time productions. Put another way, the

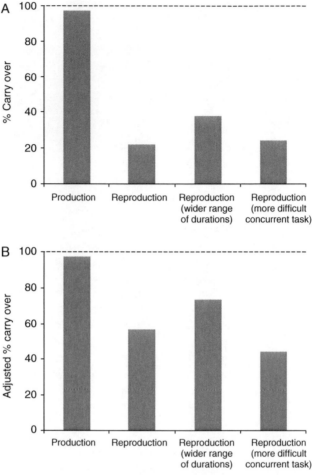

Fig. 9.3 A) Percentage carryover, calculated as the effect of concurrent task difficulty on time productions/reproductions (× 100) divided by its effect on the concurrent task itself. When reproducing intervals, participants might incorporate their estimate of elapsed time on a given trial with their estimate of the mean elapsed time across all trials. This could explain why subjects' reproductions did not increase one-for-one with increases in actual stimulus duration (regression to the mean). To correct for potential regression to the mean (B), we first calculated for each experiment the proportion of the range in actual stimulus durations that was captured by subjects' reproduced durations. Then we divided the percentage carryover (shown in A) by this proportion.

observed carryover onto time reproductions was only about 57% of maximum (recall that we found virtually 100% carryover in our earlier experiment on time production).

Increased variation in stimulus duration

To encourage subjects to rely on their perception of the passage of time during each stimulus presentation, rather than the average stimulus duration, we conducted a follow-up experiment with a wider range of stimulus durations (spanning 1 second rather than 0.5 seconds): 1, 1.25, 1.5, 1.75, and 2 sec. This effort appears to have been successful in that the range of time reproductions captured more of the variation in stimulus durations (52.0% versus 38.8%); that is, there appeared to be less regression to the mean.

Another concern regarding our previous experiment is that the difficult brightness discrimination, which produced 15.8% errors, was overly difficult. We therefore increased slightly the brightness difference used in the difficult condition, which brought error rates (3.1%) back into the range typical of most experiments with speeded responses (where the primary dependent measure is response time, not accuracy). Nevertheless, the manipulation still had a substantial effect on response times, as discussed later. A further benefit of a more subtle difficulty manipulation is that it reduces the likelihood that subjects are aware of the different conditions and deliberately compensate for them by adjusting their time estimates away from the perceived duration. To further reduce any such concerns over a deliberate compensation, we also eliminated the trial-by-trial feedback on timing performance. Without this feedback, subjects are less likely to become aware that their time estimates deviate systematically in certain conditions.

Without trial-by-trial feedback, subjects began to more severely underestimate the stimulus duration; the mean reproduced time was 1304ms (SD = 253ms), compared to the actual mean duration of 1500ms. Most critically, however, the difficulty manipulation had a 95-ms effect on brightness judgements, but only a 36-ms effect on time reproductions. Thus, the carryover was only 37.9%. In the preceding section we noted that subjects might integrate perceived time with a stable estimate of the average time; if so, 100% carryover would not occur, even if timing were subject to a central bottleneck. In this experiment, 52% of the variation in actual stimulus duration (from 1 to 2 seconds) was reflected in time reproductions. Even taking possible regression into account, the observed 37.9% carryover effect was only 73% percent of the 'carryover' of actual variation in stimulus duration.

Time reproduction with a more difficult concurrent task

Our initial experiments using time reproductions suggested that subjects could perceive stimulus duration (albeit imperfectly) even while central attentional mechanisms were busy with another task. A potential concern, however, is that the brightness discrimination (even the most difficult version) was not sufficiently demanding to fully engage central attentional mechanisms. In particular, it is possible that the stage sensitive to our difficulty manipulation relies more on perceptual processing mechanisms than central attentional mechanisms.

To address this issue, we used a much more demanding concurrent task that required subjects to map eight alphanumeric stimuli (1, 2, 3, 4, A, B, C, D) onto four response fingers. The mean response time for this task was 873ms, compared to only 481ms for the brightness discrimination. We varied the difficulty of this task via a stimulus–response (S–R) compatibility manipulation (e.g. Van Selst, Ruthruff, and Johnston, 1999; Ruthruff, Pashler and Hazeltine, 2003). The letters were mapped compatibly onto the four fingers, and the digits incompatibly, or vice versa (counterbalanced across subjects). Numbers and digits were randomly intermixed within blocks to avoid confounding difficulty effects with overall task load. Importantly, it seems clear that the manipulated stage (response selection) is central in this case, rather than perceptual. We found that mean response time was 763ms in the compatible condition (per cent error = 1.6%) and 987ms in the incompatible condition (per cent error = 7.3%). Thus, the mean effect size was 224ms.

The mean reproduced interval (1373ms; SD = 301ms) was again shorter than the actual mean stimulus duration of 1500ms. The key finding, however, is that only 24.1% of the difficulty effect on the S–R compatibility task carried over onto time reproductions. In contrast, 54.8% of the actual variation in stimulus duration was reflected in the time reproductions; as the actual duration increased from 1 to 2 seconds, the reproduced duration increased from 1093ms to 1641ms. Thus, the observed 24.1% carryover of difficulty effects represents only 44% of the 'carryover' from actual variation in stimulus duration. Even though the difficult S–R compatibility task clearly requires central mechanisms for an extended period of time, it appears that subjects were simultaneously able to keep track of the elapsed time (albeit imperfectly).

Conclusions

In this chapter, we posed the question of whether mental timing mechanisms can operate even while central attention is occupied with a demanding concurrent task. As we described earlier, previous literature seems generally inconclusive on this issue. Recent investigations in our lab suggest that when subjects actually *produce* time intervals in parallel with a concurrent task, timing mechanisms are subject to a central processing bottleneck. On the other hand, when subjects merely note stimulus duration in order to *reproduce* it shortly afterwards, mental timing is affected only to a rather modest degree by a concurrent speeded task. These results therefore refute the suggestion that timing is wholly subject to the same discrete central bottleneck as other types of effortful mental processes (such as response selection, memory encoding, and mental rotation). To put it simply, there must exist some mechanism(s) capable of perceiving time that are not completely disabled while central mechanisms are devoted to a concurrent task. It is an open question whether such mechanisms are functionally dedicated to timing or have other functions (see Ivry and Schlerf, 2008).

Models of time perception

A widely cited model of time perception proposes the existence of an autonomous pacemaker and an accumulator that counts the ticks (see, e.g. Gibbon, Church, and Meck, 1984; Ulrich, Nitschke, and Rammsayer, 2006). It is often suggested that, under dual-task conditions, attention must be divided between the concurrent task and the counting. The result is that many counts are missed and perceived time is foreshortened. Such a model potentially explains the present findings with time reproductions (i.e. mild disruption of timing during a concurrent task) if one adds the proviso that the accumulator benefits from central attention but is not entirely disabled without it. To account for the bottleneck in timing performance we found with time productions, one could add the plausible assumption that people can strategically disable this counting mechanism when it suits them. That is, perhaps the demanding nature of the time production paradigm encourages people to break performance down into two phases: performance of the concurrent task, followed by time production of the remaining time interval. Time reproduction, meanwhile, is easier because it merely requires online recording of an estimate of the elapsed time (actual reproduction of the estimated time can be delayed until well after the concurrent task has finished).

The present results could also be reconciled by proposing a combination of explicit and implicit time perception mechanisms. Suppose that the explicit timing mechanism—the one that is subject to bottleneck-type interference—is the most accurate timing mechanism. However, the implicit timing mechanism—which is not subject to the central bottleneck—can also provide useful temporal information, albeit with a lower resolution. People might be able to utilize the latter, less-precise mechanism when central attention is occupied by a concurrent task and thus not lose track of time completely.

References

Bratzke, D., Ulrich, R., Rolke, B., and Schröter, H. (2008). Motor limitation in dual-task processing with different effectors, *Quarterly Journal of Experimental Psychology, 61*, 1385–99.

Brown, S. W. (1985). Time perception and attention: the effects of prospective versus retrospective paradigms and task demands on perceived duration. *Perception & Psychophysics*, **38**, 115–24.

Brown, S. W. (1997). Attentional resources in timing: interference effects in concurrent temporal and nontemporal working memory tasks. *Perception & Psychophysics*, **59**, 1118–40.

Byrne, M. D. and Anderson, J. R. (2001). Serial modules in parallel: the psychological refractory period and perfect time-sharing. *Psychological Review*, **108**, 847–69.

Carrier, L. M. and Pashler, H. (1995). Attentional limits in memory retrieval. *Journal of Experimental Psychology: Learning, Memory, & Cognition*, **21**, 1339–48.

Champagne, J. and Fortin, C. (2008). Attention sharing during timing: modulation by processing demands of an expected stimulus. *Perception & Psychophysics*, **70**, 630–9.

Fortin, C., and Rousseau, R. (1998). Interference from short-term memory processing on encoding and reproducing brief durations. *Psychological Research*, **61**, 269–76.

Gibbon, J., Church, R. M., and Meck, W. H., (1984). Scalar timing in memory. *Annals of the New York Academy of Sciences*, **423**, 52–77.

Gottsdanker, R. (1979). A psychological refractory period or an unprepared period? *Journal of Experimental Psychology: Human Perception and Performance*, **5**, 208–15.

Green, C., Johnston, J. C., and Ruthruff, E. (2007). Recognition of pictures may not require central attentional resources. *Proceedings of the 29th Annual Cognitive Science Society*, pp.317–22. Austin, TX: Cognitive Science Society.

Hazeltine, E., Teague, D., and Ivry, R. B. (2002). Simultaneous dual-task performance reveals parallel response selection. *Journal of Experimental Psychology: Human Perception and Performance*, **28**, 527–45.

Hicks, R. E., Miller, G. W., and Kinsbourne, M. (1976). Prospective and retrospective judgments of time as a function of amount of information processed. *American Journal of Psychology*, **89**, 719–30.

Johnston, J. C. and McCann, R. W. (2006). On the locus of dual-task interference: Is there a bottleneck at the stimulus classification stage? *Quarterly Journal of Experimental Psychology*, **59**, 694–719.

Jolicoeur, P. (1999). Concurrent response selection demands modulate the attentional blink. *Journal of Experimental Psychology: Human Perception and Performance*, **25**, 1097–113.

Kahneman, D. (1973). *Attention and effort*. Englewood Cliffs, NJ: Prentice-Hall.

Ivry, R. B. and Shlerf, J. E. (2008). Dedicated and intrinsic models of time perception. *Trends in Cognitive Sciences*, **12**, 273–80.

Lejeune, H. (1998). Switching or gating? The attentional challenge in cognitive models of psychological time. *Behavioural Processes*, **44**, 127–45.

Lien, M.-C., and Proctor, R. W. (2002). Stimulus-response compatibility and psychological refractory period effects: Implications for response selection. *Psychonomic Bulletin and Review*, **9**, 212–38.

Lien, M.-C., Ruthruff, E., Hsieh, S.-L., and Yu, Y.-T. (2007). Parallel central processing between tasks: Evidence from lateralized readiness potentials. *Psychonomic Bulletin and Review*, **14**, 133–41.

Luck, S. J. (1998). Sources of dual-task interference: Evidence from human electrophysiology. *Psychological Science*, **9**, 223–7.

Maquestiaux, F., Lague-Beauvais, M., Ruthruff, E., and Bherer, L. (2008). Bypassing the central bottleneck after single-task practice in the psychological refractory period paradigm: evidence for task automatization and greedy resource recruitment. *Memory & Cognition*, **36**, 1262–82.

Mattes, S. and Ulrich, R. (1998). Directed attention prolongs the perceived duration of a brief stimulus. *Perception and Psychophysics*, **60**, 1305–17.

McCann, R. S. and Johnston, J. C. (1992). Locus of the single-channel bottleneck in dual-task interference. *Journal of Experimental Psychology: Human Perception and Performance*, **18**, 471–84.

Miller, J., Ulrich, R., and Rolke, B. (2009). On the optimality of serial and parallel processing in the psychological refractory period paradigm: effects of the distribution of stimulus onset asynchronies. *Cognitive Psychology* **58**, 273–310.

Navon, D. and Miller, J. (2002). Queuing or sharing? A critical evaluation of the single-bottleneck notion. *Cognitive Psychology*, **44**, 193–251.

Osman, A. and Moore, C. M. (1993). The locus of dual-task interference: Psychological refractory effects on movement-related brain potentials. *Journal of Experimental Psychology: Human Perception & Performance*, **19**, 1292–312.

Pashler, H. (1984). Processing stages in overlapping tasks: evidence for a central bottleneck. *Journal of Experimental Psychology: Human Perception and Performance*, **10**, 358–77.

Pashler, H. (1994). Dual-task interference in simple tasks: data and theory. *Psychological Bulletin*, **116**, 220–44.

Pashler, H. and Christian, C.L. (1994). Bottlenecks in planning and producing vocal, manual and foot responses (Center for Human Information Processing Technical Report). La Jolla, CA: University of California, San Diego, Center for Human Information Processing. (Available from http://www.pashler.com/manuscripts.html)

Pashler, H. and Johnston, J. (1989). Chronometric evidence for central postponement in temporally overlapping tasks. *Quarterly Journal of Experimental Psychology*, **41A**, 19–45.

Pashler, H. and Johnston, J. C. (1998). Attentional limitations in dual-task performance. In H. Pashler (Ed.) *Attention*, pp.155–89. Hove: Psychology Press/Erlbaum (UK) Taylor & Francis.

Rammsayer, T. and Ulrich, R. (2005). No evidence for qualitative differences in the processing of short and long temporal intervals. *Acta Psychologica*, **120**, 141–71.

Rogers, R. D. and Monsell, S. (1995). Costs of a predictable switch between simple cognitive tasks. *Journal of Experimental Psychology: General*, **124**, 207–31.

Ruthruff, E. and Pashler, H. (2001). Central and peripheral interference in RSVP displays. In K. Shapiro (Ed.), *The Limits of Attention: Temporal Constraints on Human Information Processing*, pp.100–23. New York: Oxford University Press.

Ruthruff, E. and Pashler, H. (2008). Does mental timing require central attention? Unpublished manuscript.

Ruthruff, E., Miller, J. O., and Lachmann, T. (1995). Does mental rotation require central mechanisms? *Journal of Experimental Psychology: Human Perception and Performance*, **21**, 552–570.

Ruthruff, E., Pashler, H., and Hazeltine, E. (2003). Dual-task interference with equal task emphasis: graded capacity-sharing or central postponement? *Perception and Psychophysics*, **65**, 801–16.

Ruthruff, E., Van Selst, M., Johnston, J. C., and Remington, R. W. (2006). How does practice reduce dual-task interference: Integration, automatization, or simply stage-shortening? *Psychological Research*, **70**, 125–42.

Ruthruff, E., Allen, P. A., Lien, M.-C., and Grabbe, J. (2008). Visual word recognition without central attention: Evidence for greater automaticity with greater reading ability. *Psychonomic Bulletin & Review*, **15**, 337–43.

Schumacher, E. H., Seymour, T. L., Glass, J. M., Fencsik, D., Lauber, E., Kieras, D. E., et al. (2001). Virtually perfect time sharing in dual-task performance: Uncorking the central attentional bottleneck. *Psychological Science*, **12**, 101–8.

Sigman, M. and DeHaene, S. (2005). Parsing a cognitive task: a characterization of the mind's bottleneck. *PLoS Biology*, **3**, e37.

Tomasik, D., Ruthruff, E., Allen, P. A., and Lien, M.-C. (2009). Non-automatic emotion perception in a dual-task situation. *Psychonomic Bulletin & Review*, **16**, 282–8.

Tombu, M. and Jolicoeur, P. (2002). All-or-none bottleneck versus capacity sharing accounts of the psychological refractory period phenomenon. *Psychological Research*, **66**, 274–86.

Tombu, M. and Jolicoeur, P. (2003). A central capacity sharing model of dual-task performance. *Journal of Experimental Psychology: Human Perception and Performance*, **29**, 3–18.

Ulrich, R., Ruiz Fernández, S., Jentzsch, I., Rolke, B., Schröter, H., and Leuthold, H. (2006). Motor limitation in dual-task processing under ballistic movement conditions. *Psychological Science*, **17**, 788–93.

Ulrich, R., Nitschke, J., and Rammsayer, T. (2006). Crossmodal temporal discrimination: assessing the predictions of a general pacemaker–counter model. *Perception and Psychophysics*, **68**, 1140-52.

Van Selst, M. V., Ruthruff, E., and Johnston, J. C. (1999). Can practice eliminate the psychological refractory period effect? *Journal of Experimental Psychology: Human Perception and Performance*, **25**, 1268–83.

Welford, A. T. (1952). The "psychological refractory period" and the timing of high-speed performance: a review and a theory. *British Journal of Psychology*, **43**, 2–19.

Zakay, D. (1998). Attention allocation policy influences prospective timing. *Psychonomic Bulletin & Review*, **5**, 114–18.

Zakay, D. and Block, R. A. (1996). The role of attention in time estimation processes. In M. A. Pastor and J. Artieda (Eds.) *Time, internal clocks and movement*, pp.143–64. Amsterdam: Elsevier.

Zakay, D. and Block, R. A. (1997). Temporal cognition. *Current Directions in Psychological Science*, **6**, 12–16.

Zakay, D., Nitzan, D., and Glicksohn, J. (1983). The influence of task difficulty and external tempo on subjective time estimation. *Perception & Psychophysics*, **34**, 451–6.

Acknowledgements

This work was supported by grants from the National Institute of Mental Health (R01-MH45584, H. Pashler, PI, and P50 MH066286, Keith Nuechterlein, PI) and the National Science Foundation (Grant BCS-0720375, H. Pashler, PI; Grant SBE-0542013, G. Cottrell, PI).

Chapter 10

Attention underlies subjective temporal expansion

Peter Ulric Tse

Perhaps you have noticed that events sometimes seem to slow down transiently. I first noticed this as a schoolboy, eager for class to be over. I noticed that when I first looked at the analogue clock, whose second hand jumped each second, that it seemed that the second hand had stopped, at least initially (see Yarrow, Chapter 12, this volume). After an inordinately long time it seemed to move again, and return to its usual pace. Now I notice this when I come home at night, and cannot initially tell whether the red light on my answering machine is blinking or not, because the first blink seems so inordinately long (compare Rose and Summers, 1995; Kanai and Watanabe, 2006). This temporal expansion has also happened to me in circumstances where my attention has suddenly been brought into focus, as when I swerve to miss a deer that has jumped onto the road, or as I watch myself helplessly skid into the back of another car. Why does this illusion of conscious experience occur? This chapter explores this question by summarizing key findings of Tse and colleagues (Tse, Sheinberg, and Logothetis 2004), and then discussing them in terms of more recent findings from the time-perception literature.

The perception of duration is rooted in the perceptual processing of events. In cases of prospective duration judgements (i.e. when observers know that the experiment is about judging durations), when no concurrent processing of stimuli is required, the ratio of judged duration to real duration generally *increases* as a function of both the number of stimuli that occur over an interval (e.g. Frankenhauser, 1959; Fraise, 1963; Ornstein, 1969; Thomas and Brown, 1974) and the complexity of those stimuli (e.g. Schiffman and Bobko, 1974; Avant, Lyman, and Lee, 1975; Thomas and Weaver, 1975). However, when observers must process non-durational information about stimuli during prospective tasks, or when they must perform a concurrent task, the ratio of judged to real time generally *decreases* as a function of the amount of information processed (e.g. Katz, 1906; Hülser, 1924; Quasebarth, 1924; Underwood and Swain, 1973; Hicks and Brundige, 1974; Hicks, Miller, and Kinsbourne, 1976; Thomas and Cantor, 1978; Zakay and Tsal, 1989; Grondin and Macar, 1992; Zakay, 1993; Macar, Grondin, and Casini, 1994; Predebon, 1996). Duration estimations therefore follow opposite trends in prospective experiments that involve concurrent processing and those that do not. In the absence of concurrent processing, subjective time expands whereas in its presence, it typically contracts. Here I explore the temporal dynamics of subjective temporal expansion (henceforth referred to as just 'temporal expansion') and describe the role of attention in this illusion.

An extensive literature provides evidence for the hypothesis that attention plays a role in the perception of duration (e.g. James, 1890; Katz, 1906; Mattes and Ulrich, 1998). Building on earlier models (Creelman, 1962; Treisman, 1963), Thomas (Thomas and Brown, 1974; Thomas and Cantor 1978; Thomas and Weaver, 1975) and Hicks (Hicks, Miller, and Kinsbourne, 1976; Hicks et al., 1977) proposed an attentional allocation/distraction model according to which attention can increase (or decrease) the perceived duration of a unit of objective time. If attention is distracted by non-temporal information processing, less capacity is available for processing temporal information (Kahneman, 1973), and duration judgements will tend to decrease or become less reliable (Brown, 1985; Brown, Chapter 8, this volume). If attention is not distracted from temporal information processing, then more capacity is available for processing temporal information, and duration judgements will tend to increase. In agreement with Fraisse (1963), these authors argue that the prospective judgement of time requires attention to the passage of time. Concurrent processing entails a relative underestimation of clock time because the observer must attend to the distracting task rather than to the passage of time. When not paying attention to cues for the passage of time, the observer misses more such cues, causing underestimations of clock time. Fraisse (1984) found evidence supporting this model (Thomas and Cantor, 1978). In particular, the easier a concurrent task, the more observers tend to overestimate an interval, presumably because when a distracting task is easy, observers are able to attend more to duration.

According to these models there is a 'counter' that keeps track of the number of units of temporal information processed for a given perceived event (Treisman, 1963; Thomas and Weaver, 1975).[1] These models argue that the number of units of temporal information that are counted decreases when attention is distracted from processing the duration of an interval. According to these models, attention increases duration judgements when duration per se is attended because fewer temporal cues are missed. However, the data of Tse and colleagues (2004) suggest that it is also possible that the number of units of temporal information processed is boosted above baseline when an observer orients to an improbable event. If attending to a stimulus boosts information processing of that stimulus, then the counter would count more units, and subjective time would expand (but see Eagleman, Chapter 11, this volume). The 'missed temporal cues' and 'attentional boost' interpretations are not mutually exclusive. Both could contribute to distortions in perceived duration and both are compatible with the notion of a counter or some other as yet unknown neural mechanism that measures the amount of information processed per unit objective time in order to calculate the duration of perceived events. That is, on both accounts, that of Thomas and Weaver (1975) or Tse et al. (2004), if the amount of information processed per unit objective (i.e. clock) time, particularly information about duration per se, increases or decreases, the perceived duration of an event changes accordingly.

The majority of research in the time literature therefore supports, dare I say, a 'standard attentional model' of time perception according to which paying more (less) attention to the duration of an event increases (decreases) its perceived duration (Brown, Chapter 8, this volume). Questions remain, however. Is the expansion in perceived duration really an attentional effect, or is it simply a consequence of the amount of information processed? If attention increases the amount of information processing brought to bear on a stimulus, it might be difficult to separate these two possibilities. However, a strictly attentional account would make at least four predictions that a (non-attentional) speeded information-processing account would not. First, at least 80–150ms are required before attention can be allocated to a new stimulus (e.g. Nakayama and Mackeben, 1989; Hikosaka, Miyauchi, and Shimojo, 1993). If it can be shown that there is an expansion of perceived duration for objective durations above ~120ms, but a contraction for durations below ~80ms (because attention is not yet fully allocated to the stimulus), then this would support an attentional account. Second, attention is commonly believed to have two components, one transient (or exogenous) and one sustained (or endogenous) (e.g. Nakayama

---

[1] In the literature on duration perception the terms 'unit,' 'cue,' and 'pulse' are used equivalently in the context of clock/counter models.

and Mackeben, 1989). These two attentional components have different temporal dynamics, and this difference should manifest itself in duration-estimation data. Third, attention is a central process, and should therefore exert its effects in the visual and auditory modalities in a similar fashion. Lastly, there is extensive evidence that attention cannot be applied to the pattern of low-level retinal activation itself. Rather, attention can only be allocated over information that has been processed by grouping, shape formation, and other processes that operate pre-attentively (e.g. He and Nakayama, 1992; Baylis and Driver, 1995; Rensink and Enns, 1995). Temporal expansion should therefore not be a function of image novelty per se but instead should be a function of the novelty of pre-attentively processed information.

Tse and colleagues (2004) carried out a series of experiments to test these predictions. Their experiments explored the role of attentional orienting in the subjective expansion of time by testing both visual and auditory stimuli within an oddball paradigm. In an oddball paradigm the observer responds to a low-probability stimulus that occurs within a train of high-probability stimuli. An oddball paradigm was used because: (1) a 'transient' or 'exogenous' component of attention is allocated automatically to the abrupt onset of a new stimulus (e.g. Nakayama and Mackeben, 1989; Remington, Johnston, and Yantis, 1992), and (2) a large literature shows that detection of an oddball typically leads to marked changes in event-related potentials that are believed by many researchers to be highly sensitive to attentional mechanisms (e.g. the P3 is highly dependent on attention; Polich, 1986; Garcia-Larrea, Lukaszewicz, and Mauguiere, 1992; Potts et al., 1996). Since observers tend to orient and thus attend to an oddball quite automatically, an oddball paradigm offers certain advantages over experimental paradigms that manipulate 'willed,' 'sustained,' or 'endogenous' attention to stimuli. In particular, since the present research focuses on the temporal dynamics of temporal expansion, an oddball paradigm afforded us good control over the timing of observers' allocation of attention.

The goal was to describe the objective temporal dynamics of distortions in subjective time as events are experienced in the present. Some researchers have called the amount of experience sustainable within a short-term memory store the 'psychological present,' (Fraisse, 1963; Michon, 1978) and argue that it has an upper limit of 5 seconds and an average value of 2–3 seconds (Fraisse 1984). We therefore limited our research to an examination of distortions in the 75–4000ms range; longer durations most likely involve memory processes beyond those of short-term memory, and temporal expansion is an illusion of how long something seems to last now, not of how long something seems to have lasted minutes or years after the event.

Subjective temporal expansion of an oddball stimulus

Experiment 1 tested how the subjective duration of oddball stimuli compared to that of standard stimuli. The oddball stimulus was a solid black disk that grew smoothly in size, whereas the standard was a solid black disk that did not move, and was the same size as the initial size of the oddball. It was determined how long a visually expanding oddball would have to last in objective duration in order to have the same subjective duration as stationary standards. An oddball event of variable clock duration was placed in a temporal sequence of standards, each of which lasted 1050ms. The observers' task was to say whether the moving oddball stimulus lasted longer or shorter than the standards. In order to obtain a psychometric function, the oddball was presented at nine objective durations (450, 525, 600, 675, 750, 825, 900, 975, 1050ms) around a central duration in randomized order. So that observers could not know when the oddball would appear, a variable number of standards appeared between two oddballs. Observers were told that all standards were of constant duration, which was the case. Standards were available both before and after oddball presentation and observers were encouraged to use both these standards in making their judgement of duration relative to the standard; they could respond until the start of the second standard following an oddball. All stimuli were separated by an interstimulus interval that varied randomly around 1050ms in the range 950–1150ms. The irregular temporal spacing of stimuli ensured that observers responded to the duration of stimuli per se, rather than the rhythm or beat that would be created if the interstimulus interval were held constant. The point at which the observer responded 'longer' on half the trials was taken to be the point of subjective equality obtained from Weibull fitted curves. The average point of subjective equality was 675ms Thus an oddball (an expanding solid disc) lasting 675ms was judged to feel, on average, as long in duration as a standard lasting 1050ms. This was the strongest example of subjective temporal expansion found using the oddball paradigm.

Temporal dynamics of temporal expansion

In Experiment 2, the hypothesis was tested that observers overestimate durations only after a temporal delay which corresponds to the number of milliseconds necessary for attention to be allocated to a new stimulus after onset of that stimulus. Again, a dynamically growing oddball of variable clock duration was placed within a train of standard events of constant clock duration. The observers' task was to say whether the oddballs lasted longer or shorter than the standard events. By repeating the procedure for standards of different durations, it was possible to determine the points of subjective equality between oddballs and standards around different durations. For each of the standard durations tested (75, 135, 225, 375, 525, 1050, 2100ms), the oddball was tested at nine objective durations around a central duration chosen to span a range that would permit the plotting of a psychometric function.

The ratio of 'perceived to real' durations was obtained by dividing the veridical duration of the standard by the subjective duration for the oddball as shown in the following formula: temporal expansion factor = (standard duration)/(point of subjective equality of oddball). The averaged data (arithmetic mean) for the visual expanding oddball among non-expanding standards is shown in Figure 10.1A. Note that there is no overestimation of duration for the 75-ms case. Indeed, there is *underestimation* for the oddball at this low standard duration. However, already by 135ms, there is considerable overestimation of the oddball's duration.

According to the standard attentional model, subjective durations are a function of the amount of temporal information processed over a perceived stimulus per unit objective duration. If an increase of information processing occurs, subjective durations will seem longer than they might otherwise. These results support the standard attentional model. Interestingly, time does not appear to expand subjectively until 75–120ms after stimulus onset. This result is consistent with the view that duration overestimation is a function of the allocation of attention, because attention presumably takes some time to allocate to the oddball target after it is detected.

But why would there be a reverse effect, or subjective temporal contraction, for the 75-ms case (compare Nakajima, ten Hoopen, and van der Wilk, 1991; Nakajima et al., 1992)? If attention boosts the amount of information processed, then the allocation of attention will boost perceived durations. However, it takes time to allocate attention. One possibility is that there is a momentary decrease in the amount of temporal information processed, perhaps because attention cannot be allocated to a stimulus while it is being shifted to that stimulus. This decrease relative to the baseline rate of information processing would be experienced as a subjective contraction of time. Another possibility is that some information about a stimulus is lost before attention can be fully allocated to a stimulus. Information loss would lead to a relative shortening of perceived duration. Another possibility is that when the oddball target is detected at this brief duration, attention may only be allocated after the target stimulus has disappeared. After the blank interstimulus

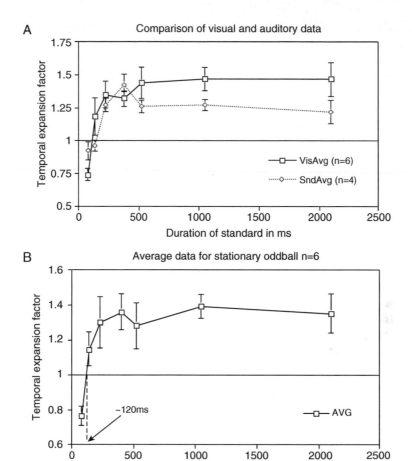

Fig. 10.1 A) A comparison of the temporal dynamics of subjective temporal expansion for both the visual (VisAvg) and auditory (SndAvg) domains. B) Average data for a non-expanding (stationary) oddball among expanding standards using the method of constant stimuli, with standard errors of the mean indicated by error bars.

interval, a standard stimulus appears on the screen. Because attention is now allocated to *this* stimulus, it is this standard disc that undergoes temporal expansion. In relative terms, this standard will seem to last longer than the target that preceded it, and observers may therefore respond 'shorter' for the target more often than not. Another possible contributing factor may be that the blank interstimulus interval after oddball disappearance gets expanded. This may make the oddball, in retrospect, seem shorter. The temporal dynamics of attentional allocation may therefore contribute to subjective temporal contraction in more than one way.

An interesting observation about the curve shown in Figure 10.1A is that it has a dip centred at 375ms, and a local peak at 225ms. This peak and dip pattern is more consistent in the individual data (not shown). Of six observers, only one did not demonstrate a peak followed by a dip then followed by a rise in the temporal expansion factor. Indeed, because the dip occurs at different times for different observers, the size of the peak and dip is somewhat attenuated in the averaged data shown in Figure 10.1A. Assuming attention is fully allocated to a stimulus only

~75–120ms or more after the onset of that stimulus, this local peak would occur at ~100ms after attentional allocation. Thus this local peak happens in the neighbourhood of 175–220ms after cue onset.

If this peak-dip-rise pattern reflects real underlying processes, it is consistent with the existence of transient and sustained components of attention (Nakayama and Mackeben, 1989; see also Olivers, Chapter 4, this volume). The transient component has a sudden onset, followed by a rapid decline, and the sustained component rises more slowly, but does not fade as rapidly. According to Nakayama and Mackeben (1989), the transient component peaks in the neighbourhood of 100ms after cue onset and begins to rapidly decline approximately 200ms after cue onset. The transient-peak in their data therefore tends to occur more rapidly than the peak in our data[2]. In contrast, the sustained component of attention does not peak and decline, but instead increases logarithmically with time. If attentional effects are due to the superposition or summation of these two types of attention, one transient, fast, and involuntary, and the other slow, sustained, and voluntary, then there may be a point where the effects of the former have begun declining before the effects of the latter have become strong. Such a point would look very much like the dip that we see in our data.

In summary, the data shown in Figure 10.1A are consistent with a model of time estimation based on attention according to which: 1) the amount of temporal expansion increases with the amount of information about duration processed and 2) attention enhances such information processing. Our data are consistent with the notion that attention takes in the order of 75–120ms to engage once an oddball stimulus has been detected. The data from individual observers suggest that a transient component of attention peaks within approximately 100ms following initial engagement. As the transient component weakens, a sustained component of attention becomes dominant. It may be that the transient component induces a burst of temporal information processing that is greater than the rate of information processing that occurs during the sustained component phase. Therefore the temporal expansion factor hits a peak with the peak of the transient component, but stays above unity because of enhanced information processing due to the sustained component of attention.

Temporal expansion for a stationary oddball

In the experiments described earlier, the occurrence of the oddball was confounded with the occurrence of expanding motion. Another potentially confounding factor was the rate or velocity of radial expansion, which depended on the duration of the oddball, because the ball had to grow from its initial to its final size within the time afforded by the allotted duration. Brown (1995; Chapter 8, this volume) has shown that a moving stimulus tends to undergo more temporal expansion than a stationary stimulus of identical objective duration, and that faster speeds tend to lengthen perceived time more than slower speeds. Similarly, Fraisse (1963) argued that judged duration is a function of the number of perceived changes. Since a radially expanding stimulus has more perceived changes per unit objective duration than a stationary stimulus, the temporal expansion observed might be a consequence of change perception, rather than attentional orientation to an oddball. To address these potential confounds, the oddball in Experiment 3 was a stationary ball placed among a sequence of expanding standards.

----

[2] The reason for this is unclear, but may be due to the differing nature of the two experimental paradigms. Their task is an attentional response to cue onset, whereas ours involves making a duration judgement based on novelty detection under conditions of sustained endogenous attention to the stimuli, necessitating a comparison between the oddball and the standards, which may cost additional time.

It might be that the pattern of results shown in Figure 10.1A is not a consequence of the target being an oddball so much as it is a consequence of the target being a more salient stimulus. Thus, in this experiment, the roles of target and standard in Experiment 2 were reversed so that the oddball was a stationary disc among expanding standards.

The results are shown in Figure 10.1B. Although the magnitude of temporal expansion was less than in the two previous experiments (~1.2 here versus ~1.6 for Experiment 1 and ~1.45 for Experiment 2 at 1050ms; compare Figure 10.2B), the overall pattern of results is very similar. Again, temporal expansion occurs beyond ~75–120ms and there is a peak-dip-rise pattern, although the peak occurs later in this case than in Experiment 2. This trend is also discernible in the individual data.

Although we cannot say with certainty what delays the peak in temporal expansion in Figure 10.1B relative to Figure 10.1A, it is not solely the motion of the oddball that induces temporal expansion. Rather, it is the fact that the target stimulus is an oddball to which the observer must respond that underlies temporal expansion. It could be that attentional orienting to a moving stimulus is faster than it is to a non-moving stimulus. An extensive recent literature has shown that exogenous attention is allocated automatically and rapidly to a sudden onset or motion (Jonides and Yantis, 1988; Yantis and Jonides, 1990; Remington, Johnston, and Yantis, 1992; Yantis and Egeth, 1999; Tse, Irwin et al., 2000; Sheinberg, and Logothetis, 2001). Moreover, if attention is already at an elevated level because the standards are moving, the boost in attention afforded by the stationary oddball's novelty may take longer to rise to its peak level.

It is likely that oddball motion contributed to the magnitude of temporal expansion in the case of the expanding oddball, because the oddball was salient not only due to its relative novelty, but also due to its motion. In the converse experiment, where standards moved, and the oddball did not, however, it is likely that the inherent salience of the moving standards diminished the strength of temporal expansion. This weakening of temporal expansion might have had at least two non-exclusive causes. First, more attention may have been allocated to the standards, raising the 'baseline' level of processing from which orienting to the oddball occurred. Second, the oddball may have drawn less attention to itself, because of its relatively lower salience.

Temporal expansion for colour, form, and size oddballs

In other experiments, we determined whether temporal expansion occurs for various other types of oddball stimuli, presented within a series of 1050-ms standards. We tested a red stationary disc as an oddball among black stationary discs of the same size; a circle among squares; a square among circles; and a large disc among small discs. The results for these oddballs are compared to those for the expanding and stationary oddballs from the previous experiments in Figure 10.2.

The strongest effect occurs for an expanding oddball among stationary standards (Experiment 1), where inter-observer variability was also the lowest. The weakest effect occurs for a stationary oddball among expanding standards (Experiment 2). The other four cases are intermediate, but generally support the notion that whenever an observer must detect and respond to an oddball stimulus, its subjective duration will expand. The same data have been replotted in Figure 10.2B in terms of the temporal expansion factors found in the various conditions.

Temporal expansion for an auditory oddball

If the curve shown in Figure 10.1A is due to the effects of a central process such as attention, rather than a specifically visual process, then repeating Experiment 2 using a sound analogue of the standards and expanding oddball should result in a similar curve. Alternatively, if the process is specifically visual, then we might expect a different pattern of results. This experiment used two

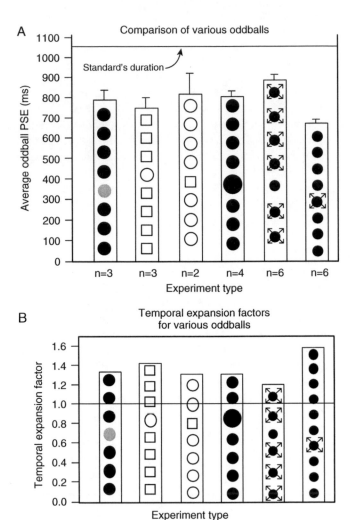

Fig. 10.2 A) Points of subjective equality (PSE) for six types of oddball/standard combination. The pattern within the bars of this bar graph is meant to indicate the type of standard and oddball stimuli used. For the sake of comparison, the final two bars illustrate the results from Experiments 1, 2, and 3. The rightmost bar indicates an expanding oddball among stationary standards. The second bar from the right indicates the stationary oddball among the expanding standards of Experiment 2. The new data are shown in the four bars starting at the left. The leftmost bar was a red stationary oddball among black stationary standards. The next bar to the right shows data for a disc oddball among square standards, and the next bar shows the inverse case. The fourth bar shows data for a large oddball (radius 100 pixels) among smaller standards (radius 30 pixels). The number of observers used in each case is indicated at the base of each bar. Error bars indicate standard errors of the mean. B) The same data now in terms of temporal expansion factors.

types of tones presented with stereo headphones; the standard tone was a pure sinusoidal tone set at middle C and the oddball tone was a smoothly rising tone that started at 20 half-notes below middle C and rose to 30 half-notes above middle C. Special care was taken to control the timing of this oddball. In all other respects, the experiment was identical to Experiment 2, and used the method of constant-duration standards and random inter-trial intervals.

Of particular interest is the relationship of the averaged data for this auditory experiment and the curve for its visual analogue. To make the relationship of these two curves apparent, they have been overlaid in Figure 10.1A. Even though there is more temporal expansion for the visual case at longer durations, the basic pattern of results is similar for the visual and auditory conditions. Indeed, the auditory data are virtually identical to the visual data for a stationary oddball among expanding standards (Figure 10.1B). We therefore conclude that temporal expansion is due to a central process, such as attention, that can express itself similarly in both the visual and auditory channels. We would predict that the temporal dynamics visible in Figure 10.1A would be present even if the stimuli were presented haptically, or in some modality other than vision or audition. However, we predict that subjective expansion of time would be undermined if attention were diverted, or even damaged as in neglect or Balint's patients.

Our data partly corroborate those of Nakajima and colleagues (Nakajima et al., 1991; Nakajima, ten Hoopen, and van der Wilk, 1992; see Allan and Gibbon, 1994), who reported that empty durations seem relatively shorter than a preceding 50-ms standard when the duration of the test stimulus is less than 120–160ms. However, they do not find temporal expansion beyond 160ms as we do, but report that 'time-shrinking' merely disappears. This could be because they were studying empty intervals, whereas we are studying intervals filled with events. Subjective temporal expansion may not be as strong an effect for empty intervals because there is nothing to attend to in empty intervals.

Note that both the visual and auditory curves in Figure 10.1A suggest that temporal expansion begins to occur in the neighbourhood of 120–150ms. This is consistent with the hypothesis that a brief span of time is required before attention can be allocated to a stimulus following stimulus onset. In addition, note that the auditory curve also has a peak that is suggestive of a transient component. However, its peak occurs 150ms after the local peak at 225ms for the visual curve. This trend is not an artefact of averaging data across observers. In Figure 10.1A, the peak occurs (for five of the six observers who do have a peak) between 135ms and 375ms, with four of the six observers demonstrating a peak at or before 225ms. In contrast, all four observers in the auditory condition demonstrate a peak at 375ms. The reason for this is unclear, but may be due to differences in the temporal dynamics of the transient and sustained components of attention in different sensory modalities. On the other hand, the peak and dip in the visual data shown in Figure 10.1B, where the oddball is a stationary disc among expanding standards, occurs at the same durations (375ms and 500ms respectively) as for the auditory data. Thus, slight differences in the locations of the peak and dip may be less important than the fact that there is a peak and dip in both the auditory and visual sense modalities. We take the existence of a peak and dip followed (at least in the visual cases shown in Figures 10.1A and 10.1B) by a rise, to be suggestive of a transient and sustained component of attention with differing temporal dynamics, as described in Nakayama and Mackeben (1989).

Conclusions

We used an oddball paradigm to explore distortions in subjective time, under the assumption that observers orient or attend to a low-probability stimulus more than they do to a high-probability stimulus. The goal was to probe the objective temporal dynamics of temporal expansion as well as to determine whether the effect is truly attentional.

The data presented here support the traditional view (e.g. Creelman, 1962; Treisman, 1963; Thomas and Weaver, 1975) of time perception according to which perceived duration is a function of the amount of information processed per unit objective time, and also support the standard view that attention can influence the perception of duration (e.g. James, 1890;

Katz, 1906; Creelman, 1962; Treisman, 1963; Fraisse, 1963, 1984; Thomas and Brown, 1974; Thomas and Cantor 1975, 1978; Thomas and Weaver, 1975; Hicks, Miller, and Kinsbourne, 1976; Hicks et al., 1977; Brown, 1985; Mattes and Ulrich, 1998). According to the standard attentional model of time perception that has emerged through these papers, there is a 'counter' that keeps track of the number of units of temporal information processed for a given perceived event (Treisman, 1963; Thomas and Weaver, 1975). These models argue that some proportion of the units of temporal information is typically missed, especially when other tasks distract attention from monitoring the temporal markers. An increase of attention to the duration judgement itself results in fewer temporal cues being missed, therefore lengthening the apparent duration. These two factors account for the general pattern of reported distortions in the experience of duration.

However, the data described earlier (Tse et al., 2004) require a modification to the standard attentional model of time perception. Specifically, the engagement of attention by an unexpected event may not simply reduce missed information but actually increase the rate of information processing brought to bear on a stimulus. More units are detected during the event and it therefore seems to last longer, but this occurs because there are more units detected, not because fewer are missed. The previous hypothesis assumed that attention affected sensitivity, leading to fewer missed cues in a stream of constant rate. Alternatively, it could be that sensitivity remains unchanged by attention but the rate of information processing increases. These interpretations are not mutually exclusive. Both could contribute to distortions in perceived duration and both are compatible with the notion of a counter that measures the amount of information processed in order to calculate the duration of perceived events. For either reason, an attended stimulus may appear to last longer than a less attended stimulus that lasts the same objective duration. The data presented here do not distinguish between these possible mechanisms of enhanced information processing.

An increased rate of information processing might favour an 'early' view of attentional action, where, for example, sensory neurons actually increase their rate of firing when acted upon by neuronal circuitry that realizes attentional allocation. Conversely, increased sensitivity, but constant information processing rate, might predict that early neurons whose receptive fields lie within an attended region would not demonstrate a rate of firing above non-attended baseline. Of course, increased sensitivity in the form of lowered firing threshold would tend to make a neuron fire more than when threshold was not lowered, suggesting that the mechanism that increases sensitivity to processed information could be inextricably linked to the mechanism that increases the rate of firing and rate of information processed.

It may be impossible to establish beyond all doubt that temporal expansion is caused by attentional allocation, and not by some other process associated with the onset of an oddball. Nonetheless, four properties of the discussed data suggest that temporal expansion is indeed a result of attentional allocation to the oddball. First, temporal expansion does not begin until at least ~75–120ms after stimulus onset. This may be due to the time it takes attention to be allocated to a stimulus after its onset. Second, the temporal rise-dip-rise dynamics of temporal expansion are consistent with the summation of effects from transient and sustained components of attention. Third, approximately the same temporal dynamics are evident for both visual and auditory modalities (Figure 10.1A), suggesting that the mechanism that underlies temporal expansion is central rather than peripheral. Fourth, evidence that temporal expansion is central in origin was found in another experiment (Tse et al., 2004; experiment 7), not described here, where it was shown that the effect can be found with high-level category novelty rather than just image novelty. While none of these experiments can prove beyond a shadow of a doubt that temporal expansion is attentional in origin, the evidence strongly implicates an attentional account.

The predictions of traditional counter-based theories (Creelman, 1962; Treisman, 1963; Thomas and Weaver, 1975) and the results described here can be accounted for within a simple unified model. In line with the standard counter-based models, duration information about an event is lost to the extent that one is not attending to that event. The data described here update the standard attentional model insofar as processing of duration information may also get a boost when one attends to a stimulus. This could account for the temporal dynamics of the oddball-induced expansion in subjective time reported here. Subjective time never gets 'out of sync' with objective time, despite its expansion and contraction, because the 'rate' of subjective time per unit objective time may be flexible, as diagrammed in Figure 10.3. It may speed up when one orients to an oddball, and may slow down to the extent that one is not attending to a stimulus. More than one unit of subjective time can occupy a single unit of objective time because a unit of subjective time is a function of the amount of perceptual information processed, and this amount can presumably vary per unit objective time. An oddball stimulus would then seem to last longer than a standard stimulus of equal objective duration because it triggers an increase in perceptual information processing.

This simple model allows us to make several predictions, which can be tested in the future. First, the degree of subjective temporal expansion should increase with the 'oddness' or improbability of an oddball (as long as the oddballs are all in the temporal expansion domain, i.e. longer in duration than ~150ms corresponding to the point where the curves cross zero in Figures 10.1A and B). For example, an oddball that occurs once every ten standards should appear to last longer than an oddball that occurs once every three standards. A corollary of this would be that an oddball can only be so 'odd,' since there is presumably an upper limit on how much and how long attention can boost information-processing resources above baseline, rooted ultimately in a physical limit, such as the maximum firing rate of neurons. Another prediction would be that stimuli that last longer than ~150ms should seem to last longer when they appear in unlikely rather than likely locations, contexts, or times. A related prediction is that temporal expansion should be enhanced by more salient oddballs. Indeed, the difference between the temporal expansion in experiments 1 and 2 is probably due to the fact that an expanding oddball is more salient than a stationary one. Another prediction is that temporal expansion should be triggered across

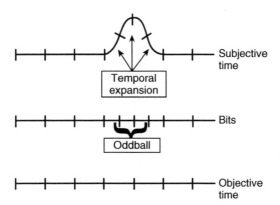

Fig. 10.3 When an oddball occurs, more information is processed over the stimulus per unit objective time. If subjective time is gauged in terms of the amount of perceptual information processed, subjective time will seem to expand relative to objective time, as shown at the top of the figure, indicated 'temporal expansion'.

modalities, if it is a central attentional effect. For example, an unexpected and very loud noise should make a visual stimulus appear to last longer. This raises interesting questions. When temporal expansion occurs for a moving stimulus, it may seem to move 'in slow motion'. Indeed, temporal expansion may underlie the experience of slow motion during an attention-demanding event, such as skidding into the back of a car. But would temporal expansion in the visual domain lead to an analogue of slow motion in the auditory domain? Would, for example, pitches become deeper? Or would a given pitch just seem to last longer?

In unpublished data that is currently being collected in my lab we are checking for such cross-modal effects. So far we have found that a constant-tone sound standard does *not* seem to last longer or have a different pitch relative to other sound standards, when a visual stimulus with simultaneous onset and offset as the sound standards undergoes temporal expansion. All sound standards had the same onsets and offsets as visual standards and oddballs, and subjectively had the same duration even when one of them co-occurred with a visual oddball that underwent temporal expansion. Such 'splitting' of temporal expansion seems counterintuitive, because we think of time perception as subjectively unified. This raises the possibility that independent visual and auditory processes, attentional or otherwise, underlie temporal expansion in their respective domains. Still, this preliminary finding seems bizarre. How can two events, one auditory and the other visual, that start and stop at the same times, not feel like they have the same subjective duration? We are carrying out experiments to try to get to the root of this puzzle.

Finally, it is interesting to ask why we have evolved to experience events in a subjective time that can expand and contract relative to the presumed regular flow of objective time. One possibility is that just as attention can enhance the spatial acuity of the visual system (Nakayama and Mackeben, 1989; Mackeben and Nakayama, 1993; Shiu and Pashler, 1995) attention can also enhance the temporal resolution of visual processing (Correa and Nobre, 2008). Since heightened spatial or temporal resolution is presumably expensive, the visual system may only invoke heightened processing for stimuli of probable interest or importance. By making novel or important events run 'in slow motion' they may be processed in greater depth per unit objective time than 'normal' events, and afford greater consideration of possible courses of action than normally would be the case in the absence of temporal expansion.

References

Allan, L. G. and Gibbon, J. (1994). A new temporal illusion or the TOE once again? *Perception & Psychophysics,* **55**(2), 227–9.

Avant, L. L., Lyman, P. J., and Antes, J. R. (1975). Effects of stimulus familiarity on judged visual duration. *Perception & Psychophysics,* **17**, 253–62.

Baylis, G. and Driver, J. (1995). One-sided edge assignment in vision: 1. Figure-ground segmentation and attention to objects. *Current Directions in Psychological Science,* **4**(5), 140–6.

Brown, S. W. (1985). Time perception and attention: The effects of prospective versus retrospective paradigms and task demands on perceived duration. *Perception & Psychophysics,* **38**(2), 115–24.

Brown, S. W. (1995). Time, change, and motion: the effects of stimulus movement on temporal perception. *Perception & Psychophysics,* **57**(1), 105–16.

Correa, A. and Nobre, A. C. (2008) Spatial and temporal acuity of visual perception can be enhanced selectively by attentional set. *Experimental Brain Research,* **189**(3):339–44.

Creelman, C. D. (1962). Human discrimination of auditory stimuli. *Journal of the Acoustical Society,* **34**, 582–93.

Fraisse, P. (1963). *The Psychology of Time.* New York: Harper and Row.

Fraisse, P. (1984). Perception and estimation of time. *Annual Review of Psychology,* **35**, 1–36.

Frankenhauser, M. (1959). *Estimation of time*. Uppsala, Sweden: Almqvist and Wiksell.

Garcia-Larrea, L., Lukaszewicz, A.-C., and Mauguiere, F. (1992). Revisiting the oddball paradigm, non-target vs. neutral stimuli and the evaluation of ERP attentional deficits. *Neuropsychologia, 30*(8), 723–41.

Grondin, S. and Macar, F. (1934). Dividing attention between temporal and nontemporal tasks: a performance operating characteristic -POC- analysis. In F. Macar, V. Pouthas, and W. Friedman (Eds.) *Time, action and cognition: Towards bridging the gap*, pp.119–28. Dordrecht: Kluwer.

He, Z. J. and Nakayama, K. (1992). Surfaces versus features in visual search. *Nature, 359*, 231–3.

Hicks, R. E. and Brundige, R. M. (1974). Judgments of temporal duration while processing verbal and physiognomic stimuli. *Acta Psychologica, 38*, 447–53.

Hicks, R. E., Miller, G. W., and Kinsbourne, M. (1976). Prospective and retrospective judgments of time as a function of amount of information processed. *American Journal of Psychology, 89*, 719–30.

Hicks, R. E., Miller, G. W., Gaes, G., and Bierman, K. (1977). Concurrent processing demands and the experience of time-in-passing. *American Journal of Psychology, 90*, 431–46.

Hikosaka, O., Miyauchi, S., and Shimojo, S. (1993). Focal visual attention produces illusory temporal order and motion sensation. *Vision Research, 33*, 1219–40.

Hülser, C. (1924). Zeitauffassung und Zeitschaetzung verschieden ausgefüllter Intervalle unter besonderer Berücksichtigung der Aufmerksamkeitsablenkung. *Archiv der gesamten Psychologie, 49*, 363–78.

Irwin, D. E., Colcombe, A. M., Kramer, A. F., and Hahn, S. (2000). Attentional and oculomotor capture by onset, luminance and color singletons. *Vision Research, 40*, 1443–58.

James, W. (1890). *The Principles of Psychology*. New York: Dover.

Jonides, J. and Yantis, S. (1988). Uniqueness of abrupt visual onset in capturing attention. *Perception & Psychophysics, 43*, 346–54.

Kahneman, D. (1973). *Attention and effort*. Englewood Cliffs, NJ: Prentice-Hall.

Kanai, R. and Watanabe, M. (2006). Visual onset expands subjective time. *Perception & Psychophysics, 68*(7), 1113–23.

Katz, D. (1906). Experimentelle Beitrage zur Psychologie des Vergleichs im Gebiete des Zeitsinns. *Zeitschrift für Psychologie, Physiologie der Sinnesorgane, 42*, 302–40.

Macar, F., Grondin, S., and Casini, L. (1994). Controlled attention sharing influences time estimation. *Memory & Cognition, 22*, 673–86.

Mackeben, M. and Nakayama, K. (1993). Express attentional shifts. *Vision Research, 33*(1) 85–90.

Mattes, S. and Ulrich, R. (1998). Directed attention prolongs the perceived duration of a brief stimulus. *Perception & Psychophysics, 60*, 8, 1305–17.

McKee, S. P., Klein, S. A., and Teller, D. Y. (1985). Statistical properties of forced-choice psychometric functions: implications of probit analysis. *Perception & Psychophysics, 37*(4), 286–98.

Michon, J. A. (1965). Studies in subjective duration. II: subjective time measurement during tasks with different information content. *Acta Psychologica, 24*, 205–19.

Michon, J. A. (1978). The making of the present: A tutorial review. In J. Requin (Ed.) *Attention and Performance, VII*. Hillsdale, NJ: Erlbaum.

Nakayama, K. and Mackeben, M. (1989). Sustained and transient components of focal visual attention. *Vision Research, 29*(11), 1631–47.

Nakajima, Y., ten Hoopen, G., and van der Wilk, R. G. H. (1991). A new illusion of time perception. *Music Perception, 8*, 431–48.

Nakajima, Y., ten Hoopen, G., Hilkhusen, G., and Sasaki, T. (1992). Time-shrinking: A discontinuity in the perception of auditory temporal patterns. *Perception & Psychophysics, 51*(5), 504–7.

Ornstein, R. E. (1969). *On the experience of time*. Baltimore: Penguin Books.

Polich, J. (1986). Attention, probability, and task demands as determinants of P300 latency from auditory stimuli. *Electroencephalography & Clinical Neurophysiology, 63*(3), 251–9.

Potts, G. F., Liotti, M., Tucker, D. M., and Posner, M. I. (1996). Frontal and inferior temporal cortical activity in visual target detection: Evidence from high spatially sampled event-related potentials. *Brain Topography*, **9**(1), 3–14.

Predebon, J. (1996). The relationship between the number of presented stimuli and prospective duration estimates: The effect of concurrent task activity. *Psychonomic Bulletin & Review*, **3**, 376–9.

Quasebarth, K. (1924). Zeitschaetzung und Zeitauffassung optisch und akustisch ausgefüllter Intervalle. *Archiv der gesamten Psychologie*, **49**, 379–432.

Remington, R. W., Johnston, J. C., and Yantis, S. (1992). Involuntary attentional capture by abrupt onsets. *Perception & Psychophysics*, **51**(3), 279–90.

Rensink, R. A. and Enns, J. T. (1995). Preemption effects in visual search: evidence for low-level grouping. *Psychological Review*, **102**(1), 101–30.

Rose, D. and Summers, J. (1995). Duration illusions in a train of visual stimuli. *Perception*, **24**, 1177–87.

Schiffman, H. R. and Bobko, D. J. (1974). Effects of stimulus complexity on the perception of brief temporal intervals. *Journal of Experimental Psychology*, **103**, 156–9.

Shiu, L.-P. and Pashler, H. (1995). Spatial attention and vernier acuity. *Vision Research*, **35**(3) 337–43.

Thomas, E. A. C. and Brown, T. (1974). Time perception and the filled-in duration illusion. *Perception & Psychophysics*, **16**, 449–58.

Thomas, E. A. C. and Cantor, N. E. (1978). Interdependence between the processing of temporal and non-temporal information. In J. Raquin (Ed.) *Attention and performance VIII* (pp. 43–62). Hillsdale, NJ: Erlbaum.

Thomas, E. A. C. and Weaver, W. B. (1975). Cognitive processing and time perception. *Perception & Psychophysics*, **17**, 363–7.

Treisman, M. (1963). Temporal discrimination and the indifference interval: Implications for a model of the "internal clock." *Psychological Monographs*, **77**, 1–31.

Tse, P. U., Sheinberg, D. L., and Logothetis, N. K. (2003). Attentional enhancement opposite a peripheral flash revealed by change blindness, *Psychological Science*, **14**, 2, 1–8.

Tse, P. U., Rivest, J., Intriligator, J., and Cavanagh, P. (2004). Attention and the subjective expansion of time. *Perception & Psychophysics*, **66**(7), 1171–89.

Underwood, G. and Swain, R. A. (1973). Selectivity of attention and the perception of duration. *Perception*, **2**, 101–5.

Yantis, S. and Egeth, H. E. (1999). On the distinction between visual salience and stimulus-driven attentional capture. *Journal of Experimental Psychology: Human Perception and Performance*, **25**(3), 661–76.

Yantis, S. and Jonides, J. (1990). Abrupt visual onsets and selective attention: voluntary versus automatic allocation. *Journal of Experimental Psychology: Human Perception and Performance*, **16**(1), 121–34.

Zakay, D. (1993). Time estimation methods: do they influence prospective duration estimates? *Perception*, **22**, 91–101.

Zakay, D. and Tsal, Y. (1989). Awareness of attention allocation and time estimation accuracy. *Bulletin of the Psychonomic Society*, **27**, 209–10.

Chapter 11

Duration illusions and predictability

David M. Eagleman

The separation in time between two events—say, the onset of an amber traffic light and its subsequent change to red—is conventionally assumed to be directly perceivable: that is, the subjective duration is thought to be a faithful report of the objective duration. But research in recent decades has shattered this conception. In its place, we now know that perceived duration is subject to illusory distortions of many sorts (Eagleman, 2008).

To appreciate subjective duration and its illusions, we here turn to illusions that are easily reproduced in the laboratory. As a first example, the first stimulus in a train of repeated presentations is perceived to have a longer duration than successive stimuli (Pariyadath and Eagleman, 2007), by as much as 50% in trains of visual stimuli (Rose and Summers, 1995; Kanai and Watanabe, 2006) and as much as 15% in trains of auditory stimuli (Hodinott-Hill et al., 2002). In a related phenomenon, a novel or 'oddball' stimulus presented within such a repeated train appears to last longer in duration than the repeated stimulus (Tse et al., 2004; Ulrich et al., 2006; Pariyadath and Eagleman, 2007).

What explains these duration illusions? Several authors have suggested that the duration distortion results from increased attention or arousal triggered by the appearance of the first stimulus (Rose and Summers, 1995; Kanai and Watanabe, 2006) or the oddball stimulus (Ranganath and Rainer, 2003; Tse et al., 2004; Ulrich et al., 2006). For the specific role of attention, Tse and colleagues (2004; Tse, Chapter 10, this volume) have appealed to the pacemaker-accumulator model of timing (Treisman, 1963; Gibbon et al., 1997). In this model, an increase in attention caused by the appearance of an oddball stimulus causes a transient hastening of the tick rate of the internal clock. As a result, the accumulator collects a larger number of ticks per unit time—and subjective duration is thus presumably slowed during the oddball.

Although such an attention-allocation model has been proposed in several papers, we were uncertain whether it could explain all the data, and we therefore set out to test it directly. In one experiment, we attempted to increase the size of the duration distortion by employing more emotionally salient oddballs (such as guns, growling dogs, and spiders) instead of the standard, neutral oddballs (such as geometric shapes or photographs of everyday objects) (Pariyadath and Eagleman, 2007). The surprising result was that the size of the duration distortion was no larger when the neutral oddballs were replaced by emotionally charged and attention-grabbing oddballs. This result suggested to us two possibilities: either the duration dilation is caused by attentional mechanisms but saturates at approximately 15%, or the duration dilation is not fundamentally an attentional effect (Pariyadath and Eagleman, 2007).

The second possibility led us to begin considering a new hypothesis: the duration dilation may result from violations of predictability rather than attention. Note that unpredictability and attention are related concepts—for example, something unpredictable can draw attention—but they are not equivalent. One can imagine, for example, paying no attention to the unpredictable patterns of static on the television, or directing endogenous attention to the perfectly predictable clanking of a furnace. To explore the possibility that predictability, not attention, lies at the heart of duration distortions, we turned to the electrophysiology literature on familiarity and repetition.

Note that while duration dilations of unexpected stimuli have traditionally been considered as an expansion of subjective time (Tse et al., 2004), the results could equally well be construed as a duration *contraction* of the repeated stimuli, rather than an expansion of the first or oddball stimulus (Eagleman and Pariyadath, 2009). This change of viewpoint on the problem immediately opens a potential tie-in to the neurophysiology literature. Specifically, the amplitude of a neural response diminishes after repeated presentations of a stimulus (Fahy et al., 1993; Li et al., 1993; Rainer and Miller, 2000), an effect known as *repetition suppression* (Figure 11.1) (Henson and Rugg, 2003; Wark et al., 2007). In non-human primates, this effect has been studied extensively with single unit electrophysiology; in humans it has been demonstrated with electro-encephalography (EEG, Allison et al., 1993; Grill-Spector et al., 2006), positron emission tomography (PET, Buckner et al., 1995), magnetoencephalography (MEG, Noguchi et al., 2004; Ishai et al., 2006), and functional magnetic resonance imaging (fMRI, Henson and Rugg, 2001). Although the diminishing neural response has been interpreted as stimulus-specific fatigue, recent frameworks have interpreted repetition suppression as an increasing efficiency of representation (Desimone and Duncan, 1995; Wiggs and Martin, 1998; Grill-Spector et al., 2006). In the latter view, a more economical representation is obtained after several repetitions of a stimulus, necessitating lower metabolic costs.

We began to consider the possibility that this differential response to novel versus repeated stimuli maps onto perceived duration—i.e. a suppressed neural response corresponds to a briefer perceived duration (Pariyadath and Eagleman, 2007, 2008; Eagleman, 2008; Eagleman and Pariyadath, 2009). Note that this hypothesis is not necessarily incompatible with previous attentional models, but, as we will make a case for next, this viewpoint may have the ability to

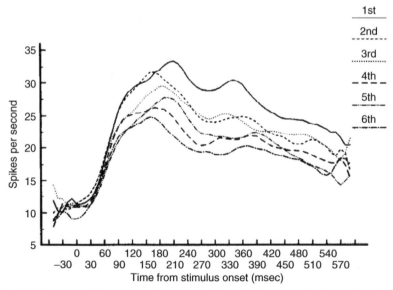

Fig. 11.1 Repetition suppression: successive presentations of the same stimulus reduce the neural response (figure reproduced with permission from Li et al, 1993). As argued in the main text, this pattern of diminishing neural response appears to parallel diminishing duration perception with repetition of a stimulus.

tie the study of duration encoding to a large neurophysiology literature of predictability and familiarity.

To explore this hypothesis further, we turned to the task of designing new paradigms to study very brief durations—conditions under which shifts in attention would be too slow to keep up. First, we noted that the oddball studies cited earlier all used stimuli in the range of hundreds of milliseconds, and we wondered whether these same principles would apply for stimuli briefer than 100ms—i.e. stimuli too brief to make explicit temporal judgements. We tested this by developing a novel variation of the traditional flicker-fusion paradigm (Pariyadath and Eagleman, 2008). Specifically, in flicker-fusion experiments, a light is rapidly flashed on and off: at a low frequency, the subject perceives flicker, while at a high frequency the light appears steady. The frequency at which the perception switches from flickering to steady is called the critical flicker-fusion threshold. Importantly, flicker experiments employ a single stimulus that is presented repeatedly (in this case, the light). Because novel and repeated stimuli engender different perceptions of duration (Pariyadath and Eagleman, 2007; Eagleman, 2008), we hypothesized that the flicker-fusion threshold would change if the rapid stimulus could be made novel with each appearance. To accomplish this, we flashed single letters of the alphabet in different locations on a computer monitor. Although only one character was present at any moment, more than one appeared to be present on screen at any given moment. This effect is due to visual persistence, the phenomenon that a briefly presented stimulus appears to last longer than the time it was physically presented (Efron, 1970; Bowen et al., 1974; Di Lollo, 1977). We named this perceived multiplicity of stimuli the *proliferation effect* (Pariyadath and Eagleman, 2008). We employed two conditions (Figure 11.2A): in the first, the same letter was presented ('Repeated'); in the second, the letter was changed each time ('Random'). Participants reported the number of stimuli that they perceived to be present on screen at any one moment of time—that is, how many characters appeared to be sharing screen time.

The number of characters perceived to be on the screen simultaneously differed significantly between the repeated and random conditions (Pariyadath and Eagleman, 2008). Fewer items were perceived to be simultaneously present in the repeated condition (Figure 11.2B), putatively due to a contraction in the visual persistence of repeated stimuli (and therefore less temporal overlap between stimuli). These results support the hypothesis that repetition has the same effect of contracting duration at both short time scales (proliferation effect) and long time scales (oddball effect).

These findings with the proliferation effect generalize across all the stimuli we tested—flashed words, non-words, photographs, and faces (Pariyadath and Eagleman, 2008)—as predicted by a framework in which subjective duration parallels repetition suppression. That is, perceptually shortened durations map onto neural responses that have been reduced by repeated presentation. Critically, note that an attentional-distortion explanation for these results would be difficult to defend, since attentional reallocation is typically thought to require longer than 120ms (Sperling, 1960; Tse et al., 2004)—far too much time to explain the distortion of the current stimuli, which were presented at 50Hz (Pariyadath and Eagleman, 2008)

The framework explains many findings in the literature

This potential relationship between subjective duration and the size of the neural response suggests a way to understand several illusions reported previously. An example is the stopped clock illusion (also known as chronostasis): the second hand of a clock sometimes appears to be momentarily immobile upon first glance before it begins to move at its expected pace (Yarrow et al., 2001, 2004; Park et al., 2003; Yarrow and Rothwell, 2003; Yarrow, Chapter 12, this volume).

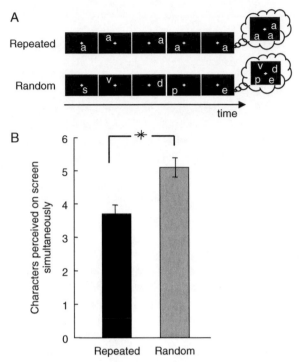

Fig. 11.2 Repeated stimuli subjectively proliferate less than random stimuli. (A) Schematic of experiment: single letters of the alphabet are flashed on screen, either repeatedly or randomly. (B) Participants report more stimuli present on screen when the letters are different than when they are repeated. (n=31, * p<0.05, paired t-tests). Error bars S.E.M. (Pariyadath and Eagleman, 2008).

The framework presented earlier suggests that the successive stimuli (i.e. positions of the second hand) are contracted in perceived duration compared to the first.

As another example, when two short stimuli are presented serially, the second tends to be underestimated in duration (Nakajima et al., 1992, 2004; ten Hoopen et al., 1995; Arao et al., 2000; Sasaki et al., 2002). Moreover, this underestimation disappears when the interval between the two stimuli increases (Wearden and Ferrara, 1993; Wearden et al., 2002; Kanai and Watanabe, 2006). We suggest that both findings belie a single phenomenon: the repetition of a stimulus contracts its perceived duration, and the repetition suppression recovers with time (Li et al., 1993).

Another finding that can be addressed is a long-standing mystery about flicker fusion. In 1974, Herrick noted that for two flashes to be perceived as being separate, they must be separated by a minimal interval (the two-flash fusion threshold). He measured this, as well as the interval for an ongoing train of flashes (the critical flicker-fusion threshold), and noticed something strange: the two-flash threshold is greater than the flicker-fusion threshold (Herrick, 1974). It seemed odd that two events, widely separated, could be perceived as a single event, while multiple events, closer together in time, could be distinguished. We note that this finding can be explained from the perspective of repetition suppression: in the two-flash case, the visual persistence of the first flash overlaps with the appearance of the second flash, making a single perceptual event, while in the ongoing train of flashes, the visible persistence of the flash putatively contracts due to repetition suppression. As a result of shorter visual persistence, a rapid train of flashes is perceived as a series of separate events (Eagleman and Pariyadath, 2009).

Note that our hypothesis also relates to a recent report of 'change-related persistence,' a phenomenon in which a moving object changes suddenly (say, in size or brightness), and at the moment of the change is perceived as two separate objects (Moore et al., 2007). Moore and colleagues (2007) proposed that visual persistence is reduced when an object is interpreted by the visual system as a single object in motion. If the object suddenly changes along some dimension, the explanation goes, it is now registered as a different object and its visual persistence expands, thus causing the perception of two objects overlapping in time. This effect is consistent with our framework, although there seems to be an advantage to framing the result in terms of repetition suppression rather than a breaking of objecthood. Specifically, the concept of novelty has degrees (something can be more or less novel than something else), while the concept of an object is binary (something either is an object or is not). We thus pitted the concepts against each other by comparing different degrees of novelty using the proliferation effect. As previously shown in Figure 11.2, we had found that more letters are perceived to be simultaneously present when they are random; expanding the experimental conditions, we found an even higher perceived number when random letters were presented in random colours (Eagleman and Pariyadath, 2009). In other words, the *degree* of novelty of the newly appearing stimuli influenced the visual persistence, suggesting that a spectral measure (such as the amplitude of neural responses) may serve as a better framework than the all-or-none concept of objecthood.

Tying the physiology to the psychophysics

Many studies in the psychophysics literature have manipulated stimulus properties (brightness, size, numerosity) in order to achieve duration distortions; these reports have never, to our knowledge, been unified under a common framework. We propose that they can all be explained with the hypothesis that stimulus manipulations which increase neural responses also increase perceived durations (Eagleman and Pariyadath, 2009). For example, objects with higher luminance (either physically or illusorily) are perceived to last longer (Brigner, 1986; Sperandio et al., 2008). On the flip side, objects with reduced visibility (e.g. stimuli during a saccade) are perceived to be briefer (Terao et al., 2008). Expanding the scope of these findings, Xuan and colleagues (2007) showed that duration can be dilated by the *magnitude* of a stimulus. By manipulating brightness, size, or numerosity, they could make higher magnitude stimuli appear to last longer (Xuan et al., 2007). The magnitude need not be physical, only perceived; for example, the illusory enlargement of a stimulus can modulate subjective duration (Ono and Kawahara, 2007). All of these findings, at least to a first approximation, map onto electrophysiological studies: stimuli that are brighter (Barlow et al., 1978; Tikhomirov, 1983; Maunsell et al., 1999), larger (Murray et al., 2006), and of higher numerosity (Roitman et al., 2007) all engender more neural activity.

As another example, motion also leads to distortions of subjective duration: moving objects appear to last longer than stationary objects (J. F. Brown, 1931). In parallel, a much larger region of neural activity is activated in response to visual motion when compared to the viewing of stationary objects (Dupont et al., 1994). Similarly, looming stimuli appear to last longer in duration than stationary or receding stimuli (Tse et al., 2004; van Wassenhove et al., 2008); in parallel, parietal areas are more active in response to inward moving radial dots than outward moving ones (de Jong et al., 1994). Finally, it has also been shown that a flickering stimulus will appear to last longer as its temporal frequency increases from 4Hz to 8Hz (Kanai et al., 2006). Strikingly, the BOLD response to flicker shows the same pattern: an increase in flicker rate leads to increasing activation in striate cortex, and the trend saturates at 8Hz (Kaufmann et al., 2000).

There are at least three further ways we know of to induce duration distortions. First, filled intervals are perceived to last longer than empty intervals of equal physical duration (Ihle and Wilsoncroft, 1983). Second, the apparent duration of a sequence appears longer with increasing pattern complexity (Roelofs and Zeeman, 1951; Schiffman and Bobko, 1974). Third, durations seem longer when they contain an increasing number of 'events' (Fraisse, 1963; Poynter, 1989; S. W. Brown, 1995). Unfortunately, there are no available physiological studies that provide a direct comparison to these psychophysical observations, although it seems likely that future experiments will bear out the prediction that more neural energy will be expended when representing a higher density of events in the same amount of time. For now, these physiology experiments remain as experimental predictions of our framework.

Models and their discontents

At what level are these proposed effects on duration implemented? Our framework of looking at the amplitudes of neural activity resonates with an emerging view that duration perception may be related to low-level properties of neurons rather than high-level cognitive algorithms. For example, the low-level view is supported by recent findings that adaptation to a flickering stimulus leads to duration distortions of subsequent stimuli in a spatially specific manner (Johnston et al., 2006; Johnston, Chapter 14, this volume). Likewise, the role of temporal frequency in duration distortions may also implicate early levels of visual processing (Kanai et al., 2006). Finally, the finding that reductions in stimulus visibility lead to compressed subjective durations (Terao et al., 2008) may be related to the connection between stimulus visibility and the transient responses of visual neurons (Macknik and Livingstone, 1998). All these findings are at least consistent with that the idea that low-level neural signatures of neurons will be a useful first place to look for duration perception.

A look at the popular models of duration perception reveals that there remain many unsolved questions. One class of model (which we will call the 'counter' models) suggests that internally generated pulses, or 'ticks', are collected up and integrated during the presence of a stimulus (Creelman, 1962; Treisman, 1963). This kind of model seeks to account for duration dilations by assuming that the collection rate of ticks can change under conditions of high arousal or attention. However, as noted earlier, this model was not supported by our finding that emotionally salient stimuli effected no change in the size of the oddball effect (Pariyadath and Eagleman, 2007). More importantly, clock-like counters have found little support in the physiology. A second class of model instead proposes that intervals can be encoded in the evolving activity patterns of neural networks (Buonomano and Mauk, 1994; Buonomano and Merzenich, 1995; Mauk and Buonomano, 2004; Buhusi and Meck, 2005; Karmarkar and Buonomano, 2007; Ivry and Schlerf, 2008). Although these state-dependent models hold theoretical appeal, their Achilles heel is that they are difficult to keep regulated when there is noise in the network. In the context of this chapter, the major challenge for the state-dependent model is to account for illusions of duration: it is difficult to speed up or slow down the passage of an evolving pattern through a neural network without spinning off into an entirely new pattern (but see Yamazaki and Tanaka, 2005, for an attempt at this in a noise-free artificial neural network). Given these challenges, it remains to be seen how the counter and state-dependent models will fare.

We have suggested that subjective duration reflects the size of neural response to a stimulus, but this hypothesis, if correct, will require a great deal of refinement. We do not currently know which activity specifically will be implicated. For example, it is possible that only certain cell types will be involved, or only certain windows of time within a spike train, or only certain brain regions. We intend to refine the theory experimentally by varying the stimulus feature that is being repeated, and concomitantly measuring both the neural response and perceived duration.

Finally, note that our framework for duration also allows us to explore issues of duration and attention in disorders such as schizophrenia. An impaired novelty response is typically found in schizophrenia, as measured by an impaired pre-pulse inhibition of the startle response (Hong et al., 2007), impaired mismatch negativity (Javitt et al., 1998; Light and Braff, 2005), diminished oddball detection (Kiehl and Liddle, 2001), and, consistent with our framework, a lowered flicker-fusion threshold (Black et al., 1975; Slaghuis and Bishop, 2001). All these findings are consistent with electrophysiology that shows a reduced or absent repetition suppression in schizophrenics, presumably due to a deficit in cortical inhibition (Daskalakis et al., 2002). That is, repetition does not reduce neural responses in schizophrenic brains as much as it does in normal brains. In our framework, this predicts that schizophrenic patients should perceive a smaller contraction in visual persistence with repetition when compared with controls. To test this, we examined schizophrenic patients with the proliferation effect, and, consistent with predictions, we found that schizophrenic patients perceive less difference between repeat and random conditions (Gandhi et al., 2007). This trend suggests the proliferation effect may have potential future use as a screening tool for schizophrenia.

Conclusions

In summary, we have presented a new framework: the subjective duration assigned to a stimulus reflects the magnitude of the neural response to the stimulus (Pariyadath and Eagleman, 2007; Eagleman, 2008; Eagleman and Pariyadath, 2009). Let us now return to the main issue, which is whether attention can, by itself, modulate subjective duration, or whether something very different is going on—something involving stimulus predictability and the concomitant amplitudes of neural responses. To review, the duration dilation during an oddball might appear to result from increased attention (Tse et al., 2004; Kanai and Watanabe, 2006; Ulrich et al., 2006), but there are at least two problems with that hypothesis: first, the oddball effect is not modulated by increased emotional salience (Pariyadath and Eagleman, 2007). Second, the proliferation effect, which demonstrates a clear effect of repetition on duration, operates at timescales much too rapid for attentional reallocation (Pariyadath and Eagleman, 2008). Thus, predictability, not attention, may be the key element in understanding duration illusions.

In the middle of all these studies hides a deep, generally unasked question: if duration judgements have some evolutionary importance, why are they so malleable? We here submit a highly speculative suggestion. While it has been previously assumed that increases in attention are responsible for increases in duration (Rose and Summers, 1995; Tse et al., 2004), we would like to at least consider the opposite hypothesis: perhaps increases in subjective duration drive attention, allowing more opportunity for the perceptual systems to 'grab onto' a stimulus. Note that the correlation between duration and attention does not specify a causal direction, so it is logically possible that the direction goes either way. If this speculation turns out to be correct, it suggests that subjective duration is not meant as an exact report of the outside world, but is meant to warp the fabric of time perception such that important (unpredicted) stimuli have more opportunity to be processed by other parts of the system. In other words, unpredictability allows the attentional machinery more opportunity to fixate on the new data in order to be better positioned to predict it upon the next encounter. Whatever refinement our framework will encounter in the future, we hope it may provide a good starting point for new experiments that can put it to the test.

To summarize, we have marshalled evidence that the subjective duration assigned to a stimulus parallels the magnitude of the neural response to the stimulus. While this appears at first blush to be consistent with an attentional model, we have suggested that the root of the explanation lies with predictability, not with attention.

References

Allison, T., Begleiter, A., McCarthy, G., Roessler, E., Nobre, A. C., and Spencer, D. D. (1993). Electrophysiological studies of color processing in human visual cortex. *Electroencephalogr Clin Neurophysiol*, **88**, 343–55.

Arao, H., Suetomi, D., Nakajima, Y. (2000). Does time-shrinking take place in visual temporal patterns? *Perception*, **29**, 819–30.

Barlow, R. B., Snodderly, D. M., and Swadlow, H. A. (1978). Intensity coding in primate visual system. *Exp Brain Res*, **31**, 163–77.

Black, S., Franklin, L. M., de Silva, F. P., and Wijewickrama, H. S. (1975). The flicker-fusion threshold in schizophrenia and depression. *N Z Med J*, **81**, 244–6.

Bowen, R. W., Pola, J., and Matin, L. (1974). Visual persistence: effects of flash luminance, duration and energy. *Vis Res*, **14**, 295–303.

Brigner, W. L. (1986). Effect of perceived brightness on perceived time. *Percept Mot Skills*, **63**, 427–30.

Brown, J. F. (1931). Motion expands perceived time. On time perception in visual movement fields. *Psychologische Forschung*, **14**, 233–48.

Brown, S. W. (1995). Time, change, and motion: the effects of stimulus movement on temporal perception. *Percept Psychophys*, **57**, 105–16.

Buckner, R. L., Petersen, S. E., Ojemann, J. G., Miezin, F. M., Squire, L. R., and Raichle, M. E. (1995). Functional anatomical studies of explicit and implicit memory retrieval tasks. *J Neurosci*, **15**, 12–29.

Buhusi, C. V. and Meck, W. H. (2005). What makes us tick? Functional and neural mechanisms of interval timing. *Nat Rev Neurosci*, **6**, 755–65.

Buonomano, D. V. and Mauk, M. D. (1994). Neural codes and distributed representations: foundations of neural computation. *Neural Comput*, **6**, 38–55.

Buonomano, D. V. and Merzenich, M. M. (1995). Temporal information transformed into a spatial code by a neural network with realistic properties. *Science*, **267**, 1028–30.

Creelman, C. D. (1962). Human discrimination of auditory duration. *J Acoust Soc Am*, **34**, 528–93.

Daskalakis, Z. J., Christensen, B. K., Chen, R., Fitzgerald, P. B., Zipursky, R. B., and Kapur, S. (2002). Evidence for impaired cortical inhibition in schizophrenia using transcranial magnetic stimulation. *Arch Gen Psychiatry*, **59**, 347–54.

de Jong, B. M., Shipp, S., Skidmore, B., Frackowiak, R. S., and Zeki, S. (1994). The cerebral activity related to the visual perception of forward motion in depth. *Brain*, **117**(5), 1039–54.

Desimone, R. and Duncan, J. (1995). Neural mechanisms of selective visual attention. *Ann Rev Neurosci*, **18**, 193–222.

Di Lollo, V. (1977). Temporal characteristics of iconic memory. *Nature*, **267**, 241–3.

Dupont, P., Orban, G. A., De Bruyn, B., Verbruggen, A., and Mortelmans, L. (1994). Many areas in the human brain respond to visual motion. *J Neurophysiol*, **72**, 1420–4.

Eagleman, D. M. (2008). Human time perception and its illusions. *Curr Opin Neurobiol*, **18**, 131–6.

Eagleman, D. M. and Pariyadath, V. (2009). Is subjective duration a signature of coding efficiency? *Phil Trans Royal Society B (Biol Sci)*, **364**, 1841–51

Efron, R. (1970). The minimum duration of a perception. *Neurophysiologia* **8**, 57–63.

Fahy, F. L., Riches, I. P., and Brown, M. W. (1993). Neuronal activity related to visual recognition memory: long-term memory and the encoding of recency and familiarity information in the primate anterior and medial inferior temporal and rhinal cortex. *Exp Brain Res*, **96**, 457–72.

Fraisse, P. (1963). *The Psychology of Time*. New York: Harper and Row.

Gandhi, S. K., Pariyadath, V., Wassef, A. A., and Eagleman, D. M. (2007). 'Timing judgments in schizophrenia.' Paper presented at the Society for Neuroscience annual meeting, San Diego, CA.

Gibbon, J., Malapani, C., Dale, C. L., and Gallistel, C. (1997). Toward a neurobiology of temporal cognition: advances and challenges. *Curr Opin Neurobiol*, 7, 170–84.

Grill-Spector, K., Henson, R., and Martin, A. (2006). Repetition and the brain: neural models of stimulus-specific effects. *Trends Cog Sci*, 10, 14–23.

Henson, R. and Rugg, M. (2001). Effects of stimulus repetition on latency of the BOLD impulse response. *NeuroImage*, 13, 683.

Henson, R. N. A. and Rugg, M. D. (2003). Neural response suppression, haemodynamic repetition effects, and behavioural priming. *Neuropsychologia*, 41, 263–70.

Herrick, R. M. (1974). Frequency thresholds for two-flash flicker and critical flicker: why they differ. *Percept Psychophys*, 15, 79–82.

Hodinott-Hill, I., Thilo, K. V., Cowey, A., and Walsh, V. (2002). Auditory chronostasis: hanging on the telephone. *Curr Biol*, 12, 1779–81.

Hong, L. E., Summerfelt, A., Wonodi, I., Adami, H., Buchanan, R. W., and Thaker, G. K. (2007). Independent Domains of Inhibitory Gating in Schizophrenia and the Effect of Stimulus Interval. *Am J Psychiatry*, 164, 61–5.

Ihle, R. C. and Wilsoncroft, W. E. (1983). The filled-duration illusion: limits of duration of interval and auditory fillers. *Percept Mot Skills*, 56, 655–60.

Ishai, A. Bikle, P. C., and Ungerleider, L. G. (2006). Temporal dynamics of face repetition suppression. *Brain Res Bull*, 70, 289–95.

Ivry, R. B. and Schlerf, J. E. (2008). Dedicated and intrinsic models of time perception. *Trends Cogn Sci*, 12, 273–80.

Javitt, D. C., Grochowski, S., Shelley, A., and Ritter, W. (1998). Impaired mismatch negativity (MMN) gneration in schizophrenia as a function of stimulus deviance, probability, and interstimulus/interdeviant interval. *Electroencephalogr Clin Neurophysiol*, 108, 143–53.

Johnston, A., Arnold, D. H., and Nishida, S. (2006). Spatially localized distortions of event time. *Curr Biol*, 16, 472–9.

Kanai, R. and Watanabe, M. (2006). Visual onset expands subjective time. *Percept Psychophys*, 68, 1113–23.

Kanai, R., Paffen, C. L., Hogendoorn, H., and Verstraten, F. A. (2006). Time dilation in dynamic visual display. *J Vis*, 6, 1421–30.

Karmarkar, U. R. and Buonomano, D. V. (2007). Timing in the absence of clocks: encoding time in neural network states. *Neuron*, 53, 427–38.

Kaufmann, C., Elbel, G. K., Gossl, C., Putz, B., and Auer, D. P. (2000). 'Gender differences in a graded visual stimulation paradigm for fMRI are limited to striate visual cortex.' In Proceedings of International Society for Magnetic Resonance in Medicine, 8: 903. Denver, Colorado.

Kiehl, K. A. and Liddle, P. F. (2001). An event-related functional magnetic resonance imaging study of an auditory oddball task in schizophrenia. *Schizophr Res*, 48, 159–71.

Li, L., Miller, E. K., and Desimone, R. (1993). The representation of stimulus familiarity in anterior inferior temporal cortex. *J Neurophysiol*, 69, 1918–29.

Light, G. A. and Braff, D. L. (2005). Mismatch negativity deficits are associated with poor functioning in schizophrenia patients. *Arch Gen Psychiatry*, 62, 127–36.

Macknik, S. L. and Livingstone, M. S. (1998). Neuronal correlates of visibility and invisibility in the primate visual system. *Nat Neurosci*, 1, 144–9.

Mauk, M. D. and Buonomano, D. V. (2004). The neural basis of temporal processing. *Annu Rev Neurosci*, 27, 307–40.

Maunsell, J. H., Ghose, G. M., Assad, J. A., McAdams, C. J., Boudreau, C.E., and Noerager, B. D. (1999). Visual response latencies of magnocellular and parvocellular LGN neurons in macaque monkeys. *Vis Neurosci*, 16, 1–14.

Moore, C. M., Mordkoff, J. T., and Enns, J. T. (2007). The path of least persistence: object status mediates visual updating. *Vis Res*, **47**, 1624–30.

Murray, S. O., Boyaci, H., and Kersten, D. (2006). The representation of perceived angular size in human primary visual cortex. *Nat Neurosci*, **9**, 429–34.

Nakajima, Y., ten Hoopen, G., Hilkhuysen, G., and Sasaki, T. (1992). Time-shrinking: a discontinuity in the perception of auditory temporal patterns. *Percept Psychophys*, **51**, 504–7.

Nakajima, Y., ten Hoopen, G., Sasaki, T., Yamamoto, K., Kadota, M., Simons, M., et al. (2004). Time-shrinking: the process of unilateral temporal assimilation. *Perception*, **33**, 1061–79.

Noguchi, Y., Inui, K., and Kakigi, R. (2004). Temporal dynamics of neural adaptation effect in the human visual ventral stream. *J Neurosci*, **24**, 6283– 90.

Ono, F. and Kawahara, J. (2007). The subjective size of visual stimuli affects the perceived duration of their presentation. *Percept Psychophys*, **69**, 952–7.

Pariyadath, V. and Eagleman, D. M. (2007). The effect of predictability on subjective duration. *PLoS ONE*, **2**, 1264.

Pariyadath, V. and Eagleman, D. M. (2008). Brief subjective durations contract with repetition. *J Vis*, **8**(16), 11.1–6

Park, J., Schlag-Rey, M., and Schlag, J. (2003). Voluntary action expands perceived duration of its sensory consequence. *Exp Brain Res*, **149**, 527–9.

Poynter, W. D. (1989). Judging the duration of time intervals: a process of remembering segments of experience. In Zakay, I. L. D. (Ed.) *Time and Human Cognition: A Life-span Perspective*, pp.305–21. Amsterdam: Elsevier.

Rainer, G. and Miller, E. K. (2000). Effects of visual experience on the representation of objects in the prefrontal cortex. *Neuron*, **27**, 179–89.

Ranganath, C. and Rainer, G. (2003). Neural mechanisms for detecting and remembering novel events. *Nat Rev Neurosci*, **4**, 193–204.

Roelofs, C. O. Z. and Zeeman, W. P. C. (1951). Influence of different sequences of optical stimuli on the estimation of duration of a given interval of time. *Acta Psychologica*, **8**, 89–128.

Roitman, J. D., Brannon, E. M., and Platt, M. L. (2007). Monotonic coding of numerosity in macaque lateral intraparietal area. *PLoS Biol*, **5**, e208.

Rose, D. and Summers, J. (1995). Duration illusions in a train of visual stimuli. *Perception*, **24**, 1177–87.

Sasaki, T., Suetomi, D., Nakajima, Y., and ten Hoopen, G. (2002). Time-shrinking, its propagation, and Gestalt principles. *Percept Psychophys*, **64**, 919–31.

Schiffman, H. R. and Bobko, D. J. (1974). Effects of stimulus complexity on the perception of brief temporal intervals. *J Exp Psychol*, **103**, 156–9.

Slaghuis, W. L. and Bishop, A. M. (2001). Luminance flicker sensitivity in positive- and negative-symptom schizophrenia. *Exp Brain Res*, **138**, 88–99.

Sperandio, I., Savazzi, S., Marzi, C. A., and Gregory, R. (2008). Does reaction time depend upon perceived or retinal stimulus size? *Perception*, **37**, 14.

Sperling, G. (1960). The information available in brief visual presentations. *Psychol Monogr*, **74**, 1–29.

ten Hoopen, G., Hartsuiker, R., Sasaki, T., Nakajima, Y., Tanaka, M., and Tsumura, T. (1995). Auditory isochrony: time shrinking and temporal patterns. *Perception*, **24**, 577–93.

Terao, M., Watanabe, J., Yagi, A., and Nishida, S. (2008). Reduction of stimulus visibility compresses apparent time intervals. *Nat Neurosci*, **11**, 541–2.

Tikhomirov, A. S. (1983). [Characteristics of the coding of light stimulus intensity by visual cortex neurons during light adaptation in the cat]. *Neirofiziologiia*, **15**, 211–17.

Treisman, M. (1963). Temporal discrimination and the indifference interval: implications for a model of the 'internal clock'. *Psychol Monogr*, **77**, 1–31.

Tse, P. U., Intriligator, J., Rivest, J., and Cavanagh, P. (2004). Attention and the subjective expansion of time. *Percept Psychophys*, **66**, 1171–89.

Ulrich, R., Nitschke, J., and Rammsayer, T. (2006). Perceived duration of expected and unexpected stimuli. *Psychol Res*, **70**, 77–87.

van Wassenhove, V., Buonomano, D. V., Shimojo, S., and Shams, L. (2008). Distortions of subjective time perception within and across senses. *PLoS ONE*, **3**, e1437.

Wark, B., Lundstrom, B. N., and Fairhall, A. (2007). Sensory adaptation. *Curr Opin Neurobiol*, **17**, 423–9.

Wearden, J. H. and Ferrara, A. (1993). Subjective shortening in humans' memory for stimulus duration. *Q J Exp Psychol B*, **46**, 163–86.

Wearden, J. H., Parry, A., and Stamp, L. (2002). Is subjective shortening in human memory unique to time representations? *Q J Exp Psychol B*, **55**, 1–25.

Wiggs, C. L. and Martin, A. (1998). Properties and mechanisms of perceptual priming. *Curr Opin Neurobiol*, **8**, 227–33.

Xuan, B., Zhang, D., He, S., and Chen, X. (2007). Larger stimuli are judged to last longer. *J Vis*, **7**, 1–5.

Yamazaki, T. and Tanaka, S. (2005). Neural modeling of an internal clock. *Neural Comput*, **17**, 1032–58.

Yarrow, K. and Rothwell, J. C. (2003). Manual chronostasis: tactile perception precedes physical contact. *Curr Biol*, **13**, 1134–9.

Yarrow, K., Johnson, H., Haggard, P., and Rothwell, J. C. (2004). Consistent chronostasis effects across saccade categories imply a subcortical efferent trigger. *J Cogn Neurosci*, **16**, 839–47.

Yarrow, K., Haggard, P., Heal, R., Brown, P., and Rothwell, J. C. (2001). Illusory perceptions of space and time preserve cross-saccadic perceptual continuity. *Nature*, **414**, 302–5.

Acknowledgements

Funding for the research was provided by National Institutes of Health grant RO1 NS053960 (DME).

Chapter 12

Temporal dilation: the chronostasis illusion and spatial attention

Kielan Yarrow

Have you ever found yourself in a busy train station, looking across from the overhead information board to the station clock to see if you can make the next train? You may recall thinking, just for a moment, that the clock was not working, as it seemed to dwell too long on the current second. Then it ticked on, and you forgot this odd experience as you rushed to get to that train. Or perhaps you have experienced the stopped clock illusion when glancing at your wrist watch, or even when returning your gaze to the blinking cursor of your word-processing display? These anecdotes are familiar to many of us. Brown and Rothwell (1997) reported that the stopped clock illusion is most common when a saccadic eye movement causes us to foveate a counter just after it advances, right at the beginning of a new one-second interval.

It is unlikely that time actually dilates whenever we move our eyes. A more plausible account suggests that it is only our experience of time that has changed, in an illusory fashion. Perceptual illusions can provide insights regarding how the brain draws inferences about the state of the world (e.g. Gregory, 1997). With this in mind, Yarrow and colleagues (2001) developed a protocol to estimate the magnitude of the stopped clock illusion, and labelled the effect 'chronostasis' to reflect the apparent dilation of time.

The experimental task was straightforward. Participants fixated a cross on one side of a computer screen, then made a saccade to a counter presented on the opposite side. The counter initially showed a zero, but eye movements were monitored, with these recordings being used to trigger a change in the display during the saccade. Hence when the eyes arrived at the counter, a new number ('1') was displayed. The display change was assumed to be masked by saccadic suppression (see following section). The new digit (the comparison stimulus) was presented for a variable duration, and followed by a short sequence of reference stimuli (the digits '2', '3', and '4') displayed for 1 second each. Participants were required to judge whether they had seen the variable-duration comparison stimulus for more or less time than the standard-duration reference stimuli that followed. Their responses were used to determine a point of subjective equality (PSE) at which the comparison stimulus seemed identical to the reference stimuli. In a control condition, participants made the same judgement, but without any saccadic eye movement. They started by fixating the '0', which advanced through the numbers 1–4, all presented at fixation. PSEs were compared between the experimental and control conditions to estimate the chronostasis effect.

The most striking finding came from an experiment in which the size of the saccadic eye movement was varied. Two experimental conditions involving a large (22°) or a very large (55°) saccade were compared with two control conditions in which the counters appeared at matched peripheral positions. To elicit such a large saccade, subjects were seated very close to the monitor in the 55° condition. On average, the smaller saccade took 72ms, and the larger one 139ms, a difference of 67ms. PSEs were lower in the experimental conditions compared with the control conditions, implying a relative overestimation of the first interval following the saccade. This finding describes the chronostasis effect. Critically, the PSE in the larger saccade condition was 69ms lower than that obtained for the smaller saccade, implying that the size of the chronostasis effect had grown linearly with the duration of the preceding saccade. It was as if the extra time taken to complete the larger saccade had been added on to the estimated duration for the post-saccadic comparison stimulus.

While more recent work has modified and improved this task in a number of ways (see Box 12.1), temporal dilation of the first interval perceived after a saccade has been a consistent finding. In the remainder of this chapter, I will first briefly review some accounts of the

Box 12.1 Control conditions for saccadic chronostasis

The first chronostasis experiments used a counter to allow comparison of the post-saccadic interval with a series of subsequent 1-second reference intervals. Because temporal biases had already been shown to arise when the first of a series of stimuli is compared with subsequent stimuli (Rose and Summers, 1995; see also Eagleman, Chapter 11, this volume) it was important to include a constant-fixation control condition. This allowed the additional effect of a saccade to be determined. While this protocol reproduces the conditions of the stopped clock illusion, it is unnecessarily complicated. Reducing the number of reference intervals from three to one simplifies the procedure (although it does not obviate the need for a control condition, as two-interval comparison tasks can also yield a bias, known as the 'time-order error'; see Hellstroem, 1985, for a review). Furthermore, reducing the reference interval from 1000ms to 500ms (or even less) reduces variance in the data, because time perception appears to follow a generalized version of Weber's law (Wearden and Lejeune, 2008).

In addition to controlling for order effects and related biases, constant fixation conditions should ideally also control for the unusual pattern of visual stimulation experienced in saccadic conditions, as this might itself give rise to changes in temporal perception. Early experiments did so only approximately. For example, in the saccade conditions of Yarrow et al. (2001) and Park et al. (2003), participants foveated a cross, then experienced a brief period of degraded visual motion during the saccade. They then foveated a '1', followed by subsequent reference digits. In control conditions, they foveated a '0', immediately followed by a '1' and subsequent reference digits.

More recent investigations have included improved control conditions, which better match the foveal saccadic experience (e.g. Yarrow et al., 2006a). These conditions match the stimulus that is fixated as the participant prepares to move their eyes, and include a short blank interval to simulate the saccade itself. This still leaves open the possible role of peripheral visual movement experienced during the saccade. However, displacing the saccade target object in a manner that approximates its retinal motion during the saccade does not produce equivalent temporal dilation, as demonstrated in an early control experiment (Yarrow et al., 2001) and subsequently replicated with an improved display (Yarrow et al., 2004a). Furthermore, a chronostasis effect can be obtained relative to such a motion control condition (Georg and Lappe, 2007) which rules out any issues of experimental power for the previously described null effects. As yet, no one has reported a control condition in which the entire visual scene moves with a saccadic time course. This is impossible to achieve using a CRT (cathode ray tube) monitor, but has been accomplished with alternative displays in experiments investigating saccadic suppression (e.g. Diamond et al., 2000).

chronostasis effect. Then, in view of the theme of this volume, I will consider the relationship between chronostasis and spatial attention.

Saccadic suppression and saccadic chronostasis

Saccadic eye movements are a ubiquitous behaviour, yet we are rarely aware of them. A moment's thought illustrates how strange this situation is. When the eye sweeps across a complex visual scene during a saccade, the retina is subjected to a rapidly changing pattern of stimulation. One question that arises is why motion detectors remain quiet in the presence of such a potent motion stimulus?

It now seems likely that an active process of 'saccadic suppression' decreases the responsiveness of visual cells, particularly in the magnocellular division that is most sensitive to motion (Ross et al., 2001; but see Castet et al., 2002). A key finding comes from experiments measuring contrast sensitivity during saccades, which decreases for luminance-modulated stimuli presented at low spatial frequencies, but not for isoluminant colour-modulated stimuli (Burr et al., 1994). Anatomically, saccadic suppression is found in single-cell recordings from extrastriate areas such as middle temporal (MT) and superior middle temporal (MST) (e.g. Thiele et al., 2002) but suppression is greater for phosphenes generated at the eye than those generated in primary visual cortex (Thilo et al., 2004) so the process must start in the lateral geniculate nucleus (LGN)(see also Reppas et al., 2002; Sylvester et al., 2005).

Active suppression is one thing, but for a fuller account of peri-saccadic visual insensitivity we should add the smearing effects of rapid retinal motion on high spatial frequency visual components, and the backwards masking effect of the post-saccadic image (Campbell and Wurtz, 1978). One question that has rarely been asked is why a suppressed or empty period should not register in temporal consciousness. Saccadic chronostasis may offer an explanation, because our experience of time is effectively stitched up to take account of the saccade. The influence of saccade duration on saccadic chronostasis suggests that time is being added on to compensate for the period of degraded vision caused by the saccade (Yarrow et al., 2001). This extra time is presumably tagged on to the beginning of the comparison interval, when the saccade is occurring. This antedating account (see also Spence, Chapter 7, this volume), then, suggests that we see the post-saccadic stimulus earlier in time than the moment of foveation (or indeed the moment the comparison stimulus first appeared physically, during the saccade) and that this illusory impression about the timing of an event subsequently influences our judgement about the interval which that event initiates.

The issue of saccadic suppression is important when explaining saccadic chronostasis, but also when measuring it, because the interpretation of experimental results requires an assumption about what can be seen during the saccade. The simplest assumption is that the change of stimulus to the variable duration comparison, which occurs during the saccade, is not registered due to saccadic suppression. Hence the duration of the comparison stimulus is often corrected before analysis to reflect the time it was foveated, rather than the time it was present on the screen. This assumption was considered reasonable based on a control experiment showing that the precise time at which the comparison stimulus changed during the saccade did not influence the magnitude of the chronostasis effect (Yarrow et al., 2001).

If the assumption is false, the chronostasis effect will have been overestimated. More critically, the dependency of chronostasis on saccade size might be artefactual, reflecting differences in the size of the corrections applied in the different saccade conditions. For this reason, one recent investigation replicated this important result, but reported effect sizes with and without a correction for saccadic suppression (Yarrow et al., 2006a). This paper demonstrated clearly that a larger saccade yields a larger chronostasis effect in a situation where the correction was carefully equated (or indeed absent). See Yarrow et al. (in press) for a fuller discussion of this issue.

Comparing accounts of saccadic chronostasis

The 'antedating' account is by no means the only explanation that has been offered for saccadic chronostasis. One early alternative posited instead that the act of making a saccade increases physiological arousal (Hodinott-Hill et al., 2002). Arousal is known to prolong subjective time, perhaps by increasing the speed at which a putative internal clock runs (e.g. Penton-Voak et al., 1996). Under this account, the events that border the post-saccadic comparison interval are not shifted, but the intervening time nonetheless dilates.

Another suggestion is that the time at which the sensory consequence of any movement, not just a saccade, is perceived to occur, shifts towards the time of the action (Park et al., 2003). This proposal builds on experimental evidence favouring so-called 'intentional binding' (Haggard et al., 2002; Buehner, Chapter 15, this volume). This is essentially a more general event-shift account. Box 12.2 discusses non-saccadic illusions that have been linked with chronostasis.

Box 12.2 Chronostasis for non-saccadic movements

Chronostasis-like effects have been reported following manual actions, and even in the absence of any movement at all. Alexander et al. (2005), building on work by Hodinott-Hill et al. (2002), investigated an illusion analogous to the stopped clock illusion, in which the repetitive tone of an engaged telephone may appear delayed when we return our attention to it. Participants heard five tones that marked out four consecutive intervals. The tones were either presented all to one ear (the control condition) or with the first tone in one ear and all subsequent tones in the other ear. The first interval seemed prolonged in comparison to the subsequent intervals when the auditory stimuli that bordered it were presented to different ears, with PSEs reduced by around 160ms compared to the control condition. Presumably, attention was refocused from one ear to the other during the comparison interval of the experimental condition, and this might explain the result. However, increasing the volume of the second tone also yielded somewhat reduced PSEs (an effect of around 50ms) even when all tones were presented to the same ear. These are interesting findings, but temporal dilation can result from a variety of mechanisms. Given the differences in the methods used to elicit auditory and saccadic chronostasis, it is not clear that they are related, or that a common explanation should necessarily be sought.

Chronostasis-like effects have also been sought where a movement is required, but not a saccadic movement. Yarrow and Rothwell (2003) asked participants to make reaching movements towards a vibrating tactile stimulus which marked out target and reference intervals. Participants overestimated the duration of the post-movement interval by 60–120ms compared to a static control condition, but the size of the effect did not change for reaches of different extents/durations. This situation is closely analogous to the saccadic case, because participants only feel the vibrator when they first touch it, leaving its state ambiguous prior to contact. Another closely analogous situation was tested by Jackson et al. (2005) who investigated chronostasis for visual stimuli in a patient with congenital ophthalmoplegia who made rapid head movements in place of saccades. No effect was obtained, although the absence of a matched control group complicates the interpretation.

Box 12.2 Chronostasis for non-saccadic movements *(continued)*

When manual movements trigger the beginning of a visual interval, results have been mixed. Park et al. (2003) initiated a digit sequence either randomly, 500ms after a key press, or immediately after a key press. PSEs for the first interval were reduced by around 70ms when the key press initiated the sequence compared to the random and delayed conditions. These authors also observed a similar effect when a vocal signal initiated the digit sequence. These results contrast with those of Yarrow and Rothwell (2003). They tested conditions in which participants judged visual intervals initiated by reaching to and/or pressing a button. PSEs for the first interval did not differ between movement and control conditions in any of three experiments, with experimental powers ranging from 0.8–0.99. Most recently, Hunt et al. (2008) found a key-press effect of around 70ms in two experiments using a digit sequence, but not in three rather similar subsequent experiments reported in the same paper. It is worth noting that the manual–visual situation, in contrast to the saccadic–visual or manual–tactile cases, introduce no ambiguity about the time at which the critical interval begins. Hence there seems less reason for misperception to occur.

Finally, and most recently, Ibbotson et al. (2007) have suggested that the rapid latency responses recorded from motion-sensitive neurons in MT and MST during a saccade (which contrast with longer latency responses in the post-saccadic epoch) may underlie the chronostasis effect. This hypothesis again has strong similarities with the original antedating account, but emphasizes a relative shift in latencies between the event that initiates the critical comparison interval and the event that terminates it.

What evidence is there to distinguish these possibilities? One class of accounts suggest a shift in the time at which the post-saccadic stimulus is perceived (hereafter referred to as event-shift accounts). A second class suggest an increase in the rate at which time is perceived to pass (hereafter referred to as rate-increase accounts). Behavioural evidence supports the former over the latter. The saccade-length effect found with interval judgements is simple to explain under an event-shift framework by assuming that the initial boundary event is shifted to a position that is constant with respect to saccade initiation. In contrast to this, it is not obvious why a larger saccade should yield a larger increase in the rate of perceived time (although the suggestion that it might is not unreasonable). Furthermore, any rate increase account makes the straightforward prediction that the size of the chronostasis effect should grow in proportion to the duration of the post-saccadic interval that is judged, because perceived time should equal clock rate multiplied by actual time. This prediction has not been verified; for the shortest post-saccadic intervals tested, the chronostasis effect was similar for intervals ranging from 100–300ms (Yarrow et al., 2004a). These data strongly constrain rate-increase accounts, implying that the rate of perceived time would have to rise sharply above baseline following a saccade, then return to baseline within 100ms.

However, the most direct evidence favouring event-shift accounts was obtained in an experiment where the typical interval comparison task was replaced with a temporal order judgement task (Yarrow et al., 2006a). Participants judged whether a brief auditory event occurred before or after they first perceived the post-saccadic target. Relative to control conditions without a saccade, the point of subjective simultaneity (PSS) between these events was shifted substantially. Participants judged the beep to be synchronous with the onset of the post-saccadic visual target when it occurred when they had only just begun to move their eyes, long before the target's physical onset on the screen. This was in direct contrast to an audio-visual PSS of the opposite sign found in control conditions, which fell in line with the typical observation that sounds must be presented *after* lights to appear simultaneous. This pattern was obtained for both short and long saccades, replicating the saccade-size effect found with interval-comparison tasks.

These behavioural data favour event-shift accounts, but leave open the question of whether the change in event time is implemented as events unfold, or subsequently, based on a retrospective assessment of the preceding saccadic episode. There are two plausible physiological mechanisms for an event shift, and both imply that the illusion reflects neural activity that is available immediately. The first mechanism, proposed by Yarrow et al. (2001), depends upon a class of cells known to shift their receptive fields prior to a saccade. The suggestion is that their neural activity is used to mark the onset of the post-saccadic stimulus. These cells, first described in the lateral intraparietal cortex, but subsequently found in regions such as frontal eye fields and superior colliculus (Duhamel et al., 1992; Walker et al., 1995; Umeno and Goldberg, 1997), respond predictively to a stimulus presented at a position their receptive field should occupy only after the saccade. Across the cell population this predictive response occurs at a range of times, including well before the saccade has even been made. Marking time based on the activity of such a population provides a qualitative fit to behavioural data from chronostasis experiments.

The second mechanism, alluded to earlier and proposed by Ibbotson et al. (2007), is based on their finding that activity in MT or MST arising in response to the mid-saccadic onset of a motion stimulus has a head start compared with activity arising in response to an identical stimulus presented after the saccade. If such activity were used to demarcate the interval of interest in chronostasis experiments, this interval would appear prolonged, because its onset occurs during the saccade whereas its offset occurs after the saccade. This suggestion is intriguing, but it is less easily reconciled with the dependency of the chronostasis illusion on saccade size than an account based on shifting receptive fields.

Of course, the neural events highlighted in each account share some common features. Both must depend upon some saccade-related input such as an efference-copy signal. Because saccadic chronostasis has been observed following express saccades (Yarrow et al., 2004b), and these saccades are commonly considered to arise without a significant contribution from cortical areas involved in saccade generation (Hopp and Fuchs, 2002), it seems likely that the relevant efference copy signal is sent just prior to saccade generation from a subcortical structure such as the superior colliculus. Appropriate pathways exist in the primate brain, including one from the superior colliculus to the frontal eye fields via the dorsal thalamus (Sparks, 1986). This pathway has been shown to carry efference copy information in a double-saccade task (Sommer and Wurtz, 2002).

Although the shift in event time that characterizes chronostasis might typically be implemented in an online fashion, there is also evidence that peri-saccadic perception may be moulded in a surprisingly flexible fashion over a longer time window. In early experiments, the saccade target was made to step to a new position during the saccade (at the same moment that it changed to its new post-saccadic form). The chronostasis illusion was eliminated when the step was perceived, and reduced when it was not (Yarrow et al., 2001). Intuitively, it only makes sense to assume that post-saccadic objects have occupied their current states throughout the saccade (and thus to add on an appropriate amount of time) if things remain much as they were. If not, it is better to make a different assumption. It is as though a veto were available to override the standard mechanism for estimating the peri-saccadic timeline of events.

Even more striking results are obtained when a saccade is made to a moving object. Under these circumstances, we might expect a backwards shift in the perceived position at which a post-saccadic stimulus is first reported to be seen, mirroring the temporal report. There is some evidence for this, at least relative to the forward shift obtained in control conditions (Yarrow et al., 2006b). However, the surprise result is that the position at which the post-saccadic stimulus is seen to terminate actually shifts forwards compared to when no saccade is made. It appears as though time added on to the beginning of a period of stimulus motion is compensated partially by an illusory elongation of trajectory at the end of stimulus motion, up to 500ms later. In this way, time, velocity, and position are made to cohere.

Chronostasis and attention

Because chronostasis occurs in the aftermath of saccades, and saccades are intimately linked with shifts of covert spatial attention (e.g. Deubel and Schneider, 1996; Moore and Armstrong, 2003), it is natural to ask if a relationship exists between chronostasis and processes of selective attention. There are a number of ways in which it is possible to envisage attention playing a role. In the previous section I alluded to physiological events that might operate as time markers for the onset of the post-saccadic stimulus. The shift of attention that is hypothesized to precede saccade initiation is a candidate for this role, although there is little data on its precise time course (but see Montagnini and Castet, 2007). A related suggestion was made by Deubel and colleagues (1999) to explain discrepancies in temporal order judgements for peri-saccadic stimuli (see Yarrow et al., 2006a, for a discussion).

One experiment that bears on this explanation was described by Yarrow and colleagues (2001). Participants began by fixating centrally, then made unspeeded saccades to either the left or right. In addition to a typical saccade condition used to measure chronostasis, a second condition included an additional central arrow cue prior to the saccade, pointing at the saccade target. Participants were required to direct their attention voluntarily in the direction indicated by this cue before beginning their saccade and then completing a duration judgement task as usual. An interleaved reaction-time task, performed every other trial, required speeded saccades to a target appearing randomly to the left or right, without any subsequent duration judgement. Again, some trials included a central arrow cue, this time equally likely to predict the upcoming target or not, but which participants were instructed to obey just as they did in the duration judgement trials. It was concluded that participants were indeed allocating their attention as directed, based on an RT cost at the unattended location in RT trials. In the duration judgement trials, the chronostasis effect was identical regardless of whether attention had been deliberately allocated to the saccade target long in advance of the saccade, or no such instruction had been given. This result suggests that shifting attention is not the critical time marker used to estimate the onset of the post-saccadic object. There are, however, a number of problems which might lead us to question such an interpretation. Most critically, the relationship between an endogenous (instructed) shift of attention and the shift of attention that automatically precedes a saccade is unknown when both processes target the same location. It is far from certain that a pre-saccadic shift of attention would not occur even when attention has already been voluntarily allocated to the saccade target.

Aside from its possible role as a temporal marker, attention will undoubtedly be tightly focused at the position where the post-saccadic stimulus appears in typical chronostasis experiments (Deubel and Schneider, 1996) and might influence judgements about time in other ways. When attention is drawn to an object, it can give rise to temporal dilation (e.g. Tse et al., 2004; Tse, Chapter 10; Brown, Chapter 8, this volume) We can, however, discount attentional modulation of the rate of perceived time as an explanation of chronostasis based on the behavioural data described in the previous section. This is a rate-increase account, and does not fit with either the constant effect size found when post-saccadic stimulus duration was manipulated or the saccade-dependent shift in the PSS found using a temporal order judgement task.

Temporal dilation is, however, not the only way in which the focus of attention can influence temporal judgements. 'Prior entry' refers to the advantage found for attended stimuli over unattended ones when they are compared in a temporal order judgement task (Spence, Chapter 7, this volume). Physiological evidence that attention affects the timing of neural activity has been somewhat mixed (e.g. McDonald et al., 2005; Vibell et al., 2007). Behaviourally, however, this speeding of attended stimuli is robust, although it may be exaggerated in tasks that encourage response biases (Spence et al., 2001). Prior entry might, therefore, be responsible for the shift in the time at which the post-saccadic stimulus is seen in chronostasis experiments.

There are, however, a number of caveats we should bear in mind when attempting to apply prior entry as an explanation of chronostasis. Firstly, chronostasis is obtained with both interval judgements and temporal order judgements, whereas prior entry has been described and explored systematically only for the latter type of task. Secondly, prior entry does not currently explain the saccade-size effect because there is no reason to believe that larger saccades invoke a greater degree of attentional modulation at the saccade target than smaller saccades. Finally, chronostasis experiments require subjects to judge time in both control and saccade conditions. There is currently no evidence that visual attention is concentrated more completely at the target of a saccade prior to the saccade, than it is at a fixed position during steady fixation. All we know is that prior to a saccade, attention is concentrated more completely at the target of a saccade than at other locations assessed at the same time. In summary, we need to make a lot of assumptions in order to explain chronostasis with prior entry.

One recent paper has attempted to move beyond such speculation and explore the relationship between chronostasis and attention directly by investigating how much of the visual scene the illusion applies to. In their first condition, Georg and Lappe (2007) had participants make a saccade to a counter, replicating the original demonstration of chronostasis. They also included a constant fixation control condition, with a moving counter (see Box 12.1). The critical new condition also involved a saccade to a target object (now a cross) but this time the counter was presented mid-way across the screen at a position intermediate between the initial fixation and saccade target positions. This permitted the authors to assess temporal dilation away from the saccade target object. No chronostasis effect was obtained for this intermediate counter.

The result appears to suggest that chronostasis does not occur for the entire visual scene, but only for the object targeted by a saccade, which is known also to be the target of covert attention (e.g. Deubel and Schneider, 1996). It is noteworthy, however, that this result is the exact opposite of that found in an experiment I carried out around the same time, in collaboration with John Rothwell, Patrick Haggard, and Doeschka Ferro. This experiment has not been published, so I present the details here.

Participants were required to saccade towards a letter target that might appear either alone, or accompanied by additional letters arrayed beyond the target letter in a semicircle. There were three possible arrays: target alone, five letters, or nine letters. The five-letter condition is shown in the inset to Figure 12.1, which schematizes the procedure. In saccade conditions, participants pressed a button to reveal the target array in peripheral vision. After 500ms, they had to react to a change of colour at the initial fixation cross by saccading to the middle target letter, then maintaining their fixation at this point. Any one of the letters in the array could change colour during the saccade, signifying that the duration for which that letter was presented in its terminal colour should be judged on an absolute scale. The dependent variable was mean judgement error. A further manipulation varied the degree of advanced knowledge about the letter that would form the basis of the subsequent judgement. On half of all trials, a red outline box cue appeared for 100ms around the letter that would change colour (at the same moment the array appeared) disappearing 400ms before the signal to make a saccade. The same factors were manipulated in control conditions, but subjects fixated a cross while the letter array first appeared in peripheral

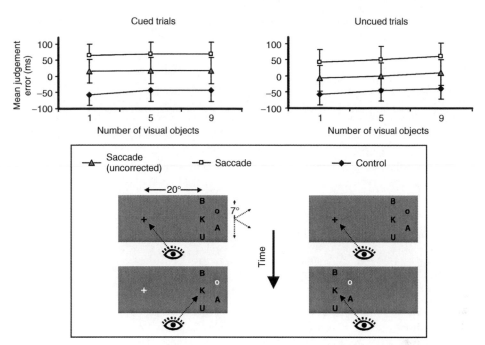

Fig. 12.1 Mean judgement errors in all 12 conditions of an experiment investigating the spatial extent of saccadic chronostasis. Both corrected and uncorrected values are shown for saccade conditions (see section entitled "saccadic suppression and saccadic chronostasis" for explanation of these terms) alongside results from a constant fixation control task. Durations were selected randomly on each trial from a uniform distribution with a range from 250–750 ms, and participants made absolute duration estimates with a range from 0 to 1000 ms. The mean judgement error is the mean difference between subjects' absolute duration estimates and stimulus display times. Positive values denote overestimations. Error bars show standard error of the mean. The inset schematises the experimental task, with the saccade task shown on the left and the control task shown on the right. The schematic shows black letters, with one letter turning white to indicate that its duration should be judged. In the actual experiment, stimuli were black or white fixation crosses (subtending 1° visual angle; cross turned white as an imperative stimulus), blue or red capital letters (approx. 1° visual angle; one letter turned red (here, shown as white) for duration judgement), and a red open square (2° visual angle; used to cue the location of the red letter on 50% of trials). The blue (here, shown as black) letters remained on screen after the red letter had disappeared to ensure that only the red letter could be used when estimating duration. Around 10–15% of trials were rejected and repeated, mainly because of failures to saccade and/or hold fixation according to instructions. Participants completed 45 trials in each of 12 conditions for a total of 540 pseudorandomised trials. Their heads rested in a chin/forehead rest, 41 cm from a 22" CRT colour monitor (refresh rate 120 Hz). Eye movements were recorded from both eyes (left for horizontal, right for vertical) using an infra-red eye tracker (Applied Science Laboratories Eye-trac model 310) and sampled at 200 Hz (12 bit A/D card; National Instruments DAQ 1200).

vision, then disappeared and reappeared around fixation with a time course that approximated visual input in the saccade conditions.

If chronostasis were limited to the saccade target, the effect should have been drastically reduced in the five- and nine-object conditions (because only a small minority of trials in those conditions required a judgement about the saccade target letter, whereas in most trials a peripheral letter was being judged). Figure 12.1 shows that this was not the case. The data were corrected to reflect saccadic suppression and entered into a three-factor ANOVA. There was a difference between saccade and control conditions, representing the classic chronostasis effect. The presence or absence of the cue also had an effect, and these two factors interacted, indicating that the presence of a cue had no effect in the control conditions, but elevated estimates in saccade conditions.[1] Figure 12.1 also shows the data without any correction for saccadic suppression. The pattern of significance was identical. Critically, the number of objects was not significant in either ANOVA and did not interact with the other factors. Hence the chronostasis effect extended to all the objects in an array of up to nine objects separated by up to 7° visual angle. Visual attention, by contrast, modulates performance at the target of a saccade compared to locations only 1° away (Deubel and Schneider, 1996).

Why the difference in results between this experiment and that of Georg and Lappe (2007)? It is possible that Georg and Lappe's choice of location for the second object represents a special case. Following a saccade, it would have required a shift of attention directly back along the saccade path. This shift of attention might have been unusually slow because of inhibition of return (Posner and Cohen, 1984), an RT effect that is often interpreted as a difficulty in shifting attention back to a location that has recently been visited (Lupiáñez, Chapter 2, this volume). Inhibition of return might affect duration estimates by delaying perception of the mid-trajectory object (i.e. prior entry), counteracting the typical temporal bias caused by a saccade.

Another difference between the two studies is that the study I have described here used a relatively complex semicircular array of objects rather than just two objects. Might such an array have been combined via gestalt grouping, operating like a single object and extending the temporal bias to all component objects in an artificial manner? In other unpublished work, my co-workers and I have used only two objects, with the second object presented at one of three positions 7° beyond the saccade target. We still obtained identical temporal biases when judging either this additional object or the saccade target object. However, these two objects would still be more likely to group than the two objects used by Georg and Lappe (2007) which were separated by 8°. Further research appears necessary to explain the difference in findings, as the outcome is of theoretical importance. For example, an account of chronostasis in terms of the predictive activity of cells with shifting receptive fields implies that the illusion should be obtained at multiple spatial locations (because remapping, which is typically measured in cells with somewhat peripheral receptive fields, can be assumed to occur in numerous cells which combine to form a fairly complete retinotopic map).

Conclusions

The term saccadic chronostasis describes the temporal overestimation of a stimulus seen immediately following a saccade. The effect can also be observed as a relative misperception of the time at which the post-saccadic stimulus is first seen. It seems likely that both behaviours result from a tendency to time erroneously the uncertain onset of the post-saccadic stimulus using a pre-saccadic marker. The most plausible physiological marker suggested so far is the activity of a class of cells which shift their receptive fields ahead of a saccade in order to gain a head start when

---

[1] This small but reliable effect appears to contrast with the result of Yarrow et al. (2001) described earlier (no effect on temporal estimates for an endogenous cue directing attention to a single target). Because of the many differences between the two studies, it is difficult to draw any strong inferences about the reason for the diverging effects.

responding at their new position. However, the nature of the illusion also suggests explanations in terms of mechanisms of spatial attention. At this point, the exact role played by such mechanisms in generating saccadic chronostasis is unclear. Prior entry and attention-based temporal dilation are not particularly convincing explanations for the illusion, but there is some controversy regarding the spatial extent of chronostasis and its relationship with the shift of attention that precedes a saccade. Further research may help resolve these issues. Whichever explanation wins out, I hope this review will give you pause for thought the next time you glance at your broken watch, or catch the gaze of someone who's been looking at you for a little too long!

References

Alexander, I., Thilo, K. V., Cowey, A., and Walsh, V. (2005). Chronostasis without voluntary action. *Experimental Brain Research,* **161,** 125–32.

Brown, P. and Rothwell, J. C. E. (1997). Illusions of time. *Society for Neuroscience Abstracts, 27th Annual Meeting,* **23,** 1119.

Burr, D. C., Morrone, M. C., and Ross, J. (1994). Selective suppression of the magnocellular visual pathway during saccadic eye movements. *Nature,* **371,** 511–13.

Campbell, F. W. and Wurtz, R. H. (1978). Saccadic omission: why we do not see a grey-out during a saccadic eye movement. *Vision Research,* **18,** 1297–303.

Castet, E., Jeanjean, S., and Masson, G. S. (2002). Motion perception of saccade-induced retinal translation. *Proceedings of the National Academy of Science, U S A,* **99,** 15159–63.

Deubel, H. and Schneider, W. X. (1996). Saccade target selection and object recognition: evidence for a common attentional mechanism. *Vision Research,* **36,** 1827–37.

Deubel, H., Irwin, D. E., and Schneider, W. X. (1999). The subjective direction of gaze shifts long before the saccade. In W.Becker, H. Deubel, and T. Mergner (Eds.) *Current Oculomotor Research: Physiological and Psychological Aspects,* pp.65–70. New York: Plenum.

Diamond, M. R., Ross, J., and Morrone, M. C. (2000). Extraretinal control of saccadic suppression. *Journal of Neuroscience,* **20,** 3449–55.

Duhamel, J. R., Colby, C. L., and Goldberg, M. E. (1992). The updating of the representation of visual space in parietal cortex by intended eye movements. *Science,* **255,** 90–2.

Georg, K. and Lappe, M. (2007). Spatio-temporal contingency of saccade-induced chronostasis. *Experimental Brain Research,* **180,** 535–9.

Gregory, R. L. (1997). *Eye and Brain: The Psychology of Seeing, 5th edn.* Princeton, NJ: Princeton University Press.

Haggard, P., Clark, S., and Kalogeras, J. (2002). Voluntary action and conscious awareness. *Nature Neuroscience,* **5,** 382–5.

Hellstroem, A. (1985). The time-order error and its relatives: mirrors of cognitive processes in comparing. *Psychological Bulletin,* **97,** 35–61.

Hodinott-Hill, I., Thilo, K. V., Cowey, A., and Walsh, V. (2002). Auditory chronostasis: hanging on the telephone. *Current Biology,* **12,** 1779–81.

Hopp, J. J. and Fuchs, A. F. (2002). Investigating the site of human saccadic adaptation with express and targeting saccades. *Experimental Brain Research,* **144,** 538–48.

Hunt, A. R., Chapman, C. S., and Kingstone, A. (2008). Taking a long look at action and time perception. *Journal of Experimental Psychology: Human Perception and Performance,* **34,** 125–36.

Ibbotson, M. R., Price, N. S., Crowder, N. A., Ono, S., and Mustari, M. J. (2007). Enhanced motion sensitivity follows saccadic suppression in the superior temporal sulcus of the macaque cortex. *Cerebral Cortex,* **17,** 1129–38.

Jackson, S. R., Newport, R., Osborne, F., Wakely, R., Smith, D., and Walsh, V. (2005). Saccade-contingent spatial and temporal errors are absent for saccadic head movements. *Cortex,* **41,** 205–12.

McDonald, J. J., Teder-Salejarvi, W. A., Di, R. F., and Hillyard, S. A. (2005). Neural basis of auditory-induced shifts in visual time-order perception. *Nature Neuroscience*, **8**, 1197–202.

Montagnini, A. and Castet, E. (2007). Spatiotemporal dynamics of visual attention during saccade preparation: independence and coupling between attention and movement planning. *Journal of Vision*, **7**, 8–16.

Moore, T. and Armstrong, K. M. (2003). Selective gating of visual signals by microstimulation of frontal cortex. *Nature*, **421**, 370–3.

Park, J., Schlag-Rey, M., and Schlag, J. (2003). Voluntary actions expands perceived duration of its sensory consequence. *Experimental Brain Research*, **149**, 527–9.

Penton-Voak, I. S., Edwards, H., Percival, A., and Wearden, J. H. (1996). Speeding up an internal clock in humans? Effects of click trains on subjective duration. *Journal of Experimental Psychology: Animals Behavior Processes*, **22**, 307–20.

Posner, M. I. and Cohen, Y. (1984). Components of visual orienting. In H. Bouma and D. Bouwhuis (Eds.) *Attention and Performance X: Control of language processes*, pp. 531–56. Hove: Erlbaum.

Reppas, J. B., Usrey, W. M., and Reid, R. C. (2002). Saccadic eye movements modulate visual responses in the lateral geniculate nucleus. *Neuron*, **35**, 961–74.

Rose, D. and Summers, J. (1995). Duration illusions in a train of visual stimuli. *Perception*, **24**, 1177–87.

Ross, J., Morrone, M. C., Goldberg, M. E., and Burr, D. C. (2001). Changes in visual perception at the time of saccades. *Trends in Neurosciences*, **24**, 113–21.

Sommer, M. A. and Wurtz, R. H. (2002). A pathway in primate brain for internal monitoring of movements. *Science*, **296**, 1480–2.

Sparks, D. L. (1986). Translation of sensory signals into commands for control of saccadic eye movements: role of primate superior colliculus. *Physiological Reviews*, **66**, 118–71.

Spence, C., Shore, D. I., and Klein, R. M. (2001). Multisensory prior entry. *Journal of Experimental Psychology: General*, **130**, 799–832.

Sylvester, R., Haynes, J. D., and Rees, G. (2005). Saccades differentially modulate human LGN and V1 responses in the presence and absence of visual stimulation. *Current Biology*, **15**, 37–41.

Thiele, A., Henning, P., Kubischik, M., and Hoffmann, K. P. (2002). Neural mechanisms of saccadic suppression. *Science*, **295**, 2460–2.

Thilo, K. V., Santoro, L., Walsh, V., and Blakemore, C. (2004). The site of saccadic suppression. *Nature Neuroscience*, **7**, 13–14.

Tse, P. U., Intriligator, J., Rivest, J., and Cavanagh, P. (2004). Attention and the subjective expansion of time. *Perception and Psychophysics*, **66**, 1171–89.

Umeno, M. M. and Goldberg, M. E. (1997). Spatial processing in the monkey frontal eye field. I. Predictive visual responses. *Journal of Neurophysiology*, **78**, 1373–83.

Vibell, J., Klinge, C., Zampini, M., Spence, C., and Nobre, A. C. (2007). Temporal order is coded temporally in the brain: early event-related potential latency shifts underlying prior entry in a cross-modal temporal order judgment task. *Journal of Cognitive Neuroscience*, **19**, 109–20.

Walker, M. F., Fitzgibbon, E. J., and Goldberg, M. E. (1995). Neurons in the monkey superior colliculus predict the visual result of impending saccadic eye movements. *Journal of Neurophysiology*, **73**, 1988–2003.

Wearden, J. H. and Lejeune, H. (2008). Scalar properties in human timing: Conformity and violations. *Quarterly Journal of Experimental Psychology*, **61**, 569–87.

Yarrow, K. and Rothwell, J. C. E. (2003). Manual chronostasis: tactile perception precedes physical contact. *Current Biology*, **13**, 1134–9.

Yarrow, K., Haggard, P., Heal, R., Brown, P., and Rothwell, J. C. E. (2001). Illusory perceptions of space and time preserve cross-saccadic perceptual continuity. *Nature*, **414**, 302–5.

Yarrow, K., Haggard, P., and Rothwell, J. C. (2004a). Action, arousal, and subjective time. *Consciousness and Cognition*, **13**, 373–90.

Yarrow, K., Johnson, H., Haggard, P., and Rothwell, J. C. E. (2004b). Consistent chronostasis effects across saccade categories imply a subcortical efferent trigger. *Journal of Cognitive Neuroscience,* **16**, 839–47.

Yarrow, K., Whiteley, L., Haggard, P., and Rothwell, J. C. (2006a). Biases in the perceived timing of perisaccadic visual and motor events. *Perception and Psychophysics,* **68**, 1217–26.

Yarrow, K., Whiteley, L., Rothwell, J. C., and Haggard, P. (2006b). Spatial consequences of bridging the saccadic gap. *Vision Research,* **46**, 545–55.

Yarrow, K., Haggard, P., and Rothwell, J. C. (In press). Saccadic chronostasis and the continuity of subjective visual experience across eye movements. In R. Nijhawan and B. Khurana (Eds.) *Space and Time in Perception and Action.* Cambridge: Cambridge University Press.

Chapter 13

Space-time in the brain

Concetta Morrone and David Burr

How do we sense time? It has long been thought that the brain counts the ticks of some centralized clock, in the same way that a computer is controlled by a clock in its central processing unit. However, recent studies are beginning to challenge this idea. Much evidence suggests that visual events are not timed by a single clock, but by many independent clocks, each selective to a particular region of space. And, more generally, that space and time are not separate for the brain, but to a certain extent are analysed together.

There is one obvious sense in which time and space are intrinsically intertwined, namely motion perception. Motion necessarily involves changes in space over time (e.g. Burr, 2003) so the two must be considered together in order to sense it. However, although time is an intrinsic component of motion perception, it does not have to be sensed *directly* for motion to be perceived, and therefore usually not considered to involve perception of time.

The time that we sense consciously lags behind the time associated with the processing of the sensory information: we know that the impulse response of a visual event usually lasts in the order of 100ms. Measuring intervals below the critical flicker frequency is very easy for the visual system because this can be measured by the change in firing rate of visual neurons. Nevertheless, we are able to measure the duration of visual events 5–10 times longer, with the same relative accuracy, well after all traces of response activity have disappeared. Surprisingly, in analogy with motion mechanisms, it seems that even for these long intervals 'brain-time' depends not only on time but also on space. In this chapter we will consider recent work by our group studying the perception of the *event duration*. We discuss evidence showing that the perception of event duration—at least over the sub-second range—is strongly linked to our perception of space. Thus, the mechanisms that measure event duration must be inherently intertwined with those responsible for the representation of space. We present three main lines of evidence for this claim: adaptation, estimation of event duration during saccades, and the effect of attention on event duration.

Motion adaptation affects perceived event duration

Many factors can alter the apparent duration of an event. For example, if attention is directed to a particular item in a serial stream, it will appear to be of longer duration than the others (Rose and Summers, 1995; Enns, Brehaut, and Shore, 1999; Tse et al., 2004). Similarly, apparent duration of visual stimuli has long been known to depend on stimulus speed (Roelofs and Zeaman, 1951; Kanai et al., 2007); faster moving stimuli appear to last longer than slower moving stimuli. Recently, Johnston, Arnold, and Nishida (2006) have shown that adaptation can also affect apparent duration (Johnston, Chapter 14, this volume). After adapting to a fast moving grating, stimuli displayed to the adapted region of the retina appeared shorter than those displayed elsewhere. The reason for the altered duration is still unclear, but, whatever the mechanism by which adaptation causes underestimation of duration, it is clear that the effects are spatially specific.

We pursued further the adaptation of event duration and showed that it was spatially selective in external, or world coordinates (Burr, Tozzi, and Morrone, 2007). We used a technique introduced by Melcher (2005), where subjects stare at a fixation point left of centre, while a fast-drifting grating (1 cycle/degree, 20Hz) moves within a window to the upper right of the fixation point (see Figure. 13.1A). After extensive adaptation, the fixation point—and the subject's gaze—moves to the right. A test grating, drifting at 10Hz, is then displayed for 600ms in one of three possible positions: in the same position the adaptor had occupied on the screen (*spatiotopic* condition); in the same position the adaptor occupied relative to fixation (*retinotopic* condition); or in a completely different position, below left of fixation (*control*). In separate sessions, the fixation dot did not move, and the test was presented in the same retinotopic and spatiotopic position as the adaptor (*full* adaptation). One second after the presentation of the test, a *probe* grating (of variable duration) was presented to the lower left of fixation, and subjects were required to report whether it seemed of shorter or longer duration than the test. Psychometric curves were calculated, from which the point of subjective equality (PSE) was estimated from the median. In order to ensure that the changes in apparent duration were not merely a result of the apparent slowing of the grating after adaptation, the physical speed of the probe was adjusted to match the apparent speed of the test (in practice this was necessary only for the retinotopic and full adaptation conditions).

Figure 13.1B shows the perceived durations for the four conditions, averaged over five observers. In the control condition, the average duration was about 600ms, close to the real physical duration of the stimulus. Interestingly, the average perceived duration for the retinotopic condition was also around 600ms, not significantly different from the control, while for the spatiotopic condition the average duration was 440ms, similar to the full adaptation condition. This suggests that under these conditions, with probe speed matched to the apparent speed of the test, the adaptation is primarily spatiotopic. In another control condition, probes of the same physical speed as the test were used, yielding retinotopic-specific adaptation, similar in strength to the spatiotopic effect (bars at right).

These results suggest that at least two mechanisms are involved in adaptation of duration, one retinotopic and the other spatiotopic. As mentioned earlier, apparent duration of visual stimuli is known to increase with increasing speed (Kanai et al., 2007), and adaptation to fast stimuli decreases apparent speed of subsequently viewed stimuli (Thompson, 1981; Wohlgemuth, 1911). Thus the retinotopically selective decrease in apparent duration, which occurred only when the apparent speed of the test and probe were not matched (so the probe seemed to drift more quickly than the test), is probably an indirect consequence of the adaptor causing a reduction in the neural representation of speed, rather than direct action on neural timing mechanisms. Spatiotopic adaptation, on the other hand, occurred for both the speed-matched probes (which in practice changed little) and the 10-Hz probes, suggesting that its effects do not depend on changes in apparent speed (that are probably mediated by lower-level mechanisms), but reflect direct action on the neural mechanisms of interval judgement, or their afferents. Further studies showed that *dichoptic* adaptation (adapt one eye, test the other) was spatiotopically but not retinotopically selective also suggesting that spatiotopic adaptation occurs at a higher level than retinotopic adaptation, as there is no anatomical convergence of eye input before V1, with strong functional interactions occurring only at later stages (Macknik and Martinez-Conde, 2004).

The fact that the adaptation was spatiotopic is interesting. In the macaque, early visual areas, including primary and secondary visual cortex, have strong retinotopicity unaffected by eye position, while some higher-order areas of parietal cortex seem to encode position in spatiotopic rather than retinotopic coordinates (Galletti, Battaglini, and Fattori, 1995; Duhamel et al., 1997;

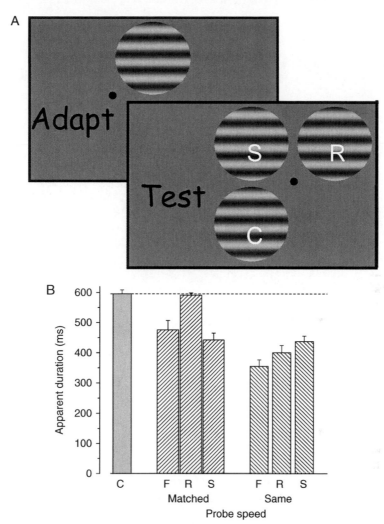

Fig. 13.1 A) Illustration of the setup to study the spatial selectivity of adaptation effects on event duration. Subjects stare at the black fixation while observing a fast-drifting grating within a window to the upper right of it. They then make a saccade to the dot at right, and observe a test grating displayed for 600ms in one of three possible positions: in the same position the adaptor had occupied on the screen (*spatiotopic* (S) condition), to the same position the adaptor occupied relative to fixation (*retinotopic* (R) condition), or to a completely different position, below left of fixation (*control* (C) condition). They then reported whether a probe grating of variable duration presented to the lower left of fixation appeared shorter or longer than the test. B) Effects of adaptation on apparent duration. The bar graphs show the matched duration (point of subjective equality of test and probe match) in the control (C), full (F), retinotopic (R) and spatiotopic (S) conditions. The bars on the left show results when the apparent speed of the probe was matched to that of the test, those on the right when the physical speeds were the same. In both cases, after spatiotopic-specific adaptation perceived duration was reduced from 600ms to 450ms. There was a similar effect for retinotopic-specific adaptation when the physical speed was the same, but none when the apparent speed was matched.

Snyder et al., 1998). The lateral intraparietal area (area LIP) does not seem to be truly spatiotopic, but its receptive fields are strongly affected by eye movements in a way to give it a transient spatiotopicity (Duhamel, Colby, and Goldberg, 1992). This area has been shown to be involved with event timing of sub-second intervals (Leon and Shadlen, 2003; Janssen and Shadlen, 2005), making it a plausible candidate for the spatiotopic-specific adaptation of duration. Transcranial magnetic stimulation (TMS) studies (Bueti, Bahrami, and Walsh, 2008) have also implicated this area in duration judgement in humans. All this fits well with our present results, implicating parietal areas like LIP in event duration timing.

Saccades affect event duration

Other evidence for the strong interconnection of space and time, and for the involvement of area LIP, comes from testing the effects of saccadic eye-movements on the perception of duration. Saccades are ballistic movements of the eyes made to reposition our gaze, sometimes deliberately, but normally automatically and unnoticed. Not only do the actual eye movements escape notice, but so does the image motion they cause, and the fact that gaze itself has been repositioned. Besides being interesting in their own right, saccades provide a fascinating window through which to study perception. Saccades cause many transient but bizarre effects on perception (Ross et al., 2001; see also Yarrow, Chapter 12, this volume): motion perception is severely dampened, probably because of selective suppression of the magnocellular system (Burr, Morrone, and Ross, 1994); and visual space is grossly distorted, compressed towards the saccadic landing point (Ross, Morrone and Burr, 1997; Morrone, Ross, and Burr, 1997). The spatial distortion occurs selectively for verbal reports, not for action (Burr, Morrone, and Ross, 2001).

More recently, we have shown that saccades cause not only a compression of space but also of time (Morrone, Ross, and Burr, 2005). Subjects were asked to compare the apparent separation of pairs of bars presented near saccadic onset with a probe pair presented 2 seconds later. The physical separation of the bars was 100ms, but when presented near saccadic onset, they were judged to be equal to probes of only 50ms, a compression of 50%. Figure 13.2A shows the time course of the compression. As with spatial compression, the effect was maximal near saccadic onset, and followed very tight temporal dynamics, falling off before and after the saccade. Interestingly, although the durations were judged to be shorter, the precision of these judgements actually *improved* during saccades, as shown by the steeper psychometric functions (see Morrone et al., 2005, for full experimental details). Importantly, the compression effects occurred only for visual stimuli, not for auditory clicks. Time and space are linked in vision, but this does not necessarily cross over to the other senses.

Even more surprisingly, for certain intervals of stimulus presentation, not only was duration misjudged, but temporal order was inverted. In a further experiment, subjects were asked to estimate the temporal order of the bars (which were always presented in random order). Figure 13.2C shows a psychometric function (probability of judging first bar as first as a function of temporal separation) for stimuli presented just before saccadic onset, within the narrow range −70ms to −30ms. The psychometric function is far from conventional, and actually *triphasic*, running smoothly in the opposite direction to reality for bar separations within the range −50ms to +50ms: as if time had reversed. Only for very large separations (greater than 100ms or so) is temporal order perceived correctly.

We have also studied the effects of saccades using an auditory marker technique (Binda et al 2009). Subjects were required to report whether a bar, flashed at various times relative to saccadic onset, was perceived before or after a tone. As saccades do not affect the perception of sounds (Harris and Lieberman, 1996), these measurements allowed us to calculate the time visual

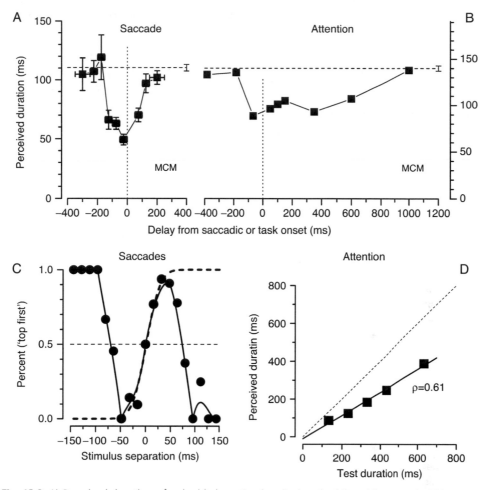

Fig. 13.2 A) Perceived duration of a double-bar stimulus displayed while subjects made 30° horizontal saccades, plotted as a function of delay from saccadic onset (mean time of the two bars). For a period of about 150ms either side of saccadic onset, the perceived duration of the 100-ms interval was considerably reduced (roughly halved). The dashed horizontal line shows the estimate of duration for bars displayed during fixation. Vertical bars refer to standard errors, calculated by the bootstrap method, and horizontal bars to the width of the averaging bin.
B) Perceived duration of a double-bar stimulus relative to the onset of an attention-grabbing task. Subjects maintained fixation on a central fixation point and performed two tasks: identify which of two laterally positioned circles abruptly expanded (at an unpredictable time); and whether a pair of horizontal bars (similar to those used in the saccade experiment, displayed with 140-ms separation) seemed shorter or longer than the probe. The shift in attention to identify the expanding circles caused a strong compression in perceived duration, but was less extreme than that caused by saccades, and lasted for much longer. The dashed horizontal line shows the estimate of duration for bars displayed without the double task. C) Psychometric functions of temporal order judgements for pairs of bars presented within a critical peri-saccadic interval −70ms to −30 ms. The function is inverted over the range of ±50-ms bar separation, suggesting that the bars are perceived in the reverse order of their actual presentation. D) Perceived duration of bar-pairs presented near the onset of a double task (identify expanding circle), as a function of the physical separation of stimulus bars. The data are well fitted by a line passing through 0 (of slope 0.61), suggesting that the effect of attention on stimulus duration is multiplicative.

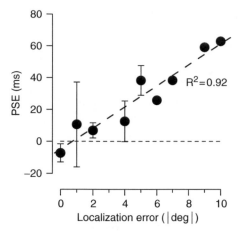

Fig. 13.3 Relationship between spatial and temporal mislocalization. Subjects were required to make simultaneous spatial and temporal judgements about a briefly flashed stimulus presented around the time of saccades. They reported its apparent position, and also the temporal order with respect to an auditory probe, from which temporal mislocalization was calculated. Temporal mislocalization (PSE) is plotted against spatial mislocalization, averaged over hundreds of trials. The linear regression between the two variables accounts for 92% of the variance.

stimuli are perceived when presented during saccades. We showed that stimuli presented near saccadic onset were strongly delayed, by about 100ms. Furthermore, this delay predicted the apparent inversions described earlier. Although both the delay and the time of inversion were idiosyncratic for each individual observer, in all cases the delay well predicted the inversion. This suggests that the mechanism generating the inversion during saccades is robust and specific to the visual stimuli and insensitive to the particular task. Given the precise and sharp tuning dynamics, the effects are consistent with the start of a deterministic hard-wired phenomenon. Soon after the inversion, perceived time is delayed with respect to physical time, and this is consistent with the increased latencies of the neuronal response of LIP or V3A at the time they change or 'remap' their receptive field properties (Nakamura and Colby, 2002). Both inversion and delay of perceived time may be associated with the onset and rapid phase of remapping.

As mentioned earlier, saccades affect both space and time: they cause briefly presented stimuli to appear displaced and contracted, and change both the perceived duration onset-time of brief stimuli. The time courses for both effects are similar. In a recent study (Binda et al., 2009), we measured both spatial and temporal mislocalizations in the same experiment: subjects were required to report the apparent position of a briefly flashed bar, and also to pinpoint it in time, relative to a brief sound. There was a good deal of variability in the amount of spatial and temporal mislocalization, but the two attributes varied together. Figure 13.3 plots the temporal mislocalization against the spatial mislocalization, for all collected data. Mislocalizations in space and time clearly occur together, with covariance $R^2 = 0.92$. Whatever causes the spatial mislocalization also causes temporal mislocalization. Space and time are tightly linked.

Event duration during shifts in attention

As mentioned earlier, there is much evidence showing how attention can affect apparent duration (Rose and Summers, 1995; Enns et al., 1999; Tse et al., 2004). LIP is also strongly affected by attention (Gottlieb, Kusunoki, and Goldberg, 1998; Ben Hamed et al., 2002), so it seemed conceivable that covert shifts in spatial attention, that often precede eye-movements (Deubel and Schneider, 1996), could also affect apparent duration, in a similar way to overt eye movements. We have recently investigated this possibility by asking subjects to maintain fixation on a central fixation point and judge which of two laterally positioned circles had undergone a slight expansion (Cicchini and Morrone, 2009). Two distinct horizontal bars, similar to those used in the saccade experiment, were displayed with 430-ms separation. As in the previous saccade tasks, subjects were required to compare the apparent interval separating these bars to a later probe interval. The results, shown in Figure 13.2B, were similar to those obtained with overt saccades. The covert shift in spatial attention caused a strong compression in perceived duration. The compression was less extreme (to about 70% instead of 50% of its original value), and followed broader dynamics.

We measured the effect of spatial attention on apparent duration for various bar separations. Figure 13.2D shows the average results for two subjects. The effect of attention is multiplicative, reducing apparent duration by a constant proportion at all measured durations. The best fitting regression passes near zero with a slope of 0.61, suggesting that covert shifts of spatial attention cause intervals over the range of 100–1000ms to be perceived as 60–70% of their actual duration. This is different from that observed with overt saccades, which had little effect on durations greater than about 200ms (unpublished observations). So while there are certainly similarities between the effects of attention and saccades on event duration, the two do not act in an identical manner. In a control experiment, we measured the effect of attention on the apparent duration of a bar displayed twice to the same location. In this case, attention had no effect on apparent duration, showing again the interaction of time and space.

Conclusions

The results of these three lines of experiments collectively show that, at least for duration judgements of visual stimuli in the sub-second range, space and time are intrinsically interconnected. Adaptation to duration is spatially selective, in external spatial coordinates; and the temporal distortions that occur during saccades are closely linked to contemporaneous spatial distortions. What do these results tell us about the mechanisms and neural substrate of the perception of event duration?

The fact that spatial and temporal localization errors co-vary suggests that both functions may be mediated by a common mechanism. A simple framework for keeping track of time could be to measure within a layer of connected neurons the spatial extent of a propagation wave generated by the event. If these connected neurons also represent space, at any instant the most active neuron will code the spatial localization of the event, and the spread of the activity in the layer will code the time lapsed from event onset. The analogy is similar to the waves generated when throwing a stone in a lake: the centre of the ripples localizes the impact point, the diameter or number of the ripples the time lapsed. An ideal observer with access to the layer information can decode it to derive the position and time of one or more events.

Within this simple framework, we can add a remapping process that considers that, around the time of saccades, the diffusion is not homogeneous in space, but strongly biased towards the representation of the saccadic target. Given that in our model the diffusion is fast with respect to the impulse response of the neurons and the dissipation constant, the neuronal spread will generate an oblique 'comet' in a space–time plot, with peaks delayed in time and shifted in space, towards the saccadic target. This schema predicts most of the distortions, including the compression, given that the tail activity of two stimuli will be confusable with stimuli that are physically closer in space and in time. The approach also predicts inversion, if the neuronal receptive fields have a centre-surround antagonism.

All the results tend to implicate parietal areas in the perception of visuospatial event duration. One possible candidate is area LIP, where recent physiological evidence in macaques (Leon and Shadlen, 2003; Janssen and Shadlen, 2005) shows that single neurons are strongly modulated during timing tasks. Area LIP is not strictly spatiotopic, but its receptive fields are strongly affected by saccades in such a way as to give it a transient spatiotopicity (Duhamel et al., 1992), making it a plausible candidate for the spatiotopic-specific adaptation of duration. The fact that the receptive fields undergo saccade-induced changes is also consistent with the fact that time is grossly distorted during saccades. Although the effect of saccades on the temporal encoding of these neurons has not yet been measured, it is conceivable that it changes dramatically around the time of saccades, as these neurons shift receptive fields. LIP is also strongly affected by attention (Ben Hamed et al., 2002, Gottlieb et al., 1998), consistent with the fact that shifts in attention also reduce apparent duration. But the reduction occurs only for stimuli presented to different spatial positions.

TMS studies (Bueti et al., 2008) have also implicated this area in duration judgement about moving visual stimuli in humans. Interestingly, they also implicate area MT in the timing of visual events. Spatiotopic selectivity has not studied extensively in humans, but recent functional magnetic resonance imaging (fMRI) results suggest that the portion of hMT+ that was thought to be retinotopic is in fact spatiotopic (d'Avossa et al., 2007), and this could well be true of other parietal areas. Interestingly, an fMRI study that manipulated attentional allocation to distinct stimulus features (Coull et al., 2004) showed that when attention was directed to a duration task temporal-parietal circuitry was activated, together with fronto-striatal circuitry (considered a major network of time mechanisms: Buhusi and Meck, 2005). When attention was directed to a colour task, no part of this network showed a correlation with the attentional allocation. Interestingly the Talairach coordinates of the temporal areas overlap partially with those of the MT+ complex. All this fits well with our present results, suggesting that the spatially selective visual neural mechanisms implicated in visual event timing probably reside in temporal and parietal cortex, and with evidence of spatiotopicity of these time mechanisms.

All these results suggest that sub-second visual events are timed not by a centralized clock, but by neural mechanisms that are spatially selective (in real-world coordinates). One recently suggested possibility (Karmarkar and Buonomano, 2007) is that cortical networks of neurons are inherently able to tell time as a result of time-dependent changes in network state, like reading the state of ripples on a pond. If these neurons were spatially tuned and adaptable, then stimulation with high temporal frequencies may slow down the dynamics of the network, leading to an under-estimation of event duration.

Of course this leaves open the question of whether spatially localized timers can be monitored simultaneously (recent evidence: Giora, Morgan, and Solomon, 2006, suggesting that they can not). But mechanisms of this sort could be the basis for timing specific perceptual events that occur in specific spatial positions: when watching a field of fireflies, we have a very clear idea of both the duration and the spatial position of any given flash, and this does not change if we make a saccade between flashes (provided the flash is not peri-saccadic). As humans saccade on average three times per second, it is certainly advantageous that the spatial selectivity of interval-timing mechanisms is grounded in external rather than retinal coordinates.

References

Ben Hamed, S., Duhamel, J.R., Bremmer, F., and Graf, W. (2002). Visual receptive field modulation in the lateral intraparietal area during attentive fixation and free gaze. *Cereb Cortex*, 1(3), 234–45.

Binda, P., Cicchini, G.M., Burr, D.C., and Morrone, M.C. (2009). Spatio-temporal distortions of visual perception at the time of saccades. *J. Neurosc.*, in press.

Bueti, D., Bahrami, B., and Walsh, V. (2008). Sensory and association cortex in time perception. *J Cogn Neurosci,* **20**(6), 1054–62.

Buhusi, C.V., and Meck, W.H. (2005). What makes us tick? Functional and neural mechanisms of interval timing. *Nat Rev Neurosci,* **6**(10), 755–65.

Burr, D., Tozzi, A., and Morrone, M.C. (2007). Neural mechanisms for timing visual events are spatially selective in real-world coordinates. *Nat Neurosci,* **10**(4), 423–5.

Burr, D.C. (2003). Motion perception: elementary mechanisms. In M.A. Arbib (Ed.) *The Handbook of Brain Theory and Neural Networks: Second Edition,* pp.672–6. Cambridge: MIT Press.

Burr, D.C., Morrone, M.C., and Ross, J. (1994). Selective suppression of the magnocellular visual pathway during saccadic eye movements. *Nature,* **371**, 511–13.

Burr, D.C., Morrone, M.C., and Ross, J. (2001). Separate visual representations for perception and action revealed by saccadic eye movements. *Curr Biol,* **11**(10), 798–802.

Cicchini, G.M. and Morrone, M.C. (2009). Shifts in spatial attention affect the perceived duration of events. *J Vis.* **9**(1):1–13.

Coull, J.T., Vidal, F., Nazarian, B., and Macar, F. (2004). Functional anatomy of the attentional modulation of time estimation. *Science,* **303**(5663), 1506–8.

D'Avossa, G., Tosetti, M., Crespi, S., Biagi, L., Burr, D.C., and Morrone, M.C. (2007). Spatiotopic selectivity of BOLD responses to visual motion in human area MT. *Nat Neurosci,* **10**(2), 249–55.

Deubel, H., and Schneider, W.X. (1996). Saccade target selection and object recognition: evidence for a common attentional mechanism. *Vision Res,* **36**(12), 1827–37.

Duhamel, J., Bremmer, F., BenHamed, S., and Graf, W. (1997). Spatial invariance of visual receptive fields in parietal cortex neurons. *Nature,* **389**, 845–8.

Duhamel, J.R., Colby, C.L., and Goldberg, M.E. (1992). The updating of the representation of visual space in parietal cortex by intended eye movements. *Science,* **255**(5040), 90–2.

Enns, J.T., Brehaut, J.C., and Shore, D.I. (1999). The duration of a brief event in the mind's eye. *J Gen Psychol,* **126**(4), 355–72.

Galletti, C., Battaglini, P.P., and Fattori, P. (1995). Eye position influence on the parieto-occipital area PO (V6) of the macaque monkey. *European J Neuroscience,* **7**, 2486–501.

Giora, E., Morgan, M.J., and Solomon, J.A. (2006). Parallel processing is much harder for temporal duration than for spatial length. *J Vision,* **6**, 1012.

Gottlieb, J.P., Kusunoki, M., and Goldberg, M.E. (1998). The representation of visual salience in monkey parietal cortex. *Nature,* **391**(6666), 481–84.

Harris, L.R. and Lieberman, L. (1996). Auditory stimulus detection is not suppressed during saccadic eye movements. *Perception,* **25**(8), 999–1004.

Janssen, P. and Shadlen, M.N. (2005). A representation of the hazard rate of elapsed time in macaque area LIP. *Nat Neurosci,* **8**(2), 234–41.

Johnston, A., Arnold, D.H., and Nishida, S. (2006). Spatially localized distortions of event time. *Curr Biol,* **16**(5), 472–9.

Kanai, R., Paffen, C. (2006). L., Hogendoorn, H., and Verstraten, F.A. Time dilation in dynamic visual display. *J Vis,* **6**, 1421–30.

Karmarkar, U.R. and Buonomano, D.V. (2007). Timing in the absence of clocks: encoding time in neural network States. *Neuron,* **53**(3), 427–38.

Leon, M.I. and Shadlen, M.N. (2003). Representation of time by neurons in the posterior parietal cortex of the macaque. *Neuron,* **38**(2), 317–27.

Macknik, S.L. and Martinez-Conde, S. (2004). Dichoptic visual masking reveals that early binocular neurons exhibit weak interocular suppression: implications for binocular vision and visual awareness. *J Cogn Neurosci,* **16**(6), 1049–59.

Melcher, D. (2005). Spatiotopic transfer of visual-form adaptation across saccadic eye movements. *Curr Biol,* **15**(19), 1745–8.

Morrone, M.C., Ross, J., and Burr, D.C. (1997). Apparent position of visual targets during real and simulated saccadic eye movements. *J Neuroscience,* **17**, 7941–53.

Morrone, M.C., Ross, J., and Burr, D. (2005). Saccadic eye movements cause compression of time as well as space. *Nat Neurosci,* **8**(7), 9504.

Morrone, M.C., Binda, P., and Burr, D.C. (2008). Spatiotopic selectivity for location of events in space and time *J Vis,* **8**, 819.

Nakamura, K. and Colby, C.L. (2002). Updating of the visual representation in monkey striate and extrastriate cortex during saccades. *Proc Natl Acad Sci U S A,* **99**(6), 4026–31.

Roelofs, C.O. and Zeaman, W. (1951). Influence of different sequences of optical stimuli on the duration of a given interval of time. *Acta Psychol (Amst),* **8**, 89–128.

Rose, D. and Summers, J. (1995). Duration illusions in a train of visual stimuli. *Perception,* **24**(10), 1177–87.

Ross, J., Morrone, M.C., and Burr, D.C. (1997). Compression of visual space before saccades. *Nature,* **384**, 598–601.

Ross, J., Morrone, M.C., Goldberg, M.E., and Burr, D.C. (2001). Changes in visual perception at the time of saccades. *Trends Neurosci,* **24**, 131–21.

Snyder, L.H., Grieve, K.L., Brotchie, P., and Andersen, R.A. (1998). Separate body- and world-referenced representations of visual space in parietal cortex. *Nature,* **394**(6696), 887–91.

Thompson, P. (1981). Velocity after-effects: the effects of adaptation to moving stimuli on the perception of subsequently seen moving stimuli. *Vis Res,* **21** (3), 337–45.

Tse, P., Intriligator, J., Rivest, J., and Cavanagh, P. (2004). Attention and the subjective expansion of time. *Percept Psychophys,* **66**, 1171–89.

Wohlgemuth, A. (1911). On the after-effect of seen movement. *Br J Psychol, Monogr, Suppl,* **1**, 1–117.

Acknowledgements

Supported by the European Union Framework Programme 6 and 7: 'MEMORY' and ERCl advanced grant 229445 'STANIB'.

Chapter 14

Modulation of time perception by visual adaptation

Alan Johnston

Significant progress has been made in the last 50 years in understanding the components of the visual process. Specialized systems for encoding form, motion, and colour have been identified and linked to anatomically separate brain regions. To a large extent these neural systems can be thought of as autonomous computational machines that deliver, continuously and in parallel, some local interpretation of the visual input such as the orientation of a local contour, the colour of a patch, or the velocity of a moving dot.

Progress has been less certain in understanding processes that encode ordinal information such as which event precedes another[1] or metric information such as length or duration. Although the perception of spatial extent could in principle be encoded instantaneously since the start point and end points of the line are always present, the encoding of duration has to be time-dependent, since the duration of an event is not defined until the event is over (Morgan, Giora, and Solomon, 2008). Indeed, Morgan et al. have demonstrated a set-size effect for duration perception. In a task in which subjects have to judge whether a target was longer or shorter than a standard in a set of temporally overlapping standards, they found temporal discrimination accuracy decreased with the number of elements. This indicates an attention-limited component of the duration judgement task. A similar set-size effect was found for line-length discrimination judgements when the lines grew or shrank over time such that line length was not signalled until the end of the dynamic event. These experiments highlight the fact that generic attentional control process are required to recover simple properties such as duration and length but leave open the issue of which representations these process operate upon. The identification of such temporal representations in the visual domain will be the main focus of this chapter.

The 'stopwatch' model

The judgement of duration is generally thought to be accomplished entirely by means of a generic, central timing mechanism, which can be applied to all events. The classical integrator or stopwatch model (Creelman, 1962; Treisman, 1963) has many positive features as a candidate timing device. It can be applied to a range of temporal scales. It distinguishes the physical time interval, when the stopwatch is started and stopped, from the rate signal (ticks per second) that is integrated over the interval. The only signal that needs to be sent to the clock is the start point and end point of the interval. Since the rate signal is internally generated, it can be used to time any event, including empty events. There are only two ways in which such a clock could make errors in

---

[1] How we encode temporal order, or judge the simultaneity of events that are sufficiently separated in space or sensory modality to be processed by separate neural systems, has been the subject of considerable debate and is reviewed in detail elsewhere (Nishida and Johnston, 2010)

determining duration. The start and stop points might be incorrect or the rate signal might be set incorrectly. Scalar expectation theory (SET) (Wearden, 1999) distinguishes between these two by noticing that errors resulting from changes in clock rate should be proportional to the interval length, conforming to Weber's law, whereas effects due to stopping or starting errors should be additive. Typically, changes in perceived duration are attributed to a speeding or slowing of the clock rate. However, the benefits of the internal clock model also seed its demerits. Distortions of time perception have to be explained as influencing this generic variable, leading to explanations of changes in time perception as mediated by changes in domain-independent state variables such as arousal or attentiveness.

A visual clock

Perceived duration has been found to be influenced by state variables such as body temperature (Wearden and Penton-Voak, 1995), disease, pharmalogical intervention (Buhusi and Meck, 2005) and arousal, for example, as generated by life-threatening events (Stetson, Fiesta, and Eagleman, 2007). In these cases, the modality of stimulation or the content of the interval per se should not be expected to be an important factor.

On average a long interval may be expected to contain more events than a short interval. Although more generally associated with time estimation (>5 seconds) than time perception (Fraisse, 1984) a number of authors have proposed that the apparent duration of an interval should be related to the number of events or the number of stimulus changes within the interval (Fraisse, 1963, 1984; S. W. Brown, 1995; Tse et al., 2004; Kanai et al., 2006; Brown, Chapter 8; Tse, Chapter 10; Eagleman, Chapter 11; this volume). Kanai and colleagues (2006) reported that perceived duration increases with the temporal frequency (i.e. the number of cycles passing a point per second) rather than the speed of a drifting sine grating. The speed is the temporal frequency (cycles/second) divided by the spatial frequency (cycles/degree). Subjects reproduced intervals in the sub-second range using a button press. They first replicated a classic finding (J. F. Brown, 1931) that a moving object appears to last longer than a static object of the same duration. They then went on to show the amount of time dilation depended on the temporal frequency, not the speed, of motion. Similar results were also found for flickering Gaussian blobs, which varied in luminance over time but did not move. Kanai and colleagues support the view that the number of events or changes in the stimulus determines its duration, with the caveat that this cannot be definitive since the effects on duration saturate at a temporal frequency of around 4–8Hz. Time dilation for motion is generally explained by recruiting the idea that motion involves multiple position change events. However, this is debatable. Motion is clearly seen in random-dot kinematograms[2] (Julesz, 1971) indicating that a sense of motion does not depend on the sense of position change, and there is no means of enumerating how many spatial change events have occurred in a smoothly moving sequence.

The internal clock model has also been used to explain the effects of attention on duration perception (Taatgen, van Rijn, and Anderson, 2007). When two stimuli are presented, the attended one appears to last longer (Thomas and Weaver, 1975). The general proposal is that when attention is distracted by a different task, clock ticks are missed, leading to an apparent reduction in unattended duration. In an exogenous attention paradigm, a low-probability 'oddball' in a sequence

---

[2] Random dot kinematograms are constructed by spatially shifting a section of an image made by randomly assigning pixels to be black or white. On any single frame of the sequence the moving region is invisible. However given a sequence of frames the location of the moving region is visible even though it is impossible to identify a position shift for each individual dot. In this case form derives from motion.

of high-probability items appears longer than the high-probability items of the same objective duration (Tse et al., 2004; Tse, Chapter 10, this volume). Tse and colleagues supplement the missing-ticks proposal with an increase in the number of units of temporal information to explain how an oddball can appear to last longer in situations where there is no competition from another stream of events. However, a problem that would need to be solved in this approach is how to segment an arbitrary sequence into a number of events.

If one directly compares intervals with high temporal frequencies and those with low temporal frequencies it is difficult to discount the possibility that the visual stimulus differences have general, rather than specific, influences on time perception. Looking at visual flicker, or listening to tones presented at low or high rates, might decrease or increase arousal or attentiveness and thereby increase the clock rate. In addition, when comparisons are made between intervals that do not contain identical stimuli, there may be stimulus-dependent neural latency effects at onset or offset that contribute to apparent duration. These problems can be circumvented to some degree by using adaptation. Adapting the system using click-trains (Treisman et al., 1990; Wearden, Philpott, and Win, 1999) or a flickering white circle (Droit-Volet and Wearden, 2002) has been shown to increase apparent duration. Droit-Volet and Wearden presented their subjects (children aged 3, 5, or 8 years) with a flickering (5 seconds; 7Hz) or static white circle, which was followed by a blue circle in the same location lasting 200–800ms or 400 and 1600ms depending on conditions. There were seven durations in each range. Their subjects responded to these durations by indicating, on each trial, whether the interval was long or short. Essentially they reported whether the duration of the blue circle on a given trial appeared to be a one of the longer or one of the shorter durations of the set. They found that after flicker adaptation, the blue circle was judged to last longer, as compared to the static adaptor condition, for all ages. They interpret the finding as demonstrating flicker caused an increase in pacemaker speed. Again this change could be attributed to non-specific effects such as arousal.

To test whether adaptation can alter expressly visual rather than non-specific mechanisms, Johnston, Arnold, and Nishida (2006) adapted a region of the near visual periphery on one side of fixation to drifting sine gratings or Gaussian blobs whose luminance varied sinusoidally over time. After a 15-second adaptation period, a sub-second interval of 10-Hz drift (motion) or luminance modulation (flicker) was presented sequentially to the adapted and non-adapted sides of the visual field. Observers were asked to report which interval lasted longer. The duration of the interval on the non-adapted side was varied from trial to trial to generate a psychometric function. The point of subjective equality provided a measure of relative duration. They found that apparent duration of a 10-Hz motion stimulus on the adapted side was reduced after adaptation to a 20-Hz drift, but only slightly reduced or unaffected after 5-Hz adaptation. A similar result was found for the flicker stimulus. Adapting to motion or flicker may have non-specific effects, but any non-specific effect will not contribute to the comparison between adapted versus non-adapted regions of the visual field.

The observation that the perceived duration of identical intervals can vary after adaptation of a localized region of the visual field cannot be explained with reference to a generic central clock. Neither can it be explained with reference to the influence of state changes, such as changes in arousal or attention on the clock rate. In any case adapting to high frequencies, which might be thought to increase arousal and, consequently, clock rate and therefore, ultimately, duration in fact *reduce* apparent duration. Similarly, increased attention is expected to dilate the interval rather than compress it. If the change in apparent duration was a result of attending more to the adapted region then we should expect the same amount of apparent time compression in the 5-Hz condition as in the 20-Hz condition, but this was not the case. These 5-HZ and 20-Hz adaptors shift the apparent frequency of a 10-Hz test pattern by about the same amount (around 3-Hz shift away from the adaptor). An account of the duration effect based on differential attention to the adapter would have to explain why there was not a similar asymmetry for perceived temporal frequency. The test patterns are presented sequentially, so there is no competition and little reason to expect time compression is due to 'missed ticks'. In addition, we have demonstrated that time compression occurs even in the case of invisible (60-Hz) flicker (Johnston et al., 2008). In this paradigm, since the adapter is invisible, it is not possible for observers to tell which side of the visual field is being adapted.

As introduced earlier, adaptation can also change the apparent temporal *frequency* of the test patterns (Johnston et al., 2006). Adapting to a high temporal frequency (20-Hz) drifting grating reduced the apparent frequency of a 10-Hz test grating in the adapted region of visual space and adapting to low temporal frequency (5Hz) had the reverse effect, increasing the apparent temporal frequency of the 10-Hz test. This raises the issue of whether the changes in apparent duration are mediated by changes in apparent temporal frequency. The proposal that the number of stimulus events or changes determines duration would predict that the reduced temporal frequency after 20-Hz adaptation should deliver temporal compression. However, there are a number of reasons to discount this idea of mediation via temporal frequency. First the changes in apparent temporal frequency are bidirectional whereas adaptation introduces only a reduction in apparent duration (apart from in one special case[3]; Johnston et al., 2008). Second, there is only a very small, <1Hz, decrease in temporal frequency after adaptation to 10-Hz drift, nevertheless the apparent duration of a 10-Hz test grating still appears compressed (Johnston et al., 2006). Third, we also measured temporal compression for test patterns in which the comparison stimulus was reduced in temporal frequency to match the apparent temporal frequency of the test in the adapted region. Time compression was unaffected. Fourth, the induced changes in temporal frequency at around 10Hz only reduced apparent temporal frequency to 7Hz, and Kanai et al. (2006) showed that the effects of temporal frequency on duration saturated at around 4–8Hz, i.e. we would not expect a change in temporal frequency from 10Hz to 7Hz to have an effect on apparent duration. Fifth, dyslexics show a different pattern to controls when asked to judge duration but are not different to controls after the same exposure to the adapter when asked to judge temporal frequency (Johnston et al., 2008). Sixth, we have shown duration compression for interleaved 5-Hz, which induce limited or no compression, and 20-Hz adapters, which induce significant compression, with duty cycles chosen to null any changes in apparent temporal frequency (Ayhan, Bruno, and Johnston, 2008; Bruno, Ayhan, and Johnston, 2008). Thus, there is ample evidence that the effects of adaptation on duration and temporal frequency can be dissociated.

It is worth noting that we also observed an additional effect. The apparent number of cycles of the modulated Gaussian blob was reduced after high temporal frequency adaptation (Johnston, Arnold, and Nishida, 2003). Again, this effect does not mediate the apparent duration compression, as there is still compression for drifting test gratings for which the apparent number of cycles at a point is not a salient variable.

Adaptation may alter the perception of the onset and offset of the interval. For example, the onset might appear to be delayed after adapting to high temporal frequencies with little effect on offset. However, we found that the apparent compression was proportional to the length of the interval (Johnston et al., 2006), which may be interpreted as an influence on pacemaker rate, rather than a subtraction from the length of the interval, which is what would be expected if adaptation introduces some processing delay at onset. We also measured the apparent onset

---

[3] Johnston et al. (2008) found that dyslexic participants showed an increase in apparent duration after 5-Hz adaption.

and offset times relative to an auditory tone and found little effect of adaptation on apparent onset or offset.

We can summarize then by saying that adaptation to high temporal frequencies generates a spatially localized compression of the apparent duration of drifting or flickering stimuli and that this is not a consequence of alteration of the apparent time of onset or offset of the interval or a consequence of any change in apparent temporal frequency which is concurrently observed. This implies separate encoding of duration, temporal frequency, and apparent number of cycles.

The neural basis of apparent interval compression

One can ask where duration is encoded in the brain, but the answer is likely to be complex. Brain imaging studies have highlighted the involvement of a number of areas, which are likely to be active depending upon stimulus and task (Nobre and O'Reilly, 2004). We should also be mindful of the earlier discussion that the timing mechanism may require a visual routine that makes timing information explicit, which is flexible and under cognitive control. This process, which individuates and selects the visual events the subject is required to time, is expected to act on earlier representations. Indeed, there are a number of reasons to believe that adaptation-based time compression may derive from changes occurring early in the visual pathway.

The first observation is that adaptation-based compression of apparent time is not orientation specific. Rotating the test grating 90° with respect to the adapting grating has virtually no effect on the strength of the apparent compression (Johnston et al., 2006). Neurons in the visual pathway up to the input layers of visual cortex have a centre-surround receptive-field geometry. Thus the lack of orientation specificity is consistent with a pre-cortical site for adaptation, although it remains a possibility that the site might be cortical but contain neurons that pool over orientation-tuned units. The second issue is the spatial specificity of the adaptation effect. If the mechanism is early, since receptive fields are small, we should expect relatively narrow spatial tuning functions. In fact adaptation-based time compression appears well localized to the adapted area (Ayhan et al., 2008). The third point is that compression occurs for invisible (60-Hz) flicker (Johnston et al., 2008). The fact that the adaptor is invisible is interesting but not critical, since visibility per se is not a criterion for distinguishing between subcortical and cortical processing. However, neurons in the retina and lateral geniculate nucleus (LGN) respond to frequencies about 20Hz higher than is the case in the visual cortex (Hawken, Shapley, and Grosof, 1996). The absent or poor response of cortical cells to 60-Hz stimulation indicates a subcortical locus for the adaptation effect.

It used to be thought that contrast adaptation only occurred in the cortex, however this has been recently overturned by evidence of contrast adaptation in the mammalian retina (Baccus and Meister, 2002) and more recently in the primate (Chander and Chichilnisky, 2001; Solomon et al., 2004). Solomon and colleagues (2004) have shown that magnocellular (M) cells in the LGN show slow adaptation at high temporal frequencies (45Hz) but not at low temporal frequencies (1Hz). These adaptation effects occur at frequencies higher than the typical upper limit for cortical cells. Concurrently recorded S potentials, action potentials which reflect ganglion cell input, show this slow adaptation is retinal in origin. Magnocellular cells also show a fast contrast-gain adaptation (Shapley and Victor, 1978; Mante, Bonin, and Carandini, 2008) in which the contrast response function is shifted to the right (towards higher contrasts). This results in a higher threshold contrast but greater variation in response to contrast at high contrasts (i.e. reduced saturation). Contrast gain reduces the responsivity of the cell and sharpens and advances the temporal impulse response (Benardete and Kaplan, 1999). Parvocellular (P) cells in the LGN and retina do not show any substantive fast or slow contrast adaptation. There exist a number of parallels between contrast adaptation in the magnocelluar pathway up to the LGN and adaptation-based time compression. They both occur selectively at high temporal frequency, and can occur for temporal frequencies beyond those likely to stimulate the visual cortex. Both are independent of the relative orientation of adapter and test, and both are induced by luminance modulation and drifting gratings.

Slow adaptation induces a drop in the maintained discharge rate of neurons after adaptation rather then a decline in firing rate during the adaptation period. There is also a change in the contrast gain as indicated by a right-shift in the neuron's contrast response function. The size of the post-adaptation drop in the discharge rate and the magnitude of the contrast-gain shift tend to be correlated (Solomon et al., 2004). We have shown that slow adaption delivers time compression and hypothesized that this is mediated by a change in the temporal impulse response associated with contrast-gain control. As a test of the magnocellular basis of time compression, we investigated whether one can also get effects of fast adaptation (contrast-gain control) on time perception (Bruno and Johnston, 2007). Subjects were presented with a sequence that contained five intervals in total. The first and last intervals contained a high-contrast (90%) and the middle interval contained a low-contrast (10%) drifting sine grating. In other blocks the first and last intervals contained a low-contrast (10%) grating and the middle interval was occupied by a high-contrast (90%) grating. Two intermediate-contrast (50%) intervals, in positions 2 and 4, were the test intervals. Subjects reported which of the two 50% contrast intervals lasted longer. The duration of one of the two intermediate contrast intervals was varied over trials to generate a psychometric function. The point of subjective equality provided a measure of relative perceived duration. The gratings drifted at 2Hz, 4Hz, 10Hz, and 20Hz in separate blocks. On each trial the stimulus location varied within an annulus centred on fixation to avoid slow adaption. The adaption intervals were 1.5 seconds and the standard test interval was 500ms. We found an apparent temporal compression of the interval following the high-contrast adapter relative to the low-contrast context, but only for high (10 or 20-Hz) temporal frequencies. No similar change in temporal perception occurred when stimuli with equiluminant chromatic contrast were used, confirming our prediction that adaptation-based temporal compression is based on magnocellular adaptation.

The inferior parietal cortex has been identified as an area that may be specialized for temporal processing (Battelli, Pascual-Leone, and Cavanagh, 2007). Leon and Shadlen (2003) and Janssen and Shadlen (2005) have shown that in the lateral intraparietal region of the primate brain, some neurons' firing rates increase over time consistent with the probability that the primate will make an eye-movement response to a location within its receptive field (Goldberg et al., 2006). It is clear from this work that these neurons reflect the likelihood that the animal will respond and this likelihood varies over time. However, it does not necessarily indicate that the parietal lobe is specialized for time perception, just that it has access to an accurate time signal, which modulates the likelihood of a response. A similar time-dependent change of firing rate can be observed in neurons in rat V1 (Shuler and Bear, 2006) prior to the administration of a reward, and in V4 cells during the allocation of attention to detect an orientation change (Ghose and Maunsell, 2002). Therefore, temporal dependence in neural firing is not specific to the eye-movement system in the lateral intraparietal cortex.

However, Morrone, Ross, and Burr (2005) report that perceived time, like perceived space (Ross et al., 2001) appears compressed around the time of a saccade (Morrone and Burr, Chapter 13, this volume). Morrone and Burr asked subjects to report the duration of the interval defined by the presentation of two bars, one above and one below the point of fixation. These green flanking bars were equiluminant with a central red background, to reduce the sense of apparent motion that might otherwise be induced by the temporally offset presentation and to ensure the temporal impulse response triggered by onset or offset would be monophasic. A 'test' stimulus was presented just before the saccade, and was compared against a test pattern presented 2 seconds after the saccade. The duration of the test stimulus was 100ms, and the comparison stimulus varied in duration around 100ms from trial to trial. Subjects reported which interval lasted longer. They found that, when test stimulus was presented 50–100ms before saccade onset, a 50-ms comparison stimulus appeared to match the duration of the 100-ms test stimulus. The effect disappeared when the test stimulus was presented 200ms or more before the saccade. Interestingly the precision of the judgement, measured by the slope of the psychometric function, also increased with compression. They did not find any compression for auditory intervals presented just before a saccade, which was taken as evidence that this is a purely visual effect. When asked to report the temporal order of bars presented 20–75ms prior to the saccade, the order appeared reversed. This occurred for small temporal separations of 20–70ms, but not for longer ones (over 75ms).

Temporal compression around saccades may relate to magnocellular suppression. Terao and colleagues (2008) used the same interval-duration discrimination task as Morrone and Burr (Morrone et al., 2005), but instead of introducing a saccade they presented the flanking bars within a sequence of high-frequency random dynamic luminance flicker. They also found that the interval defined by the two bars appeared compressed. Thus the saccade itself is not essential to compression and therefore compression cannot uniquely be identified with remapping of receptive fields around the time of the saccade. Terao and colleagues suggested that both the high-frequency flicker and the saccade may result in magnocellular suppression (Johnston et al., 2006). Magnocellular suppression may be the key factor in compression, but this does not provide a ready explanation for the reversal of temporal order. Kitazawa and colleagues (2007) report a less complete reversal of temporal order prior to a saccade and also, surprisingly, that tactile temporal order can reverse just before a saccade prompting a multisensory explanation for the effect.

The study by Johnston and colleagues (2006) measured adaptation with the visual fixation held constant; therefore it was impossible to say whether the adaptation-induced time compression was retinotopic or spatiotopic. Burr, Tozzi, and Morrone (2007) investigated this issue by changing fixation between adaptation and test (Morrone and Burr, Chapter 13, this volume). After adapting part of the upper right portion of the visual field, fixation is shifted to the right. The test pattern can then be presented at the same retinal location as the adapter or at the same location in head-centred space or at another position (in the lower left field) that remained unadapted. They compared apparent duration of an interval of flicker in the upper field with one in the lower field that was unaffected by adaptation. They reported that when changes in apparent frequency were compensated, by changing the temporal frequency of the comparison, there was no retinotopic effect but there was a clear spatiotopic effect. The presence of a spatiotopic effect was taken as evidence of the involvement of parietal mechanisms involved in coordinate transformation between retinal and head-centred spatial representations required to maintain the sense of a stable world under saccadic eye movements.

Since we previously found that compensation for changes in temporal frequency made little difference to the amount of apparent time compression, the lack of a retinotopic effect in the Burr ct al. (2007) paradigm was surprising. Adaptation-based compression can be demonstrated for stimuli matched in apparent temporal frequency, when the adaptor and test are of the same temporal frequency (10Hz) (Johnston et al., 2006), and when 20-Hz and 5-Hz adapters are interleaved with a duty cycle chosen to eliminate any effects of adaptation on the apparent temporal frequency of the test (Bruno et al., 2008). We therefore adapted a region of the retina, with mixed adapters, while tracking a fixation spot with the eye. This meant that many spatiotopic locations (across the whole screen) were adapted for only a very short time, while the retinal location was adapted to the same degree as in the standard paradigm. We found a robust time-compression effect indicating that there is indeed a significant retinotopic component to adaptation-based time compression without any change in apparent temporal frequency (Bruno et al., 2008). Motion-based adaptation effects tend to be only weakly modulated by gaze direction (Nishida et al., 2003). We were unable to find any significant spatiotopic component to adaptation-based time compression using two different paradigms, one resembling the method used by Nishida and colleagues (2003) and one resembling the method used by Burr and colleagues (2007). It is not clear at present why we have this discrepancy, but craniotopic effects may be more fragile that the retinotopic effect.

The application of transcranial magnetic stimulation (TMS) over the right inferior parietal cortex (IPC) has been shown to degrade temporal duration discrimination both for visual and auditory modalites (Bueti, Bahrami, and Walsh, 2008). TMS applied over the left V5/MT degraded duration discrimination but only for visual stimuli. There was no change in perceived duration in any other site (left IPC, vertex) stimulated. TMS over V5/MT was equally effective for intervals defined by moving or static patterns, which was interpreted as indicating that TMS added noise to the encoding of the onset and offset of the patterns. Interestingly patients with lesions in the right inferior parietal lobe have problems individuating items resented in a rapid sequence (Battelli et al., 2007). In an experiment in which subjects had to identify one of six spots flickering in opposite phase to the others, controls and left parietal patients could succeed with temporal frequencies of up to 7Hz, whereas right parietal patients' temporal frequency limit was around 3Hz (Battelli et al., 2003, 2007). Battelli and colleagues identify the inferior parietal lobule as part of the 'when' pathway, which computes temporal order. Although the perception of temporal order differs from other temporal properties such as duration, it seems possible that the inferior parietal lobule may be the locus of visual routines for processes that are necessary for individuation and analysis of temporal events. However, we have also seen that low-level magnocellular processes contribute to duration perception. How can we link low-level magnocellular adaptation to duration perception?

A content-dependent clock

The 'stopwatch model' proposes a content-independent clock, which is regulated according to the current arousal or attentive state of the observer. However, to explain how time perception might depend upon the content of the visual stimulus, we need to consider how to construct a content-dependent clock. Simply adding up events will not give a good estimate of duration in general since events can be temporally dense or sparse. Here a content-dependent version of the stopwatch model is proposed.

It is likely that time processing uses the same early temporal mechanisms required for temporal change and motion processing. The general consensus is that there is evidence for two or perhaps three temporal filters in human vision. These temporal filters describe how the visual system integrates the luminance signal over time. They can be thought of as temporal weighting functions that are entirely analogous to a neuron's spatial receptive field. Just like spatial receptive fields, temporal receptive fields can come in different forms. The forms of the temporal filters for human vision were measured psychophysically by Hess and Snowden (1992). Johnston and Clifford (1995) showed they were well fitted by a Gaussian curve in log time and its first and second derivatives (Figure 14.1C). It is worth noting here that all three filters are fitted to Hess and Snowden's contrast sensitivity data by setting the point at which the log Gaussian peaks and adjusting one parameter (the spread of the filter). The form of the three filters is fully determined by the process of differentiation, i.e. once the parameter setting for the log Gaussian is chosen, the

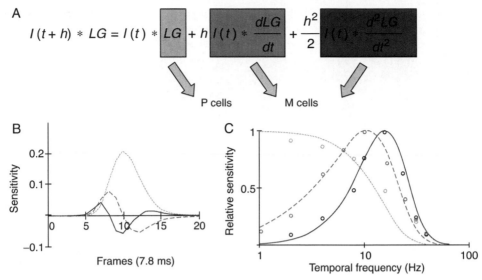

Fig. 14.1 (See also Pate 5) A) Taylor's series can be used to predict the value of a function (the image brightness, $I(t)$), in the neighbourhood around a point, in time, t. Temporal derivatives of the image brightness are calculated at a point, t, by convolving ($*$) the image brightness with the derivatives of Gaussians in log time. Throughout the figures dotted line indicates the temporal blur kernel (the log Gaussian, LG), dashed line indicates the first derivative and solid grey line indicates the second derivative of the log Gaussian. The excursion parameter, h, indicates the point $(t+h)$ at which the value of the function is to be predicted. The parameter, h, can take on a range of values. B) The temporal tuning functions for human vision. The data are from Hess and Snowden (1992) and the fitted functions, the Gaussian in log time (dotted line) and its first (dashed line) and second (solid grey line) derivatives, are from Johnston and Clifford (1995). All data for each of the three functions are fitted by adjusting just one parameter (see Johnston and Clifford, 1995, for details). The band-pass filters (dashed and solid grey lines) correspond to the tuning curves of magnocellular neurons and the low-pass temporal filter (dotted line) is representative of parvocellular neuron's temporal tuning curves C) The impulse responses for the filters, calculated as the inverse Fourier transform of the corresponding (matching line-style) frequency sensitivity curves in B.

other two filters are found by calculating the first and second derivative and normalizing. The zero-order filter is normalized to sum to 1.0.[4]

Temporal differentiation can be accomplished by convolving a temporal signal with the temporal differentiating filters. This simultaneously blurs and differentiates the signal. The zero-order filter has the low-pass temporal property characteristic of parvocellular neurons. The derivative filters have the band-pass property associated with magnocellular neurons (Figure 14.1B and C). The relationship between the temporal impulse response and the frequency response of the filters is shown in Figure 14.1B and C.

---

[4] For reference the zero order filter is:

$$LG = \left(\sqrt{\pi}\,\tau\alpha e^{\frac{t^2}{4}}\right)^{-1} e^{-\left(\frac{\ln\left(\frac{t}{\alpha}\right)}{\tau}\right)^2},$$

where t is time, α is the time at which the filter peaks and τ is the spread of the filter.

Johnston and colleagues (2006) found that adaptation to the temporal frequency of sinusoidal flicker could alter perceived temporal frequency as well as duration. For sine functions, temporal frequency can be recovered from the ratio of band-pass to low-pass filters (Smith and Edgar, 1990). It is in fact simplest to use the zero-order and second-derivative filters since their outputs have the same phase and the ratio only depends upon frequency, ω.

$$I(t) = \sin(\omega t),$$

$$\frac{dI(t)}{dt} = \omega \cos(\omega t) \text{ and}$$

$$\frac{d^2 I(t)}{dt^2} = -\omega^2 \sin(\omega t).$$

We can explain the change in apparent temporal frequency with adaptation by referring to Figure 14.1C. The low-pass (dotted line) and second band-pass (solid line) filters cross over at about 10Hz. After adapting to 20Hz the band-pass filter will be reduced in sensitivity. After adaptation, 10-Hz stimulation will give a larger response in the low-pass channel—the signature of a lower than 10-Hz temporal frequency. The opposite change will arise after adaptation at lower frequencies. Since changes in perceived duration can be dissociated from changes in perceived temporal frequency, we cannot use the same mechanism to explain changes in apparent duration. Changing the filter characteristics cannot of itself generate time compression or dilation since changing the temporal scale can only increase or decrease the temporal blur, which for a sine wave simply changes the signal amplitude, and shifting the peak of the zero-order filter can only change the temporal phase of the output. We previously linked time compression to the sharpening of the temporal impulse response (Johnston et al., 2006). Here we describe how sharpening of the temporal impulse of temporal differentiating filters can generate compression in a content-dependent clock.

One can exploit the derivative properties of the temporal filters (Figure 14.1) to construct a Taylor-series approximation (Figure 14.1A) of the image brightness. The Taylor series allows the reconstruction of a function from a sum of terms based on the derivatives of the function at a point. The advantage of this procedure for biological vision is that it extends the representation of visual information to before and after the immediate present. The visual system can also use it as a simple way of predicting forwards (or backwards) in time. The parameter, h, in the Taylor series determines the direction and amount of predicted displacement. We can substitute a range for h, instead of an instantaneous value, to predict a displaced temporal sequence (Figure 14.2B). This construction would allow a forward or reverse prediction of the image brightness though time. Spatial differentiating filters allow the same trick to be played in the spatial domain.

We can now build a content-sensitive clock in the following way (Figure 14.2A). First, predict the current image brightness sequence forward for, let's say, 30ms using the magnocellular signal and store it in a temporal buffer. Next, cross-correlate the current parvocellular-based sequence with the stored sequence. The new input has to be filtered by the zero-order kernel otherwise the phase of the signal will be quite different from the stored signal. After 30ms of comparing prediction and input, the cross-correlation should peak and, at that point we determine that 30ms has passed and reset the prediction. The number of 30-ms resettings, which we could think of as clock ticks, are then accumulated as in the standard stopwatch model until the stimulus has completed, at which point the stimulus duration is read out. Note that the parameter that determines the time shift is 'h', which only multiplies the magnocellular outputs. The magnocellular pathway controls the temporal prediction.

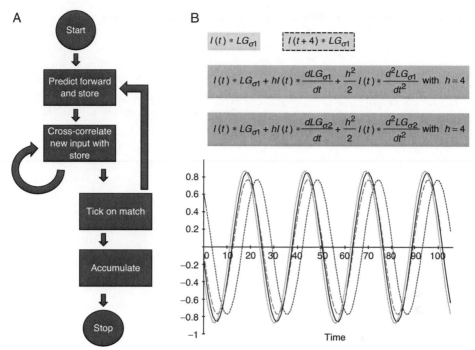

Fig. 14.2 (See also Plate 7) A) A content-dependent clock. The free-running pacemaker from the standard clock model is replaced with a 'predict and compare' circuit. The Taylor series is used to predict an image-based temporal sequence at some future time at a point or region in space. This forward prediction is stored. The new input is cross-correlated with the stored data in a temporal buffer. When the cross-correlation peaks, the clock ticks, the tick is accumulated, and the prediction is reset. The interval over which the prediction is made could vary, and if it does vary, the number of ticks may be scaled by the length of the interval over which the prediction is made (e.g. 10 × 30-ms ticks). B) The dotted line is the profile of a filtered (by the log Gaussian) sine function. The dashed line is the dotted line time shifted forward by 4 temporal units. The solid black line is the prediction constructed from the Taylor expansion. The predicted signal is slightly increased in amplitude at this frequency, however the temporal shift is quite accurate. The solid grey line is the prediction, with a sharpened temporal impulse response in the M cell filters, as a response to temporal adaptation. The advance in the filter leads to a phase advance in the derivative functions, which would have the same effect as predicting forward with a larger excursion parameter.

Only magnocellular neurons show significant adaptation to contrast. However, changes in magnocellular sensitivity after adaptation cannot explain time compression. A relatively lower magnocellular signal, as a result of adaptation, would have the same effect as a smaller value of the excursion parameter, h, leading to more resetting, more ticks, and a longer duration. A higher magnocellular signal should lead to compression. Thus, an analysis based on sensitivity appears to provide a prediction that is opposite to our observations.

However, we have argued that an account based on filter sensitivity needs to be reserved for the explanation of changes in apparent temporal frequency. A change in sensitivity is just one aspect of contrast-gain control, the other is that the phase of signals carried by magnocellular neurons are advanced though adaptation (Benardete and Kaplan, 1999). This phase shift is seen in magnocellular but not parvocellular neurons (Benardete and Kaplan, 1999). This phase shift will shift the predicted sine wave forward in time, which is equivalent to having a larger h parameter. This should lead to resetting after a longer delay, leading to fewer ticks, and therefore time compression. The greater the magnocellular phase advance relative to the parvocellular phase, the greater the time compression. Although this forward model, or 'predict and compare' strategy, could be applied generally to time perception, in the current context the key theoretical elements that link duration perception to the magnocellular pathway are the identification of a role for the magnocellular system in generating a forward prediction through a Taylor expansion, the recognition of the role of magnocellular cells as temporal differentiators, which is also central to their role in motion computation (Johnston, McOwan, and Benton, 1999, 2003; Johnston, McOwan, and Buxton, 1992), the magnocellular system's greater sensitivity to adaptation in comparison to the parvocellular system, the dual change in sensitivity and sharpening of the impulse response, and, specifically, the phase advance caused by the shortening of the temporal impulse response as a result of temporal frequency adaptation and contrast gain control.

The proposal of a content-dependent clock, one in which the pacemaker tick depends on there being variation in contrast in the field, is subject to criticism that time perception would be impossible with one's eyes shut or when there is no change in the visual field. If a content-independent clock is necessary, a content-dependent clock would appear to be redundant. However, the proposal is that there are many clocks that could work on a 'predict and compare' strategy. The evidence from functional imaging is that temporal judgements involve a network of sensory and motor areas. Indeed it may be that there are no purely abstract temporal areas and all temporal processing piggybacks on to sensory-motor and cognitive systems. Counting can be seen in this context as a prediction to say the word 'one' in 1 second. When the mental act matches the forward model, one second has elapsed.

References

Ayhan, İ., Bruno, A., and Johnston, A. (2008). Adaptation induced temporal compression is highly space specific. *J Vision*, **8**(6), 480.

Baccus, S. A. and Meister, M. (2002). Fast and slow contrast adaptation in retinal circuitry. *Neuron*, **36**(5), 909–19.

Battelli, L., Cavanagh, P., Martini, P., and Barton, J. J. (2003). Bilateral deficits of transient visual attention in right parietal patients. *Brain*, **126**(10), 2164–74.

Battelli, L., Pascual-Leone, A., and Cavanagh, P. (2007). The 'when' pathway of the right parietal lobe. *Trends Cogn Sci*, **11**(5), 204–10.

Benardete, E. A. and Kaplan, E. (1999). The dynamics of primate M retinal ganglion cells. *Vis Neurosci*, **16**(2), 355–68.

Brown, J. F. (1931). On time perception in visual movement fields. *Psychologische Forschung*, **14**, 233–48.

Brown, S. W. (1995). Time, change, and motion: the effects of stimulus movement on temporal perception. *Percept Psychophys*, **57**(1), 105–16.

Bruno, A. and Johnston, A. (2007). Contrast gain changes affect the perceived duration of visual stimuli. *J Vision*, **7**(9), 376a.

Bruno, A., Ayhan, İ., and Johnston, A. (2008). Retinotopic adaptation can influence the apparent duration of a visual stimulus. *J Vis*, **8**(6), 364a.

Bueti, D., Bahrami, B., and Walsh, V. (2008). Sensory and association cortex in time perception. *J Cogn Neurosci*, **20**(6), 1054–62.

Buhusi, C. V., and Meck, W. H. (2005). What makes us tick? Functional and neural mechanisms of interval timing. *Nat Rev Neurosci*, **6**(10), 755–65.

Burr, D., Tozzi, A., and Morrone, M. C. (2007). Neural mechanisms for timing visual events are spatially selective in real-world coordinates. *Nat Neurosci*, **10**(4), 423–5.

Chander, D. and Chichilnisky, E. J. (2001). Adaptation to temporal contrast in primate and salamander retina. *J Neurosci,* **21**(24), 9904–16.

Creelman, C. (1962). Human discrimination of auditory duration. *J Acoust Soc Am,* **34**, 582–93.

Droit-Volet, S. and Wearden, J. (2002). Speeding up an internal clock in children? Effects of visual flicker on subjective duration. *Q J Exp Psychol B,* **55**(3), 193–211.

Fraisse, P. (1963). *The Psychology of Time.* New York: Harper and Row.

Fraisse, P. (1984). Perception and estimation of time. *Annu Rev Psychol,* **35**, 1–36.

Ghose, G. M. and Maunsell, J. H. (2002). Attentional modulation in visual cortex depends on task timing. *Nature,* **419**(6907), 616–20.

Goldberg, M. E., Bisley, J. W., Powell, K. D., and Gottlieb, J. (2006). Saccades, salience and attention: the role of the lateral intraparietal area in visual behavior. *Prog Brain Res,* **155**, 157–75.

Hawken, M. J., Shapley, R. M., and Grosof, D. H. (1996). Temporal-frequency selectivity in monkey visual cortex. *Vis Neurosci,* **13**(3), 477–92.

Hess, R. F. and Snowden, R. J. (1992). Temporal properties of human visual filters: number, shapes and spatial covariation. *Vision Res,* **32**, 47–60.

Janssen, P. and Shadlen, M. N. (2005). A representation of the hazard rate of elapsed time in macaque area LIP. *Nature Neuroscience,* **8**(2), 234–41.

Johnston, A. and Clifford, C. W. (1995). A unified account of three apparent motion illusions. *Vision Res,* **35**(8), 1109–23.

Johnston, A., Arnold, D. H., and Nishida, S. (2003). The effects of temporal adaptation on the perception of flicker duration. *Perception,* **32**, 46–7.

Johnston, A., Arnold, D. H., and Nishida, S. (2006). Spatially localized distortions of event time. *Curr Biol,* **16**(5), 472–9.

Johnston, A., McOwan, P. W., and Benton, C. P. (1999). Robust velocity computation from a biologically motivated model of motion perception. *Proc R Soc Lond B,* **266**, 509–18.

Johnston, A., McOwan, P. W., and Benton, C. P. (2003). Biological computation of image motion from flows over boundaries. *J Physiol Paris,* **97**(2–3), 325–34.

Johnston, A., McOwan, P. W., and Buxton, H. (1992). A computational model of the analysis of some first-order and second-order motion patterns by simple and complex cells. *Proc R Soc Lond B,* **250**, 297–306.

Johnston, A., Bruno, A., Watanabe, J., Quansah, B., Patel, N., Dakin, S., et al. (2008). Visually-based temporal distortion in dyslexia. *Vision Res,* **48**(17), 1852–8.

Julesz, B. (1971). *Foundation of Cyclopean Perception.* Chicago: The University of Chicago Press.

Kanai, R., Paffen, C. L. E., Hogendoorn, H., and Verstraten, F. A. J. (2006). Time dilation in dynamic visual display. *J Vis,* **6**(12), 1421–30.

Kitazawa, S., Moizumi, S., Okuzumi, A., Saito, F., Shibuya, S., Takahashi, T., et al. (2007). Reversal od subjective temporal order due to sensory and motor interactions. In P. Haggard, M. Kawato, and Y. Rosetti (Eds.) *Attention and Performance XXII.* Oxford: Oxford University Press.

Leon, M. I. and Shadlen, M. N. (2003). Representation of time by neurons in the posterior parietal cortex of the macaque. *Neuron,* **38**(2), 317–27.

Mante, V., Bonin, V., and Carandini, M. (2008). Functional mechanisms shaping lateral geniculate responses to artificial and natural stimuli. *Neuron,* **58**(4), 625–38.

Morgan, M. J., Giora, E., and Solomon, J. A. (2008). A single "stopwatch" for duration estimation, a single "ruler" for size. *J Vis,* **8**(2), 14.11–18.

Morrone, M. C., Ross, J., and Burr, D. (2005). Saccadic eye movements cause compression of time as well as space. *Nat Neurosci,* **8**(7), 950–4.

Nishida, S. and Johnston, A. (2010). Time marker theory of cross-channel temporal binding. In R. Nijhawan and B. Khurana (Eds.) *Problems of Space and Time in Perception and Action.* Cambridge: Cambridge University Press.

Nishida, S., Motoyoshi, I., Andersen, R. A., and Shimojo, S. (2003). Gaze modulation of visual aftereffects. *Vision Res,* **43**(6), 639–49.

Nobre, A. C. and O'Reilly, J. (2004). Time is of the essence. *Trends Cogn Sci,* **8**(9), 387–9.

Ross, J., Morrone, C. M., Goldberg, M. E., and Burr, D. C. (2001). Changes in visual perception at the time of saccades. *Trends Neurosci,* **24**(2), 113–21.

Shapley, R. M. and Victor, J. D. (1978). The effect of contrast on the transfer properties of cat retinal ganglion cells. *J Physiol,* **285**, 275–98.

Shuler, M. G. and Bear, M. F. (2006). Reward timing in the primary visual cortex. *Science,* **311**(5767), 1606–9.

Smith, A. T. and Edgar, G. K. (1990). The influence of spatial frequency on percieved temporal frequency and percieved speed. *Vision Res,* **30**, 1467–74.

Solomon, S. G., Peirce, J. W., Dhruv, N. T., and Lennie, P. (2004). Profound contrast adaptation early in the visual pathway. *Neuron,* **42**(1), 155–62.

Stetson, C., Fiesta, M. P., and Eagleman, D. M. (2007). Does time really slow down during a frightening event? *PLoS ONE,* **2**(12), e1295.

Taatgen, N. A., van Rijn, H., and Anderson, J. (2007). An integrated theory of prospective time interval estimation: the role of cognition, attention, and learning. *Psychol Rev,* **114**(3), 577–98.

Terao, M., Watanabe, J., Yagi, A., and Nishida, S. (2008). Reduction of stimulus visibility compresses apparent time intervals. *Nat Neurosci,* **11**(5), 541–2.

Thomas, E. A. C. and Weaver, W. B. (1975). Cognitive processing and time perception. *Percept Psychophys,* **17**(4), 363–7.

Treisman, M. (1963). Temporal discrimination and the indifference interval. Implications for a model of the "internal clock". *Psychol Monogr,* **77**(13), 1–31.

Treisman, M., Faulkner, A., Naish, P. L., and Brogan, D. (1990). The internal clock: evidence for a temporal oscillator underlying time perception with some estimates of its characteristic frequency. *Perception,* **19**(6), 705–43.

Tse, P. U., Intriligator, J., Rivest, J., and Cavanagh, P. (2004). Attention and the subjective expansion of time. *Percept Psychophys,* **66**(7), 1171–89.

Wearden, J. H. (1999). "Beyond the fields we know . . . ": exploring and developing scalar timing theory. *Behav Process,* **45**(1–3), 3–21.

Wearden, J. H. and Penton-Voak, I. S. (1995). Feeling the heat: body temperature and the rate of subjective time, revisited. *Q J Exp Psychol B,* **48**(2), 129–41.

Wearden, J. H., Philpott, K., and Win, T. (1999). Speeding up and (. . . relatively . . .) slowing down an internal clock in humans. *Behav Process,* **46**(1), 63–73.

Acknowledgement

I would like to thank the Leverhulme Trust for financial support.

Chapter 15

Temporal binding

Marc J. Buehner

'What's the time, Ireneo?'
Without looking up, without stopping, Ireneo replied: 'In ten minutes
it will be eight o'clock...'
Jorge Luis Borges: Funes, the Memorious (*Ficciones Part Two*)

Borges' fictional character Funes the Memorious is often cited in introductions to cognitive science as an example of how useful it is to have categories and abstract thought. For Ireneo Funes had infallible perception and memory, yet, according to the narrator in Borges' story 'was not very capable of thought'. Funes would recall everything that occurred to him, everything he heard or read with absolute detail, but with no abstraction whatsoever. Not only that, but he felt the need to keep these impressions distinct and separated in his memory. He rejected generic terms like *dog* because so many different kinds of dogs of varying sizes, form, and colour could not, according to Funes, possibly all be designated the same. What's more, Funes felt 'disturbed by the fact that a dog at 3:14 pm (seen in profile) should have the same name as the dog at 3:15 pm (seen from the front)'.

This latter part of Funes' ability (or affliction) reflects an absence of object constancy—the automatic understanding that objects remain constant despite variations in the retinal image—or, more generally, undue attention to the proximal stimulus, combined with a failure to register the distal stimulus. Borges' illustrations of Funes' fixation on specific instances is limited to singular events, but we can extrapolate that Funes would have likewise lacked the ability to appreciate generic *event sequences*; getting ready for bed (brushing his teeth, undressing etc.) would—to Funes—be a completely new and different experience every day. Most of us, however, exploit routine and similarity to construct an event schema or script, which we use to recognize, plan, and execute meaningful event sequences (for the classic reference see Schank and Abelson, 1977). An important component of such event scripts or schemata is the temporal position and order (see Spence, Chapter 7, this volume) of component events. In Schank and Abelson's well cited restaurant script, for instance, one does not order food before sitting down, pay before one has eaten, and starters always come before main courses. In addition to order, the temporal spacing between events is also important: In the restaurant example, if we had to wait more than one hour for our starters after ordering, we would recognize that something is amiss. More generally, the time elapsing between individual events often serves as a useful guide to inform us whether they belong together: We understand that thunder follows lightning *within a given timeframe* but would not attribute rumbling noises we hear today to lighting we observed yesterday.

This chapter is concerned with our ability to group together events occurring over time and to recognize that they belong together, a facility to appreciate—unlike Funes—that not all occurrences are isolated experiences on their own, but that some go together with others that happen later on or have already taken place earlier. This grouping together of separate events occurring at different time points into one coherent and meaningful event *sequence* is what *temporal binding* is all about, although the phrase most often refers only to the sensory consequences that come as a result of binding (which I shall discuss in more detail later on). The hypothesis to be explored is that binding is a two-way street that serves to resolve mutual ambiguities: Not only are things that occur in close temporal succession good candidates for belonging together, but things that belong together might also be good candidates for occurring in close temporal succession.

Resolving ambiguities in event and time perception

But what are the ambiguities that need to be resolved? In the first instance—event segmentation—it is obvious that our perceptual input is not carved into semantically meaningful units *a priori*. As Funes' example shows, the world is a continuous flux of events, and the art of abstraction is to detect meaningful patterns, recognize the invariants, and ignore irrelevant detail; in short, to come up with a stable yet flexible representation of events. Recent theoretical developments (Zacks et al., 2007) suggest that the process of discretizing the event stream into meaningful units recruits both lower level perceptual processes and higher level cognitive resources, such as event models and schemata. Moreover, event segmentation can occur at various levels of granularity, depending on the task demands: taking a plate, washing it, rinsing it, and putting it in the draining rack can be parsed either at the level of the various subunits just described, as one event (washing plates), or even as one subunit of a larger event (washing plates before moving on to pots and pans). The event-prediction model proposed by Zacks and colleagues specifies that event boundaries are most likely driven by prediction errors: while affairs are fairly predictable (by a currently active event model), the event is perceived to be ongoing; once the evidence deviates from what is expected, prediction errors occur, and an event boundary will be identified, which in turn will lead to the activation of a new event model.

Predictability therefore plays a fundamental role in event segmentation. One of the key concepts that licenses prediction and explanation is causality: if we know what causes what, we can utilize this information to forecast what is to come, why it is happening, and what to do if things turn out unexpectedly. How exactly we can know that one thing causes another is of course no trivial matter. Just as we cannot perceive event boundaries directly, we do not perceive causality directly (cf. Buehner and Cheng, 2005); both have to be inferred from available evidence, though the inference may frequently be spontaneous and automatic. In the case of causality, cognitive science still draws upon David Hume's (1739/1888) tenets: causal beliefs are formed in the mind based on three empirical cues—temporal priority, constant conjunction, and contiguity in space and time. In other words, the cause has to precede the effect, it should produce the effect regularly, and, if it does so, it should happen soon after and close by. There are of course exceptions to these principles, where people can recognize causal relations over long temporal distances, but this typically requires more cognitive processing power (see Buehner and May, 2002, 2003), and consequently immediate cause–effect pairings are generally privileged. In short, people are good at recognizing a causal connection between events that follow one another regularly and immediately. Temporal contiguity therefore promotes the recognition of a causal connection, which in turn may aid event segmentation.

The second ambiguity to be resolved by temporal binding—perception of temporal intervals—is equally compelling. It is self evident that the perception and evaluation of temporal intervals is inherently ambiguous. We don't have a sensory modality dedicated to perceive time.

Consequently, time 'perception' always requires computation and indeed comparison relative to some reference standard held in memory. As with all perceptual processes, there is a component of error and noise in the system. According to a Bayesian account of perception (cf. also Kersten et al., 2004) ambiguities in the input can be resolved by probabilistic integration of perceptual properties with prior knowledge. For time perception this means that higher-level knowledge about which things 'go together' would bias impressions of temporal distance, such that the same objective interval would subjectively appear shorter if its constituent events are related than if they are not. Causality again might play a decisive role here. Not only is it a key concept that licenses prediction (see earlier), it also is a powerful tool that links things together (there is a reason why Mackie, 1974 referred to causation as 'the cement of the universe'). Thus, events marked by a causal relationship might appear closer in time than events not marked this way (Eagleman and Holcombe, 2002).

Evidence of temporal binding in action-outcome learning

Evidence for ambiguity resolution via temporal binding has only been reported fairly recently, but the field has been very active since, trying to pinpoint exactly when binding occurs, and what its determinants are. The majority of research in this area comes from Patrick Haggard and colleagues. Haggard, Clark, and Kalogeras (2002b, see also Haggard et al., 2002a) used the Libet clock paradigm (Libet et al., 1983) to assess temporal binding. In this paradigm, participants are looking at a standard 12-figure clock face containing only one hand, which completes a full rotation every 2.56s. Their task is to report the position of the clock hand when certain things happen (Figure 15.1). Haggard, Clark, and Kalogeras firstly established baseline measures by asking participants to report (on separate trials) the position of the hand when they heard a tone, and when they pressed a key. In the latter case, participants were instructed to press whenever they felt like it, and to avoid trying to press at predetermined clock hand positions. The reported times of when participants felt they executed the action or heard the tone were compared to the actual times to obtain a baseline measure of judgement error or accuracy. Of central interest, however, were the operant conditions, in which a participant's action was followed by a tone 250ms later. On these trials, participants were cued to report the subjective time of *either* their action or the consequent tone (it would not have been feasible to report both). Haggard, Clark, and Kalogeras found that subjective perception of action and tone had shifted towards one another, relative to baseline. More specifically, operant actions were perceived to have occurred later than their baseline equivalents, while consequent tones were perceived to have occurred earlier than baseline tones. Two control conditions suggested that this temporal-attraction effect requires that the first marker of the inter-event interval is a voluntary action: no attraction was found between an involuntary muscle twitch (induced via transcranial magnetic stimulation [TMS] of the motor cortex) and a subsequent tone. Instead, in this case there was a repulsion effect, so that the twitch and tone were respectively perceived earlier and later relative to baseline. A third condition linked a sham TMS (in other words a simple click noise) with a subsequent tone, and judgements of both events were accurate with respect to baseline.

An additional experiment, which considered the subjective time of a tone only (brought about by an earlier keypress as before), investigated the extent of the binding effect in relation to the temporal interval between action and outcome. Haggard, Clark, and Kalogeras (2002) considered intervals of 250ms, 450ms, and 650ms, and found that the size of the binding effect decreased as the action-outcome interval increased. Furthermore, the effect was strongest when the interval was kept constant over repeated trials; it decreased or disappeared when the three intervals were presented in random alteration over trials. Haggard, Clark, and Kalogeras (2002) concluded that

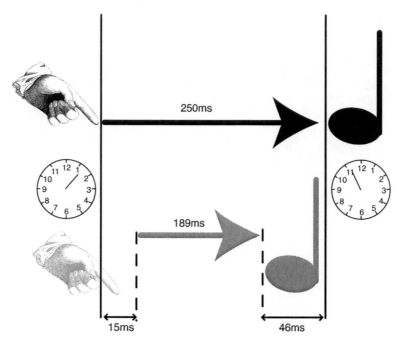

Fig. 15.1 A schematic depiction of the temporal attraction effect found by Haggard, Clark and Kalogeras (2002) using the Libet clock paradigm: key presses are followed by tones after an interval (here 250ms). Participants report (on separate trials) the subjective timestamps of their actions and the tones by reporting the position of a fast-moving clock hand. Comparing these timestamps to baseline judgement error (derived from single-event trials involving only actions not followed by tones, or tones not preceded by actions) reveals that subjective awareness of actions and outcomes are shifted together in time. For the 250ms example, awareness of the action is delayed by 15ms, and awareness of the tone is advanced by 46ms. Combining these two shifts suggests that the subjective interval between action and outcome is 189ms. Note that perception of the interval is not directly measured.

'the brain contains a specific cognitive module that binds intentional actions to their effects to construct a coherent conscious experience of our own agency.' (p.385). Presumably, the purpose of this intentional, or efferent, binding is to strengthen the association between our actions and their consequences (see also Haggard et al., 2002a), or, to return to Funes, to facilitate the construction of meaningful mental representations of event structures. Importantly, Haggard, Clark, and Kalogeras also pointed out two limitations of this effect, which parallel general constraints of associationism: firstly, temporal attraction was modulated by temporal contiguity—the amount of perceptual shifts decreased as the action-outcome interval increased. Secondly, the strength of the effect critically relied on the predictability of the interval. These findings illustrate the hypothesized two-way structure of temporal binding: If an action repeatedly and reliably produces an outcome, and does so with good contiguity, then a strong association between action and outcome is formed (in line with Hume's principles of association and causation). At the same time, once this association has taken place, the temporal interval between action and outcome subjectively shortens, which in turn would further strengthen the action-outcome association.

Predictability modulates the extent of binding not only with respect to whether the action-outcome interval can be anticipated, but also with respect to how frequently the action produces the effect. Engbert and Wohlschläger (2007) demonstrated that the subjective perception of actions which produced an effect two-thirds of the time was shifted towards the effect when compared to actions which produced the same effect one-third of the time. Critically, this difference was found only when the action genuinely produced the effect. In a control experiment, where the computer instigated both a passive movement of the finger, and the subsequent tone, perception of when the passive movement occurred remained stable regardless of whether it was followed by the tone two-thirds or one-third of the time. This indicates that predictability on its own is not sufficient to elicit temporal binding; what matters is that a meaningful relation (such as that between action and outcome) is at the heart of the predictability.

Moore and Haggard (2007) examined the role of predictability even further. They reported an experiment where an action produced a tone after 250ms either 75% or 50% of the time. Critically, they examined the subjective perception of actions that successfully produced the effect (i.e. were followed by it) separately from actions that failed to produce the effect. Interestingly, the extent to which subjective perception of the action was shifted towards the tone was identical on trials where the action produced the tone, regardless of whether—in general—actions produced the effect 50% or 75% of the time. In other words, no matter how reliably the action produced the tone, if it did so, awareness of this action was shifted in time towards the effect by the same amount for both the 50% and 75% condition. In contrast, the shift on unsuccessful trials (i.e. those where the action was not followed by the tone) differed between the 50% and 75% conditions, such that action awareness in the latter case was delayed to a larger extent than in the former case. Moore and Haggard interpreted these results to identify two component processes contributing to temporal binding: A predictive and a postdictive process. When actions reliably produce an effect, a predictive process kicks in, so that subjective perception of the time of an action shifts toward the time of its expected outcome, even when the outcome does not occur. When actions do not reliably produce effects, prediction is poor. Expectations about action outcome are absent or weak, and very little or no binding happens. The postdictive process, in contrast, affects both reliable and unreliable actions. If an action does produce an effect, it will be attracted towards it, regardless of how often effects follow actions.

Intentional or causal binding?

The evidence reviewed so far suggests that temporal binding follows the same constraints that apply to causal learning: the size of the effect is dependent on regularity (how reliable the action produces the outcome) and contiguity (shorter intervals result in more binding). Moreover, mere association is not sufficient for binding to occur—the constituent events have to be linked by a meaningful relation, which, at least in Engbert and Wohlschläger's (2007) case, can best be characterized as one of instrumental causation. Yet, other strands of work have linked the binding effect to slightly different literatures, namely that of intentionality and consciousness.

For instance, in their original study, Haggard, Clark, and Kalogeras (2002) contrasted intentional actions with involuntary (TMS-induced) muscle-twitches. Binding was found in the former, and repulsion in the latter. More importantly, Wohlschläger and collagues (2003) have reported a series of studies, which linked temporal binding to the mirror-neuron system, and thus directly to attribution of intentional action plans. They used the Libet clock paradigm to examine subjective awareness of: (a) self-generated, voluntary key presses; (b) observations of such key presses performed by the experimenter rather than by the participant; and (c) machine actions. All three types of events were always followed by a tone 250ms later. The experimental setup consisted of a lever, which the participant or the experimenter operated in (a) and (b). In (c), the lever was pulled down by a solenoid attached to the lever's fulcrum. The results showed that action awareness was identical in (a) and (b), and that both were different to (c). More specifically, both self-executed actions and observations of these same actions performed by the experimenter were subjectively perceived to occur later (i.e. closer in time to the subsequent tone), compared to machine actions also followed by the tone. Put simply, conditions involving self- and other-generated actions evidenced signs of temporal binding, while conditions involving machine action did not. Wohlschläger and colleagues interpreted these results in light of Dennett's intentional stance, and suggested that the critical difference between self- and other-generated actions relative to machine actions was that the former involved an intentional action plan, which was either available via introspection (in the self-generated action) or via theory of mind (in other-generated action). The absence of such an intentional action plan in the machine (or at least attribution of such a plan to the machine) presumably led to the absence of binding.

There is an alternative interpretation of these results, however, which is more general, and in line with the causal principles outlined at the beginning of this chapter. In Wohlschläger et al.'s (2003) experiments both the self- and other-generated conditions clearly involved a causal relation that would have been obvious to the participant: They were introduced to the experimental setup and learnt that pressing the lever generated the tone. This causal relation was independent of who actually pressed the lever. In the machine action condition, however, the causal relations were less obvious. Participants were instructed that the lever would move automatically, presumably controlled by the computer. This was then followed by the tone, which participants knew was generated by the computer. Thus, whereas the action of pressing down the leaver was necessary in the self and other conditions to generate the tone, it was not in the machine condition. A normative causal analysis of the machine condition suggests that the automatic depression of the lever and the subsequent delivery of the tone were both effects of a common cause—the experimental protocol implemented in the computer. More specifically, the direct causal connection between (automatic) lever press and tone was lost in the machine condition.

Unfortunately, Wohlschläger et al.'s (2003) design conflated manipulations of causal status with the presence of intentionality, such that both a causal and an intentional theory of temporal binding equally explain the results. A similar argument can be made about Haggard, Clark and Kalogeras's (2002) TMS and sham-TMS conditions: in both conditions, it would have been obvious that the computer scheduled both the TMS discharge and the consequent beep, and again no binding would be predicted based on the lack of a causal relation between the two. Thus, the evidence reviewed so far does not allow a disambiguation between the intentional and the causal account of temporal binding.

Note, however, that the causal and intentional accounts are not mutually exclusive. Instead, the causal account of binding is a more general and comprehensive theory, and the intentional account is a special subcategory of it. Every situation that involves intentional actions resulting in real-world consequences is also an instance of a causal relationship. Naturally, however, there are many causal relationships which do not involve intentional action plans (such as those between natural events, or indeed those involving machines). Likewise, intentional actions are often followed by other events, but do not necessarily cause them.

We have recently tried to distinguish the causal and intentional accounts of temporal binding using a novel method based on reaction times rather than Libet clock judgements (see Buehner and Humphreys, 2009). The basic premise was to create an experimental paradigm where intentional actions were always followed by a sensory event (tone), but where the causal relation linking the action to the tone was varied. More specifically, we created a within-subjects design comprising of two conditions that appeared absolutely identical on the surface, and deployed the same actions and stimuli. The critical difference was whether—in a prior training phase—participants had learnt that this action produced the tone. Participants performed a stimulus-anticipation task. They were presented with a Go signal, leading into Target 1, which was followed, after an interval of 500ms, 900ms, or 1300ms, by Target 2. Both Targets were tones. In the non-causal Baseline conditions, participants were first passively exposed to the inter-target interval by listening to the tone sequence. They were then asked to press a key (Response 1) to coincide with Target 1 (which was still followed by Target 2). In the final, experimental phase, they were asked to anticipate both Target 1 and 2 with differential key-presses (Response 1 and 2). In the Causal Control condition, participants first learnt that Response 1 generates Target 2 after the appropriate interval. They were then asked to perform Response 1 in anticipation of Target 1, just as in the Baseline condition. In the final condition, they had to synchronize Response 1 and 2 with Target 1 and 2. Thus, the critical final experimental condition was identical in the Baseline and Causal groups, save the difference that Target 2 occurs automatically as part of the experimental protocol in the former, but is contingent on Response 1 in the latter. Figure 15.2 outlines the basic design.

What would the presence of a causal link between action and outcome mean for the timing of responses? If temporal binding is a function of causality, then Target 2 should be attracted towards Response 1 in the Causal condition. Because we are using Response 2 as a measure of when Target 2 is expected, we would thus predict that participants perform Response 2 earlier (with respect to Target 2) in the Causal relative to the Baseline condition. This is exactly what we found, at all three intervals. Note that from an intentional perspective, Causal and Baseline conditions are identical: both contain two responses intentionally planned in anticipation of an external stimulus. The critical difference is that in one condition, Response 1 causes the

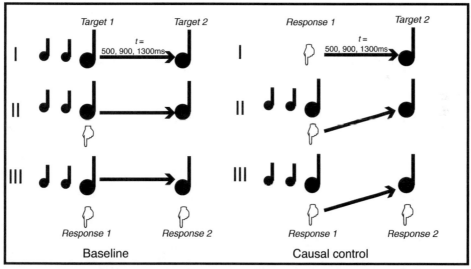

Fig. 15.2 A schematic depiction of the stimulus anticipation task used by Buehner and Humphreys (2009). Participants first (top row) learn about an inter-event interval, which either involves two tones and thus no causal connection, or an action (Response 1) producing a tone, and thus a causal link. They then (middle row) synchronize an action to a signal (Target 1). At Baseline, Target 1 is followed by Target 2 as before, and in Causal Control Response 1 still produces Target 2 as before. In the final, experimental, phase (bottom row), participants synchronize both Response 1 to Target 2, and a new Response 2 to Target 2. Baseline and Causal Control thus both involve two actions executed in anticipation of an external stimulus, but only the latter deploys a causal relation, such that the second stimulus is caused by the earlier response.

subsequent tone, whereas that same tone happens regardless of whether or when the response takes place in the other condition. The paradigm we reported thus successfully disambiguated intentionality from causality. Results suggest that causality drives temporal binding over and above intentionality.

A different way to tease apart causality and intentionality, of course, is to improve Wohlschläger et al.'s (2003) design and compare machine action to self- or other-generated action, but ensuring that the machine is clearly perceived to be causing the subsequent event in the machine-action condition. This would require a different setup, one where the causal machine is distinct and independent of the remaining experimental setup. If binding critically relies on awareness of intentional action, or draws upon the mirror-neuron system, then machine actions should not be attracted to subsequent events caused by the machine. In contrast, for the causal account, binding should still occur. Preliminary results from our laboratory involving machines as independent causal agents suggest that binding also occurs in intention-free, causal situations (Buehner, 2009).

Binding for action or binding for perception?

Regardless of whether one prefers the causal or the intentional binding approach, there are two perspectives one can take on temporal binding, which I have not distinguished so far. One is centered on the level of the constituent events, and the other on the interval between them. All the experimental paradigms I have reviewed thus far have focused on individual events: the Libet-clock method explicitly asks participants to provide subjective time stamps of when things happen, and the stimulus-anticipation method concerns preparation of motor responses to coincide with specific stimuli. Yet, the theoretical underpinnings of temporal binding I have offered at the beginning of this chapter all concern intervals between events. Naturally, it is possible to infer a subjective shortening of an inter-event interval based on a subjective shifting together in time of the events marking the interval. Notice, however, that the Libet-clock paradigm can only measure awareness of one event on any given trial. The temporal contraction of the interval between events is reconstructed post-experimentally by considering separately the judgement error of the action and the outcome. This is at best a very indirect method. A more direct way to measure changes in people's perception of time would be to employ well established paradigms from psychophysics, such as magnitude estimation.

Humphreys and Buehner (in press) compared people's estimations of *operant* intervals—between an action and a subsequent tone—to estimates of equivalent *observational* intervals—between a click (equivalent to the noise associated with the action on operant intervals) and subsequent tone. Across five experiments, Humphreys and Buehner compared temporal estimates of intervals ranging from 150–4000ms. Operant intervals were reliably perceived to be shorter than their observational counterparts, and, surprisingly, this difference remained stable at intervals in excess of 1 second, and up to intervals more than six times the length of the maximum intervals previously reported to support temporal binding. A further surprising element of these results was that the size of the binding effect increased as the intervals increased. Haggard, Clark, and Kalogeras (2002), in contrast, reported that temporal binding was reduced when the interval increased from 250ms to 450ms and 650m.

How can these contradictory findings be reconciled? One suggestion is to consider what is being measured in the various tasks. As outlined earlier, studies using the Libet clock measure subjective awareness of events, whereas the study by Humphreys and Buehner (in press) measured estimates of temporal intervals. The former judgement takes place online, while the latter takes place retrospectively. Moore and Haggard (2007) have argued that online judgements of awareness involve both predictive and postdictive components. Predictive components are thought to be related to an internal forward model of action control; they are short-lived in nature and most likely do not outlast the execution of the action. Postdictive, inference-based components, on the other hand, are not constrained in this way but come online only once the evidence has become available in its entirety (i.e. at the end of the inter-event interval). Thus, the survival of temporal binding across such long intervals in a magnitude-estimation task could be based on the retrospective, inferential nature of the task. This would mean that the temporal binding observed when considering interval estimates is largely based on cognition, whereas binding in studies of event awareness and motor planning is based both on cognition and action control. Inspection of Moore and Haggard's (2007) data suggests that the bulk of the binding in action-awareness studies is done by the predictive, action-control component, with the retrospective component adding only a little boost. More specifically, binding based on a successful prediction of the effect is not further augmented by sensory evidence that the effect has, in fact, occurred; this evidence only makes a difference when prediction is weak and would have lead to little or no binding. If binding in awareness paradigms is largely rooted in predictions from a forward model of motor planning, this could explain why it can only operate over such short timescales. In contrast, binding in explicit interval-estimation tasks most likely arises from postdictive elements, which are not limited to short timescales. The discrepancy between the temporal limitations of binding thus may reflect the different contributing processes.

The distinction between predictive and postdictive components could explain the survival of temporal binding over long intervals reported by Humphreys and Buehner (in press), but it does not address why the size of the binding effect increased as a function of interval length. Results of this kind typically indicate differences in internal clock speed (see Penton-Voak et al., 1996). It is well established that arousal, task demands, and stimulus modality can all influence the rate of the pacemaker. Could it be that the internal clock slows down while causal relations unfold? Alternatively, it could be that causal and non-causal intervals have different attentional affordances. It is commonly assumed that the reason why time flies when we are having fun is because we are paying less attention to time passing (Brown, Chapter 8, this volume). Mapping this assumption to causal binding would suggest that people pay less attention to time passing during causal episodes, perhaps because the events marking the intervals (i.e. causes and effects) themselves are more meaningful than those delineating non-causal, arbitrary intervals, and consequently draw more attention. Future research is needed to shed light on these different possibilities.

Conclusions

I began this chapter with the hypothesis that temporal binding is a two-way street: information about temporal proximity helps us recognize that things are causally related; at the same time, knowing that things are causally related makes them appear more proximal to one another. Support for this bi-directional relation between temporal contiguity and causality comes from a variety of experimental paradigms, including studies of action awareness and explicit interval estimation. This two-way relation fits well with a Bayesian approach of sensory integration (cf. Eagleman and Holcombe, 2002, Moore and Haggard, 2007), according to which prior knowledge and beliefs are integrated with sensory evidence to form coherent representations of the world around us. Both components—priors and evidence—are weighted according to their reliability. If the evidence is ambiguous (as it often is in time perception) prior beliefs that promote temporal contiguity (e.g. belief in a causal relation) can adjust the representation accordingly. If the beliefs are weak or unreliable (e.g. when the causal relation is weak), no, adjustments are minor or absent. At the same time, of course, sensory representations of the world around us are the very foundations on which we build our understanding of the world, including that of causality, and as such, our priors are constantly adjusted as beliefs change. Subjective experience of time thus simultaneously shapes our experience of the world, and is shaped by these experiences. Funes, with his unsurpassed capacity for noticing, naming, and remembering singular detail would have felt deeply disturbed by this duality of time. Perhaps this is why he tried to pinpoint time so exactly and without reference to an external clock.

References

Borges, J. L. (1993/1944). *Ficciones,* London: David Campbell Publishers.

Buehner, M. J. (2009). 'Causality and the perception of time.' Presentation given at Tzu Chi University, Hualien, Taiwan, and National Yang Ming University, Taipei, Taiwan.

Buehner, M. J. and Cheng, P. W. (2005). Causal learning. In Holyoak, K. J. and Morrison, R. (Eds.) *Handbook of Thinking & Reasoning.* Cambridge: Cambridge University Press.

Buehner, M. J. and Humphreys, G. R. (2009). Causal binding of actions to their effects. *Psychological Science,* **20**(1), 1221–28.

Buehner, M. J. and May, J. (2002). Knowledge mediates the timeframe of covariation assessment in human causal induction. *Thinking and Reasoning,* **8**, 269–95.

Buehner, M. J. and May, J. (2003). Rethinking temporal contiguity and the judgement of causality: effects of prior knowledge, experience, and reinforcement procedure. *The Quarterly Journal of Experimental Psychology A, Human Experimental Psychology,* **56**, 865–90.

Eagleman, D. M. and Holcombe, A. O. (2002). Causality and the perception of time. *Trends in Cognitive Sciences,* **6**, 323–5.

Engbert, K. and Wohlschläger, A. (2007). Intentions and expectations in temporal binding. *Consciousness and Cognition,* **16**, 255–64.

Haggard, P., Aschersleben, G., Gehrke, J., and Prinz, W. (2002a). Action, binding, and awareness. In Prinz, W. and Hommel, B. (Eds.) *Common Mechanisms in Perception and Action: Attention and Performance.* Oxford, Oxford University Press.

Haggard, P., Clark, S., and Kalogeras, J. (2002b). Voluntary action and conscious awareness. *Nature Neuroscience,* **5**, 382–5.

Hume, D. (1739/1888) A treatise of human nature. In Selby-Bigge, L. A. (Ed.) *Hume's treatise of human nature.* Oxford: Clarendon Press.

Humphreys, G. R. and Buehner, M. J. (in press). Magnitude estimation reveals temporal binding at super-second intervals. *Journal of Experimental Psychology: Human Perception and Performance.*

Kersten, D., Mamassian, P., and Yuille, A. (2004). Object perception as Bayesian inference. *Annual Review of Psychology,* **55**, 271–304.

Libet, B., Gleason, C. A., Wright, E. W., and Pearl, D. K. (1983). Time of conscious intention to act in relation to onset f cerebral activity (readiness-potential): the unconscious initiation of a freely voluntary act. *Brain,* **106**, 623–42.

Mackie, J. L. (1974). *The Cement of the Universe: A study on Causation.,* Oxford: Clarendon Press.

Moore, J. and Haggard, P. (2007). Awareness of action: inference and prediction. *Consciousness & Cognition,* **17**, 136–44.

Penton-Voak, I. S., Edwards, H., Percival, A., and Wearden, J. H. (1996). Speeding up an internal clock in humans? Effects of click trains on subjective duration. *Journal of Experimental Psychology: Animal Behavior Processes,* **22**, 307–20.

Schank, R. C. and Abelson, R. P. (1977) Scripts, plans, goals and understanding: an inquiry into human knowledge structures, Hillsdale, NJ: Erlbaum.

Wohlschläger, A., Haggard, P., Gesierich, B., and Prinz, W. (2003). The perceived onset time of self- and other-generated actions. *Psychological Science,* **14**, 586–91.

Zacks, J. M., Speer, N. K., Swallow, K. M., and Braver, T. S. (2007). Event perception: a mind-brain perspective. *Psychological Bulletin,* **133**, 273–93.

Acknowledgement

Preparation of this chapter has been supported by EPSRC grant EP/C004469/1.

Section 3

Directing attention in time enhances perception and action

Temporal predictions inherent in the temporal structure of events

Chapter 16

Behavioural adaptation to redundant frequency distributions in time

Annika Wagener and Joachim Hoffmann

Every object or event stands in temporal and spatial relation to adjacent objects or events. These relations are by no means random: objects or events appear at certain locations and at certain moments in time more frequently than at other locations and times. For instance, taps are normally assembled above sinks and not beside them and water consumption increases more during halftime of a football match than during its playing time.

Numerous experiments have shown that redundant distributions of stimuli in space involuntarily affect stimulus processing. In particular, target stimuli are processed more quickly if they are presented at locations where they frequently appeared in the past compared to locations where they rarely appeared (e.g. Meyers and Rhoades, 1978; Miller, 1988; Chun and Jiang, 1998, 2003; Hoffmann and Kunde, 1999; Olson and Chun, 2002; Hoffmann and Sebald, 2005). The finding suggests that orienting of spatial attention to a location is accompanied by an automatic readiness to process those stimuli that have been frequently experienced at a particular location. In other words, it has been assumed that covariation between locations and stimuli incidentally lead to location-specific target expectancies (Hoffmann and Kunde, 1999). In the present chapter, we will discuss to what extent repeated temporal relations between stimuli automatically lead to preferential treatment of those stimuli that have frequently been experienced at some given point in time.

Surprisingly, the issue of stimulus-specific temporal expectation has rarely, if ever, been explored until now, although numerous studies with the 'foreperiod paradigm' have already indicated a dynamic adaptation of implicit temporal expectations to the point in time at which target stimuli are presented. In this chapter, we will briefly review the main findings of the foreperiod paradigm and subsequently report three experiments exploring the extent to which such implicit temporal expectations might involuntarily become linked to those stimuli that are preferentially presented at particular points in time.

Foreperiod effects

In a typical foreperiod experiment, a ready signal is initially presented. After a certain delay—the 'foreperiod'—another target stimulus is presented to which participants have to respond as quickly as possible. This stimulus arrangement resembles the start of a sprint, where the go-signal regularly follows a preceding ready signal and, like athletes in a sprint, participants in a foreperiod experiment are assumed to strive to be maximally ready to react at the point in time at which the target is presented. The first studies employing this design aimed to define the foreperiod that would result in the fastest responses, i.e. the point in time at which the readiness to react would reach its maximum (e.g. Woodrow, 1914). For this purpose, the length of the foreperiod was

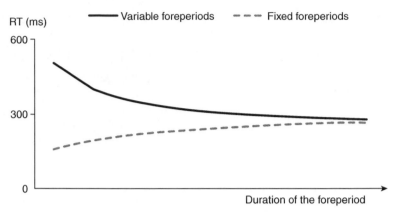

Fig. 16.1 Schematic drawing of fixed and variable foreperiod effects.

systematically varied in consecutive blocks of trials. The results revealed that there was no single 'optimal' foreperiod, but rather reaction times (RTs) tended to increase with the duration of the foreperiod. This increase of RTs with the duration of the foreperiod has been confirmed in many follow-up studies and is known as the fixed-foreperiod effect. However, if the foreperiod was not fixed within a block of trials, but instead varied from trial to trial in an unpredictable manner, the reverse pattern was observed: response times decreased systematically as the foreperiod increased (see Niemi and Näätänen, 1981, for a comprehensive review). This is called the variable-foreperiod effect (Los, Chapter 21; Vallesi, Chapter 22, this volume). Thus, responses are slower the longer the *expected* delay before target appearance, but responses are faster the longer the *unpredictable* delay before target appearance (see Figure 16.1 for a schematic drawing of both foreperiod effects; for empirical data see Mattes and Ulrich, 1997).

Both foreperiod effects stimulated several theoretical accounts. For example, the fixed-foreperiod effect was thought to be due to a continuous slowing down of the readiness to react. According to this proposal, the readiness to react is high immediately after the ready signal and, because it takes effort to maintain a high state of readiness, this readiness decays over time. Accordingly, RTs increase the longer the foreperiod lasts (e.g. Alegria, 1975; Gottsdanker, 1975; for a review see Niemi and Näätänen, 1981; Vallesi, and Shallice, 2007). Another account relates the increasing RTs to the accuracy of duration judgements. According to this account, participants try to tailor response readiness to the point in time at which the target signal is to be expected. It is well known that short durations are more accurately estimated than longer ones, the so-called 'scalar property of variance' (e.g. Gibbon, 1977; Gibbon et al., 1984; Allan and Gibbon, 1991; Wearden and Lejeune, 2008). Accordingly, if in a block of trials the foreperiod is long, response readiness more frequently misses the point in time at which the target is presented than if the current foreperiod is short, simply because the estimate of presentation time, on average, deviates more strongly from the real presentation time. As a result, RTs increase the longer the duration of the predictable foreperiod (see Los, Chapter 21; Vallesi, Chapter 22, this volume).

Two different accounts have also been proposed to explain the variable-foreperiod effect. First it was assumed that the effect was due to adaptation to hazard functions, i.e. to the continuous increase in conditional probability of target presentation at a certain time given that the target had not yet occurred (e.g. Bertelson and Tisseyre, 1968; Näätänen, 1970). Imagine, for example, an experiment in which four different foreperiods are used with equal frequency. Initially, the probability for the presentation of a target after each of the four foreperiods is 0.25. However, once the shortest foreperiod has elapsed only three possible foreperiods remain, each of which have a probability of target presentation of 0.33. Finally, after the third foreperiod has passed, the target must occur at the longest foreperiod, i.e. the probability for its occurrence increases to 1.0. Participants most likely adjust to this 'hazard function' by continually enhancing their response readiness the longer the foreperiod lasts. In agreement with this account, the foreperiod effect almost disappears if target presentations are made equally probable after each of the foreperiods by inserting corresponding blank trials in which no target at all is presented (e.g. Näätänen, 1970).

Another theoretical account for the variable-foreperiod effect attributes the decrease of RTs with the duration of the foreperiod to a sequential modulation of temporal expectations. According to this notion, participants tend to expect the same foreperiod in a current trial as had been experienced in the preceding trial (Los, Chapter 21, this volume). If the foreperiod of the preceding trial is indeed repeated, the current temporal expectation is fulfilled and responses are fast. Likewise, if the expected foreperiod has elapsed without a target being presented, participants can re-orient their temporal expectations to the next possible presentation time so that response speed remains largely unaffected (e.g. Alegria, 1975; Thomas, 1967). However, if the foreperiod is shorter than expected, the presentation of the target comes as a surprise and RTs are correspondingly lengthened. Thus, responses only tend to be delayed if the foreperiod in the current trial is shorter than the foreperiod in the preceding trial and, because this happens more frequently in trials with short foreperiods, RTs tend to increase the shorter the current foreperiod is (Woodrow, 1914; Karlin, 1959; Baumeister and Joubert, 1969). In agreement with this notion, the foreperiod effect is largely diminished if trials in which the current foreperiod are shorter than the preceding one are excluded from data evaluation (Alegria and Delhaye-Rembaux, 1975). Moreover, Los and Agter (2005) recently varied the frequencies of short and long foreperiods and found that frequencies of transitions between short and long foreperiods, without changes in sequential modulation, had a great impact on RTs.

In any case, the given experimental evidence suggests that temporal expectations adapt to experienced presentation times by an adjustment of the response readiness to a fixed point in time for expected target presentation, to a time related to conditional probabilities of target presentation, or to a time that varies as a function of the foreperiod of the preceding trial. In all studies reported so far, the main concern was the adjustment of temporal expectations to the experienced foreperiods, irrespective of the target stimulus or the required response. Thus, the extent to which temporal expectations might be adjusted not only to certain points in time but also to likely processing demands at the corresponding points in time, still remains unexplored.

In this chapter, we will describe an initial set of experiments that go beyond the foreperiod effects discussed earlier by exploring the effects of covariation between foreperiods and other stimulus properties. Imagine a situation in which different stimuli appear after different foreperiods. Each stimulus and each foreperiod occurs equally often so that neither the stimulus nor the foreperiod is predictable. However, a particular stimulus is more probable after a certain foreperiod than after other foreperiods. Accordingly, the point in time at which a stimulus is presented carries information about the likely identity of the current stimulus. As reported earlier, covariations between stimuli and *locations* lead to very effective adaptation of stimulus-specific processing capacities to stimulus-specific locations. The question arises of whether redundant assignments of stimuli to foreperiods will result in comparable adaptation: is processing of a stimulus selectively facilitated if it appears at its likely point in time?

Temporal expectations for visual stimuli

We investigated the impact of a covariation between two foreperiods and two visual targets on performance in a choice reaction-time task (Wagener and Hoffmann, 2009a). Targets comprised a circle or square presented in the centre of the screen after a short (600-ms) or a long (1400-ms) foreperiod. Participants responded as quickly as possible to target identity by pressing either a left or a right button. Both targets and both foreperiods were equally often presented in random order. However, after the short foreperiod one of the targets was more likely whereas after the long foreperiod the other target was more likely. Accordingly, when a target appeared after a certain foreperiod, it could either be the target that typically appeared at this point in time or the target that appeared infrequently after this foreperiod. In this sense, the point in time at which a target appeared (the foreperiod) delivered information about the likely identity of the current target as well as the likely required response. If this temporal information is used, responses to temporally probable or 'valid' targets should be faster and/or less error prone than responses to temporally less probable or 'invalid' targets. Note that although both foreperiods were equally likely, they differed with respect to their predictability in the course of a trial: During the short foreperiod, the point in time at which the target appeared was indeed unpredictable as both foreperiods were equally likely. However, once the short foreperiod had passed, it became certain that the target had to appear at the late point in time so that the target, which often appeared late, consequently became predictable.

The data showed that the response to the temporally valid target is faster and less error prone than to the temporally invalid target at each of the two points in time (Figure 16.2). This temporal

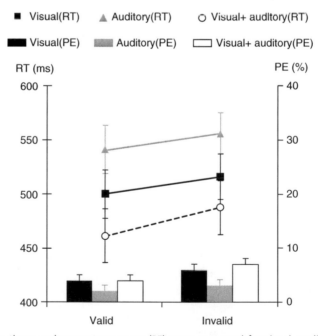

Fig. 16.2 Reaction times and percentage errors (PE) were measured for visual, auditory, or audiovisual targets. RTs were faster for valid compared to invalid targets across all three experiments. Compound audiovisual stimuli produced larger validity effects than auditory or visual stimuli alone.

'validity benefit' suggests that participants not only oriented non-specific attention to points in time but also assigned stimulus- and/or response-specific processing resources to those points in time at which the corresponding stimulus-response coupling was most likely to occur.[1]

We have already mentioned that the forthcoming presentation time and target remain unpredictable until after the short foreperiod has elapsed. Thereafter, stimulus presentation is certain to occur at the late point in time and consequently the corresponding late-valid target becomes most likely. Accordingly, participants generally responded more quickly and with fewer errors to targets that were presented at the late point in time—the variable foreperiod effect. Furthermore, averaged data reflect the different predictability of the early-valid and the late-valid target. Comparing the difference in RTs and error rates between predicted and unpredicted target type at each of the intervals, the validity benefit for the late-valid target (20ms, 2.8%) is larger than for the early-valid target (12ms, 1.2%). Although this interaction does not reach significance, it nevertheless suggests that there is both: (1) increased predictability that any event will occur at a given time (as the first foreperiod remains unoccupied), and (2) increased probability that a specific event will occur.

Temporal expectations for auditory stimuli

It may be assumed that the temporal validity effect should be even greater with acoustic stimuli. For example, Wearden and colleagues (1998) found that the duration of acoustic stimuli is perceived more accurately than that of visual stimuli. They explained their findings by assuming that the on- and offset of acoustic stimuli could be assessed with less variability than those of visual stimuli. If participants were able to assess the onset of a stimulus more accurately, they should be even better prepared for stimulus presentation at a given point in time. Therefore, the processing of acoustic stimuli appearing at an expected time should be facilitated even more than that of visual stimuli.

We tested this claim by replicating the temporal validity effect with acoustic stimuli. After one of two foreperiods (500ms or 1500ms), one of two tone pitches (660Hz: note E, high pitch tone; and 440Hz: note A, low pitch tone) served as targets (Wagener and Hoffmann, 2009b). The participant's task was to respond as quickly as possible to the presentation of a tone. Unbeknownst to the participants, one foreperiod usually preceded one tone and the other foreperiod preceded the other (valid trials: 80%). In 20% of the trials (invalid trials), the combination of preceding foreperiods and tones were switched.

The results replicated the findings of the experiment with visual stimuli: participants made fewer errors and responded more quickly during temporally valid trials compared to temporally invalid ones (Figure 16.2). The size of the temporal validity effect averaged over the two foreperiods (15ms) was almost the same as that in experiments with visual stimuli (16ms) (Wagener and Hoffmann, 2009b). Again, there was a significant foreperiod effect as participants responded more quickly to targets appearing after long foreperiods than to targets after short foreperiods. Although there was no significant interaction of foreperiod duration with temporal validity, the averaged data nevertheless suggest a smaller validity effect after the short foreperiod (7ms) than

---

[1] In other experiments we also found temporal validity effects for locations, i.e. targets presented at locations that were frequently associated with a certain point in time were detected more quickly than targets appearing at locations that were seldom used at this moment (Wagener and Hoffmann, 2009a). Similar to the time-specific target expectancies described in the current experiment, participants also seem able to build time-specific location expectancies under suitable conditions.

after the long one (21ms), indicating an effect of higher target predictability after the long compared to the short foreperiod.

Temporal expectations for compound visual and auditory stimuli

It is well established that responses are speeded when participants respond to redundant combinations of two targets instead of responding to only one target (e.g. Miller, 1982; Grice et al., 1984; Diederich and Colonius, 1987). This 'redundant target effect' is presumably the result of at least two mechanisms (Gondan et al., 2005). Presentation of two stimuli may provide more excitation (more energy) in the nervous system than presentation of a single stimulus and therefore speed up stimulus processing (e.g. Bernstein et al., 1969). In addition, each of the two imperative stimuli may coactivate the required response, so that the response threshold is reached more quickly than if it is triggered by only one target. Correspondingly, we would expect faster responses with compound stimuli than with single stimuli.

In contrast to response speed, predictions regarding the temporal validity effect are less obvious. If the temporal validity effect is primarily based on facilitating the execution of the currently most likely response, redundant targets should result in validity effects of comparable size to single targets. The speeding of responses to temporally valid targets should be one and the same regardless of whether the target is a single stimulus or a compound of two stimuli. If, however, the temporal validity effect is primarily based on an acceleration of stimulus processing, an increase in the validity effect can be expected provided that temporal expectations include both elements of the currently most likely stimulus compound.

To test which explanation holds true, we compared the results described earlier to those of an experiment employing compound visual-auditory stimuli (Wagener and Hoffmann, 2009b). The compound targets consisted of two fixed combinations of the same visual and auditory stimuli that were used for the experiments with only visual and only auditory stimuli. As in the experiments with single stimuli, one stimulus compound was preferentially presented after a short (500-ms) foreperiod and the other after a long (1500-ms) foreperiod. Besides a general acceleration in response speed, participants once again responded more quickly and with fewer errors if the stimulus compounds appeared at their more likely point in time than if they appeared at the less likely point in time (Figure 16.2). For mean RTs, this temporal validity effect was substantially more pronounced than in experiments with visual or auditory stimuli only (27ms compared to 16ms and 15ms respectively). Although the comparison must be taken with caution, as it is based on different groups of participants, the doubling of the RT validity effect suggests that temporal expectations comprise both sensory elements of the currently likely compound stimulus. If the expected compound is presented, both targets are processed more quickly and the assigned response is executed earlier, as compared to when the currently non-expected compound is presented.

Interestingly, the tendency to respond more quickly to targets appearing after the long foreperiod than to targets after the short foreperiod, i.e. the variable-foreperiod effect, was significantly reduced in the experiment with compound stimuli compared to experiments with single stimuli. As already noted, the variable-foreperiod effect in these experiments is very likely due to the fact that target presentation after the long foreperiod becomes 100% certain as soon as the short foreperiod has passed without a target being presented. The absence of the variable-foreperiod effect with compound stimuli suggests that participants did not prepare for the predictable presentation of a likely target. One explanation for this finding could be that participants might have been at ceiling with their response speed when responding to the temporally valid compound stimuli.

Conclusions

It is well established that stimuli occurring at their most likely spatial locations are responded to more quickly and more accurately than the same stimuli appearing at non-likely locations (e.g. Miller, 1988; Musen, 1996; Hoffmann and Kunde, 1999). The experiments described here investigated to what extent redundant distributions of stimuli in time would result in comparable behavioural effects. To this end, either a short or a long foreperiod preceded one of two different targets. Though each foreperiod and target type was equally likely, their combination was highly predictable, so that each target type was most likely to appear at a given presentation time. The experiments used either only visual targets (squares and circles), only auditory targets (a high and a low pitch tone), or a fixed combinations of both shapes and tones.

All experiments provided evidence for a behavioural adaptation to redundancies in the temporal distribution of targets. After each of the foreperiods, targets were processed more quickly and more accurately if they were likely to occur at this point in time than if they were unlikely at this point in time. Numerous experiments have already shown an automatic adaptation of temporal expectations to experienced foreperiods—the so-called foreperiod effects (cf. Niemi and Näätänen, 1981). Moreover, recent experiments have also shown that temporal expectations can be voluntarily oriented to points in time which were either explicitly or implicitly cued as being likely (e.g. Coull and Nobre, 1998; Coull et al., 2000; Griffin et al., 2002; Albinet and Fezzani, 2003; Doherty et al., 2005; Correa and Nobre, 2008; Correa, Chapter 26; Nobre, Chapter 27; Coull, Chapter 31, this volume). The present results go beyond these findings by showing that temporal expectations may selectively facilitate those perceptual and/or motor processes that are likely to be required at a certain point in time. Analogously to location-specific target expectancies (Hoffmann and Kunde, 1999), one may speak of temporal expectation for specific targets according to the frequencies with which these targets have been experienced at the current point in time.

In the present experiments, the two targets required different responses, so that, at a given point in time, not only a particular target but also the assigned response was more likely than the alternative target-response coupling. Accordingly, any time-specific improvement in performance may index the processing of the currently likely target and/or to the generation of the currently likely response. The data from our experiment with compound visual and auditory stimuli, however, provide a hint that modulation of stimulus processing contributes to the observed effects of temporal validity. Combined audio-visual targets produced a temporal validity effect of almost double the size to that produced by visual or auditory stimuli alone. This substantial enhancement of the temporal validity effect by a duplication of the targets suggests that temporal expectation affected stimulus processing, as well as the conversion of given sensory information into response selection. This conclusion is in line with recent findings showing a facilitation at the level of stimulus processing and response selection at cued, and hence predictable, presentation times (e.g. Müller-Gethmann et al., 2003; Bausenhart et al., 2006; Rolke and Ulrich, Chapter 17; Correa, Chapter 26, this volume).

In all reported experiments, a target presented at the late point in time was certain to occur as soon as the short foreperiod had passed without a target being presented. Additionally, the target that was most frequently presented at the late point in time also became most likely and so, in turn, predictable. Accordingly, responses to late targets were faster and less error prone, and the benefits for late-valid targets were empirically larger, than for early-valid targets in experiments with only one kind of stimuli. However, temporal validity effects were also always present at early points in time, when targets were unpredictable. Furthermore, in the experiment with compound stimuli, the validity effect was significantly enhanced while the foreperiod effect was significantly reduced, compared to experiments with only one kind of stimuli. This data pattern suggests dissociable effects of temporal predictability related to the particular association between a temporal interval and a target type (as measured by validity effects) and temporal predictability as a result of the passage of time (as measured by short/long foreperiod differences) (see also Coull, Chapter 31, this volume for neural evidence of a dissociation).

Finally, the matter of awareness about these temporal associations is to be considered. In our experiments, participants were informed about the existence of a relationship between foreperiods and the frequency of targets only after the experiments were over. Although we did not conduct the experiments in order to compare implicit and explicit covariation, we nevertheless questioned our participants as to whether they had correctly identified the covariation between the duration of the foreperiods and the frequency with which the targets were presented. In all of our experiments a majority of participants reported not to have noticed the experienced covariation. Nevertheless, all experiments showed reliable behavioural effects of unequal target frequencies at each of the two foreperiods. Thus, temporal target expectation does not seem to require a conscious recognition of temporal target frequencies but may rather emerge as an automatic consequence of the frequent co-occurrence of a certain point in time and a certain target/response episode. However, if one compares, across experiments, the size of the temporal validity effect for the small group of 14 participants who correctly indicated the covariation with that produced by the remaining 34 participants who had no explicit knowledge about the frequency manipulation, the explicit sample somewhat outperform the implicit sample (24ms and 3.3 % errors versus 18ms and 1.7% errors respectively). It will be interesting to investigate this issue in the future. For now, we conclude that explicit awareness is not necessary.

In summary, we assume that the observed target-specific effects of temporal validity are based on associations between the critical points in time at which targets appear and the task-relevant features of the targets that are frequently experienced at these points in time, such as target identity and required response. The formation of these time-target/response associations primarily depend on the frequencies with which certain points in time co-occur with certain target features but their formation is certainly also influenced by the predictability of the corresponding points in time and the corresponding target features. In any case, once associated, the encoding of the current presentation time facilitates the encoding of its associated parts. Accordingly, targets, and/or responses that frequently appear, and/or are reliably to be expected, at a particular point in time are processed more effectively. The underlying mechanisms might be comparable to the mechanism of trace conditioning in animals (cf. Gibbon, 1977; Gallistel and Gibbon, 2000; Woodruff-Pak and Disterhoft, 2008) and, indeed, variable-foreperiod effects in experiments with human subjects have already been simulated by equivalent conditioning models (cf. Machado, 1997; Los and van den Heuvel, 2001; Los, Chapter 21, this volume). However, whether these models can be adapted to explain the present findings of temporal processing benefits for those targets and/or responses that appear frequently at the current point in time is a matter of future research.

References

Albinet, C. and Fezzani, K. (2003). Instruction in learning a temporal pattern on an anticipation-coincidence task. *Perceptual and Motor Skills*, **97**, 71–9.

Alegria, J. and Delhaye-Rembaux, M. (1975). Sequential effects of foreperiod duration and conditional probability of the signal in a choice reaction time task. *Acta Psychologica*, **39**, 321–8.

Alegria, J. (1975). Sequential effects of foreperiod duration: Some strategical factors in tasks involving time uncertainty. In P. M. A. Rabbit and S. Dornic (ed.) *Attention and Performance*, pp.1–10. London: Academic Press.

Allan, L. G. and Gibbon, J. (1991). Human bisection at the geometric mean. *Learning and Motivation*, **22**, 39–58.

Baumeister, A. A. and Joubert, C. E. (1969). Interactive effects on reaction time of preparatory interval length and preparatory interval frequency. *Journal of Experimental Psychology*, **82**, 393–5.

Bausenhart, K. M., Rolke, B., Hackley, S. A., and Ulrich, R. (2006). The locus of temporal preparation effects: Evidence from the psychological refractory period paradigm. *Psychonomic Bulletin and Review*, **13**, 536–42.

Bernstein, I. H., Clark, M. H., and Edelstein, B.A. (1969). Effects of an auditory signal on visual reaction time. *Journal of Experimental Psychology*, **80**, 567–9.

Bertelson, P. and Tisseyre, F. (1968). The time-course of preparation with regular and irregular foreperiods. *Quaterly Journal of Experimental Psychology*, **20**, 297–300.

Chun, M. M., and Jiang, Y. (1998). Contextual cueing: implicit learning and memory of visual context guides spatial attention. *Cognitive Psychology*, **36**, 28–71.

Chun, M. M., and Jiang, Y. (2003). Implicit, long-term spatial contextual memory. *Journal of Experimental Psychology: Learning, Memory, and Cognition*, **29**, 224–34.

Correa, Á. and Nobre, A.C. (2008). Spatial and temporal acuity of visual perception can be enhanced selectively by attentional set. *Experimental Brain Research*, **189**, 339–44.

Coull, J. T., and Nobre, A. C. (1998). Where and when to pay attention: the neural systems for directing attention to spatial locations and to time intervals as revealed by both PET and fMRI. *Journal of Neuroscience*, **18**, 7426–35.

Coull, J. T., Frith, C. D., Büchel, C., and Nobre, A. C. (2000). Orienting attention in time: behavioral and neuroanatomical distinction between exogenous and endogenous shifts. *Neuropsychologia*, **38**, 808–19.

Diederich, A. and Colonius, H. (1987). Intersensory facilitation in the motor component: A reaction time analysis. *Psychological Research*, **49**, 23–29.

Doherty, J. R., Rao, A., Mesulam, M. M., and Nobre, A. C. (2005). Synergistic effect of combined temporal and spatial expectations on visual attention. *The Journal of Neuroscience*, **25**, 8259–66.

Gallistel, C. R. and Gibbon, J. (2000). Time, rate, and conditioning. *Psychological Review*, **107**, 289–344.

Gibbon, J. (1977). Scalar expectancy theory and Weber's law in animal timing. *Psychological Review*, **84**, 279–325.

Gibbon, J. Church, R. M., and Meck, W. H. (1984). Scalar timing in memory. In J. Gibbon and L.G. Allan (Eds.) *Annals of the New York Academy of Sciences: Timing and time perception*, pp.52–77. New York: New York Academy of Sciences.

Gondan, M., Niederhaus, B., Rösler, F., and Röder, B. (2005). Multisensory processing in the redundant target effect: a behavioral and event-related potential study. *Perception and Psychophysics*, **67**, 713–26.

Gottsdanker, R. (1975). The attaining and maintaining of preparation. In P. M. A. Rabbit and S. Dornic (Eds.) *Attention and Performance*, pp.33–42. London: Academic Press.

Grice, G. R., Canham, L., and Boroughs, J. M. (1984). Combination rule for redundant information in reaction time tasks with divided attention. *Perception & Psychophysics*, **35**, 451–63.

Griffin; I. C., Miniussi, C., and Nobre, A. C. (2002). Multiple mechanisms of selective attention: Differential modulation of stimulus processing by attention to space and time. *Neuropsychologia*, **40**, 2325–40.

Hoffmann, J., and Kunde, W. (1999). Location-specific target expectancies in visual search. *Journal of Experimental Psychology: Human Perception and Performance*, **25**, 1127–41.

Hoffmann, J., and Sebald, A. (2005). When obvious covariations are not even learned implicitly. *European Journal of Cognitive Psychology*, **17**, 449–80.

Karlin, L. (1959). Reaction time as a function of foreperiod duration and variability. *Journal of Experimental Psychology*, **58**, 185–91.

Los, S. A. and Agter, F. (2005). Reweighting sequential effects across different distributions of foreperiods: Segregating elementary contributions to nonspecific preparation. *Perception & Psychophysics*, **67**, 1161–70.

Los, S. A. and Van den Heuvel, C. E. (2001). Intentional and unintentional contributions of nonspecific preparation during reaction time foreperiods. *Journal of Experimental Psychology: Human Perception and Performance*, **27**, 370–86.

Machado, A. (1997). Learning the temporal dynamics of behavior. *Psychological Review*, **104**, 241–65.

Mattes, S. and Ulrich, R. (1997). Response force is sensitive to the temporal uncertainty of response stimuli. *Perception and Psychophysics*, **59**, 1089–97.

Meyers, L. S. and Rhoades, R. W. (1978). Visual search of common scenes. *Quarterly Journal of Experimental Psychology*, **30**, 297–310.

Miller, J. (1982). Divided attention: evidence for coactivation with redundant signals. *Cognitive Psychology*, **14**, 247–79.

Miller, J. (1988). Components of the location probability effect in visual search tasks. *Journal of Experimental Psychology: Human Perception and Performance*, **14**, 453–71.

Müller-Gethmann, H., Ulrich, R., and Rinkenauer, G. (2003). Locus of the effect of temporal preparation: Evidence from the lateral readiness potential. *Psychophysiology*, **40**, 597–611.

Musen, G. (1996). Effects of task demands on implicit memory for object-location associations. *Canadian Journal of Experimental Psychology*, **50**, 104–13.

Näätänen, R. (1970). The diminishing time-uncertainty with the lapse of time after the warning-signal in reaction-time experiments with varying fore-periods. *Acta Psycologica*, **34**, 399–419.

Niemi, P., and Näätänen, R. (1981). Foreperiod and simple reaction time. *Psychological Bulletin*, **89**, 133–62.

Olson, I. R., and Chun, M. M. (2002). Perceptual constraints on implicit learning of spatial context. *Visual Cognition*, **9**, 273–302.

Thomas, E. A. (1967). Reaction-time studies: the anticipation and interaction of response. *British Journal of Mathematical & Statistical Psychology*, **20**, 1–29.

Vallesi, A. and Shallice, T. (2007). Developmental dissociations of preparation over time: Deconstructing the variable foreperiod phenomena. *Journal of Experimental Psychology: Human Perception and Performance*, **33**, 1377–88.

Wagener, A. and Hoffmann, J. (2009a). Temporal cueing of target identity and target location. *Journal of Experimental Psychology*, (in press).

Wagener, A. and Hoffmann, J. (2009b). [Comparison of temporal validity with visual, auditory, and visual-auditory targets]. Unpublished raw data.

Wearden, J. H. and Lejeune, H. (2008). Scalar properties in human timing: conformity and violations. *The Quarterly Journal of Experimental Psychology*, **61**, 569–87.

Wearden, J. H., Edwards, H., Fakhri, M., and Percival, A. (1998). Why 'sounds are judged longer than light': application of a model of the internal clock in humans. *The Quarterly Journal of Experimental Psychology*, **51B**, 97–120.

Woodrow, H. (1914). The measurement of attention. *Psychological Monographs*, **5**, 1–158

Woodruff-Pak, D. S. and Disterhoft, J. F. (2008). Where is the trace in trace conditioning? *Trends in Neurosciences*, **31**, 105–12.

Acknowledgements

This research was funded through Deutsche Forschungsgemeinschaft Grant HO 1301-13-1 warded to Joachim Hoffmann.

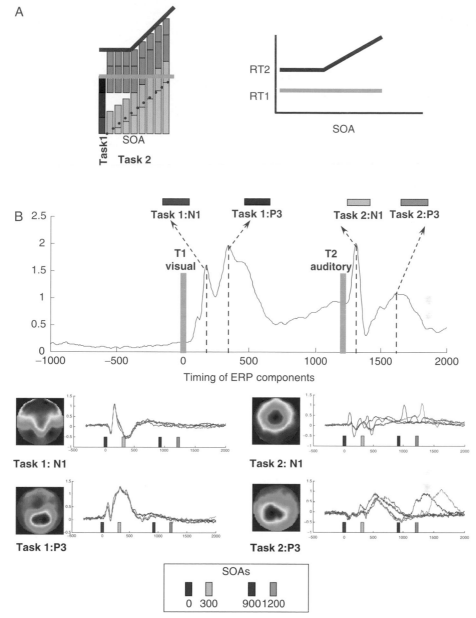

Plate 1 (See also Fig. 5.1) A) Left panel: scheme of the main PRP effect. The vertical axis labels response time. The leftmost column indicates the first task, and each colored box within the columns represents a different stage of processing: *For Task 1: Perceptual (P)* (green), *Central (C)* (red) and *Motor (M)* (blue) components and for Task 2 P (light green), C (orange) and M (cyan). The pale grey boxes for Task 2 indicate stimulus onset asynchrony (SOA). Right panel: the expected dependence of the bottleneck model for RT2 and RT1 as a function of increasing SOA. B) Identifying the response components (N1 and P3), for each task when performed at the longest SOA (1200ms) outside of the interference regime. B) Time-course of the components: components of Task 1 (left panels) are utterly unaffected by SOA. The N1 component of Task 2 (top right panel) tightly follows the stimulus presentation, as would be expected by a P-component. The P3 component of Task 2 (bottom right) reflects a bottleneck for short SOAs as would be expected by a C-component.

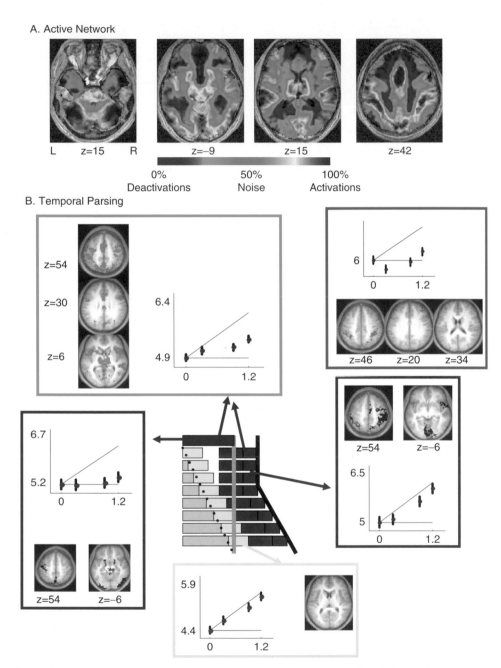

Plate 2 (See also Fig. 5.2) A) Networks activated (red) and deactivated (blue) during dual-task performance as identified by a phase coherence analysis. B) Parsing the brain network into distinct dynamic processing stages, according to their phase profile.

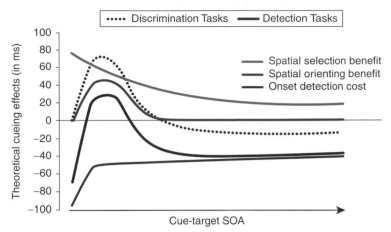

Plate 3 (See also Fig. 2.3) Theoretical cueing effects (in black) usually observed for detection and discrimination tasks as a function of cue-target stimulus onset asynchrony. The coloured lines represent different cue-triggered processes underlying the cueing effects: spatial orienting of attention (blue), onset detection cost (red), and spatial selection benefit (green). The different cueing effects for the two tasks are computed as differential contributions of each process to detection and discrimination tasks. Basically, whereas onset detection processes contribute mostly to detection tasks, spatial selection processes are tapped mainly by discrimination tasks.

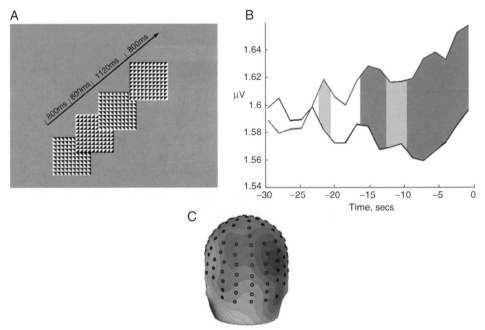

Plate 4 (See also Fig. 6.1) A) Continuous Temporal Expectancy Task (CTET). During this test of vigilant attention, participants were asked to monitor a continuous stream of checker stimuli centrally presented and flickering at a rate of 25Hz. Standard stimuli were presented for 800ms and participants were required to monitor for the occurrence of target stimuli defined by their longer duration (1120ms) relative to other stimuli. Target detection was indicated by a speeded button press. B) Alpha amplitude calculated for the 30 seconds preceding a target onset and averaged separately for correctly (hit, blue) and incorrectly (miss, red) detected targets. Significant alpha-band divergences emerged up to 20 seconds before a lapse of attention. C) Scalp topography showing that the increase in alpha-power prior to a miss was most prominent over right inferior parietal scalp sites.

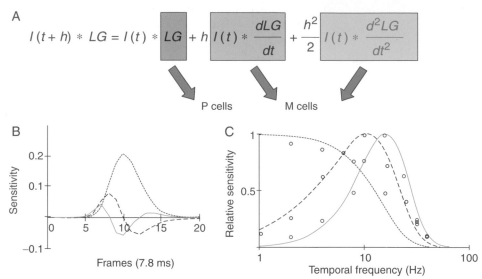

A

$$I(t+h) * LG = I(t) * \boxed{LG} + h\,\boxed{I(t) * \frac{dLG}{dt}} + \frac{h^2}{2}\boxed{I(t) * \frac{d^2LG}{dt^2}}$$

P cells   M cells

B

Sensitivity

0.2

0.1

0   5   10   15   20

−0.1

Frames (7.8 ms)

C

Relative sensitivity

1

0.5

1   10   100

Temporal frequency (Hz)

Plate 5 (See also Fig. 14.1) A) Taylor's series can be used to predict the value of a function (the image brightness, $I(t)$), in the neighbourhood around a point, in time, t. Temporal derivatives of the image brightness are calculated at a point, t, by convolving (∗) the image brightness with the derivatives of Gaussians in log time. Throughout the figures red dotted line indicates the temporal blur kernel (the log Gaussian, LG), blue dashed line indicates the first derivative and solid green line indicates the second derivative of the log Gaussian. The excursion parameter, h, indicates the point ($t+h$) at which the value of the function is to be predicted. The parameter, h, can take on a range of values. B) The temporal tuning functions for human vision. The data are from Hess and Snowden (1992) and the fitted functions, the Gaussian in log time (red line) and its first (blue line) and second (green line) derivatives, are from Johnston and Clifford (1995). All data for each of the three functions are fitted by adjusting just one parameter (see Johnston and Clifford, 1995, for details). The band-pass filters (blue and green lines) correspond to the tuning curves of magnocellular neurons and the low-pass temporal filter (red line) is representative of parvocellular neuron's temporal tuning curves C) The impulse responses for the filters, calculated as the inverse Fourier transform of the corresponding (matching line-colour) frequency sensitivity curves in B.

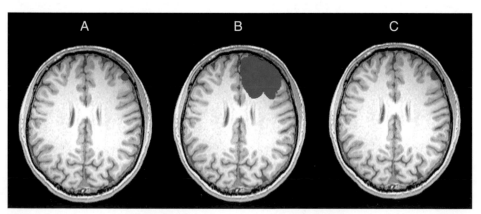

A   B   C

Plate 6 (See also Fig. 22.1) Approximate locations (in red) of the right lateral prefrontal region involved in the variable-foreperiod effect in three different studies. A) The right dorsolateral prefrontal area stimulated by TMS in Vallesi et al. 2007b (coordinates were taken from the fMRI study by Lewis and Miall, 2003); B) Pre-surgical tumour location in the group of right lateral prefrontal patients tested in Vallesi et al. 2007a; C) Cluster in the right dorsolateral prefrontal cortex activated in the variable versus fixed foreperiod contrast in the fMRI study by Vallesi et al. (2009). To allow comparison across studies, the regions are superimposed to the same axial slice (MNI z: 26) of an individual subject's standardized brain.

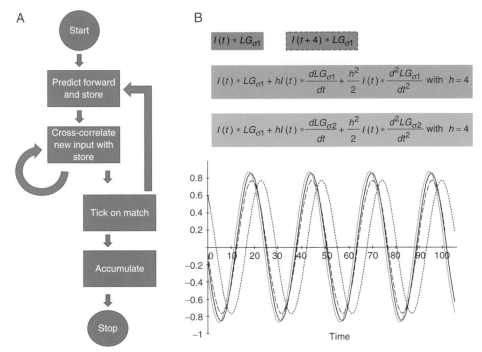

Plate 7 (See also Fig. 14.2) A) A content-dependent clock. The free-running pacemaker from the standard clock model is replaced with a 'predict and compare' circuit. The Taylor series is used to predict an image-based temporal sequence at some future time at a point or region in space. This forward prediction is stored. The new input is cross-correlated with the stored data in a temporal buffer. When the cross-correlation peaks, the clock ticks, the tick is accumulated, and the prediction is reset. The interval over which the prediction is made could vary, and if it does vary, the number of ticks may be scaled by the length of the interval over which the prediction is made (e.g. 10 × 30-ms ticks). B) The red, dotted line is the profile of a filtered (by the log Gaussian) sine function. The red, dashed line is the dotted line time shifted forward by 4 temporal units. The solid blue line is the prediction constructed from the Taylor expansion. The predicted signal is slightly increased in amplitude at this frequency, however the temporal shift is quite accurate. The green line is the prediction, with a sharpened temporal impulse response in the M cell filters, as a response to temporal adaptation. The advance in the filter leads to a phase advance in the derivative functions, which would have the same effect as predicting forward with a larger excursion parameter.

A   Temporal orienting task

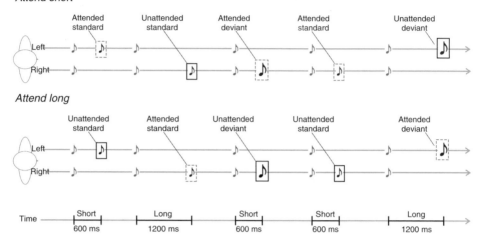

B   ERP effects of temporal orienting

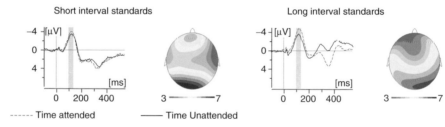

Plate 8 (See also Fig. 28.1) Schematic drawing of the temporal orienting task (A) and grand average ERPs time locked to attended and unattended standards (B). A) Musical notes represent onset (grey) and offset (black) of short and long intervals. The Attend Short condition is displayed above the Attend Long condition. Each offset marker is indicated as being either attended (dashed green marking) or unattended (black marking). The timing of the on- and offset markers and the interval durations are marked in a timeline along the bottom. B) Grand average ERPs for standards at the attended (dashed green) versus unattended (black) time. ERPs to the short interval standards (left) are shown at a representative fronto-central electrode. ERPs to the long interval standards (right) are shown at a representative frontal electrode. Next to each waveform, the normalized topography (mean = 5, SD = 2) of the N1 effect is shown (top view). Blue shadings indicate relatively more negative amplitudes for the attended than the unattended condition; red shadings indicate relatively more positive amplitudes for the attended than the unattended condition. Here, and in the following figures, the time epoch used for statistical analyses of the displayed effect is shaded grey, all traces are aligned with respect to a 100-ms pre-stimulus baseline, and Negativity is up.

A   Combined temporal and spatial orienting task

Attend short and left

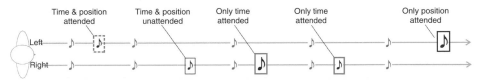

Attend Long and right

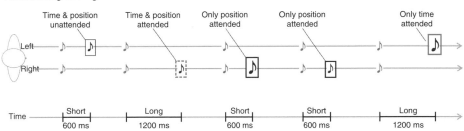

B   ERP effects of temporal and spatial orienting

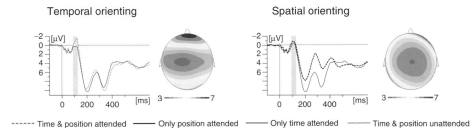

Plate 9 (See also Fig. 28.2) Schematic drawing of the combined temporal and spatial orienting task (A) and grand average ERPs time locked to attended and unattended standards (B). A) Two of the four possible conditions are shown for illustrative purposes: the Attend Short and Left condition is displayed above the Attend Long and Right condition. Each offset marker is indicated as being 'time and position attended' (dashed green marking), 'time attended' (solid green marking), 'position attended' (bold black marking), or 'time and position unattended' (fine black marking). The timing of the on- and offset markers and the interval durations are marked in a timeline along the bottom. B) Grand average ERPs for standards of short intervals at an attended (green line) versus unattended (black line) time point for the unattended position (left) and grand average ERPs for standards of short intervals at an attended (bold line) versus unattended (fine line) location for the unattended time point (right). ERPs are shown at a contralateral central electrode cluster. Next to each waveform, the normalized topography (mean = 5, SD = 2) of the N1 effect is shown (top view). Blue shadings indicate relatively more negative amplitudes for the attended than the unattended condition; red shadings indicate relatively more positive amplitudes for the attended than the unattended condition. In the topographic maps, electrodes ipsilateral to stimulation are on the left, electrodes contralateral to stimulation are on the right.

A   Uni-modal effects of temporal orienting

Auditory stimuli, audition attended

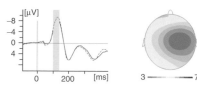

Tactile stimuli, touch attended

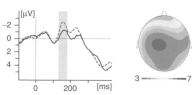

B   Cross-modal effects of temporal orienting

Auditory stimuli, touch attended

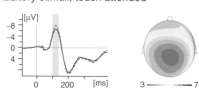

Tactile stimuli, audition attended

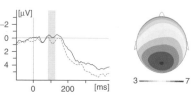

----- Time attended, touch   —— Time unattended, touch   ----- Time attended, audition   —— Time unattended, audition

Plate 10 (See also Fig. 28.3) Grand average ERPs to attended (dashed green lines) and unattended (black lines) standards for the uni-modal (A) and cross-modal (B) effects of temporal orienting. A) Left panel: ERPs to auditory stimuli, audition attended. Right panel: ERPs to tactile stimuli, touch attended. B) Left panel: ERPs to auditory stimuli, touch attended. Right panel: ERPs to tactile stimuli, audition attended. ERPs to auditory stimuli are shown at a contralateral central cluster. ERPs to uni-modal and cross-modal effects in the tactile modality are shown at an ipsilateral central and a contralateral parietal cluster, respectively. Next to each waveform, the normalized topography (mean = 5, SD = 2) of the depicted effect is shown (top view). Blue shadings indicate relatively more negative amplitudes for the attended than the unattended condition; red shadings indicate relatively more positive amplitudes for the attended than the unattended condition. Electrodes ipsilateral to stimulation are on the left, electrodes contralateral to stimulation are on the right.

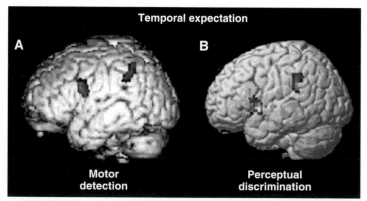

Plate 11 (See also Fig. 31.2) Using temporal expectancies to optimize behaviour activates a left fronto-parietal network, whether expectancies are established (A) endogenously by predictive pre-cues in a speeded motor detection task (Coull and Nobre, 1998) or (B) exogenously by predictable stimulus motion in a perceptual discrimination task (Coull et al., 2008).

Chapter 17

On the locus of temporal preparation: enhancement of premotor processes?

Bettina Rolke and Rolf Ulrich

Anticipating events and adapting behaviour accordingly is a fundamental ability that does not only apply to humans but also to other organisms, such as insects (Matheson, 2008). When we are required to act upon future events, we usually initiate covert preparatory processes to optimize our performance. As an everyday example, consider a table-tennis player who is trying to return a drive from his opponent. When his opponent begins to execute the drive, our table-tennis player will be heavily engaged in preparatory processes to increase the likelihood of a successful return. Preparation allows him to perform the backswing at the right moment and in the right direction. Without anticipation and preparation, it is impossible to successfully return a hard drive with an approach speed of 150km/hour or even faster (e.g. Muster, 1986; Bootsma and van Wieringen, 1990).

Because anticipation and preparation are fundamental cognitive abilities, psychologists have sought to unravel the covert processes that are related to these abilities (Woodrow 1914; Leonhard, 1953). In general, successful preparation is strongly associated with our ability to anticipate future events. Anticipation reduces our uncertainty about future events and enables an internal state that improves our ability to deal with these events in an optimal way. Thus preparation may be characterized by the processes that produce optimal adjustment for perceiving and responding to future events. There exists a continuing interest in uncovering these processes and their neuronal correlates (see Nobre et al., 2007).

Experimental approaches to the study of temporal preparation

Research on preparation relies strongly on chronometric methods. In particular, reaction-time (RT) paradigms have often been used by cognitive psychologists to investigate the covert processes associated with anticipation and preparation (e.g. A. F. Sanders, 1998). Within this field of research, two kinds of preparation have been differentiated and usually addressed independently, namely event and temporal preparation (Requin et al., 1991). In brief, event preparation is related to the reduction of future response alternatives. For example, if a goalkeeper has advance information that the penalty taker will kick the ball into the lower left corner, the goalkeeper can reduce the number of possible alternatives to just one, and thus prepare for this event. Event preparation has been studied in choice RT tasks that convey partial advance information about the forthcoming event (e.g. Rosenbaum, 1980; Miller, 1982; Schröter and Leuthold, 2009). RT usually decreases as the amount of advance information increases.

Second and most relevant to this chapter, temporal preparation is related to the reduction of temporal uncertainty, that is, uncertainty not about *what* response to produce but about *when* to produce it. Participants respond especially quickly to a stimulus when the temporal occurrence of this stimulus can be anticipated (Woodrow 1914). This benefit on RT has been repeatedly demonstrated and shown to be a robust phenomenon (Teichner, 1954; Klemmer, 1956; Bevan et al., 1965; Niemi and Näätänen, 1981). The effect has been investigated in studies that employ warning signals and manipulate the foreperiod duration, that is, the time interval between the warning signal and a subsequent imperative response signal. The duration of the foreperiod and the distribution of foreperiods influence RT.

The foreperiod effect depends on whether the foreperiod duration varies randomly from trial to trial (*variable foreperiod condition*) or remains constant within a block of trials and only varies across blocks (*constant foreperiod condition*) (see also Wagener and Hoffman, Chapter 16; Los, Chapter 21; Vallessi, Chapter 22, this volume). In the constant foreperiod condition, mean RT usually increases progressively as foreperiod increases. In the variable condition, however, mean RT usually decreases as foreperiod increases (Drazin, 1961; Bertelson and Tisseyre, 1968). These two foreperiod effects are well established and they can be observed in both simple and choice RT tasks (Bertelson and Boons 1960; Mattes and Ulrich, 1997; A. F. Sanders, 1998). Since the warning signal conveys no information about the response, these effects reflect a state of non-specific preparation, sometimes referred to as *temporal preparation* (Müller-Gethmann et al., 2003; Rolke and Hofmann, 2007; Los and Schut, 2008).

The traditional view of temporal preparation presupposes that participants intentionally prepare for the moment when the imperative signal is delivered (Los and Van den Heuvel, 2001). Central to this view is the assumption that a high preparatory state can be maintained only for a brief duration, that is, 0.1–0.3 seconds (Alegria, 1974; Gottsdanker, 1975). Accordingly, individuals need to synchronize this brief preparation period with the moment of imperative signal presentation, because optimal performance can only be achieved when the imperative signal occurs during this period. However, the individual's strategy for anticipating the imperative moment, that is, the moment of imperative signal presentation (Los and van den Heuvel, 2001), differs between the constant foreperiod condition and the variable one. In the constant condition, the individual's ability to predict the imperative moment deteriorates as foreperiod is lengthened, because the accuracy of time estimation typically deteriorates for longer intervals (e.g. Grondin, 2001). This impairs the synchronization of the preparation period with the imperative moment at longer foreperiods (Näätänen et al., 1974). Accordingly, RT increases with increasing foreperiod length in the constant condition. Because it takes some time to attain an optimal preparatory state, the function relating RT to foreperiod sharply decreases from 0 to about 300ms and increases thereafter (e.g. Müller-Gethmann et al., 2003). In the variable foreperiod condition there are several critical moments at which the imperative signal may occur. If the imperative signal occurs with equal probability at each critical moment, the conditional probability of imperative signal presentation during a single trial increases gradually as time goes by (Niemi and Näätänen, 1981), producing an increasing hazard function. This growth of expectancy is assumed to enhance the preparatory state, producing short RTs at long foreperiods in the variable condition (Niemi and Näätänen, 1981; Sollers and Hackley, 1997; see Los and Van den Heuvel, 2001; Los et al., 2001; Los and Heslenfeld, 2005, for a novel approach within the variable foreperiod domain).

The traditional approach to the study of temporal preparation has been extended in recent studies. One important extension is the *temporal orienting paradigm*. It employs either informative symbolic cues (e.g. Miniussi et al., 1999; Correa et al., 2005; Correa, Chapter 26; Nobre, Chapter 27, this volume) or blockwise instructions (e.g. Lange et al., 2003; Lange and Röder, Chapter 28, this volume) to induce expectancy of a certain foreperiod duration. An explicit cue might consist of the word 'early' or 'late', indicating after which of two foreperiods (long or short) the imperative signal will appear. Temporal orienting paradigms are useful because they allow both the investigation of the effects of directing attention to moments in time and the assessment of variable foreperiod effects (e.g. Los and Van den Heuvel, 2001). One restriction of these paradigms is that only two to three clearly distinguishable foreperiods can be experimentally employed, and effects of temporal orienting can often only be assessed after the short foreperiod, because invalidly cued long foreperiods offer the opportunity to reorient preparation (Miniussi et al., 1999; however, see Correa et al., 2004). Thus, in contrast to traditional paradigms, an analysis of the time course of preparatory processes is difficult to assess with temporal orienting procedures.

A powerful procedure for assessing the time course of the effective preparation period was proposed by Los and Schut (2008). These authors note that there are various possibilities when temporal preparation starts and when it ends. According to the traditional view, preparation starts with the onset or offset of the warning signal, and terminates with the onset of the impera- tive signal. Los and Schut provide clear evidence against this notion. They have explored the effec- tive time course of preparation by determining its starting and endpoint. Their results indicate that when both warning signal and foreperiod durations are short, preparation begins already with the onset of the warning signal. Most interestingly, they have revealed that preparation does not stop with the onset of imperative signal but rather proceeds in parallel with imperative signal encoding. This conclusion is supported by the underadditive interaction between imperative signal intensity and foreperiod duration. More specifically, if the luminance of the imperative stimulus is low, foreperiod duration has less impact on RT than when its luminance is high. This underadditive effect suggests that temporal preparation can operate on post-perceptual processes during the encoding of imperative signal.

Motor locus of temporal preparation

RT reflects the duration of the whole processing stream from stimulus input until the response. Thus it is difficult to estimate the duration of the single processing stages that contribute to over- all RT effects. Nevertheless, various approaches have been developed to address this question. The notion that temporal preparation shortens the duration of specific stages within the processing stream from stimulus input to the associated response is ubiquitous in the literature. Knowing which stage of information processing is speeded by temporal preparation (e.g. motor stages) contributes to a better understanding of its mechanisms. Like Los and Schut (2008), a number of studies have addressed this issue (for reviews see Hackley and Valle-Inclán 2003; Müller- Gethmann et al., 2003).

A standard approach for localising this effect is the additive-factor method (Sternberg, 2001; Hunt et al., Chapter 1, this volume). For example, some studies using this method (e.g. A. F. Sanders 1980, 1998; Spijkers, 1990) have shown that motor variables such as instructed muscle tension and response complexity interact with foreperiod to modulate RT (Burle et al., Chapter 18, this volume). This result corroborates the notion of a motor locus. These studies, however, employed aiming movements, whereas most RT studies use simple key-press responses. Therefore, it is difficult to generalize these results to the bulk of RT studies. Nevertheless, several studies are consistent with this motor view; for example, factors that are supposed to influence earlier, premotor processing like stimulus quality (Frowein and Sanders, 1978), stimulus-response- compatibility (e.g. Posner et al., 1973; Los and Schut 2008), and the number of response alternatives (e.g. Alegria and Bertelson 1970) usually do not alter the foreperiod effect on RT.

Two notable exceptions do not fit, however. First, Broadbent and Gregory (1965) reported a larger foreperiod effect when the stimulus-response design was compatible than when it was incompatible. This finding suggests that temporal preparation may (also) change the duration of the response selection stage, a stage that is usually conceived as a premotor stage (e.g. Miller and

Ulrich, 1998). Second, and more crucially, Niemi and Lehtonen (1982) observed that a weak visual imperative signal produced a stronger foreperiod effect than a strong one. Because a manipulation of visual intensity should influence the duration of early processes only (e.g. Miller et al., 1999), this interaction indicates that temporal preparation may also speed up very early processes. Thus, at least some studies using the additive-factors method cast doubt on an exclusively motor locus of temporal preparation. Furthermore, the interferences based on the additive-factor method rely on the assumption that information processing proceeds through serial, discrete stages (see McClelland 1979; but see Miller et al., 1995).

To probe the state of the motor system under various conditions of temporal preparation, several researchers have supplemented RT data with additional measurements. First, it has been demonstrated that response force decreases with the level of temporal preparation (e.g. Mattes and Ulrich, 1997). Reflex studies have shown that temporal preparation modulates spinal excitability during the foreperiod interval (Brunia and Boelhouwer, 1988; Requin et al., 1991). Similar results were found for motor-evoked potentials that were evoked by transcranial magnetic stimulation of the cortical area associated with a response hand muscle (Hasbroucq et al., 1999; Tandonnet et al., 2003; 2006; Burle et al., Chapter 18, this volume). Finally, the amplitude of the contingent negative variation is associated with the degree of temporal preparation (Loveless, 1973; Van der Lubbe et al., 2004; Praamstra, Chapter 24; Pouthas and Pfeuty, Chapter 30, this volume). All these studies employing motor correlates have favoured the motor view of temporal preparation. These markers are clearly sensitive to temporal preparation as they indicate that temporal preparation modulates the readiness of the motor system. Nevertheless, it is a moot point whether these correlates of preparation are also responsible for the effect of temporal preparation on RT. Usually the correlations between these measures and RT are close to zero or low. Accordingly, Jennings et al. (1998) have concluded that temporal preparation does not constitute a unitary process, but should rather be viewed as a multicomponent process. It might be quite plausible that only a subset of all these processes contribute to the foreperiod-RT effect.

Non-motor locus of temporal preparation

As outlined earlier, earlier studies have tended to favour a motor locus for the effect of temporal preparation on RT. This view, however, has changed over the last years. We will review some findings that argue against an exclusively motor locus, and describe studies demonstrating that temporal preparation may operate even at the perceptual level (Correa, Chapter 26; Nobre, Chapter 27; Lange and Röder, Chapter 28, this volume).

Premotor locus

Bausenhart et al. (2006) employed the psychological refractory period paradigm (PRP; Pashler and Johnston, 1998), which allows effects to be traced back to motoric and premotoric processing stages. Two choice RT tasks were employed. The first was a colour discrimination task; the second required tone discrimination. As a critical manipulation, the authors varied stimulus-onset asynchrony (SOA) between the presentation of the first (S1) and the second stimulus (S2). The standard PRP finding is that reaction times for S2 (RT2) increases dramatically as the SOA between S1 and S2 decreases. To account for this pattern of results, a bottleneck model of the PRP effect was proposed. This model assumes that at least three different processing stages add to the overall RT for each single task. These stages represent a central processor, which receives its input from perceptual processes, and a motor process, which executes the response. The main assumption of the model is that the central response selection constitutes a single-channel bottleneck process, which cannot serve both tasks simultaneously (e.g. Pashler 1994; see also Sigman, Chapter 5; Ruthruff and Pashler, Chapter 9, this volume). The pre- and post-bottleneck processes, however, proceed without interference and in parallel to all other processes. Because of the bottleneck process, response selection for S2 cannot begin until the response selection process for S1 has finished, and RT2 is prolonged by this 'waiting time' at short SOAs. In fact, this bottleneck model explains the pattern of results typically obtained in a PRP experiment. Moreover, it exhibits the effect-propagation property. This property is produced when suboptimal preparation prolongs, for example, perceptual processing of S1. Because of this prolongation, initiation of the central bottleneck process by S1 is delayed. Since central processing of S2 must wait until the central processor is finished with S1, RT2 is similarly prolonged by this length of time, i.e. the effect propagates from S1 processing to S2 processing. Crucially, however, this effect propagation can only occur at short SOAs. At long SOAs, processing of S1 is nearly finished when processing of S2 starts and any effect of suboptimal preparation has no consequences for S2 (see Miller and Reynolds, 2003).

Bausenhart et al. (2006) took advantage of this effect-propagation property to assess the locus of temporal preparation (see Figure 17.1). Specifically, Bausenhart and colleagues expanded the PRP paradigm by manipulating temporal preparation for the first task. The authors hypothesized that if temporal preparation affects early processes of S1, effect-propagation on RT2 should be observed at short but not long SOAs. If, however, temporal preparation operates on late processes, no such effect propagation should be observed for RT2, because motor processing of S2 is uninfluenced by S1 processing. Bausenhart and colleagues found that the effect of temporal preparation propagated completely from the first to the second task at short SOAs. As outlined earlier, this pattern of results supports the notion that temporal preparation speeds premotoric processing levels.

The premotoric locus of temporal preparation is supported by electrophysiological approaches that used the lateralized readiness potential (LRP) as a chronophysiological measure for localizing the effect of temporal preparation on RT (Smulders, 1993; Hackley and Valle-Inclán, 1998; 1999; Müller-Gethmann et al., 2003). This potential allows RT to be bisected into an early and late phase. Specifically, when the RT task involves a choice between two hands, an asymmetric readiness potential develops during the RT interval with greater negativity over the hemisphere contralateral to the responding hand. The time when the onset of asymmetry begins marks LRP onset. This onset is believed to reflect the moment in time when response selection for one hand is finished. Thus, the LRP provides an electrophysiological marker indexing the end of central processing and the beginning of hand-specific motor processes. Since LRP onset can be measured relative to the onset of the response signal (stimulus-locked) or to the onset of the overt response (response-locked), two different intervals emerge. The stimulus-locked LRP indexes the duration of processes occurring before the onset of hand-specific response activation, i.e. premotoric processes, and the response-locked LRP indexes the duration of processes occurring after the onset of hand-specific response activation, i.e. motor processes. In order to chart the effect of temporal preparation, Müller-Gethmann and colleagues (2003) conducted blocked foreperiod experiments. Shorter foreperiods reduced RT and the stimulus-locked LRP latency, but not the response-locked LRP latency. These results therefore demonstrate that temporal preparation shortens the early but not the late portion of RT. Thus, this study supports the conclusion that temporal preparation facilitates the speed of premotoric processes (similar results were obtained by Hackley and Valle-Inclán, 1998; 1999; but see Tandonnet et al., 2003 for a critique on this approach).

Whereas the PRP study and the LRP studies partitioned RT into a premotoric and a motoric part, and provided strong evidence for a premotoric locus for the temporal preparation effect,

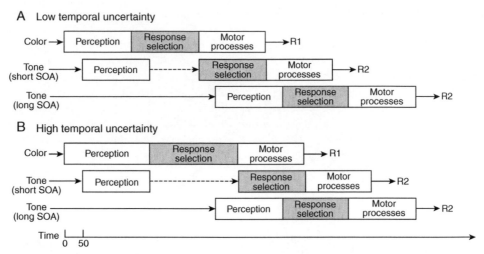

Fig. 17.1 Illustration of effect propagation. This figure depicts dual-task processing in accordance with the bottleneck model for trials with short and long SOAs and for trials with low (A) and high (B) temporal uncertainty, i.e. high and low temporal preparation, respectively. (A) The upper sequence illustrates the duration of perceptual processing, response selection, and motor processing for Task 1. The durations of these stages do not depend on the SOA. The middle sequence shows the same processing sequence for Task 2 after a short SOA. Note that response selection for Task 2 cannot begin until response selection for Task 1 has finished; this waiting period is represented by the dashed line. The third sequence depicts Task 2 processing with a long SOA. Here response selection for Task 2 can immediately begin after Task 2 perception has finished. (B) The lower sequence is identical to the one in (A) except that, due to high temporal uncertainty, longer pre-motor processing emerges in Task 1. Comparison of (A) and (B) illustrates that an increase in RT1 (i.e. the temporal interval between the onset of the first stimulus and the onset of the response, R1, to this stimulus) associated with higher temporal uncertainty would completely propagate to RT2 (i.e. the temporal interval between the second stimulus and the associated response R2) at a short SOA. At a long SOA, however, this effect on RT1 would no longer be propagated to RT2. Reproduced with permission from Bausenhart, K. M., Rolke, B., Hackley, S. A., and Ulrich, R. (2006). The locus of temporal preparation effects: evidence from the psychological refractory period paradigm. *Psychonomic Bulletin & Review*, **13**, 536–42.

they could not exactly localize the effect within premotoric stimulus processing stages. Specifically, premotoric processing includes both central and perceptual processing stages. Either one, or both, of these stages might benefit from temporal preparation. Hackley et al. (2007) therefore aimed to isolate the temporal preparation effect within premotoric processing. These authors collected the LRP as a marker for the onset of motor processes, but in addition measured the visual N2pc component. This event-related component might be viewed as the perceptual analogue of the LRP. It is the second major deflection in the visual evoked potential and exerts maximum amplitude contralateral to the hemifeld containing a predefined target (pc = posterior and contralateral to visual target). The N2pc is taken as a marker of the perceptual selection of a task-relevant, target stimulus. Therefore, one can take the time interval extending from stimulus onset to the onset of the N2pc to index the duration of early perceptual processing. By using the N2pc and the LRP, Hackley and colleagues trisected RT into three time segments. The time period between stimulus onset and the onset of the N2pc corresponded to 'perceptual' processing.

The time between the onsets of the N2pc and the stimulus-evoked LRP corresponded to 'central' processing. The time between the onsets of the response-evoked LRP and the key press corresponded to motor processing. Within a blocked foreperiod paradigm, and in line with Müller-Gethmann et al. (2003), the authors showed that a short foreperiod reduced stimulus-locked LRP latency, but not response-locked LRP latency. However, they failed to find any significant influence of foreperiod duration on N2pc latency. Thus, Hackley et al. (2007) concluded that the effect of temporal preparation is mainly restricted to the middle interval, implying that late perceptual stages or response selection benefits from temporal preparation.

Perceptual locus

The electrophysiological approaches so far seem to support a premotoric locus for the temporal preparation effect. Moreover, the study of Hackley et al. (2007) restricts the influence of temporal preparation to central rather than perceptual processing stages. These chronophysiological studies indicate that some processing stages are speeded by temporal preparation and that this speeding can be measured by electrophysiological latency markers. Several other authors, however, used a different electrophysiological approach, and employed amplitude measures of ERPs to localize temporal preparation effects (Lange et al., 2003, 2006; Correa et al., 2006a; L. D. Sanders and Astheimer 2008; Lange and Röder; Chapter 28; Nobre, Chapter 27, this volume). Although amplitude measures do not directly reveal the duration of processing stages, they nevertheless can be used to localize effects of temporal preparation within information processing. The idea is that the time point when a potential is evoked can be used to infer processing stages, which are engaged in a specific task. Specifically, if ERPs with a relative short latency (100–200ms), i.e. 'early' potentials (N1, P1), are modulated by experimental manipulations, it seems likely that relatively early processing stages are involved.

Several authors used this electrophysiological approach and in the beginning failed to find any effect of temporal preparation on early perceptual ERP potentials (e.g. Miniussi et al., 1999; Griffin et al., 2001; Nobre, Chapter 27 this volume). Other authors, however, questioned this view and particularly Correa et al. (2006a) argued that specific tasks demands might be the key factor that determine whether temporal preparation affects perception or not. The authors found that temporally attended target letters within a temporal cueing paradigm evoked a larger P1 component than unattended target letters. Since perceptual task demands were relatively high in their study, Correa et al. hypothesized that temporal preparation modulates early visual processing only for perceptually demanding tasks.

At the same time, behavioural studies provided converging evidence for this notion (Correa, Chapter 26, this volume). In one of these studies, Correa, et al. (2005) embedded a predefined target letter within a rapidly presented stream of distractor stimuli. Since all stimuli were presented at the same spatial position, they masked each other and constituted temporal noise. In each trial, a visual cue indicated whether the target was likely to appear early or late. Detection performance for the targets, which were presented at the expected time interval, was higher than detection performance of targets that occurred at an unexpected time interval. This result indicates that temporal preparation modulates processing at a perceptual processing level. This conclusion was also reached by Martens and Johnson (2005) who used a similar account. These authors investigated the influence of temporal preparation on the attentional blink phenomenon (Raymond et al., 1992), i.e. an impairment to identify a second target if it appears shortly after the presentation of a first target. Specifically, analogous to the task of Correa et al. (2005) a stream of digit distractors was presented at the same spatial position and participants were required to identify two target letters. Cueing the temporal onset between both targets reduced the magnitude of the attentional blink. This indicates that temporal cues might be useful in both distinguishing

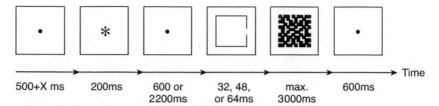

Fig. 17.2 A single trial from the perceptual masking study in the constant foreperiod condition. The warning signal (asterisk) occurred 800ms or 2400ms before target onset and provided a cue for temporal preparation. The Landolt square was displaced by a noise mask consisting of a random dot pattern. Participants had to judge whether the gap of the square was either on the right or on the left side. Reproduced with permission from Rolke, B. and Hofmann, P. (2007). Temporal uncertainty degrades perceptual processing. *Psychonomic Bulletin & Review*, **14**, 522–6.

relevant from irrelevant information and selecting targets within a temporal stream of distractors. Therefore, the two studies agree that temporal preparation improves perceptual stimulus processing in the presence of distractors, that is, in difficult perceptual tasks.

In two recent studies, Rolke and Hofmann (2007) and Rolke (2008) showed that temporal preparation affects perceptual tasks without distractors. These authors isolated the perceptual stimulus processing stage by employing a backward pattern-masking procedure that selectively influences perceptual processing (Turvey, 1973; Breitmeyer, 1984). Following a brief occurrence of the target, a random visual noise pattern was presented (see Figure 17.2). The task of the participants was to judge whether a small spatial gap within the target stimulus, a Landolt-square, was either on the right or on the left side of this square. Temporal preparation for the occurrence of the target stimulus was manipulated within a blocked foreperiod paradigm. Since discrimination performance of the gap detection task was impaired as foreperiod length increased, the authors concluded that temporal preparation enhances processing at a perceptual level. Furthermore, in the study of Rolke (2008), this beneficial effect of temporal preparation on perceptual processing was replicated for letter stimuli. This latter result indicates that not only single feature analysis benefits from temporal preparation, but also higher-level visual perceptual analysis.

The benefit of temporal preparation on perceptual processing occurs not only in the visual modality but also in the auditory modality. Substantiating earlier work (Treisman and Howarth, 1959; Howarth and Treisman, 1961; Loveless, 1975), recent studies show that tone perception is enhanced by temporal preparation. For example, Bausenhart et al. (2007) employed a psychophysical approach and required a pitch-discrimination task for tones that were masked by white noise. The durations of the target tones were adapted to the performance level of each participant, so that 75% correct discrimination responses were obtained. The results show that temporal preparation reduces the tone duration necessary to reach the threshold level. In other words, if participants were better temporally prepared, they needed shorter tone durations for pitch discrimination than when they were temporally unprepared. Whereas this result was obtained in a blocked foreperiod context and at a behavioural level, other authors have used temporal orienting tasks and additionally collected ERPs to investigate temporal preparation effects on auditory perception (Lange et al., 2003; L. D. Sanders and Astheimer 2008; Lange and Röder, Chapter 28, this volume). In line with the visual studies mentioned earlier, which show effects on early visual ERPs, these studies report a modulation of early auditory ERPs as a function of temporal preparation. Thus, studies on auditory perception also support the interpretation that temporal preparation influences perceptual, as well as central and motor stages.

Mechanism of temporal preparation

As reviewed earlier, recent studies strongly support the conclusion that temporal preparation affects the speed of premotor processes, which is in contrast with the traditional view of an exclusively motor locus. To account for the motor and perceptual effects on temporal preparation, some models have been suggested. For example, Näätänen (1971) proposed a response-preparation model in which he employs the hypothetical construct of 'motor readiness'. Motor readiness is conceived as the difference between excitatory motor commands and inhibitory motor commands (see also Burle et al., Chapter 18, this volume). It is assumed that the participant establishes a criterion (i.e. the motor action limit), and when motor readiness reaches this limit, an overt response is triggered. Motor readiness fluctuates due to ongoing central correcting commands that maintain the desired level of motor preparation. Response speed depends on the momentary distance between motor readiness and the motor action limit at the moment of stimulus delivery. If this distance is small, fast responses will result. Importantly, if participants expect the stimulus, they will adjust motor readiness so that it is close to the motor limit. According to this model, temporal preparation influences RT, because the temporal accuracy of the adjustment process depends on the predictability of stimulus occurrence. When stimulus predictability increases with increasing temporal preparation, the adjustment of motor readiness can be timed more accurately and as a consequence, response speed increases. This model is in line with foreperiod effects on motor correlates, e.g. response force (see Mattes and Ulrich, 1997). In addition, it is also in line with the increasing amount of no-go-responses in catch trials when participants are temporally prepared, because the probability for incorrect responses are assumed to increase with increasing motor readiness (e.g. Steinborn et al., 2008). However, since this model restricts the influence of temporal preparation to motor processing, it does not provide any explanation for the more recently reported perceptual effects.

To explain the effect of temporal preparation on perceptual processing, Rolke and Hofmann (2007) have suggested that temporal preparation allows the target to be detected and to be perceptually processed after shorter onset latency (*early onset hypothesis*). According to this hypothesis, temporal preparation accelerates the detection of stimulus onset (see also Simon and Slaviero 1975; Grosjean et al., 2001, for a similar suggestion). More specifically, Rolke and Hofmann assumed that physical stimulation is conveyed into some internal activation that is accumulated over time (see Figure 17.3). As soon as the accumulated information reaches the criterion value, a decision is made and a motor response can be initiated (Grice, 1968; Luce, 1986). The hypothesis furthermore assumes that the accumulation process starts earlier under high temporal preparation. If the task requires a difficult perceptual analysis of a briefly presented target that might be confused with distractors, or runs the risk of being erased by a backward mask, identification of a stimulus critically depends on the available processing time. Since the limited time interval for accumulating target information is prolonged by an earlier start of the accumulation process, the perceptual identification of the stimulus is based on a greater amount of accumulated evidence. Therefore, the early onset hypothesis predicts an enhanced perceptual processing performance when temporal preparation is high and thus explains the recent data on perceptual processing. In addition, this hypothesis might also account for some effects of temporal preparation on later processing stages, because the early perceptual benefit might propagate to later stages.

Although the early onset hypothesis originated from backward masking studies, it has received additional support from temporal discrimination research. For example, Grondin and Rammsayer (2003; see also Mo and George, 1977) investigated whether temporal preparation affects the perceived duration of empty temporal intervals delimited by auditory or visual markers. When temporal preparation was high, intervals were judged to last longer than intervals for

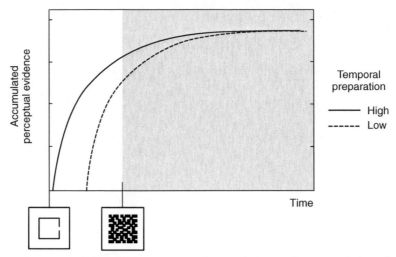

Fig. 17.3 An illustration of the early onset model. The graph depicts the accumulation of perceptual evidence as a function of time. According to the model, accumulation of perceptual evidence starts earlier under high than low temporal preparation. When a mask (random dot pattern mask) is presented after the stimulus (Landolt square), the accumulation of stimulus information will be terminated. In this case, less information is available for the perceptual decision processes under low temporal preparation.

which temporal preparation was low. Exactly this pattern of results is expected if one assumes that temporal preparation leads to an earlier onset of the accumulation process of critical perceptual events. Specifically, the first marker of the interval might be detected more quickly when participants are temporally prepared. Since the influence of temporal preparation is likely to be reduced for the second marker, this produces the impression of relatively long intervals. Furthermore, two recent studies (Correa et al., 2006b; Bausenhart et al., 2008; Correa, Chapter 26, this volume) assessed the influence of temporal preparation on the temporal resolution of visual stimulus processing. Participants were required to indicate which of two stimuli occurred earlier than the other (temporal order judgement). When participants were able to predict the moment of stimulus occurrence accurately, judgements of temporal order improved. These results suggest that temporal preparation enhances the temporal resolution of the visual system. Moreover, the results are compatible with the early-onset hypothesis, if one assumes that the earlier accumulation process of the first stimulus causes the beneficial performance. Therefore, several lines of evidence provide support for the early-onset hypothesis of temporal preparation, although this hypothesis does not deny the existence of an additional effect of temporal preparation on motor processing.

More direct support for the suggestion that temporal preparation reduces the time needed to detect a stimulus (i.e. perceptual latency) comes from a recent study by Seifried et al. (2009). These authors employed a clock paradigm—sometimes also called the *rotating spot method* (e.g. Sanford 1971, 1974; Haggard et al., 2002; Pockett and Miller 2007; see also Wundt, 1911; Buehner, Chapter 15, this volume)—to measure perceptual latency. The participants in this experiment attended to a revolving clock hand and at some time an auditory stimulus was presented. After each trial, participants indicated the position of the clock hand at the onset of the tone. The difference between perceived position and actual clock hand position at the time of tone onset was used to infer the perceptual latency of tone onset. In order to assess whether temporal preparation influences perceptual latency, the authors combined the clock paradigm with a constant foreperiod paradigm. The results showed that temporal preparation associated with short foreperiods decreases perceptual latency. Thus, this study provides rather direct evidence supporting the idea that temporal preparation speeds perceptual processing.

Conclusions

Temporal preparation is a ubiquitous and fundamental feature of human behaviour. It is linked to our ability to anticipate future events and to adjust our behaviour accordingly in order to optimize performance. Since it is not associated to a specific action pattern, temporal preparation even occurs when one does not know in advance the action that is required by an imperative signal. Early studies disclosed the properties of temporal preparation at a behavioural level. More recent cognitive and neuroscience research, however, aims to understand the hidden processes underlying temporal preparation. A first step towards this goal is to unravel the stages within the stimulus-response chain that benefit from this preparation. Early studies mostly suggested that temporal preparation operates exclusively at late stages within this chain, that is, on the motor system. Recent studies however, have shaken this prevailing view. There is now ample evidence that temporal preparation also operates on premotoric levels by speeding up the duration of these processes. This speeding may not only shorten RT but also enable a more accurate analysis of incoming sensory information.

References

Alegria, J. (1974). The time course of preparation after a first peak: some constraints of reacting mechanisms. *Quarterly Journal Experimental Psychology*, **26**, 622–32.

Alegria, J. and Bertelson, P. (1970). Time uncertainty, number of alternatives and particular signal-response pair as determinants of choice reaction time. *Acta Psychologica*, **33**, 36–44.

Bausenhart, K. M., Rolke, B., Hackley, S. A., and Ulrich, R. (2006). The locus of temporal preparation effects: evidence from the psychological refractory period paradigm. *Psychonomic Bulletin & Review*, **13**, 536–42.

Bausenhart, K. M., Rolke, B., and Ulrich, R. (2007). Knowing when to hear aids what to hear. *Quarterly Journal of Experimental Psychology*, **60**, 1610–15.

Bausenhart, K. M., Rolke, B., and Ulrich, R. (2008). Temporal preparation improves temporal resolution: evidence from constant foreperiods. *Perception & Psychophysics*, **70**, 1504–14.

Bertelson, P. and Boons, J. P. (1960). Time uncertainty and choice reaction time. *Nature*, **187**, 531–2.

Bertelson, P. and Tisseyre, F. (1968). The time-course of preparation with regular and irregular foreperiods. *Quarterly Journal of Experimental Psychology*, **20**, 297–300.

Bevan, W., Hardesty, D. L., and Avant, L. L. (1965). Response latency with constant and variable interval schedules. *Perceptual and Motor Skills*, **20**, 969–72.

Bootsma, R. J. and van Wieringen, P.C.W. (1990). Timing an attacking forehand drive in table tennis. *Journal of Experimental Psychology: Human Perception and Performance*, **16**, 21–9.

Breitmeyer, B. G. (1984). *Visual Masking: An Integrative Approach*. New York: Oxford University Press.

Broadbent, D. E. and Gregory, M. (1965). On the interaction of S-R compatibility with other variables affecting reaction time. *British Journal of Psychology*, **56**, 61–7.

Brunia, C. H. M. and Boelhouwer, A. H. W. (1988). Reflexes as a tool: a window in the central nervous system. In P. K. Ackles, J. R. Jennings, and M. G. H. Coles (Eds.) *Advances in Psychophysiology*, Vol. 3, pp.1–67. Greenwich, CT: JAI Press.

Correa, A., Lupiáñez, J., Milliken, B., and Tudela, P. (2004). Endogenous temporal orientation of attention in detection and discrimination tasks. *Perception & Psychophysics*, **66**, 264–78.

Correa, A., Lupiáñez, J., and Tudela, P. (2005). Attentional preparation based on temporal expectancy modulates processing at perceptual-level. *Psychonomic Bulletin & Review*, **12**, 328–34.

Correa, A., Lupiáñez, J., Madrid, E., and Tudela, P. (2006a). Temporal attention enhances early visual processing: a review and new evidence from event-related potentials. *Brain Research*, **1076**, 116–28.

Correa, A., Sanabria, D., Spence, C., Tudela, P., and Lupiáñez, J. (2006b). Selective temporal attention enhances the temporal resolution of visual perception: evidence from a temporal order judgment task. *Brain Research*, **1070**, 202–5.

Drazin, D. H. (1961). Effects of foreperiod, foreperiod variability, and probability of stimulus occurrence on simple reaction time. *Journal of Experimental Psychology*, **62**, 43–50.

Frowein, H. W. and Sanders, F. (1978). Effects of visual stimulus degradation, S-R cpompatibility, and foreperiod duration on choice reaction time and movement time. *Bulletin of the Psychonomic Society*, **12**, 106–8.

Gottsdanker, R. (1975). The attaining and maintaining of preparation. In P. M. A. Rabbitt and S. Dornic (Eds.) *Attention and Performance*, Vol. 5, pp.33–49. London: Academic Press.

Grice, G. (1968). Stimulus intensity and response evocation. *Psychological Review*, **75**, 359–73.

Griffin, I. C., Miniussi, C., and Nobre, A. (2001). Orienting attention in time. *Frontiers in Bioscience*, **6**, 660–71.

Grondin, S. (2001). From physical time to the first and second moments of psychological time. *Psychological Bulletin*, **127**, 22–44.

Grondin, S. and Rammsayer, T. (2003). Variable foreperiods and temporal discrimination. *Quarterly Journal of Experimental Psychology*, **56**, 731–65.

Grosjean, M., Rosenbaum, D. A., and Elsinger, C. (2001). Timing and reaction time. *Journal of Experimental Psychology: General*, **130**, 256–72.

Hackley, S.A. and Valle-Inclán, F. (1998). Automatic alerting does not speed up late motoric processes in a reaction-time task. *Nature*, **391**, 786-788.

Hackley, S.A. and Valle-Inclán, F. (1999). Accessory stimulus effects on response selection: Does arousal speed decision making? *Journal of Cognitive Neuroscience*, **11**, 321–9.

Hackley, S.A. and Valle-Inclán, F. (2003). Which stages of processing are speeded by a warning signal? *Biological Psychology*, **64**, 27–45.

Hackley, S. A., Schankin, A., Wohlschläger, A., and Wascher, E. (2007). Chronometric localization of temporal preparation effects via trisected reaction time. *Psychophysiology*, **44**, 334–38.

Haggard, P., Clark, S., and Kalogeras, J. (2002). Voluntary action and conscious awareness. *Nature Neuroscience*, **5**, 382–5.

Hasbroucq, T., Kaneko, H., Akamatsu, M., and Possamaï, C.-A. (1999). The time-course of preparatory spinal and cortico-spinal inhibition: An H-reflex and transcranial magnetic stimulation study in man. *Experimental Brain Research*, **124**, 33–41.

Howarth, C. I. and Treisman, M. (1961). Lowering of an auditory threshold by a near threshold warning signal. *Quarterly Journal of Experimental Psychology*, **13**, 12–18.

Jennings, R. J., van der Molen, M. W., and Steinhauer, S. R. (1998). Preparing the heart, eye, and brain: foreperiod length effects in a nonaging paradigm. *Psychophysiology*, **35**, 90–8.

Klemmer, E. T. (1956). Time uncertainty in simple reaction time. *Journal of Experimental Psychology*, **51**, 179–84.

Lange, K., Krämer, U. M., and Röder, B. (2006). Attending points in time and space. *Experimental Brain Research*, **173**, 130–40.

Lange, K., Rösler, F., and Röder, B. (2003). Early processing stages are modulated when auditory stimuli are presented at an attended moment in time: an event-related potential study. *Psychophysiology*, **40**, 806–17.

Leonhard, J. A. (1953). Advance information in sensorimotor skills. *Quarterly Journal of Experimental Psychology*, **5**, 141–9.

Los, S. A. and Heslenfeld, D. J. (2005). Intentional and unintentional contributions to nonspecific preparation: Electrophysiological evidence. *Journal of Experimental Psychology: General*, **134**, 52–72.

Los, S. A. and Schut (2008). The effective time course of preparation. *Cognitive Psychology*, **57**, 20–55.

Los, S. A. and Van den Heuvel, C. E. (2001). Intentional and unintentional contributions to nonspecific preparation during reaction time foreperiods. *Journal of Experimental Psychology: Human Perception and Performance*, **27**, 370–86.

Los, S. A., Knol, D. L., and Boers, R. M. (2001). The foreperiod effect revisited: conditioning as a basis for nonspecific preparation. *Acta Psychologica*, **106**, 121–45.

Loveless, N. E. (1973). The contingent negative variation related to preparatory set in reaction time situation with variable foreperiod. *Electroencephalography and Clinical Neurophysiology*, **35**, 369–74.

Loveless, N. E. (1975). The effect of warning interval on signal detection and event-related slow potentials of the brain. *Perception & Psychophysics*, **17**, 565–70.

Luce, R. D. (1986). *Response times: Their role in inferring elementary mental organization*. New York: Oxford University Press.

Martens, S. and Johnson, A. (2005). Timing attention: cuing target onset interval attenuates the attentional blink. *Memory & Cognition*, **33**, 234–40.

Matheson, T. (2008). Motor planning: insects do it on the hop. *Current Biology*, **18**, R742–R743.

Mattes, S. and Ulrich, R. (1997). Response force is sensitive to the temporal uncertainty of response stimuli. *Perception & Psychophysics*, **59**, 1089–97.

McClelland, J. L. (1979). On the time relations of mental processes: an examination of systems of processes in cascade. *Psychological Review*, **86**, 287–330.

Miller, J. (1982). Discrete versus continuous models of human information processing: In search of partial output. *Journal of Experimental Psychology: Human Perception and Performance*, **8**, 273–96.

Miller, J. and Reynolds, A. (2003). The locus of redundant-targets and notargets effects: Evidence from the psychological refractory period paradigm. *Journal for Experimental Psychology: Human Perception and Performance*, **29**, 1126–42.

Miller, J. and Ulrich, R. (1998). Locus of the effect of the number of alternative responses: Evidence from the lateralized readiness potential. *Journal of Experimental Psychology: Human Perception and Performance*, **24**, 1215–31.

Miller, J., van der Ham, F., and Sanders, A. F. (1995). Overlapping stage models and reaction time additivity: Effects of the activation equation. *Acta Psychologica*, **90**, 11–28.

Miller, J., Ulrich, R., and Rinkenauer, G. (1999). Effects of stimulus intensity on the lateralized readiness potential. *Journal of Experimental Psychology: Human Perception and Performance*, **25**, 1454–71.

Miniussi, C., Wilding, E. L., Coull, J. T., and Nobre, A. C. (1999). Orienting attention in time: Modulation of brain potentials. *Brain*, **122**, 1507–18.

Mo, S. S. and George, E. J. (1977). Foreperiod effect and time estimation and simple reaction time. *Acta Psychologica*, **41**, 47–59.

Müller-Gethmann, H., Ulrich, R., and Rinkenauer, G. (2003). Locus of the effect of temporal preparation: Evidence from the lateralized readiness potential. *Psychophysiology*, **40**, 597–611.

Muster, M. (1986). *Tischtennis. Lernen und Trainieren*. Bad Homburg: Limpert Verlag GmbH.

Näätänen, R. (1971). Non-aging fore-periods and simple reaction time. *Acta Psychologica*, **35**, 316–27.

Näätänen, R., Muranen, V., and Merisalo, A. (1974). Timing of expectancy peak in simple reaction time situation. *Acta Psychologica*, **38**, 461–70.

Niemi, P. and Lehtonen, R. (1982). Foreperiod and visual stimulus intensity: a reappraisal. *Acta Psychologica*, **50**, 73–82.

Niemi, P. and Näätänen, R. (1981). Foreperiod and simple reaction time. *Psychological Bulletin*, **89**, 133–62.

Nobre, A. C., Correa, A., and Coull, J. T. (2007). The hazards of time. *Current Opinion in Neurobiology*, **17**, 1–6.

Pashler, H. (1994). Dual-task interference in simple tasks: Data and theory. *Psychological Bulletin*, **116**, 220–44.

Pashler, H. and Johnston, J.C. (1998). Attentional limitations in dual-task performance. In H. Pashler (Ed.) *Attention*, pp.155–89. East Sussex: Psychology Press.

Pockett, S. and Miller, A. (2007). The rotating spot method of timing subjective events. *Consciousness and Cognition*, **16**, 241–54.

Posner, M. I., Klein, R., Summers, J., and Buggie, S. (1973). On the selection of signals. *Memory & Cognition*, **1**, 2–12.

Raymond, J. E., Shapiro, K., L., and Arnell, K. M. (1992). Temporary supression of visual processing in an RSVP task: An attentional blink ? *Journal of Experimental Psychology, Human Perception and Performance*, **18**, 849–60.

Requin, J., Brener, J., and Ring, C. (1991). Preparation for action. In J. R. Jennings and M. G. H. Coles (Eds.), *Handbook of Cognitive Psychophysiology: Central and Autonomic Nervous System Approaches*, pp.357–448. New York: John Wiley.

Rolke, B. (2008). Temporal preparation facilitates perceptual identification of letters. *Perception & Psychophysics*, **70**, 1305–13.

Rolke, B. and Hofmann, P. (2007). Temporal uncertainty degrades perceptual processing. *Psychonomic Bulletin & Review*, **14**, 522–6.

Rosenbaum, D. A. (1980). Human movement initiation: Specification of arm, direction, and extent. *Journal of Experimental Psychology: General*, **109**, 444–74.

Sanders, A. F. (1980). Some effects of instructed muscle tension on choice reaction time and movement time. In R. Nickerson (Ed.) *Attention and Performance VIII* (pp.59-74). Hillsdale, NJ: Lawrence Erlbaum.

Sanders, A. F. (1998). *Elements of human performance: Reaction processes and attention in human skill.* Mahwah, NJ: Lawrence Erlbaum.

Sanders, L. D. and Astheimer, L. B. (2008). Temporally selective attention modulates early perceptual processing: Event-related potential evidence. *Perception & Psychophysics*, **70**, 732–42.

Sanford, A. J. (1971). Effects of changes in the intensity of white noise on simultaneity judgments and simple reaction time. *Quarterly Journal of Experimental Psychology*, **23**, 296–303.

Sanford, A. J. (1974). Attention bias and the relation of perception lag to simple reaction time. *Journal of Experimental Psychology*, **102**, 443–6.

Schröter, H. and Leuthold, H. (2009). Motor programming of rapid finger sequences: Inferences from movement-related brain potentials. *Psychophysiology*, **46**, 388-401.

Seifried, T., Ulrich, R., Bausenhart, K.M., Rolke, B., and Osman, A. (submitted). Temporal preparation decreases perceptual latency: evidence from a clock paradigm.

Simon, R. J., and Slaviero, D. P. (1975). Differential effects of a foreperiod countdown procedure on simple and choice reaction time. *Journal of Motor Behavior*, **7**, 9–14.

Smulders, F. T. (1993). *The selectivity of age effects on information processing: Response times and electrophysiology.* Amsterdam: University of Amsterdam.

Sollers, J. J. and Hackley, S. A. (1997). Effects of foreperiod duration on reflexive and voluntary responses to intense noise bursts. *Psychophysiology*, **34**, 518–26.

Spijkers, W.A. (1990). The relation between response-specificity, S-R compatibility, foreperiod duration and muscle tension in a target aiming task. *Acta Psychol (Amst)*, **75**(3): 261–77.

Steinborn, M., Rolke, B., Bratzke, D., and Ulrich, R. (2008). Sequential effects within a short foreperiod context: further support for the conditioning account of temporal preparation. *Acta Psychologica*, **129**, 297–307.

Sternberg, S. (2001). Separate modifiability, mental modules, and the use of pure and composite measures to reveal them. *Acta Psychologica*, **106**, 147–246.

Tandonnet, C., Burle, B., Vidal, F., and Hasbroucq, T. (2003). The influence of time preparation on motor processes assessed by surface Laplacian estimation. *Clinical Neurophysiology*, **114**, 2376–84.

Tandonnet, C., Burle, B., Vidal, F., and Hasbroucq, T. (2006). Knowing when to respond and the efficiency of the cortical motor command: A Laplacian ERP study. *Brain Research*, **1109**, 158–63.

Teichner, W. H. (1954). Recent studies of simple reaction time. *Psychological Bulletin*, **51**, 128–49.

Treisman, M. and Howarth, C. I. (1959). Changes in threshold level produced by a signal preceding or following the threshold stimulus. *Quarterly Journal of Experimental Psychology*, **11**, 129–42.

Turvey, M. T. (1973). On peripheral and central processes in vision: Inferences from an information-processing analysis of masking with pattern stimuli. *Psychological Review*, **80**, 1–52.

Van der Lubbe, R. H., Los, S. A., Jaskowski, P., and Verleger, R. (2004). Being prepared on time: on the importance of the previous foreperiod to current preparation, as reflected in speed, force and preparation-related brain potentials. *Acta Psychologica*, **116**, 245–62.

Woodrow, H. (1914). The effect upon reaction time of variation in the preparatory interval. In J. Angell, H. Warren, J. Watson and S. Franz (Eds.) *The Psychological Monographs*, pp.16–65. Princeton, NJ: Psychological Review Company.

Wundt, W. (1911). *Grundzüge der physiologischen Psychologie* [Main features of physiological psychology]. (6. umgearbeitete Auflage, Bd. 3). Leipzig: Engelmann.

Chapter 18

Excitatory and inhibitory motor mechanisms of temporal preparation

Boris Burle, Christophe Tandonnet, and
Thierry Hasbroucq

About a century ago, Woodrow (1914) provided the first empirical demonstration that time orientation is critical for information processing. Following his pioneering studies, the influence of temporal preparation has classically been explored in the framework of the reaction time (RT) paradigm by studying the effects of warning signals, which provide information about timing of the forthcoming stimulus. The duration of the interval, termed 'foreperiod', that separates the warning signal from stimulus presentation has a potent influence on the participant's perform- ance (for a review, see Requin et al., 1991; Wagener and Hoffman, Chapter 16; Los, Chapter 21; Vallesi, Chapter 22, this volume). The duration of the foreperiod can be manipulated either between or within blocks. These two types of manipulation may produce opposite effects, and hence deserve to be discussed separately, although some common mechanisms encompass the two designs. When the foreperiod is manipulated between block, RT generally gets longer as the foreperiod increases, although the minimum RT is obtained for foreperiods of around 500ms (below this interval, it is likely that there is insufficient time for preparation to be established, see Bertelson and Tisseyre, 1969; Alegria, 1980).

When manipulated within block, the foreperiod can have one of n durations (n typically being between 2 and 6) each with equal objective probability. In such a situation, the effect of foreperiod is opposite to that described earlier: RT decreases non-linearly as foreperiod increases, before finally reaching an asymptote (see Niemi, 1979).

Niemi and Näätänen (1981) explained this discrepancy (see also Durup and Requin, 1970) by arguing that motor preparation varies as a function of participants' *expectancy* regarding stimulus onset. Importantly, expectancies are established differentially for between- and within- blocks situations. In between-block designs, expectancy is determined only by the subjective estimate of the possible moment of stimulus onset: since preparation is optimal for only a few milliseconds (Alegria, 1975) the participants estimate this moment and attempt to synchronize their level of preparation to it. However, the absolute accuracy of temporal estimation decreases as the time elapsed since warning signal presentation lengthens (Weber's law, see Gibbon, 1977). The participants are therefore less precise in their estimate of long, as compared to short, foreperiods and thus, on average, are less prepared at the time of stimulus presentation (Requin et al., 1991).

In within-block designs, just as for between-block designs, the participants estimate the possible moment of stimulus presentation. However, an additional factor comes into play in such a design: the *conditional* probability of stimulus onset, which evolves as a function of time elapsed since warning signal presentation. Consider three possible foreperiods, say 0.5, 1.0, and 1.5 seconds. If the three foreperiods have the same *objective* probability (which is often the case), their *conditional* probabilities change with time. At 0.5 seconds, there is a 1 in 3 chance that the stimulus will appear. If it does not appear at this interval, the probability that it will appear at 1 second becomes 1 in 2. Finally, if the signal did not appear at either 0.5 or 1 second, it is certain to appear at 1.5 seconds, putting its probability at 1. Since participants prepare as a function of the probability of stimulus occurrence, the preparation induced by these changing conditional probabilities increases as foreperiod lengthens. The level of preparation induced by the accuracy of time estimation over lengthening delays on the one hand, and by changing conditional probabilities over time on the other, are thus acting in opposing directions, and the actual outcome depends on the relative strength of these two sources of preparation (Durup and Requin, 1970). Although such a general framework explains *why* performance is altered by temporal preparation, it does not account for *how* temporal preparation affects information processing. A first step in providing an explanatory hypothesis was proposed by Näätänen (1971) and later elaborated by Niemi and Näätänen (1981).

These authors proposed a simple scheme relating foreperiod duration to RT performance. Subjects increase their neural activity according to their expectancies relative to the time of presentation of the forthcoming stimulus and to the conditional probability of this event. When this preparatory neural activity bypasses a threshold—termed 'motor action limit'—an overt response is triggered. RT depends on the difference between the motor action limit and the level of neural activity attained during the foreperiod. If this difference is large RT is long, when the difference is small RT is short. While participants are expecting the stimulus to appear, they attempt to adjust neural activity close to the motor action limit. Given the variations in expectancies described earlier, the difference between the current level of activity and the motor action limit will be inversely proportional to the level of expectancy.

In order to study temporal preparation per se, between-block designs are more appropriate, at least initially, since expectancy (supposedly) relies on only one process, namely time estimation. We will therefore first concentrate on between-block manipulations, and review the neurophysiological correlates of preparation in such conditions. We shall then broaden our discussion by proposing new perspectives for deciphering the neural mechanisms underlying within-block designs.

The 'motor action limit' model clearly relates temporal preparation to motor processes. This relationship was first studied behaviourally. We briefly review this literature before then describing more recent, complementary neurophysiological approaches, which reveal that temporal preparation does not only involve an increase in neural activity but also varies as a function of a subtle interplay between response activation and inhibition.

Temporal preparation effects during reaction time

Behavioural overview

A widely held assumption in cognitive psychology is that information processing involves several computations, generally termed 'stages'. Based on logical considerations, three sets of stages—perceptual, central, and motor—are generally distinguished (see e.g. Van der Molen et al., 1991). This is simply because the nervous system must first identify the stimulus (perceptual stage), then associate a response to this stimulus (central stage), and, finally, implement the selected response (motor stage). In order to understand how temporal preparation affects information processing, several authors have sought to determine which processing stage(s) it affects. This was first addressed with the additive factor method (Sternberg, 1969, 2001). In essence, the additive factor method relies on analysing statistical interactions between manipulated factors: if the effects of the manipulated factors are additive on RT (i.e. if their joint effect is equal to the sum of the two individual main effects) then the factors are likely to affect different stages; conversely, if the effects interact in an overadditive way (i.e. if the joint effect is larger than the sum of the two individual effects) then the factors are likely to affect at least one stage in common (see Hunt et al., Chapter 1, this volume). In a meta-analysis based on this logic, Sanders (1998) pointed out that the effect of foreperiod duration was additive with the effects of all factors manipulated thus far, with the exception of instructed muscle tension and movement specificity, two factors that alter the 'motor adjustment' stage in Sanders' terminology. Sanders therefore concluded that temporal preparation specifically affected motor processing.

Since then, several authors have provided clear evidence for an effect of temporal preparation on perceptual processes (Correa et al., 2005, 2006; Rolke and Hofmann, 2007; Correa, Chapter 26; Rolke and Ulrich, Chapter 17; Lange and Röder, Chapter 28, this volume), rendering the claim that the effect is specifically motor less tenable. While non-motor effects are undisputable, the motor system remains nonetheless a key target of temporal preparation.

Temporal preparation and the motor command

Although behavioural analyses have provided valuable information, even this short review indicates their limits, namely that inner operations are inferred from overall performance. Furthermore, knowing which processing operations are affected by temporal preparation provides limited information on *how* they are affected. To deepen our understanding of temporal preparation, we have investigated these effects with different neurophysiological techniques (see Figure 18.1). Our approach was based on a 'backward' analysis of the response processes implemented in an RT task. In essence, we looked for neural indices that preceded the behavioural response and whose sensitivity to temporal preparation could be assessed. We started with indices close in time to the overt response, then stepped back towards higher brain processes. The first index we analysed was the electromyographic (EMG) activity of muscles involved in

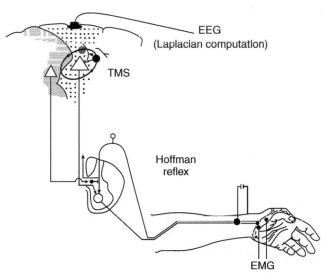

Fig. 18.1 Motor cortex and corticospinal track along with a representation of the four techniques used in the series of experiments: electroencephalography (EEG), transcranial magnetic stimulation (TMS), Hoffman (H) reflex, and electromyography (EMG).

response execution. We bisected the overall RT into two periods as a function of the onset of muscle contraction (Hasbroucq et al., 1995). The time interval between the stimulus and the onset of EMG activity is classically termed 'premotor time', while the time interval between the onset of EMG activity and the mechanical response is termed 'motor time' (Botwinick and Thompson, 1966). Premotor time reflects the duration of all processes preceding motor execution, whereas motor time reflects peripheral motor execution. Interestingly, motor time was shown to be longer for long foreperiods than for short ones (Hasbroucq et al., 1995; Tandonnet et al., 2003). By itself, the increase in motor time explained 19% and 16% of the overall foreperiod effect in these two studies, respectively. This undoubtedly shows that response execution is affected by temporal preparation, even if some other processes are also affected. Hasbroucq et al. (1995) also analysed the EMG burst in more detail to understand the effect of temporal preparation on motor time. They reported that the initial slope of the EMG burst was steeper for short foreperiods compared to longer ones. According to models of force and/or EMG development (Meijers et al., 1976; Ulrich and Wing, 1991), such an increase in slope steepness reflects a higher degree of synchronization among the motor units involved in the genesis of the EMG burst. This indicates that the motor command sent to the muscles is more efficient in synchronizing targeted motor units when participants are more prepared, demonstrating that the very execution of the motor response is affected by temporal preparation.

After having established that motor execution was affected, the next logical step was to investigate the influence of temporal preparation on the dynamics of the motor command at the level of the primary motor cortex (M1). Electroencephalography (EEG) is the technique of choice for studying the fast dynamics of brain activity. However, most EEG studies of response preparation suffer from limitations. Volume conduction through the superficial layers of the head (dura-mater, skull, scalp), substantially worsens the spatial resolution of the EEG signal. In an attempt to circumvent this poor resolution, most research has used the so-called 'lateralized readiness potential' (LRP, initially called 'corrected motor asymmetry' by Smid et al., 1987). The LRP computation is based on a double subtraction: activity recorded by electrodes located over the M1 ipsilateral to the response is subtracted from activity recorded by electrodes located over the contralateral M1 (see Gratton et al., 1988; Coles, 1989 for more detail). A caveat of this measure is to hinder the relative contribution of each M1 (Eimer, 1999; Tandonnet et al., 2003; Vidal et al., 2003). However, the use of the surface Laplacian computation (Nunez, 1981; Babiloni et al., 2001) can effectively counteract the effects of volume conduction, and yield activities that approximate those directly measurable from the cortical surface.

In order to measure the relative contributions of contralateral and ipsilateral motor cortices to motor preparation with the best possible spatial resolution, we applied Laplacian derivations to non-subtracted EEG signals. Previous studies (Taniguchi et al., 2001; Vidal et al., 2003), have shown that when the task involves a between-hand choice, a negative wave develops about 80ms prior to EMG onset over the contralateral M1, while a positive wave simultaneously develops over the ipsilateral M1 (see also, Praamstra and Seiss, 2005). On the basis of monosynaptic reflex (Hasbroucq et al., 2000) and transcranial magnetic stimulation (TMS) studies (Burle et al., 2002) performed in similar task conditions, the negative wave can be interpreted as the response-related activation of the contralateral (i.e. involved) M1 and the positive wave as an inhibition of the ipsilateral (non-involved) M1 (for a review, see Burle et al., 2004). We thus used this activation-inhibition pattern to probe the influence of temporal preparation on the implementation of the central motor command (Tandonnet et al., 2003, 2006).

These studies revealed two main effects. First, the positive component (i.e. the inhibition of the incorrect response) was not significantly affected by preparation. By contrast, the negative component (i.e. the activation of the correct response) was affected in two ways. This wave was more tightly time-locked to EMG onset for the short than for the long foreperiod, suggesting that the build-up of the motor command was less variable across trials and/or took less time when participants were optimally prepared. Furthermore, M1 amplitude was smaller for the short foreperiod. At first sight, it may seem odd to observe reduced M1 activity for a shorter motor time (see above). However, this is likely to indicate a better (more efficient) synchronization of motor units, which leads to the more phasic muscle contraction observed in our previous EMG study (Hasbroucq et al., 1995). Furthermore, as we shall see in what follows, this potential discrepancy will be explained by data collected during the foreperiod. Indeed, the improvement in the efficiency of the motor command, as revealed by the studies reviewed earlier, results from temporal preparation-dependent mechanisms recruited during the foreperiod. Understanding how the motor command is improved requires elucidation of the neural mechanisms implemented during the foreperiod.

Changes in motor excitability during the foreperiod

Preparatory increase in neural activation

Several studies performed in the 1970s and 1980s indicate that neural preparatory mechanisms entail an increase in activation of neural structures. Notably the amplitude of long latency reflex responses (for a review, see Bonnet et al., 1981), which are considered to reflect changes in excitability of central structures, increase during the foreperiod (Bonnet and Requin, 1982; Bonnet, 1983). These findings suggest that temporal preparation induces a progressive increment of supra-spinal neural activity. Research on event related potentials (ERPs) further supports this notion. Walter et al. (1964) described a sustained negative change in brain potentials during the foreperiod: the contingent negative variation (CNV). This composite wave (see e.g. van Boxtel and Brunia, 1994a,b; Hamano et al., 1997) is a meaningful index of temporal preparation (Praamstra, Chapter 24; Pouthas and Pfeuty, Chapter 30, this volume). Indeed, as emphasized by Macar and Bonnet (1997), the CNV develops as soon as the participant attempts to associate two events, the second (e.g. the stimulus) being expected because it follows the first (e.g. the warning signal). In terms of 'threshold regulation theory' (Birbaumer et al., 1990), this development could reflect an increase in excitability of underlying neural structures, an interpretation in line with conclusions drawn from long-latency reflex investigations. Note that while long-latency reflexes and CNV data are in favour of excitatory modulations, these are inconclusive regarding which structures mediate such increases in neural activity. Modulations are likely to rely on the contribution of motor as well as non-motor neural populations.

Preparatory increases in neural suppression

In contrast, and somehow paradoxically, other results indicate that suppression plays an important role in the neural mechanisms underlying temporal preparation effects during the foreperiod. First, studies using spinal reflex techniques have shown that a subjective state of readiness induces systematic variations in the excitability of spinal nuclei. Indeed, the amplitude of monosynaptic reflexes (Hoffmann and tendinous) triggered in a response agonist decreases prior to the onset of the response signal. This reflex depression was initially interpreted as an increase in presynaptic inhibition of motoneurons' somesthetic afferents (for a review, see Schieppati, 1987), which would increase the sensitivity of the motoneuronal pool to supraspinal commands (Requin et al., 1991). Second, we have used the technique of single-pulse transcranial magnetic stimulation (TMS) in order to probe the excitability of the cortico-spinal pathway during the foreperiod (Hasbroucq et al., 1997, 1999a,b). Our results, as well as those of Touge and colleagues (1998), reveal that the size of the motor potential evoked by TMS decreases during foreperiods allowing optimal preparation as opposed to those allowing suboptimal preparation. The motor evoked potential (MEP) results from direct or transynaptic recruitment of corticospinal neurons (Terao and Ugawa, 2002). The size of the MEP reflects the degree of corticospinal excitability and hence, a decrease in MEP amplitude during the foreperiod reflects a diminution of excitability in the corticospinal pathway. Initially, this decrease was interpreted as resulting from an adaptive mechanism, increasing the sensitivity of motor structures to the forthcoming voluntary command. Such a mechanism was conceived as an active filtering of task-unrelated afferents to the corticospinal tract that would facilitate the implementation of the voluntary command by increasing its signal-to-noise ratio. Direct measures of motor-unit discharge through single-unit recordings during the foreperiod provide further support for this view. Indeed, Duclos and colleagues (2008) reported that the inter-spike interval lengthens as time elapses during the foreperiod, reflecting a decrease in excitability, although this decrease could not be correlated with performance. Second, they also reported that the variability of motor-unit discharge was lower towards the end of the foreperiod. This may indicate a dampening of background noise as participants get prepared.

Touge and colleagues (1998), however, suggested another interpretation, namely that the suppression revealed by MEP depression serves to hold back response execution during the foreperiod. Using single-cell recording techniques in monkeys, Prut and Fetz (1999) observed that a large part of the preparatory modulation of spinal interneuron activity was inhibitory and interpreted this in line with the suggestion of Touge et al. (1998). According to Prut and Fetz, inhibitory modulations are part of a general braking mechanism suppressing the tendency to initiate a response during the foreperiod. Such braking would be implemented both at the spinal and central level, and would be released during the RT, after the occurrence of the response signal. This notion was further promoted by McMillan and colleagues (2006, p.241) who proposed that: '[…] it is possible that this [MEP depression] may reflect a global descending influence to the spinal motor neuron pool, to prevent movement […]'. In the next section, we propose an alternative interpretation on the basis of more recent results.

Reconciling neural activation and suppression

In an attempt to shed light on the coupling between activation and suppression, we used single-pulse TMS to simultaneously probe changes in excitability of the corticospinal tract and of M1 during different foreperiods (Davranche et al., 2007). We capitalized on the fact that, besides eliciting MEPs that index corticospinal excitability, TMS can also reveal changes in M1 excitability through modulation of the silent period that follows the MEP when the response agonists are tonically contracted (see Burle et al., 2002). While the initial part of the silent period may be a direct consequence of the MEP (refractory period of neurons involved in the MEP, pause in spindle firing, or Renshaw inhibition), the later part results from the recruitment of inhibitory interneurons within the motor cortex (Uncini et al., 1993; Schnitzler and Benecke, 1994; Terao and Ugawa, 2002). In fact, silent periods can be obtained with TMS intensities weaker than those necessary to elicit MEPs (e.g. Rossini et al., 1995), and the latency of silent-period onset elicited at such intensities is longer than that of near-threshold MEPs (Davey et al., 1994). Thus, there is a delay between the initial recruitment of corticospinal neurons (revealed by the MEP) and the recruitment of inhibitory interneurons (revealed by the late part of the silent period).

In order to generate the background EMG activity necessary for observing a silent period, Davranche and colleagues (2007) asked participants to keep their response agonist tonically contracted during task performance. The efficiency of temporal preparation was varied by employing an optimal (500-ms) and a non-optimal (2500-ms) foreperiod.

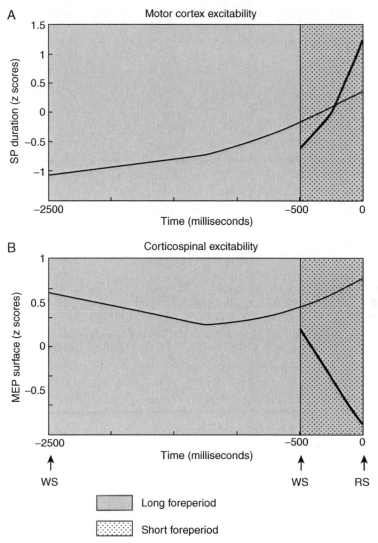

Fig. 18.2 Evolution of the excitability of the motor cortex (A) and of the corticospinal tract (B) during the short/optimal (thick lines) and long/non-optimal foreperiod (thin lines) in Davranche et al. (2007). The data are represented as fitted least-square second-degree polynomials of the silent period (SP) duration (positive values expressed as decreasing durations) and motor evoked potential (MEP) surface area. RS = response signal; WS = warning signal.

As predicted, slower RTs were observed for the longer foreperiod, consistent with the view that temporal preparation was less accurate in this condition. The MEP amplitude decreased over the course of the short foreperiod, but not over the course of the long foreperiod (Figure 18.2B), replicating previous data from our group (Hasbroucq et al., 1997). This decrease in MEP amplitude reflects inhibition of the corticospinal pathway, thereby confirming the existence of a suppression component in temporal preparation (for similar results, see Touge et al., 1998).

The silent period, however, revealed a different pattern. Indeed, its duration decreased as time elapsed and this decrement was more pronounced for the shortest foreperiod (Figure 18.2A), that is, when participants were best prepared. This modulation indicates that intracortical inhibition is removed during temporal preparation, resulting in overall activation. The neurons, to which the inhibitory interneurons recruited by TMS project, were more activated when the level of preparation was higher. This finding refines the long-latency reflex and CNV results summarized earlier, which suggested excitatory modulation of motor-induced activity that is likely to rely on contributions from both motor and non-motor neural populations. These previous results were inconclusive regarding the structures mediating such increases in neural activity. However, since TMS is relatively focal, our TMS data suggest these increases occur specifically at the level of the motor cortex. Furthermore, since the decrease in the duration of the silent period was more pronounced for the short than for the long foreperiod, the present findings demonstrate that silent-period duration is linked to RT performance and thus to the level of preparation attained in the two foreperiod conditions. Recent data using paired-pulse TMS, confirmed an increase in cortical excitability during motor preparation (Sinclair and Hammond, 2008).

The increase in corticospinal inhibition counteracts the increase in excitation of cortical neurons, which may seem odd at first sight. However, these opposing modulations concern distinct neuronal populations that influence the corticospinal pathway at different times after TMS application (e.g. Davey et al., 1994; Priori et al., 1994; Classen and Benecke, 1995; Bonhage et al., 1996). Indeed, the recruitment of corticospinal neurons (revealed by the MEP) precedes the recruitment of inhibitory interneurons (revealed by the late part of the SP).

This organization provides a clue for interpreting the functional interplay of inhibitory and excitatory modulation. Indeed, the stronger the suppression, the higher the activation can go without triggering premature responding. In other words, suppression allows a high level of cortical excitability to build up. Suppression thus appears to be the functional counterpart of activation: it secures the development of cortical excitability, preventing erroneous responding. Note that although we have outlined a tentative scheme for the interplay of excitatory and inhibitory modulations at the motor cortex level, such interplay may occur in several motor structures, from associative cortical areas to the spinal cord, regardless of their relative synaptic distance from the muscle (Alexander and Crutcher, 1990; Prut and Fetz, 1999). The preparatory modulations observed in this study could thus potentially occur at different levels of the neuroaxis. The coexistence of suppression and activation mechanisms at different levels would therefore subserve a distributed functional organization of motor preparation (Jaeger et al., 1993).

Activation, suppression, and the motor action limit

Like long-latency reflex and CNV data, the decrement of silent-period duration reflects a preparatory increase in neural activity and can be directly interpreted in terms of Näätänen's (1971) proposal. According to this proposal, neural activity increases on the basis of subjective expectancies of the time of presentation of the forthcoming stimulus. When this preparatory neural activity bypasses the motor action limit, an overt response is triggered. The SP decrement that manifests an increase in cortical activity during the RT is also compatible with such an outcome, although some additional assumptions seem necessary. Mattes and Ulrich (1997) analysed the force spontaneously generated in executing responses, and reported it to be weaker for short than for long foreperiods (see, however, van Den Heuvel and van Gemmert, 2000), indicating that the muscular contraction producing the response is weaker when a better level of preparation is attained. As stressed earlier, by estimating the surface Laplacian, we have shown that the negative wave that develops over the motor cortex during RT is smaller and better time-locked to the onset of the response when the foreperiod is short than when it is long (Tandonnet et al., 2003, 2006). These results converge with those of Mattes and Ulrich (1997) in suggesting that the amount of cortical activation that triggers muscle contraction is lower when a better level of preparation is attained. While we have interpreted this result as revealing a more efficient, and hence a more economical, motor command, another perspective, more in line with the motor action limit scheme (Näätänen, 1971), is possible. Note that this hypothesis does not negate our former proposal, but simply expands its scope. Mattes and Ulrich (1997) argued that when participants are poorly prepared and, hence, their motor-action limit is further away, they must produce a large activation in order to reach the response threshold. By itself however, this does not explain the observed force overshoot since, irrespective of the actual muscle contraction, the targeted force might be the same for both foreperiod conditions. One way to account for the overshoot is to specify how participants could estimate the increment in activation that would be required to trigger a response. In his doctoral dissertation, one of us proposed that this increment obeys Weber's law (Tandonnet, 2004). If this is the case, the representation of the required increment would be more variable when preparation is low because the distance to be covered would be larger. Since the variability of the produced force depends on the amount of force to be developed (Schmidt et al., 1979), participants could target a higher activation level when they are poorly prepared, to ensure that the response activation will be, on every trial, large enough to trigger an overt response. This would explain the higher overt force and the larger M1 activity for long compared to short foreperiods. Note that the distance to threshold might differ depending on the context: in order to avoid incorrect responses in choice compared to simple RT, this distance should be kept large. Second, this distance might also depend on the variability of the activation level: a high variability should be associated with a lower mean activation to prevent the variability from triggering a premature response. In fact, two recent studies report a decrease in variability in motor activation, either between trials in the premotor cortex (Churchland et al., 2006), or within trial as demonstrated by motor-unit discharge (Duclos et al., 2008).

We must acknowledge, however, that the results relative to neural suppression are more difficult to reconcile with this scheme. Indeed, they show that the excitability of the corticospinal tract is all the weaker when time preparation is more accurate and thus motor preparation is higher. One way to reconcile the suppression data with the motor-action limit hypothesis is to consider that it describes the level of cortical (likely M1) activity only: cortical activation would be set as close as possible to the threshold for emitting a response but, in order to avoid premature responding, the development of neural excitation would be secured by strong spinal inhibition. This inhibition would be released after stimulus presentation to allow the response to be triggered. One would thus predict a non-specific increase in corticospinal excitability shortly after stimulus onset. Indeed, we have reported such non-specific increases in MEP amplitude in the period immediately following stimulus presentation (Burle et al., 2002). The activation becomes specific only after several tens of milliseconds (Leocani et al., 2000). Note, however, that this specificity appears much stronger at the cortical level (silent-period duration) than at the corticospinal level (MEP amplitude; Burle et al., 2002).

Conclusions

Beyond time estimation in temporal preparation: the effects of conditional probabilities

In the chapter introduction, we made clear that temporal preparation can be manipulated between or within block. As indicated earlier, time estimation and conditional probabilities have opposing effects on performance, and the actual level of preparation is a balance between these two processes (Durup and Requin, 1970). Very few studies have investigated the effects of time preparation and conditional probabilities with electrophysiological techniques (see Riehle et al., 1997; van der Lubbe et al., 2004 for noticeable exceptions; Kilavik and Riehle, Chapter 19; Los, Chapter 21), and although these studies provide some insights concerning the neural effects of conditional probabilities, they provide no information as to the excitatory versus inhibitory nature of preparation under varied conditional probability conditions. We have seen above that 'pure' temporal preparation is implemented by an increase in cortical excitability counteracted by an increase in corticospinal inhibition. One may wonder whether conditional probabilities would affect cortical excitability, corticospinal suppression, or both; and how they would interact with temporal preparation at the neurophysiological level. Although we do not yet have any answers to these questions, we believe that the methodology described in this chapter paves the way towards a better understanding of how temporal preparation is affected by both 'pure time estimation' factors as well as other factors such as conditional probability. Studying the subtle interplay between the excitatory and inhibitory processes involved in temporal preparation at the motor level also reveals how preparation operates. We suggest that such an activation/suppression balance is not only implemented at the motor level but also at higher levels, and results from a general mechanism that allows neural assemblies to be preset whilst simultaneously keeping them silent before due time.

References

Alegria, J. (1975). Sequential effects of foreperiod duration: some strategical factors in tasks involving time uncertainty. In Rabbitt, P. M. A. and Dornic, S. (Eds.) *Attention and Performance V*, pp.1–10. London: Academic Press.

Alegria, J. (1980). Contrôle stratégique du choix d' instant pour se préparer à réagir. In Requin, J. (Ed.) *Anticipation et Comportement*, pp.95–105. Paris: Editions du CNRS.

Alexander, G. E. and Crutcher, M. D. (1990). Preparation for movement: neural representations of intended direction in three motor areas of the monkey. *Journal of Neurophysiology*, **64**, 133–50.

Babiloni, F., Cincotti, F., Carducci, F., Rossini, P. M., and Babiloni, C. (2001). Spatial enhancement of EEG data by surface Laplacian estimation: the use of magnetic resonance imaging-based head models. *Clinical Neurophysiology*, **112**, 724–7.

Bertelson, P. and Tisseyre, F. (1969). The time course of preparation: confirmatory results with visual and auditory warning signals. *Acta Psychologica*, **30**, 145–54.

Birbaumer, N., Elbert, T., Canavan, A. G. M., and Rockstroh, B. (1990). Slow potentials of the cerebral cortex and behavior. *Physiological Review*, **70**, 1–41.

Bonhage, S. A., Knott, H., and Ferbert, A. (1996). Effect of carbamazepine on cortical excitatory and inhibitory phenomena with paired transcranial magnetic stimulation. *Electroencephalography and Clinical Neurophysiology*, **99**, 267–73.

Bonnet, M. (1983). Anticipatory changes of long-latency stretch reflex responses during preparation for directional hand movements. *Brain Research*, **280**, 51–62.

Bonnet, M. and Requin, J. (1982). Long-loop and spinal reflexes in man during preparation for intended directional hand movement. *Journal of Neurosciences*, **2**, 90–6.

Bonnet, M., Requin, J., and Semjen, A. (1981). Human reflexology and motor preparation. In Miller, D., editor, *Exercise and sport science reviews*, pp.119–57. Philadelphia, PA: Franklin Institute Press.

Botwinick, J. and Thompson, L. W. (1966). Premotor and motor components of reaction time. *Journal of Experimental Psychology*, **71**, 9–15.

Burle, B., Bonnet, M., Vidal, F., Possama, C. A., and Hasbroucq, T. (2002). A transcranial magnetic stimulation study of information processing in the motor cortex: relationship between the silent period and the reaction time delay. *Psychophysiology*, **39**, 207–17.

Burle, B., Vidal, F., Tandonnet, C., and Hasbroucq, T. (2004). Physiological evidences for response inhibition in choice reaction time task. *Brain & Cognition*, **56**, 141–52.

Churchland, M. M., Yu, B. M., Ryu, S. I., Santhanam, G., and Shenoy, K. V. (2006). Neural variability in premotor cortex provides a signature of motor preparation. *Journal of Neurosciences*, **26**, 3697–713.

Classen, J. and Benecke, R. (1995). Inhibitory phenomena in individual motor units induced by transcranial magnetic stimulation. *Electroencephalography and Clinical Neurophysiology*, **97**, 264–74.

Coles, M. G. H. (1989). Modern mind-brain reading: psychophysiology, physiology, and cognition. *Psychophysiology*, **26**, 251–69.

Correa, Á., Lupiáñez, J., and Tudela, P. (2005). Attentional preparation based on temporal expectancy modulates processing at the perceptual level. *Psychonomic Bulletin and Review*, **12**, 328–34.

Correa, Á. Sanabria, D., Spence, C., Tudela, P., and Lupiáñez, J. (2006). Selective temporal attention enhances the temporal resolution of visual perception: evidence from a temporal order judgment task. *Brain Research*, **1070**, 202–5.

Davey, N. J., Romaiguère, P., Maskill, D. W., and Ellaway, P. (1994). Suppression of voluntary motor activity revealed using transcranial magnetic stimulation of the motor cortex in man. *Journal of Physiology (London)*, **477**, 223–35.

Davranche, K., Tandonnet, C., Burle, B., Vidal, F., and Hasbroucq, T. (2007). The dual nature of time preparation: neural activation and inhibition revealed by transcranial magnetic stimulation of the motor cortex. *European Journal of Neuroscience*, **25**, 3766–74.

Duclos, Y., Schmied, A., Burle, B., Burnet, H., and Rossi-Durand, C. (2008). Anticipatory changes in human motoneuron discharge patterns during motor preparation. *Journal of Physiology (London)*, **586**, 1017–28.

Durup, H. and Requin, J. (1970). Hypothèses sur le rôle des probabilités conditionnelles du signal d' dans le temps de réaction simple. *Psychologie Française*, **15**, 37–46.

Eimer, M. (1999). Facilitatory and inhibitory effects of masked prime stimuli on motor activation and behavioural performance. *Acta Psychologica*, 101, 293–313.

Gevins, A. S. (1989). Dynamic functional topography of cognitive tasks. *Brain Topography*, **2**, 37–56.

Gibbon, J. (1977). Scalar expectancy theory and Weber's law in animal timing. *Psychological Review*, **84**, 279–325.

Gratton, G., Coles, M. G. H., Sirevaag, E. J., Eriksen, C. W., and Donchin, E. (1988). Pre- and poststimulus activation of response channels: a psychophysiological analysis. *Journal of Experimental Psychology, Human Perception and Performance*, **14**, 331–44.

Hamano, T., Lüders, H. O., Ikeda, A., Collura, T. F.and Comair, Y. G., and Shibasaki, H. (1997). The cortical generators of the contingent negative variation in humans: a study with subdural electrodes. *Electroencephalography and Clinical Neurophysiology*, **104**, 257–68.

Hasbroucq, T., Akamatsu, M., Burle, B., Bonnet, M., and Possama, C. A. (2000). Changes in spinal excitability during choice reaction time: the H-reflex as a probe of information transmission. *Psychophysiology*, **37**, 385–93.

Hasbroucq, T., Akamatsu, M., Mouret, I., and Seal, J. (1995). Fingers pairings in two-choice reaction time tasks: does the between hands advantage reflect response preparation. *Journal of Motor Behavior*, **27**, 251–62.

Hasbroucq, T., Kaneko, H., and Akamatsu, M. P. C.-A. (1997). Preparatory inhibition of cortico-spinal excitability: a transcranial magnetic stimulation study in man. *Cognitive Brain Research*, **5**, 185–192.

Hasbroucq, T., Osman, A., Possama, C. A., Burle, B., Carron, S., Dépy, D., et al. (1999a). Cortico-spinal inhibition reflects time but not event preparation: neural mechanisms of preparation dissociated by transcranial magnetic stimulation. *Acta Psychologica*, **101**, 243–66.

Hasbroucq, T., Possama, C.-A., Bonnet, M., and Vidal, F. (1999b). Effect of the irrelevant location of the response signal on choice reaction time: an electromyographic study in humans. *Psychophysiology*, **36**, 522–6.

Jaeger, D., Gilman, S., and Aldridge, J. W. (1993). Primate basal ganglia activity in a precued reaching task: preparation for movement. *Experimental Brain Research*, **95**, 51–64.

Leocani, L., Cohen, L. G., Wasserman, E. M., Ikoma, K., and Hallet, M. (2000). Human corticospinal excitability evaluated with transcranial magnetic stimulation during different reaction time paradigms. *Brain*, **123**, 1161–73.

Macar, F. and Bonnet, M. (1997). Event-related potentials during temporal information processing. In van Boxtel, G. J. M. and Böcker, K. B. E. (Eds.) *Brain and Behavior: Past, Present, and Future*, pp.49–66. Tilburg: Tilburg University Press.

Mattes, S. and Ulrich, R. (1997). Response force is sensitive to the temporal uncertainty of response stimuli. *Perception & Psychophysics*, **59**, 1089–97.

McMillan, S., Ivry, R. B., and Byblow, W. D. (2006). Corticomotor excitability during a choice-hand reaction time task. *Experimental Brain Research*, **172**, 230–45.

Meijers, L. M. M., Teulings, J. L. H. M., and Eijkman, E. G. J. (1976). Model of the electromyographic activity during a brief isometric contraction. *Biological Cybernetics*, **25**, 7–16.

Näätänen, R. (1971). Non-aging fore-periods and simple reaction time. *Acta Psychologica*, **35**, 316–27.

Niemi, P. (1979). Stimulus intensity effects on auditory and visual reaction processes. *Acta Psychologica*, **43**, 299–312.

Niemi, P. and Näätänen, R. (1981). Foreperiod and simple reaction time. *Psychological Bulletin*, **89**, 133–61.

Nunez, P. (1981). *Electric fields of the brain*. Oxford: Oxford University Press.

Praamstra, P. and Seiss, E. (2005). The neurophysiology of response competition: Motor cortex activation and inhibition following subliminal response priming. *Journal of Cognitive Neuroscience*, **17**(3), 483–93.

Priori, A., Berardelli, A., Inghilleri, M.and Accornero, N., and Manfredi, M. (1994). Motor cortical inhibition and the dopaminergic system. Pharmacological changes in the silent period after transcranial magnetic stimulation in normal subjects, patients with parkinson's disease and drug induced parkinsonism. *Brain*, **117**, 317–23.

Prut, Y. and Fetz, E. E. (1999). Primate spinal interneurons show premovement instructed delay activity. *Nature*, **401**, 490–4.

Requin, J., Brener, J., and Ring, C. (1991). Preparation for action. In Jennings, J. and Coles, M. (Eds.) *Handbook of Cognitive Psychophysiology: Central and Autonomic Nervous System Approaches*, pp.357–448. New York: Wiley.

Riehle, A., Grün, S., Diesmann, M., and Aertsen, A. (1997). Spike synchronization and rate modulation differentially involved in motor cortical function. *Science*, **278**, 1950–3.

Rolke, B. and Hofmann, P. (2007). Temporal uncertainty degrades perceptual processes. *Psychonomic Bulletin and Review*, **14**, 522–6.

Rossini, P. M., Caramia, M. D., Iani, C., Desiato, M. T., Sciarretta, G., and Bernardi, G. (1995). Magnetic transcranial stimulation in healthy humans: influence on the behavior of upper limb motor units. *Brain Research*, **676**, 314–24.

Sanders, A. F. (1998). Elements of human performance: reaction processes and attention in human skill. Mahwah: Erlbaum.

Schieppati, M. (1987). The Hoffman reflex: A means of assessing spinal reflex excitability and descending control in man. *Progress in Neurobiology*, **28**, 345–76.

Schmidt, R. A., Zelaznik, H. N., Hawkins, B., Frank, J. S., and Quinn, J. T. (1979). Motor-output variability: a theory for the accuracy of rapid motor acts. *Psychological Review*, **86**, 415–41.

Schnitzler, A. and Benecke, R. (1994). The silent period after transcranial magnetic stimulation is of exclusive cortical origin: evidence from isolated cortical ischemic lesion in man. *Neuroscience Letters*, **180**, 41–5.

Sinclair, C. and Hammond, G. H. (2008). Reduced intracortical inhibition during the foreperiod of a warned reaction time task. *Experimental Brain Research*, **186**, 385–92.

Smid, H. G. O. M., Mulder, G., and Mulder, L. J. M. (1987). The continuous flow model revisited: perceptual and motor aspects. In Johnson, R. J., Rohrbaugh, J. W., and Parasuranam, R. (Eds.) *Current trends in event-related potential research*, pages 270–278. Amsterdam: Elsevier.

Sternberg, S. (1969). The discovery of processing stages: extension of Donder's method. *Acta Psychologica*, **30**, 276–315.

Sternberg, S. (2001). Separate modifiability, mental modules, and the use of composite and pure measures to reveal them. *Acta Psychologica*, **106**, 147–246.

Tandonnet, C. (2004). Mécanismes neuraux de la préparation à l' chez l'Homme: Contributions théoriques, méthodologiques et expérimentales. [Neural mechanisms of preparation for action in Man: Theoretical, methodological and experimental contributions]. PhD thesis, Faculté des Sciences du Sport, Université de la Méditérannée, Marseille.

Tandonnet, C., Burle, B., Vidal, F., and Hasbroucq, T. (2003). The influence of time preparation on motor processes assessed by surface Laplacian estimation. *Clinical Neurophysiology*, **114**, 2376–84.

Tandonnet, C., Burle, B., Vidal, F., and Hasbroucq, T. (2006). Knowing when to respond and the efficiency of the cortical motor command: a Laplacian ERP study. *Brain Research*, **1109**, 158–63.

Taniguchi, Y., Burle, B., Vidal, F., and Bonnet, M. (2001). Deficit in motor cortical activity for simultaneous bimanual responses. *Experimental Brain Research*, **137**, 259–68.

Terao, Y. and Ugawa, Y. (2002). Basic mechanisms of TMS. *Journal of Clinical Neurophysiology*, **19**, 322–43.

Touge, T., Taylor, J. L., and Rothwell, J. C. (1998). Reduced excitability of the cortico-spinal system during the warning period of a reaction time task. *Electroencephalography and Clinical Neurophysiology*, **109**, 489–95.

Ulrich, R. and Wing, A. M. (1991). A recruitment theory of force-time relations in the production of brief force pulses: the parallel force unit mode. *Psychological Review*, **98**, 268–94.

Uncini, A., Treviso, M.and Di Muzio, A. S. P., and Pullman, S. (1993). Physiological basis of voluntary activity inhibition induced by transcranial cortical stimulation. *Electroencephalography and Clinical Neurophysiology*, **93**, 211–20.

van Boxtel, G. J. M. and Brunia, C. H. M. (1994a). Motor and non-motor aspects of slow brain potentials. *Biological Psychology*, **38**, 37–51.

van Boxtel, G. J. M. and Brunia, C. H. M. (1994b). Motor and non-motor components of the contingent negative variation. *International Journal of Psychophysiology*, **17**, 269–79.

van Den Heuvel, C. E. and van Gemmert, A. W. A. (2000). Nonspecific motor preparation and the motor action limit. *Current Psychology Letters*, **2**, 92–111.

van der Lubbe, R. H. J., Los, S. A., Jakowski, P., and Verleger, R. (2004). Being prepared on time: on the importance of the previous foreperiod to current preparation, as reflected in speed, force and preparation-related brain potentials. *Acta Psychologica*, **116**, 245–62.

Van der Molen, M. W., Bashore, T. R.and Halliday, R., and Callaway, E. (1991). Chronopsychophysiology: mental chronometry augmented by psychophysiological time markers. In Jennings, J. and Coles, M. (Eds.) *Handbook of Cognitive Psychophysiology, Central and Autonomic Nervous System Approaches*, pp.9–178. Wiley, New York.

Vidal, F., Grapperon, J., Bonnet, M., and Hasbroucq, T. (2003). The nature of unilateral motor commands in between-hands choice tasks as revealed by surface Laplacian estimation. *Psychophysiology*, **40**, 796–805.

Walter, W. G., Cooper, R., Aldridge, V. J., McCallum, W. C., and Winter, A. (1964). Contingent negative variation. An electric sign of sensorimotor association and expectancy in the human brain. *Nature*, **203**, 380–4.

Woodrow, H. (1914). The measurement of attention. *Psychological Monographs*, **17**, 1–158.

Chapter 19

Timing structures' neuronal activity during preparation for action

Bjørg Elisabeth Kilavik and Alexa Riehle

Accurate time estimation in the anticipation of predictable events is vital for motor behaviour. Imagine the sprinter who needs to anticipate the time of the gun shot in order to make a rapid and coordinated start, or the tennis player who initiates an arm movement in relation to when (and where) the ball will arrive. Motor anticipation requires an internal representation of elapsed (or remaining) time. It has been shown that movements are initiated faster when prior knowledge is available about the time of the GO signal (Riehle at al. 1997, 2000; Roux et al., 2003; Janssen and Shadlen, 2005; see reviews in Requin et al., 1991; Riehle 2005). As a consequence, in tasks with multiple and randomly presented delay durations, the reaction time (RT) decreases with increasing delay duration, as the conditional probability of receiving a GO signal increases (hazard function). Furthermore, RTs fluctuate from trial to trial even when delay durations are held constant across trials (Riehle 2005; Renoult et al., 2006). This may be related to the imprecision of timing processes (Gibbon et al., 1997) and may thus reflect, at least partly, the variability in expecting the GO signal.

Given the strong dependency of motor preparation on time estimation and the conditional probability of the moment of GO signal occurrence, there has recently been an increased interest in their underlying neuronal correlates. In this chapter we explore different ways in which timing and probability affect neuronal activity in motor tasks. Neuronal data from motor cortex will be presented, but it is clear that very similar effects can be observed in many brain regions, such as frontal and parietal cortex, as well as subcortical structures. We will start by looking at the spiking activity of individual neurons during implicit and explicit timing. We will then describe modulation of the collective activity across multiple neurons, assessed through precise spike synchrony and local field potentials (LFPs). These data show that time is clearly represented in motor cortex, albeit in a context-dependent way.

Spiking activity in single neurons during implicit and explicit timing

To study behavioural and neural correlates of preparatory processes, instructed delay tasks are often used. These tasks typically impose a delay of fixed or variable (but often predictable) duration between an initial informative preparatory signal (PS) and a GO signal indicating that the movement should be initiated (see also Wagener and Hoffman, Chapter 16; Burle et al., Chapter 18; Los, Chapter 21; Vallesi, Chapter 22, this volume). The presence of a GO signal obviates the need to estimate delay duration explicitly in order to perform the task correctly (e.g. like the sprinter in the example given earlier). The fact that RTs are faster with prior knowledge about when the GO signal will occur indicates that information about time is exploited implicitly in order to optimize performance. To study explicit timing, on the other hand, the subject is often asked to provide an estimate of delay duration by self-timing a movement initiation (no final GO cue provided), or by associating a particular motor response with a particular delay duration (the motor response is a function of the output of the timing process).

Implicit task timing: timing as an incidental process

There is ample evidence that subjects can exploit the inherent temporal structure of task events even when it is irrelevant to task goals (implicit timing). Niki and Watanabe (1979) were the first to connect anticipatory neuronal delay activity to implicit time estimation. Since then, several studies have interpreted neuronal discharge during delays as being related to timing processes (Mauritz and Wise, 1986; Vaadia et al., 1988; Lucchetti and Bon, 2001; Ghose and Maunsell, 2002; Brody et al., 2003; Leon and Shadlen, 2003; Roux et al., 2003; Akkal et al., 2004; Janssen and Shadlen, 2005; Lucchetti et al., 2005; Roesch and Olsen, 2005; Tsujimoto and Sawaguchi, 2005; Genovesio et al., 2006; Maimon and Assad, 2006a,b; Renoult et al., 2006; Shuler and Bear, 2006; Lebedev et al., 2008; Andersen and Sheinberg, Chapter 29, this volume). Recently, we studied the neuronal correlates of timing processes in primary motor cortex (M1), while a monkey performed a simple instructed delay task (Figure 19.1A; see Bastian et al., 2003 for a description of the task). A preparatory signal provided complete information about the movement at the start of the trial. After a delay of fixed duration, the GO signal cued movement onset. Many reaction times were so short that they should be regarded as anticipations of the GO signal, rather than responses to it (see Fig. 19.1A). Thus, although not explicitly told to do so, the animal indeed estimates the delay duration. Figure 19.1A shows the spiking activity of a neuron that increased its activity strongly following the preparatory signal. However, towards the end of the delay, but well in advance of the GO signal, it stopped firing at a time that was clearly aligned to movement onset, with a constant lag being observed between firing cessation and movement onset. Thus, the activity of the neuron was modulated not only in relation to the external preparatory stimulus but also in relation to the expectancy of the GO signal.

Delay duration was identical and thus fully predictable on all trials. Nevertheless, the animal showed a considerable degree of across-trial variability in the timing of movement onset. This behavioural variability could be due to fluctuations in concentration or arousal. The anticipatory responses suggest, however, that the correlated across-trial variability in behaviour and neuronal activity instead reflects variability in interval timing. Can neuronal correlates of (variability in) time estimates be identified? A link between neuronal activity and motor behaviour has already been demonstrated, with trial-by-trial correlations between RT and firing rate of neurons in many cortical areas, for either arm reaching or saccade tasks (Kubota and Hamada, 1979; Lecas et al., 1986; Requin et al., 1990; Riehle and Requin, 1993; Hanes and Schall, 1996; Dorris et al., 1997; Dorris and Munoz, 1998; Everling and Munoz, 2000; Roitman and Shadlen, 2002; Lee and Assad, 2003; Cohen et al., 2004; Snyder et al., 2006).

Our research group has recently studied the relationship between across-trial variability of internal timing and the temporal profile of spiking activity (Renoult et al., 2006). Consider the neuron in Figure 19.1Bi, recorded while a monkey performed a task in which the GO signal could be randomly presented after either a short or a long delay, with equal probability. The animal began by expecting the GO signal at the end of the short delay (conditional probability = 0.5, expected signal, ES, the figure shows long trials). If the GO signal did not occur at the end of the expected short interval, the probability for the GO signal to occur after a long delay became 1 (see also Wagener and Hoffman, Chapter 16; Los, Chapter 21; Vallesi, Chapter 22, this volume). This neuron showed three distinct epochs of increased activity during long trials. The first epoch occurred after presentation of the preparatory signal, the second around the moment when a GO signal was expected at the end of a short delay (ES), and the third towards the end of the

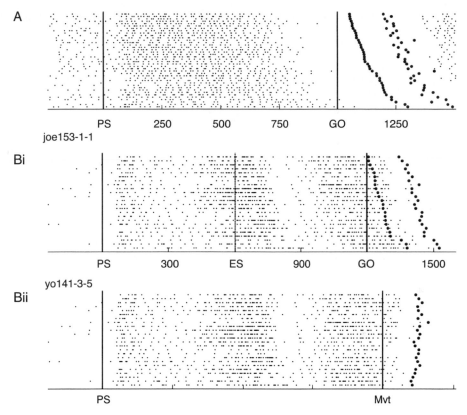

Fig. 19.1 Implicit timing and single neuron spiking activity. Raster displays of single neuron activity across multiple trials, where each line represents a behavioural trial and each dot the time of an action potential (spike). Trials are aligned (off-line) according to increasing RT (the first range of large dots after GO indicates movement onset; the second range indicates movement end). Preparatory signal (PS), movement onset (Mvt), expected signal (ES). Vertical solid lines represent signals, dotted lines internally timed events. (Unpublished data from A. Riehle, A. Bastian, F. Grammont, L. Renoult and S. Roux.)

long delay. The second and third epochs of increased activity occurred during the delay without the presentation of any external signal, thus indicating an accurate estimate of the delay duration. Whereas the phasic activity increase following PS was clearly time-locked to the stimulus, the third epoch was clearly aligned to movement onset, varying on a trial-by-trial basis. Interestingly, the second epoch around ES had an intermediate alignment. In other words, neuronal activity went from being aligned to the occurrence of an external signal (PS) to being aligned to movement onset via some intermediate alignment to an internal signal (ES). Thus, across-trial variability in the temporal profile of neuronal discharge increased throughout the delay. Renoult et al. (2006) reasoned that RT variability might indeed be an indication of across-trial variability in internal timing. To test this hypothesis they rescaled the time of each trial to the monkey's presumed internal time estimate, by making the interval between the preparatory signal and movement onset identical on all trials, thereby eliminating RT variability. They then displaced each spike in each trial according to this new time scale (Figure 19.1Bii). The overall across-trial variability was strongly reduced and no longer increased throughout the delay (Renoult et al., 2006). In this new (internal) time-scale, phasic activity overlapped from trial to trial (see Figure 19.1Bii), and was well-aligned to all trial events, both external and internal events. The authors thus concluded that 'time is a rubber-band'. Time progresses in an elastic fashion from a reset (triggered here by the preparatory signal) like a one-dimensional rubber-band that is attached to a fixed point t_0. When the rubber-band is stretched, events lying on it (internal events or spikes) are increasingly shifted in time as one moves away from t_0.

Many cortical and subcortical areas show effects of implicit task timing, as measured by phasic activity changes aligned to an expected signal onset or movement time, or by climbing activity (e.g. Niki and Watanabe, 1979; Mauritz and Wise, 1986; Lucchetti and Bon, 2001; Brody et al., 2003; Akkal et al., 2004; Janssen and Shadlen, 2005; Roesch and Olsen, 2005; Renoult et al., 2006; Praamstra, Chapter 24; Pouthas and Pfeuty, Chapter 30, this volume). As described earlier, preparatory activity in motor cortical neurons is strongly influenced by time predictability, whether they discharge tonically (like the example in Figure 19.1A) or phasically (Figure 19.1B) in anticipation of the GO signal or the movement. In addition, the modulation of neuronal discharge related to task timing seems to be highly adaptive, with only a few trials needed to realign activity when the delay duration changes (Lucchetti and Bon, 2001).

Explicit timing: timing as a task requirement

The strong effects of temporal expectation, even in situations where timing was not explicitly required, led several researchers to look for neuronal correlates of *explicit* timing using tasks where the correct estimation of elapsed time was necessary either for selecting the correct motor response (Roux et al., 2003) or for comparing delay durations (e.g. Leon and Shadlen, 2003; Sakurai et al., 2004). Other tasks required the animal to self-time his movement, with no GO signal being provided (Lee and Assad, 2003; Roux et al., 2003; Maimon and Assad, 2006a,b; Lebedev et al., 2008).

Roux et al. (2003) developed a task in which the selection of movement direction was a function of delay duration, thus requiring correct estimation of elapsed time (choice-RT task). Two spatially discrete targets of different colour were presented at the start of each trial. A non-directional GO signal was presented either after a short or a long delay, randomly and with equal probability. The monkey had previously learned to associate a specific target colour to a specific delay duration, thus the direction of movement (to one or the other coloured target) depended upon the length of the delay preceding the GO signal. Figure 19.2A shows the activity of a motor cortical neuron recorded during performance of the choice-RT task. The activity of the neuron increased slightly in anticipation of the possible occurrence of the GO signal in short delay trials (at 600ms). If the GO signal occurred after a short delay, the neuron responded to the signal with a short burst of spikes. If the GO signal did not occur after a short delay, the neuron stopped firing altogether for the remainder of the trial.

If only short trials were considered, the phasic activity after the GO signal could be interpreted as being related to processing of the GO signal or to general movement preparation, with activity being well aligned to signal occurrence; but the lack of GO-related activity on long trials, in which the monkey knew with certainty when the GO signal would occur, indicates that the activity in short trials instead seems tightly linked to temporal uncertainty of the GO signal. In this task, many neurons fired with higher frequency after a short-delay GO signal than after a long-delay one. After a short delay, the GO signal was necessary to trigger movement, due to the low probability (p = 0.5) of signal occurrence. After a long delay, however, the conditional probability of signal occurrence had turned to 1 and the time of onset of the GO signal could be predicted with certainty. In other words, the non-presentation of a GO signal at the end of a short

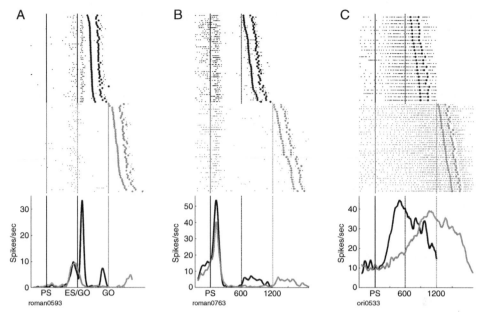

Fig. 19.2 Explicit timing and single neuron spiking activity. Upper panels are raster displays of single neuron activity across multiple trials (see Figure 19.1 for details). Bottom panels show trial-averaged activity, presented as peri-stimulus time histograms. A) Choice-RT task; B, C) SELF-task. Short trials are shown in black, long trials in grey. (Unpublished data from: A. Riehle, L. Renoult and S. Roux.)

delay provided complete information about when and where to move in long trials. Activity in many types of neurons is modulated in delay tasks (see review in Riehle, 2005), in relation to prior information about upcoming movements or as a function of movement execution. The neuron in Figure 19.2A belongs to the category of pre-processing neurons (Riehle, 2005), which process information about the upcoming movement as soon as information becomes available; but, as for many neurons encountered in this experiment, signal (and thus movement) uncertainty strongly modulated the activity. Some responded to the GO signal only after a short delay when the probability was low, whereas others changed their tonic activity when the conditional probability turned to 1 (e.g. Figure 1 in Roux et al., 2003), implying certainty regarding when and where to move.

Roux et al. (2003) also used another task, comprising the same directional and temporal parameters as the choice-RT task. However, only one PS was presented indicating both movement direction and delay duration, and no GO signal was provided. The monkey had therefore to self-initiate the movement at the (estimated) end of the delay (SELF task). The colour and position of the preparatory signal at the start of each trial provided complete information about when and where to move. The activity of a typical neuron is shown in Figure 19.2B. Similar to the neuron in Figure 19.2A, this neuron responded phasically to the signal providing complete information about movement direction and delay duration (in this case the preparatory signal at the start of the trial).

In another type of neuron that was often encountered in the SELF-task, activity increased progressively during the delay (Figure 19.2C). It is possible that such climbing (or descending) activity is part of (or reflects) a timing system, in which either the total number of emitted spikes or the instantaneous firing rate correlates with elapsed time (see also Fiorillo, Chapter 20, this volume). In line with this idea, climbing activity has been successfully used to decode elapsed time in single trials (Leon and Shadlen, 2003; Lebedev et al., 2008). Delay-related climbing activity has been proposed as a timing mechanism in several modelling approaches (Durstewitz 2003, 2004; Reutimann et al., 2004). However, Okamoto et al. (2007) suggested that graded activity resulting from averaging across trials or across neurons might instead be a result of variable transition times in bimodal activity. They presented single neuron activity from anterior cingulate cortex that displayed bimodal firing rate distributions and large across-trial variability, thus matching their proposed model well. The generality of such bimodal frequency distributions still remains to be verified in other brain areas where climbing activity has been reported.

The neurons presented in Figure 19.2B and C modulated their activity in relation to delay duration, with higher firing rates in short trials compared to long trials (see also Roesch and Olsen 2005, who relate higher firing rates in short-delay trials to the higher value of rewards expected after shorter delays). In addition, in Figure 19.2C, the slope of the climbing activity is steeper for short than for long trials. Thus, one can imagine a threshold mechanism that monitors the firing rate of such neurons and uses this to decide when 'time's up' (see also Hanes and Schall 1996). Whether this activity might be responsible for timing is not clear however.

Spike synchrony and temporal expectancy

Until now, we have described changes in activity of single neurons in relation to task timing. However, it is commonly accepted that sensorimotor functions are reflected in changes in firing rate in widely distributed populations of neurons (Riehle, 2005). This implies that networks must organize their activity in space and time, to cope with the ever-changing behavioural context. In this framework, the temporal coding hypothesis suggests that not only changes in firing rate but also precise spike timing constitute an important part of the representational substrate for perception and action. Precise spike timing here refers to spike synchronization or other precise spatiotemporal patterns of spike occurrences among neurons organized in functional groups, commonly called cell assemblies (Hebb, 1949; Aertsen et al., 1986; Gerstein et al., 1989; Abeles, 1991). The concept of cell assemblies uses synchrony as an additional dimension to firing rate, as a candidate for information processing. The observation of precise spike synchrony between pairs of neurons (Riehle et al., 1997) might be interpreted as activation of a functional cell assembly (Aertsen and Gerstein 1991). The strength of precise spike synchrony among pairs of motor cortical neurons has been shown to be modulated over time, independently of any modulation in their firing rate (Riehle et al., 1997). To indicate the end of the estimated delay duration, motor cortical neurons significantly synchronize their activity at the moment of signal expectancy, often without any detectable modulation in firing rate (Riehle et al., 1997, 2000). Thus, behavioural timing independently modulates both spike synchrony and firing rate.

Practice shapes synchrony in relation to explicit timing

Both experimental and theoretical studies point to the importance of synchronous spiking activity, particularly in a low firing-rate regime (e.g. Rudolph and Destexhe 2003). Synchrony and firing rate might be complementary coding strategies, such that increased synchrony allows for efficient computation with less activity. Assuming such a complementarity, can the interplay between synchrony and firing rate be altered by improving the behavioural performance in a timing paradigm? To study this, we quantified the strength of synchrony across pairs of neurons recorded in the previously described choice-RT task and compared it to the mean firing rate in the same neurons. We developed a measure that provides the strength of synchronous spiking activity of an entire population of neuron pairs independently of their firing rate, and did this dynamically for each moment of the behavioural trial (see Kilavik et al., 2009 for the population quantification; for the statistics see the review by Grün, 2009). This method is based on a comparison between the observed number of coincident spikes in pairs of neurons and the predicted number of coincident spikes, taking into account the instantaneous firing rates of these neurons (cf. Grün, 2009) that were summed over all pairs in a population. The difference between the numbers of observed and predicted coincident spikes yields an analytical measure, for each moment in time, indicating the statistical significance of having more (or less) synchrony than that expected by chance.

During the entire recording period, the monkey significantly improved its performance, both speeding RTs (Figure 19.3A) and reducing RT variability (Figure 19.3B), suggesting an improved estimation of the delay duration. We therefore split the population of recorded neurons into two halves, corresponding to the first and last part of the recording epoch, which spanned several months (Figure 19.3C and D). Figure 19.3C shows, in a time-resolved way along the trial, the statistical significance of synchronous spiking activity over all pairs of neurons during both epochs. Interestingly, the strength of synchrony transiently increased after the expected GO signal (ES), exceeding by far the significance level of $p = 0.01$ (dashed horizontal line), for the pairs of neurons recorded during the late sessions only (black line). This brief increase in precise synchrony might provide an internal switch signal, triggered by correct time estimation, which allows a change in movement preparation. At the same moment in time, the mean firing rate of the population decreased in late sessions compared to early sessions (Figure 19.3D). Thus, performance optimization in timing tasks might be achieved by increasing precise spike synchrony in relation to temporal expectancy, thereby boosting network efficiency, which may be accompanied by fewer spikes overall (Kilavik et al., 2009).

In summary, we find that precise spike synchrony in pairs of motor cortical neurons is strongly modulated by time estimation processes. This effect is mainly evident after excessive practice. Possibly, the representation of time might become more and more embedded in the local network dynamics as task timing becomes more strongly associated with particular motor acts. This could indicate increased local encoding of time.

Local field potentials and temporal expectancy

Finally we will focus on the activity of larger neuronal populations, as measured by LFPs. The LFP represents synaptic activity in a large population of neurons, with additional contributions from spike after-potentials or intrinsic transmembrane current changes (Mitzdorf 1985, 1994; Logothetis et al., 2007). Since the LFP sums activity around the electrode, modulations observable in the LFP must reflect activity in a sufficiently large population of neurons, possibly indicating the degree of coherent network activity (Denker at al. 2007). LFPs may be recorded from the same electrode as spikes, by low-pass filtering of the raw signal and are modulated in parallel to single neuron discharge. There is currently a great interest in understanding the relationship between the spiking activity of single neurons and the slower fluctuations of the LFP (e.g. Denker et al., 2007).

Evoked potentials

When aligning motor cortical LFPs to movement onset, a prominent feature becomes visible, called the movement-related potential (MRP). Typically it starts with a positivity (P1) prior to movement onset followed by a negativity (N1) around onset, and slower positivity and negativity (P2, N2) during and immediately after the movement (Donchin et al., 2001). The MRP is often tuned to movement direction (Mehring et al., 2003; Rickert et al., 2005; Asher et al., 2007). While early studies linked the pre-movement component (P1) to the descending motor command

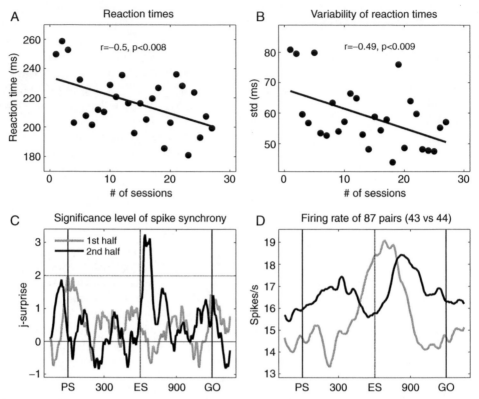

Fig. 19.3 Spike synchrony and practice in a timing task. A, B) Behavioural reaction times (A) and their variability (B) decreased significantly across sessions in a monkey performing the choice-RT task. This suggests an improved estimation of the delay duration. Lines represent linear regressions. C, D) Synchrony data were analysed by using the 'unitary event' technique (Grün et al., 2002, 2009). We developed a measure that provides the strength of synchronous spiking activity of an entire population of neuron pairs independently of their firing rate, and calculate this dynamically for each moment during the behavioural trial (Kilavik et al., 2009). In order to calculate the dynamics of the strength of precise spike synchrony, we performed our analysis by using a sliding window (size 100ms, shift 5ms) that we moved through the entire length of the trial. We determined in each trial, and for each sliding window, the number of instances of coincident firing for a temporal precision of up to 3ms and calculated the number of such coincident firing patterns that we would expect by chance if the instantaneous firing rate of the two neurons were taken into account. We then summed the result over all trials and pairs of neurons and calculated the statistical significance (joint-surprise) of the difference between numbers of observed and predicted coincident firing patterns. Whenever the significance value exceeded the threshold (dashed line, $p = 0.01$), this defined an epoch in which significantly more coincident firing activity occurred than would be expected by chance. Instances of coincident activity within such an epoch are called 'unitary events' (Grün et al., 2002). Values around zero indicate that there are as many instances of coincident firing as would be expected by chance, whereas positive (or negative) values indicate more (or less) instances of coincident firing. We split the population of recorded neurons into two halves, corresponding to the first (grey line) and last (black line) epoch of the complete recording period, which spanned several months. Time resolved statistical significance of spike synchrony for all pairs of neurons (C) and population mean firing rate (D) during both epochs is shown. Data modified from Kilavik et al., 2009.

(Gemba, et al., 1981), we recently demonstrated that it is instead related to preparatory processes. It is modulated by the level of expectancy of the GO signal, its latency, with respect to movement onset, is modulated by RT, and its frequency of occurrence varies with behavioural performance (Roux et al., 2006). Figure 19.4A shows the averaged MRP recorded in the choice-RT task, aligned to movement onset, for short (low probability of signal occurrence) and long trials (high probability). Whereas the other components of the MRP are similar for low and high probability, P1 is distinctly absent in the high-probability condition, in which the monkey has complete prior information about the movement. The P1 was also absent when the monkey performed the SELF-task, a task with no temporal uncertainty (Figure 19.4B).

Recently we found that the MRP was influenced by the delay duration itself, in a task in which two delays were successively presented in each trial and any component of temporal uncertainty was removed (two-interval task, Kilavik et al., 2007). The trial started with a time cue, indicating the delay duration of the two ensuing delays within that trial. At the end of the first delay a spatial cue was briefly presented, followed by the second delay that ended with the GO signal. Figure 19.4C shows the average MRPs in short and long trials. The amplitude of the MRP was larger when the GO signal was preceded by a long delay compared to a short delay, particularly the P1 and N1 components. This effect was observed in 90% of the LFPs, and might be related to the decreased accuracy of time estimation in long delays (RTs were longer and more variable in long trials, with fewer anticipations). We also found in two-thirds of the LFPs a significant trial-by-trial negative correlation between the size of the MRP and reaction time; the shorter the reaction time the smaller the MRP. These two results indicate a strong link between the size of the MRP and the degree of readiness to respond at the time of GO-signal occurrence.

Another intriguing feature of motor cortical LFPs has been detected in the two-interval task, namely a visual evoked potential (VEP) that was observed in response to the spatial cue. This may reflect visual processing of the cue, which is necessary for early motor preparatory processes. Interestingly, in 90% of the LFPs the VEP was also modulated by delay duration, being larger in short trials, compared to long trials (Figure 19.4D). Additionally, there was a significantly negative trial-by-trial correlation between the size of the VEP following the visual cue and the MRP around movement onset and between the size of the VEP and RT in about 10% of LFPs. Thus, we find that the larger the VEP, the smaller the MRP and the shorter the behavioural reaction time.

These results indicate a complex relationship between behavioural performance and early and late movement preparation at the population level, strongly related to task timing. Note that this was an implicit timing task. Although the monkey needed to attend in time during the first delay so as not to miss the briefly presented spatial cue, a GO signal was given at the end of the second delay obviating the need for explicit timing during the second delay. The monkey made many anticipations (extremely short RTs) in short trials, but hardly any in long trials, indicating that the short delay was estimated with better precision than the long delay (on long delay trials he awaited the final GO signal). At the same time, VEPs were larger and MRPs smaller in short trials indicating that, if the amplitude of the evoked potential is correlated with the amount of neuronal activity around the electrode tip, there was overall more neuronal activity early in the preparatory delay in short trials, but more activity around movement onset in long trials. It is therefore clear that the correlated activity in large neuronal populations, as observed in evoked field potentials, largely reflect preparatory motor processes that are strongly influenced by task timing, to a similar degree as that observed in the firing rate modulations of single neurons (Roux et al., 2006).

Oscillations

LFPs tend to oscillate, and the typically observed oscillation frequency in motor cortex is within the beta range (~15–30Hz; Berger, 1931). These oscillations are not strictly time-locked to signals

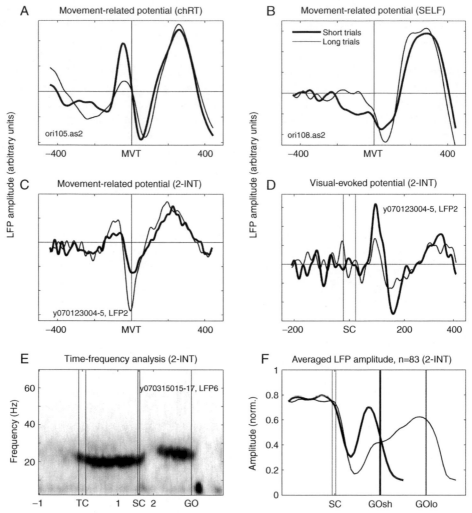

Fig. 19.4 Local field potentials (LFPs) in relation to explicit and implicit timing. Averaged movement related potentials (MRPs) in short (thick line) and long (thin line) delay trials of LFPs recorded in the choice-reaction (chRT) (A), SELF timing (B) and two-interval (INT-2) (C) tasks, aligned to movement onset (MVT). D) Averaged visual evoked potentials (VEPs) to the spatial cue in short and long delay trials in the two-interval task, aligned to the spatial cue (SC). E) Spectrogram, averaged across all long trials of a single LFP recorded in the two-interval task. F) Normalized amplitude of the main frequency of beta oscillations (see E for one representative LFP), averaged across 83 LFPs recorded in the two-interval task, for short and long delay trials, aligned to SC. Time cue (TC), GO signal on short (GOsh), and long (GOlo) trials. (Unpublished data from A. Riehle and S. Roux [chRT and SELF tasks]; B. Kilavik, A. Ponce-Alvarez and A. Riehle [2-INT task].)

or movements, but are typically strong in epochs without movements (delays) and disappear shortly before movement onset (e.g. Figure 19.4E; Kilavik et al., 2007). Motor cortical beta oscillations have been related to various phenomena, from reflecting an idling motor cortex (Jasper and Penfield 1949; Pfurtscheller et al., 1996), to being related to postural maintenance (Baker et al., 1999), or to sensorimotor and planning processes (Murthy and Fetz 1992, 1996a;

Sanes and Donoghue 1993; Donoghue et al., 1998). While it is well known that beta oscillations stop immediately prior to trained movements (e.g. Figure 19.4E), we observed recently that the time of onset of beta oscillations within a delay is modulated by the remaining delay duration. Figure 19.4F shows the average amplitude of beta oscillations for 83 LFPs recorded in the two-interval task. There was a temporary decrease in beta oscillation amplitude following the spatial cue (where we observed the VEP, described earlier; see Figure 19.4D). During the delay (between the spatial cue and the GO signal), beta oscillations again increased in strength, but this increase was faster during short compared to long trials. Thus, implicit timing (knowledge of remaining time before the movement onset) influences the onset (and strength) of oscillatory activity during the preparatory delay (see also Jones, Chapter 23; Praamstra, Chapter 24, this volume). Oscillations in LFPs that are presumably related to large-scale population dynamics therefore clearly reflect timing processes involved in movement preparation. This supports the idea that motor cortical beta oscillations are related to motor planning rather than to 'passive' processes such as idling or postural maintenance.

Conclusions

Motor preparation without timing does not exist. Timing and temporal expectancy in motor behaviour structures neuronal activity across a wide range of brain areas. This becomes clear when considering the discharge of individual neurons or network activity, as observable in the temporal coordination of spikes in pairs of neurons or the coherent local population activity seen in the LFP.

The effects of implicit and explicit timing in the activity of single neurons are very similar. Thus, it is not possible to distinguish whether different mechanisms are involved when timing is only implicitly used to improve performance, compared to when timing is a crucial component of the task. In the context of movement preparation, it might be artificial to distinguish between the two types of timing. There are indeed natural motor tasks where explicit timing is needed (particularly human behaviours such as ballet dancing and music production). However, in natural animal behaviour it is difficult to differentiate between these two notions. The concept of 'time to contact', used in hunting behaviour for instance, may be defined as explicit timing even though a hunting animal doesn't count seconds, but tries to catch the prey. Thus, one can speculate whether processes responsible for explicit timing exploit innate processes for implicit timing that allow context-dependent actions in natural behaviour. Alternatively, if the activity we observe in these areas are instead the *result* of a timing process, then it is possible that the origins of the different types of timing (implicit/explicit) are at least partly different (e.g. Coull and Nobre, 2008), whereas their ultimate effects at later stages are indistinguishable.

Indeed, the data and literature presented here indicate that time is not represented invariantly in the motor cortex, but instead is coded in a context-dependent manner by single-neuron activity or network dynamics. We have found that practice improves temporal synchrony in populations of motor cortical neurons in relation to temporal expectancy. This could favour the idea that, at least to some extent, timing is a constituent of currently active networks, and is thus a distributed brain process. On the other hand, if time estimation is a process independent of contextual features such as probability, then the signatures of time that we have described here are more likely the result of time estimation and not the time estimation process itself (see discussion in Roux et al., 2003). The question remains open whether a general, context-independent neuronal correlate of time estimation exists (e.g. Ivry and Spencer 2004; Mauk and Buonomano 2004; Ivry and Schlerf 2008).

References

Abeles, M. (1991). *Corticonics: Neural Circuits of the Cerebral Cortex*. Cambridge: Cambridge University Press.

Aertsen, A. and Gerstein, G.L. (1991). Dynamic aspects of neuronal cooperativity: fast stimulus-locked modulations of effective connectivity. In J. Krüger (Ed.) *Neuronal Cooperativity*, pp.52–67. Berlin: Springer Verlag.

Aertsen, A., Gerstein G., and Johannesma, P. (1986). From neuron to assembly: neuronal organization and stimulus representation. In G. Palm and A. Aertsen (Eds.) *Brain Theory*, pp.7–24. Berlin: Springer Verlag.

Akkal, D., Escola, L, Bioulac B., and Burbaud, P. (2004). Time predictability modulates pre-supplementary motor area neuronal activity. *Neuroreport*, **15**, 1283–6.

Asher, I., Stark, E., Abeles, M., and Prut, Y. (2007). Comparison of direction and object selectivity of local field potentials and single units in macaque posterior parietal cortex during prehension. *Journal of Neurophysiology*, **97**, 3684–95.

Baker, S. N., Kilner, J. M., Pinches, E. M., and Lemon, R. N. (1999). The role of synchrony and oscillation in the motor output. *Experimental Brain Research*, **128**, 109–17.

Bastian, A., Schöner, G., and Riehle, A. (2003) Preshaping and continuous evolution of motor cortical representations during movement preparation. *European Journal of Neuroscience*, **18**, 2047–58.

Berger, H. (1931). Über das Elektrenkephalogramm des Menschen. III. *Archiv für Psychiatrie und Nervenkrankheiten*, **94**, 16–60.

Brody, C. D., Hernández, A., Zainos. A., and Romo, R. (2003). Timing and neural encoding of somatosensory parametric working memory in macaque prefrontal cortex. *Cerebral Cortex*, **13**, 1196–207.

Cohen, Y. E., Cohen, I.S., and Gifford III, G. W. (2004). Modulation of LIP activity by predictive auditory and visual cues. *Cerebral Cortex*, **14**, 1287–301.

Coull, J. and Nobre, A. (2008). Dissociating explicit timing from temporal expectation with fMRI. *Current Opinion in Neurobiology*, **18**, 137–44.

Denker, M., Roux, S., Timme, M., Riehle, A., and Grün, S. (2007). Phase synchronization between LFP and spiking activity in motor cortex during movement preparation. *Neurocomputing*, **70**, 2096–101.

Donchin, O., Gribova, A., Steinberg, O., Bergman, H., Cardoso de Oliveira, S., and Vaadia, E. (2001). Local field potentials related to bimanual movements in the primary and supplementary motor cortices. *Experimental Brain Research*, **140**, 46–55.

Donoghue, J. P., Sanes, J. N., Hatsopoulos, N. G., and Gaal, G. (1998). Neural discharge and local field potential oscillations in primate motor cortex during voluntary movements. *Journal of Neurophysiology*, **79**, 159–73.

Dorris, M. C. and Munoz, D. P. (1998). Saccadic probability influences motor preparation signals and time to saccadic initiation. *Journal of Neuroscience*, **18**, 7015–26.

Dorris, M. C., Paré, M., and Munoz, D. P. (1997). Neuronal activity in monkey superior colliculus related to the initiation of saccadic eye movements. *Journal of Neuroscience*, **17**, 8566–79.

Durstewitz, D. (2003). Self-organizing neural integrator predicts interval times through climbing activity. *Journal of Neuroscience*, **23**, 5342–53.

Durstewitz, D. (2004). Neural representation of interval time. *Neuroreport*, **15**, 745–9.

Everling, S. and Munoz, D. P. (2000). Neuronal correlates for preparatory set associated with pro-saccades and anti-saccades in the primate frontal eye field. The *Journal of Neuroscience*, **20**, 387–400.

Gemba, H., Hashimoto, S., and Sasaki, K. (1981). Cortical field potentials preceding visually initiated hand movements in the monkey. *Experimental Brain Research*, **42**, 435–41.

Genovesio, A., Tsujimoto, S., and Wise, S.P. (2006). Neuronal activity related to elapsed time in prefrontal cortex. *Journal of Neurophysiology*, **95**, 3281–5.

Gerstein, G. L., Bedenbaugh, P., and Aertsen, A. M. H. J. (1989). Neural assemblies. *IEEE Transactions on Biomedical Engineering*, **36**, 4–14.

Ghose, G. M. and Maunsell, J. H. (2002). Attentional modulation in visual cortex depends on task timing. *Nature*, **419**, 616–20.

Gibbon, J., Malapani, C., Dale, C. L., and Gallistel, C. (1997). Toward a neurobiology of temporal cognition: advances and challenges. *Current Opinion in Neurobiology*, **7**, 170–84.

Grün, S. (2009). Data-driven significance estimation for precise spike correlation. *Journal of Neurophysiology*, **101**, 1126–40.

Grün, S., Diesmann, M., and Aertsen, A. (2002). 'Unitary events' in multiple single-neuron activity. II. Non-stationary data. *Neural Computation*, **14**, 81–119.

Hanes, D. P. and Schall, J. D. (1996). Neural control of voluntary movement initiation. *Science*, **274**, 427–30.

Hebb, D. O. (1949). *The Organization of Behavior*. New York: Wiley & Sons.

Ivry, R. B. and Schlerf, J. E. (2008). Dedicated and intrinsic models of time perception. *Trends in Cognitive Sciences*, **12**, 273–80.

Ivry, R. B. and Spencer, R. M. (2004). The neural representation of time. *Current Opinion in Neurobiology*, **14**, 225–32.

Janssen, P. and Shadlen, M. N. (2005). A representation of the hazard rate of elapsed time in macaque area LIP. *Nature Neuroscience*, **8**, 234–41.

Jasper, H. and Penfield, W. (1949). Electrocorticograms in man: effect of voluntary movement upon the electrical activity of the precentral gyrus. *Archiv für Psychiatrie und Zeitschrift Neurolgie*, **183**, 163–74.

Kilavik, B. E., Roux, S., Ponce-Alvarez, A., Confais, J., Grün, S., and Riehle, A. (2009). Long-term modifications in motor cortical dynamics induced by intensive practice. *Journal of Neuroscience*, **29**, 12653–63.

Kilavik, B. E., Ponce-Alvarez, A., and Riehle, A. (2007). Beta oscillations in monkey motor cortical LFPs are stronger during temporal attention than motor preparation. Society for Neuroscience Abstract 664.2. 37th Annual meeting of the society for Neuroscience, San Diego, USA.

Kubota, K. and Hamada, I. (1979). Preparatory activity of monkey pyramidal tract neurons related to quick movement onset during visual tracking performance. *Brain Research*, **168**, 435–9.

Lebedev, M. A., O'Doherty, J. E., and Nicolelis, M. A. (2008). Decoding of temporal intervals from cortical ensemble activity. *Journal of Neurophysiology*, **99**, 166–86.

Lecas, J. C., Requin, J., Anger, C., and Vitton, N. (1986). Changes in neuronal activity of the monkey precentral cortex during preparation for movement. *Journal of Neurophysiology*, **56**, 1680–702.

Lee, I. H. and Assad, J. A. (2003). Putaminal activity for simple reactions or self-timed movements. *Journal of Neurophysiology*, **89**, 2528–37.

Leon, M. I. and Shadlen, M. N. (2003). Representation of time by neurons in the posterior parietal cortex of the macaque. *Neuron*, **38**, 317–27.

Logothetis, N. K., Kayser, C., and Oeltermann, A. (2007). In vivo measurement of cortical impedance spectrum in monkeys: implications for signal propagation. *Neuron*, **55**, 809–23.

Lucchetti, C. and Bon, L. (2001). Time-modulated neuronal activity in premotor cortex of macaque monkeys. *Experimental Brain Research*, **141**, 254–60.

Lucchetti, C., Ulrici, A., and Bon, L. (2005). Dorsal premotor areas of nonhuman primate: functional flexibility in time domain. *European Journal of Applied Physiology*, **95**, 121–30.

Maimon, G. and Assad, J. A. (2006a). A cognitive signal for the proactive timing of action in macaque LIP. *Nature Neuroscience*, **9**, 948–55.

Maimon, G. and Assad, J. A. (2006b). Parietal area 5 and the initiation of self-timed movements versus simple reactions. *Journal of Neuroscience*, **26**, 2487–98.

Mauk, M. D. and Buonomano, D. V. (2004). The neural basis of temporal processing. *Annual Review of Neuroscience*, **27**, 307–40.

Mauritz, K. H. and Wise, S. P. (1986). Premotor cortex of the rhesus monkey: neuronal activity in anticipation of predictable environmental events. *Experimental Brain Research*, **61**, 229–44.

Mehring, C., Rickert, J., Vaadia, E., Cardosa de Oliveira, S., Aertsen, A., and Rotter, S. (2003). Inference of hand movements from local field potentials in monkey motor cortex. *Nature Neuroscience*, **6**, 1253–4.

Merchant, H. and Georgopoulos, A. P. (2006). Neurophysiology of perceptual and motor aspects of interception. *Journal of Neurophysiology*, **95**, 1–13.

Mitzdorf, U. (1985). Current source-density method and application in cat cerebral cortex: Investigation of evoked potentials and EEG phenomena. *Physiological Review*, **65**, 37–100.

Mitzdorf, U. (1994). Properties of generators of event-related potentials. *Pharmacopsychiatry*, **27**, 49–51.

Murthy, V. N. and Fetz, E. E. (1992). Coherent 25- to 35-Hz oscillations in the sensorimotor cortex of behaving monkeys. *Proceedings of the National Academy of Sciences USA*, **89**, 5670–74.

Murthy, V. N. and Fetz, E. E. (1996). Oscillatory activity in sensorimotor cortex of awake monkeys: synchronization of local field potentials and relation to behavior. *Journal of Neurophysiology*, **76**, 3949–67.

Niki, H. and Watanabe, M. (1979). Prefrontal and cingulate unit activity during timing behavior in the monkey. *Brain Research*, **171**, 213–24.

Okamoto, H., Isomura, Y., Takada, M., and Fukai T. (2007). Temporal integration by stochastic recurrent network dynamics with bimodal neurons. *Journal of Neurophysiology*, **97**, 3859–67.

Pfurtscheller, G., Stancák Jr., A., and Neuper, C. (1996). Post-movement beta synchronization. A correlate of an idling motor area? *Electroencephalography and Clinical Neurophysiology*, **98**, 281–93.

Renoult, L., Roux, S., and Riehle, A. (2006). Time is a rubberband: neuronal activity in monkey motor cortex in relation to time estimation. *European Journal of Neuroscience*, **23**, 3098–108.

Requin, J., Lecas, J. C., and Vitton, N. (1990). A comparison of preparation-related neuronal activity changes in the prefrontal, premotor, primary motor and posterior parietal areas of the monkey cortex: preliminary results. *Neuroscience Letters*, **111**, 151–6.

Requin, J., Brener, J., and Ring, C. (1991). Preparation for action. In R.R. Jennings and M.G.H. Coles (Eds.) *Handbook of Cognitive Psychophysiology: Central and Autonomous Nervous System Approaches*, pp.357–448. New York: Wiley & Sons.

Reutimann, J., Yakovlev, V., Fusi, S., and Senn, W. (2004). Climbing neuronal activity as an event-based cortical representation of time. *Journal of Neuroscience*, 24, 3295–303.

Rickert, J., Cardoso de Oliveira, S., Vaadia, E., Aertsen, A., Rotter, S., and Mehring, C. (2005). Encoding of movement direction in different frequency ranges of motor cortical local field potentials. *Journal of Neuroscience*, **25**, 8815–24.

Riehle, A. (2005). Preparation for action: one of the key functions of the motor cortex. In A. Riehle and E. Vaadia (Eds.) *Motor Cortex in Voluntary Movements: A Distributed System for Distributed Functions*, pp.213–40. Boca Raton, FL: CRC-Press.

Riehle, A. and Requin, J. (1993). The predictive value for performance speed of preparatory changes in neuronal activity of the monkey motor and premotor cortex. *Behavioural Brain Research*, **53**, 35–49.

Riehle, A., Grün, S., Diesmann, M., and Aertsen, A. (1997). Spike synchronization and rate modulation differentially involved in motor cortical function. *Science*, **278**, 1950–3.

Riehle, A., Grammont, F., Diesmann, M., and Grün, S. (2000). Dynamical changes and temporal precision of synchronized spiking activity in monkey motor cortex during movement preparation. *Journal of Physiology (Paris)*, **94**, 569–82.

Roesch, M. R. and Olson, C. R. (2005). Neuronal activity in primate orbitofrontal cortex reflects the value of time. *Journal of Neurophysiology*, **94**, 2457–71.

Roitman, J. D and Shadlen, M. N. (2002). Response of neurons in the lateral intraparietal area during a combined visual discrimination reaction time task. *Journal of Neuroscience*, **22**, 9475–89.

Roux, S., Coulmance, M., and Riehle, A. (2003). Context-related representation of timing processes in monkey motor cortex. *European Journal of Neuroscience*, **18**, 1011–16.

Roux, S., MacKay, W.A., and Riehle, A. (2006). The pre-movement component of motor cortical local field potentials reflects the level of expectancy. *Behavioral Brain Research*, **169**, 335–51.

Rudolph, M. and Destexhe, A. (2003). Tuning neocortical pyramidal neurons between integrators and coincidence detectors. *Journal of Computational Neuroscience*, **14**, 239–51.

Sakurai, Y., Takahashi, S., and Inoue, M. (2004). Stimulus duration in working memory is represented by neuronal activity in the monkey prefrontal cortex. European *Journal of Neuroscience*, **20**, 1069–80.

Sanes, J. N. and Donoghue, J. P. (1993). Oscillations in local field potentials of the primate motor cortex during voluntary movement. *Proceedings of the National Academy of Sciences USA*, **90**, 4470–4.

Shuler, M. G. and Bear, M. F. (2006). Reward timing in the primary visual cortex. *Science*, **311**, 1606–9.

Snyder, L. H., Dickinson, A. R. and Calton, J. L. (2006). Preparatory delay activity in the monkey parietal reach region predicts reach reaction times. *Journal of Neuroscience*, **26**, 10091–9.

Tsujimoto, S. and Sawaguchi T. (2005). Neuronal activity representing temporal prediction of reward in the primate prefrontal cortex. *Journal of Neurophysiology*, **93**, 3687–92.

Vaadia, E., Kurata, K. and Wise, S.P. (1988). Neuronal activity preceding directional and nondirectional cues in the premotor cortex of rhesus monkeys. *Somatosensory and Motor Research*, **6**, 207–30.

Acknowledgements

This work was supported by the French Government (ACI Cognitique 'Variability & Invariants', STIC-Santé, ANR-05-NEUR-045-01). We thank Jenny Coull and Kia Nobre for the many helpful comments on an early version of the chapter. Special thanks go to Annette Bastian, Franck Grammont, Adrián Ponce-Alvarez, Louis Renoult, and Sébastien Roux for data collection, and Marc Martin and Céline Mazenq for animal welfare.

Chapter 20

The neural basis of temporal prediction and the role of dopamine

Christopher D. Fiorillo

We currently understand the most basic aspect of how the nervous system deals with space. Different neurons and synapses are devoted to different regions of space. For example, the spatial receptive field of a photoreceptor depends on its location in the retina. Although transformed, that spatial information is propagated through the nervous system, with discrete points in space being represented by spatially discrete neurons and synapses. Sensory modalities such as colour and tone are also spatially discrete within the nervous system, since discrete neurons represent discrete parts of the frequency spectrum. By contrast, relatively little is known about how the nervous system represents time. In this chapter, I discuss a model of how individual neurons may process temporal information, which is part of a general theory of neural computation. Then I discuss experiments on dopamine neurons that provide some insight into temporal aspects of predictions at the systems and behavioural levels.

There are two basic concepts that are critical to each of the works that I will discuss, and both are of central importance to the field of reinforcement learning. First is the importance of predicting 'future reward'. If the general goal of the nervous system is to select behavioural outputs so as to maximize expected future reward, then clearly the system must predict future reward. The notion of 'future reward' intended here is a very abstract concept, but it can be thought of simply as the part of the world that is of biological relevance and therefore of interest to an animal. As discussed further in later sections, both selective attention and the dopamine signal appear to help ensure that a neuron's information is relevant to future reward.

The second fundamental concept is that of 'prediction error'. Although our conscious minds tend to focus on aspects of the world that are difficult to predict, the world actually tends to be fairly predictable. Naturally, the world is predictable only because our brains have a great deal of information about the world. At each moment in time, our information is being updated through our senses and through ongoing processing. It is useful to refer to the information that is already in the system, or in a neuron, as 'prior' information. As we know from subjective experience, events in the external world are of little interest when they are fully predicted. If an event is predictable based on prior information then, other things being equal, it is not interesting because it is not informative. Thus it makes sense that neurons should not respond when they can accurately predict their inputs, but should respond only to 'prediction errors' (Fiorillo, 2008). This concept has a long history, going back to the early work of Attneave (1954) and Barlow (1961). Although not always known by the same name, the concept of prediction error is prevalent in literature on the efficient coding of sensory information (Simoncelli and Olshausen, 2001) and in reinforcement learning (Sutton and Barto, 1998). As discussed in further detail later in this chapter, dopamine neurons signal errors in the prediction of reward (Shultz et al., 1997).

Temporal prediction in single neurons

The term 'prediction' is often used rather narrowly to refer to a high-level cognitive phenomenon of which we are consciously aware. However, information is defined by its ability to estimate or predict (Jaynes, 2003), and thus we can say that the information in a photoreceptor estimates or predicts light intensity in a particular region of space. I refer to the 'object' of a neuron's information as its 'stimulus'. Each neuron has a stimulus, although a neuron's stimulus could be easy (e.g. a sensory receptor) or difficult (e.g. a motor neuron) for us to define precisely. It has been proposed that a neuron has prior information that predicts the intensity of its stimulus, and that the neuron only responds when stimulus intensity exceeds the neuron's expectation. Thus a neuron signals prediction error (Fiorillo, 2008). Perhaps the most familiar examples come from the retina, one of the best understood parts of the nervous system.

Neurons in the retina rely on spatial and temporal correlations to predict light intensity as accurately and as early as possible. There are strong positive correlations between light intensities at neighbouring points in space and time, and there is a great deal of evidence that neurons in the retina exploit these correlations (e.g. Barlow, 1961; Srinivasan et al., 1982; Hosoya et al., 2005). For example, consider such familiar phenomena as light adaptation and surround inhibition. Adaptation results from prior information about stimulus intensity carried through time by proteins that are intrinsic to a neuron, such as voltage-activated potassium (K^+) channels. Spatial prior information would be carried through neural circuitry and would activate neurotransmitter-gated channels. A prototypical example would be GABA-gated chloride and potassium channels.

According to the model (Figure 20.1), the output of a neuron (membrane potential or firing rate) represents the difference between a neuron's current excitatory input and the prediction of that input. The prediction would depend on prior information provided by synaptic inputs as well as ion channels such as voltage-regulated potassium channels. Distinct points in space would be represented by distinct synapses. As previously proposed (Srinivasan et al., 1982), the neuron should select those synapses, and those corresponding regions of the surround, that are the best predictors of light intensity in the centre. This selection could be accomplished by an anti-Hebbian plasticity rule (Box 20.1), which strengthens those synapses that tend to inhibit the neuron at the same time that the neuron is depolarized by excitation from the centre (Hosoya et al., 2005). If the neuron signals prediction error, then an anti-Hebbian rule would strengthen those inputs that tend to minimize the error. Minimizing prediction error could instead be seen as promoting homeostasis by driving membrane voltage towards the middle of its range (see Box 20.1).

I have proposed that this same principle (anti-Hebbian selection of prior information sources) also applies to the temporal domain and to non-synaptic ion channels. Although the model is intended to apply to many types of non-synaptic ion channels, the diversity of potassium channels is particularly remarkable. Just as a synapse contributes information from a particular region of space (which depends on the pre-synaptic neuron's receptive field), a voltage-regulated channel contributes information from the past. The particular period of the past depends on the channel's kinetic properties. For example, if a channel has rapid kinetics, then it carries information from the recent past.

Because glutamate depolarizes membrane voltage, a voltage-gated channel carries information about past glutamate concentrations. Such information would be useful in predicting current glutamate concentrations if concentrations are correlated across time. An anti-Hebbian rule would tend to select those types of channels, and the corresponding periods of the past, that are the best predictors of current stimulus intensity (and thus minimize prediction errors).

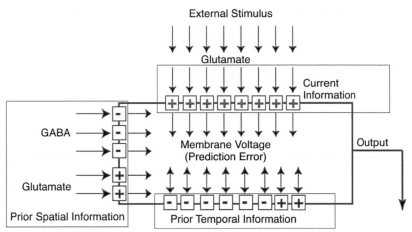

Fig. 20.1 Schematic illustration of a model neuron. Arrows indicate the direction of information flow. A neuron is proposed to receive two broad classes of inputs. Each arrow denotes an individual input (either a synapse or a class of ion channel), and the signs indicate whether an input is depolarizing or hyperpolarizing. Those inputs that contribute current information would typically come more directly from the sensory periphery and would be carried by an excitatory neurotransmitter such as glutamate (although in principle, current information could be contributed by an inhibitory neurotransmitter). The second class of inputs contributes prior information that serves to predict and cancel the excitatory influence of current information. These inputs would therefore act to drive the membrane voltage towards the middle of its range. The output or membrane voltage of the neuron would signal prediction error, the discrepancy between current and prior information. If stimulus intensity (glutamate concentration) is greater than expected, the neuron would be depolarized; if less than expected, the neuron would be hyperpolarized. Inputs contributing prior information could be either excitatory or inhibitory, and they can be further classified as either contributing prior spatial information coming from other neurons, or prior temporal information coming from voltage-regulated, non-synaptic ion channels, particularly potassium channels. There is a great diversity of potassium channels, and since these channels differ in their kinetic properties, they contribute information from different periods of the past. The neuron receives a spectrum of individual inputs, each corresponding to a discrete point in space or period of the past. The neuron selects amongst its individual inputs according to plasticity rules. The defining difference between inputs contributing current information and those contributing prior information is in the applicable plasticity rules. Those inputs contributing current information would be selected by a Hebbian type rule that tends to maximize prediction errors (although this rule may also include reward information, such as that carried by dopamine, to select those inputs that are most informative about future reward). Selection of inputs contributing prior information would occur through an anti-Hebbian rule in order to minimize prediction errors. Adapted with permission from Fiorillo, C. D. (2008). Towards a general theory of neural computation based on prediction by single neurons. *Public Library of Science ONE*, **3**, e3298.

The number of functional potassium channels of a particular type would be increased if those channels were open when the neuron were depolarized, and decreased if they were open during hyperpolarization. In this way, the neuron would learn to match the kinetics of its potassium channels to temporal patterns in its synaptic inputs. This proposal is consistent with evidence that potassium channel density is regulated to maintain homeostasis (e.g. Turrigiano et al., 1994), and it could be seen as a more sophisticated form of 'predictive' homeostasis.

Box 20.1 Working definitions of associative plasticity rules

Anti-Hebbian rule: an input to a neuron will be strengthened if its activity promotes homeostasis (opposes prediction error) by bringing the neuron's activity (membrane voltage or firing rate) towards an intermediate level. It will be weakened if it opposes homeostasis.

Hebbian rule: an input to a neuron will be strengthened if its activity opposes homeostasis (promotes prediction error) by shifting the neuron's activity (membrane voltage or firing rate) away from an intermediate level. It will be weakened if it promotes homeostasis

The best predictor of the present is often the most recent past, and likewise, many of the potassium channels expressed in neurons have fast kinetics (milliseconds). In cases of high frequency variation in stimulus intensity, a better estimate may be made by averaging over a longer period of the past, and some potassium channels activate over several seconds or longer. However, due to the complexities of channel gating, such as inactivation, a channel's state does not merely depend on an average of the most recent membrane voltages. (For a more detailed discussion of the temporal predictions made by single ion channels, see Fiorillo, 2008.) It should be noted that the proposed function of potassium channels is likely to be of limited relevance to the behavioural phenomenon of 'interval timing' (see later in this chapter), in which predictions are made over arbitrary intervals in the seconds to hours range. However, the kinetics of non-synaptic ion channels might be of more direct relevance to timing behaviour for sub-second intervals, which exhibit properties that are clearly distinct from the timing of longer intervals (Buhusi and Meck, 2005).

As far as I know, there is virtually no direct evidence for or against the proposal that potassium channel subtypes are selected through an anti-Hebbian mechanism. Very little is currently known about the rules or mechanisms by which a neuron selects amongst its potassium channels. However, it is known that a neuron somehow selectively expresses a relatively small fraction of the many types of potassium channels with which it is genetically endowed. Furthermore, the sort of molecular processes that would be required for anti-Hebbian plasticity of potassium channels (such as a coincidence detector), already has a precedent in the mechanism of Hebbian plasticity at glutamate synapses, where NMDA receptor activation triggers the insertion (or removal) of AMPA receptors into the synaptic membrane (Malinow and Malenka, 2002).

The model neuron described here would learn to predict its excitatory stimulus and to respond only to errors in prediction. Among other advantages, the signalling of prediction errors could allow a neuron to learn to respond only to the first in a stereotyped sequence of excitatory inputs, particularly if those excitatory inputs are selected through a Hebbian plasticity rule (which tends to maximize prediction errors) (see Box 20.1) (Sutton and Barto, 1981; Izhikevich, 2007; Fiorillo, 2008). The first excitatory input, or stimulus event, would be the most informative because it would predict the later events. Leaping from the cellular to behavioural level, responding to the first event would provide an animal with time to prepare appropriate behaviours in anticipation of later events.

Spectral timing models

In the model presented earlier, the membrane voltage of a generic neuron signals prediction error. This error acts to select from a spectrum of voltage-regulated ion channels that differ in their kinetic properties and thus in their prior temporal information. Such a model could therefore be referred to as a 'spectral timing model' analogous to that of Grossberg and Smajuk (1989).

The distinguishing feature of spectral timing models is their dependence on discrete components that differ in their kinetic properties. An error signal would select the component(s) with kinetics most appropriate to the input pattern. The model proposed earlier is distinctive in that some of the components are different types of ion channels, and the error signal is generated within the same neuron. Thus an entire spectrum is found within a single neuron. The model neuron also selects from amongst a spectrum of synaptic inputs, and these synaptic inputs would also tend to differ in their temporal profiles. Thus a network of the proposed model neurons could be said to implement a form of spectral timing at both the cellular and network levels.

By contrast to the model presented earlier, the spectral timing model of Grossberg and Smajuk (1989), as well as later models, were concerned solely with networks of neurons in which both the spectral components and the error signal correspond to discrete neurons. As described later in this chapter, it has been proposed that the error signal of midbrain dopamine neurons could select those spectral components in the basal ganglia that are the best predictors of reward (e.g. Schultz et al., 1997; Brown et al., 1999; Contreras-Vidal and Schultz, 1999).

Recordings of dopamine neurons in an interval-timing task

Together with Bill Newsome and Wolfram Schultz, I have studied the responses of dopamine neurons of the primate ventral midbrain (including ventral tegmental area and substantia nigra) to manipulations of reward timing (Fiorillo et al., 2008). There are several reasons that dopamine neurons are of particular interest with respect to timing. First, it is known that dopamine and its target structures in the basal ganglia are critical for timing intervals across a large range from about one second to minutes or longer (reviewed by Buhusi and Meck, 2005). Dopaminergic drugs modify interval timing, with agonists causing subjects to guess that an interval has elapsed earlier than they otherwise would ('speeding the internal clock'), and antagonists having the opposite effect.

Second, the finding that dopamine neurons encode reward prediction error inspired systems-level models that utilize this error signal for guiding behaviour. These 'reinforcement-learning' models propose that the dopamine prediction error teaches target structures such as the basal ganglia to predict both the time and magnitude of reward (a function sometimes ascribed to the 'critic') and to take actions to obtain reward (a function ascribed to the 'actor'). Although these models have the virtue of working in 'real time', they do not specify how a system should represent time, and some models have implemented an arbitrarily precise temporal representation that does not attempt to be biologically realistic—e.g. Schultz et al. (1997) but see Ludvig et al. (2008), Brown et al. (1999), and Contreras-Vidal and Schultz (1998) for more plausible accounts.

Whereas reinforcement-learning models necessarily rely on temporal predictions, the development of a biological model of timing has not been among their primary concerns. By contrast, Matell and Meck (2004) have proposed a detailed model of striatal circuitry that could explain many aspects of interval timing. Their model relies on detecting the coincident activity of multiple oscillators, rather than on selection from amongst a spectrum of different kinetic processes, but it utilizes the dopamine error signal in a similar manner for learning to time intervals. One motivation for the experiments described later in this chapter was to provide data that can guide the development of biologically realistic models of temporal prediction.

Regardless of the function of dopamine, we can use the dopamine error signal to investigate the temporal characteristics of reward prediction. Dopamine neurons briefly increase their firing rate (beyond their spontaneous rate of 3Hz) following reward events that are better than expected, and they decrease their firing rates when events are worse than expected. The increase in firing rate following reward is roughly proportional to the difference between reward value and expected reward value (Fiorillo et al., 2003; Morris et al., 2004; Bayer and Glimcher, 2005). This error signal (to events that are better than expected) provided us with a neural assay of how 'surprised' the system was upon receipt of reward. The error signal could therefore be used to measure the temporal precision of reward prediction.

When an animal has been trained with a particular temporal interval between two events, occurrence of the first event evokes an expectation of when the second event will occur. This expectation can be thought of as a probability distribution over future time (Figure 20.2A). The animal can be fairly certain that the second event will occur, but because it does not have a perfect timing ability, or because it does not trust that the current trial will be the same as the previous trials, it is uncertain about exactly when the second event will occur. There is abundant behavioural evidence that the peak of the animal's subjective expectation is very close in time to the objective end of the interval (reviewed by Gibbon et al., 1997), and in this sense animals can

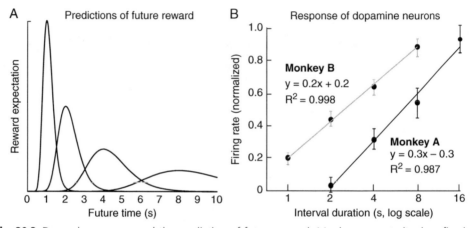

Fig. 20.2 Dopamine neurons and the prediction of future reward. Monkeys were trained on fixed intervals between conditioned stimulus onset and delivery of juice reward. A) Illustration of subjective distributions of reward expectation over future time that could emerge after extensive training on fixed stimulus-reward intervals of 1, 2, 4, and 8 seconds. Time '0' corresponds to the time of perceptual identification of the stimulus (immediately after stimulus onset). Several aspects of these distributions are supported by analysis of behaviour. First, the peak of each distribution (the most probable time of reward) matches the peak of behavioural responding, which occurred at the end of the interval on which the animal was trained. Second, the width of the distributions (their temporal uncertainty) increases as interval duration increases, and the peak expectation (at the objective end of the interval) declines as the inverse of interval duration. More precisely, these distributions are consistent with Weber's law; each is log-normal with an equivalent standard deviation measured in log units. The actual standard deviation was chosen arbitrarily. B) Mean normalized population responses of midbrain dopamine neurons to reward delivery as a function of stimulus-reward interval (26–34 neurons in monkey A, 30 in monkey B). Responses presumably increased with interval duration because the momentary expectation (at the end of the interval) declined, as illustrated in panel (A). The data was well described by a linear function of the logarithm of interval duration. I proposed that this could be explained by making several assumptions. One assumption was that subjective distributions are consistent with Weber's law, like those shown in panel (A), in which case peak expectation at the end of an interval would be inversely proportional to interval duration. Adapted from Fiorillo, C. D., Newsome, W. T. and Schultz, W. (2008). The temporal precision of reward prediction in dopamine neurons. *Nature Neuroscience*, **11**, 966–73.

make accurate temporal predictions. But how precise is the expectation, and is precision similar at the neural and behavioural levels? In principle, the expectation could be quite precise (low uncertainty), rising sharply to its peak near the end of the interval, or it could be relatively imprecise (high uncertainty), with the distribution being wider and flatter. If the neural expectation is similar to the behavioural expectation, then its precision should decline as interval duration increases (Figure 20.2A).

To establish the expectation of reward, two macaque monkeys were extensively pre-trained in a Pavlovian task in which visual stimuli were followed by juice reward. Stimulus–reward intervals of 1–16 seconds were tested. Each of four distinct visual stimuli (presented on randomly interleaved trials) was followed by juice after an interval that was exactly the same on each trial (a 'fixed' interval). Juice was delivered from a spout just in the front of the monkey's mouth. To receive the full volume of juice, the monkey had to begin licking prior to juice delivery (or some of the juice would fall to the floor). We measured licking in order to infer the animal's subjective expectation of reward. As discussed in the original paper (Fiorillo et al, 2008), it is important to recognize, first, that the monkeys clearly had an incentive for precise timing, and second, that licking behaviour does not directly reflect the monkey's subjective reward expectation.

Our observations were consistent with the behavioural literature. First, the average licking behaviour displayed the scalar or Weber property that is commonly observed with interval timing. Thus, although there was substantial variation from trial to trial, monkeys typically started licking after about half of the interval had elapsed and continued to lick until juice delivery, and this was true regardless of interval duration. Second, there was no licking on some of the trials with long stimulus–reward intervals, suggesting that the momentary expectation was lower during long intervals in comparison to shorter intervals. These observations suggest that temporal precision may be relatively low, and that it declines as interval duration increases (Figure 20.2A).

Previous studies have found that when a conditioned stimulus is repeatedly followed 1–2 seconds later by juice reward, dopamine neurons are activated by the conditioned stimulus but very little by the juice. We examined longer intervals as well. As the stimulus–reward interval was increased, the response of dopamine neurons to the conditioned stimulus decreased and the response to the reward increased. The decline in the stimulus response was anticipated by dopamine-based reinforcement-learning models, which propose that the reward value that activates dopamine neurons is the expected value of the 'discounted sum of future rewards'. A reward expected further into the future would be discounted more than an immediate reward.

The response of dopamine neurons to juice reward increased steeply with stimulus–reward interval (Figure 20.2B). The response to juice following a 16-second interval was as large as the response to the standard 'unpredicted' reward (delivered following a variable interval of 5–15 seconds), which evoked the largest response observed in this and previous studies. This result suggests that the temporal precision of reward expectation decreases sharply as interval duration increases, so that the momentary expectation at the end of a long fixed interval is relatively weak.

Responses to reward were remarkably well fitted by a linear function of the logarithm of the interval (R^2 >0.98 for the population of neurons in each monkey) (Figure 20.2B). Kobayashi and Schultz (2008) performed very similar experiments (though aimed at investigating temporal discounting of future rewards) and obtained similar results. However, they suggested that a hyperbolic function fit their data slightly better than a logarithmic function. This apparent discrepancy is likely to be due to the fact that whereas I considered only the intervals for which data were available (1–16 seconds), Kobayashi and Schultz assumed that there would be no activation of dopamine neurons to reward delivered at an interval of zero seconds (presuming that reward would be perfectly predicted, and thus there would be no prediction error). A zero-second stimulus–reward interval cannot readily be tested (due to interference from the dopamine response to the conditioned stimulus), but there are two reasons to doubt their assumption. First, regardless of past experience, the occurrence of a conditioned stimulus can never guarantee delivery of reward, and thus reward delivery may always be at least slightly better than expected, even at very short stimulus–reward intervals. Second, the properties of interval timing for short intervals (<0.5–1.0 seconds) are known to differ substantially from longer intervals (reviewed by Buhusi and Meck, 2005).

I developed a model that could account for the observed logarithmic relationship between dopamine responses and interval duration (Fiorillo et al., 2008). I will not describe the model here, but I will mention the three assumptions upon which the model was based, each of which is supported by entirely independent evidence. First, I assumed that the peak expectation of reward is inversely related to interval duration, as required for a variety of distributions of future reward that are consistent with the scalar timing property (Weber's law for timing) (Figure 20.2B). Second, I assumed that the dopamine error signal is the conventionally defined error (actual reward value minus expected value) divided by a measure of uncertainty such as standard deviation. This was previously proposed based on a study in which we manipulated reward magnitude and probability (Tobler et al., 2005). Finally, I assumed that the activity of dopamine neurons encodes a logarithmic transformation of the error signal, as implied by the Weber–Fechner law as applied to reward magnitude. Taken together, these three assumptions suggest that the dopamine error signal at the end of a familiar fixed interval should increase with the logarithm of interval duration, just as we found experimentally.

Additional experiments (Fiorillo et al, 2008) examined the temporal precision of reward expectation by varying stimulus–reward intervals. In one set of experiments, monkeys were extensively trained with a fixed stimulus–reward interval of 2.0 seconds. During physiological recordings, reward was delivered after just 1.0 second on a minority of trials. The response to early reward on these probe trials was just slightly greater than the response to juice delivered at its usual time of 2.0 seconds. However, the response was much less than the response to 'unpredicted' reward (delivered following a long and variable interval). Thus the expectation of reward appeared to be quite strong even after just half of a stimulus–reward interval had elapsed. This suggests that the expectation was spread over a large fraction of the interval, and thus temporal precision was low.

In yet another set of experiments, reward responses were examined following stimulus–reward intervals that varied from trial to trial. The distribution of intervals was flat and ranged from 1.0–3.0 seconds (or 0.5–3.5 seconds in another experiment). The animal's expectation during this variable interval should be spread over a duration of at least 2 seconds (due to averaging across previously observed intervals of differing durations). If the expectation associated with each observed interval is strong only for a brief period near the end of the interval (high precision), then introduction of variable intervals should substantially weaken the momentary reward expectation, resulting in large dopamine responses. In contrast to this high-precision hypothesis, we found that dopamine neurons were only slightly (but significantly) more activated by reward delivered after the variable interval than after a fixed 2-second interval.

In the same experiment, the activation to early reward was greater than the activation to late reward. Because reward occurred by 3 seconds on every trial, the monkeys may have learned that the absence of reward at one moment during the elapsing interval increases the likelihood that reward will occur in the next moment. The contingency over time between no reward and reward is described by the hazard function. It has been shown that the behaviour of monkeys and the firing rate of neurons in parietal cortex tracks elapsed time in a manner consistent with the hazard function (Janssen and Shadlen, 2005). Thus the expectation of reward may grow over time as the interval elapses in the absence of reward. Indeed, firing rate gradually declined as a variable interval elapsed in the absence of reward (see also Kilavik and Riehle, Chapter 19, this volume). The slight gradual decline in firing rate could reflect negative prediction errors that are small and growing over time as reward expectation increases. We also found evidence for a similar effect during short fixed CS-reward intervals, but not for longer intervals. Such an effect may be negligible for longer fixed intervals, since the reward expectation at any moment during the interval would be weaker.

In summary, we found that dopamine neurons are highly sensitive to stimulus–reward interval duration, but only weakly sensitive to variability in interval duration. We concluded that the temporal precision of reward prediction was relatively low at both neuronal and behavioural levels, and that it declined sharply with interval duration but not with variability in interval duration. These data were rather surprising to some researchers in the field, who may have thought that the temporal precision of reward prediction in dopamine neurons would be substantially higher, and that reward predictability would be strongly dependent on variability in interval duration but would have little dependence on the duration of familiar fixed intervals. However, the present results fit with a large body of behavioural data suggesting that the remarkable flexibility of interval timing, functioning over a large range of interval durations from seconds to hours, comes at the cost of precision (Gibbon et al., 1997). At the neuronal level, a lack of high precision is also implied by the expectation-related delay-period activity of many sensorimotor neurons (e.g. Ghose and Maunsell, 2002; Brody et al., 2003; Janssen and Shadlen, 2005), including dopamine neurons (Fiorillo et al., 2003). In these neurons, firing rate typically begins to increase (or decrease) gradually, shortly after the first event and continues until the second event occurs, suggesting that the neuronal expectation is characterized by high temporal uncertainty. We have come to a similar conclusion by observing the phasic prediction error of dopamine neurons following the second event. However, the low temporal precision reflected in the activity of dopamine neurons may not generalize to other types of neurons. Furthermore, there are potential limitations in using the dopamine signal to infer the temporal precision of the system's prediction(s), as discussed previously (Fiorillo et al, 2008).

The ability to make temporally precise predictions based on internal timing mechanisms may not be as advantageous as it might appear. Although the statistics of natural reward events have not been characterized, intervals that require internal timing may tend to be quite short. This is because relatively stereotyped sequences of conditioned stimuli may be prevalent, effectively providing the animal with an external 'clock.' If so, then internal timing may usually be needed only for the short intervening intervals between external stimuli (or 'ticks' of the clock). Furthermore, the repeated occurrence of very precisely timed intervals (such as those on which we trained our monkeys) may be highly unusual in more natural settings. Relatively imprecise timing could therefore suffice if the majority of recurring intervals tend to be short and variable. If, for whatever reason, a system lacks the capacity for precise internal timing of long intervals, then the accurate prediction of reward must rely on identification of external conditioned stimuli that precede reward by short intervals. The activation of dopamine neurons after long stimulus–reward intervals would be well suited for identifying shorter stimulus–reward intervals (assuming that other predictive stimuli are present in the environment). Thus our results suggest that the properties of the dopamine error signal, and the apparently low precision of the internal timing mechanisms of the dopamine reward system, would be appropriate for a world in which the majority of intervals between reward events tend to be short and variable.

Does dopamine teach the brain to predict reward?

There is strong evidence collected over several decades, particularly from pharmacological experiments, that dopamine reinforces the reward value of stimuli and actions (Wise, 2004). Within
literature on both animal and machine learning, the proper form of a reinforcement signal has
long been known to correspond to a reward prediction error (Dickinson, 1980; Sutton and Barto,
1998). Thus the finding that dopamine neurons encode a reward prediction error naturally led to
the hypothesis that dopamine reinforces stimuli and actions as described in reinforcement learning algorithms (Schultz et al., 1997). Multiple reinforcement learning models have since been
proposed based on the dopamine reward prediction error (e.g. Brown et al., 1999; Contreras-
Vidal and Schultz, 1999; Ludvig et al., 2008).

Reinforcement-learning models that utilize the dopamine error signal propose two roles for
dopamine. These distinct roles are made explicit in models that adopt an 'actor–critic' architecture (Barto, 1995). The essential function of dopamine in any such model is reinforcement,
whereby dopamine teaches target brain regions the reward value of stimuli and actions. In this
way, dopamine trains 'the actor'. The actor stores the reward values of stimuli and actions, and
selects the action with the highest value. The dopamine neurons 'criticize' the actor, and they can
be thought of as the output of a brain system which functions to predict reward. This brain system
is sometimes called 'the critic'. The difficult job of the critic is to predict reward, which means to
predict the magnitude of reward at each moment in time. The prediction of reward is then used
to compute the reward prediction error of dopamine neurons. In typical reinforcement learning
models, the reward prediction error trains both the critic and the actor (e.g. Barto, 1995; Schultz
et al., 1997; Brown et al., 1999; Contreras-Vidal and Schultz, 1999). Thus dopamine has been
proposed not only to reinforce stimuli and actions, but also to teach the brain to predict the time
and amount of reward.

There are different interpretations that might be applied to the 'prediction of reward'. There
is a sense in which the output of neurons in motor systems, and the actions of an animal, can
themselves be thought of as a prediction of future reward, and in this sense the reinforcing action
of dopamine would necessarily be involved in learning to predict reward (Fiorillo, 2008). But the
meaning of reward prediction used here and in actor–critic models, as well as in common usage,
is more closely tied to a psychological or cognitive process of the sort associated specifically with
sensorimotor regions. However, with respect to dopamine and reinforcement learning, the relevant concepts of prediction and reward do not necessarily correspond to high-level cognitive (or
conscious) processes. Furthermore, the reward value in reinforcement learning is an abstract
entity ('the sum of future rewards') that need not have any particular psychological correlate, and
which does not simply correspond to a concrete quantity such as an amount of food or money.
Given our knowledge of the dopamine system, the reward value that dopamine reinforces
(particularly in limbic regions and basal ganglia) may be best described in psychological terms as
the incentive or motivational value associated with stimuli and actions (Wise, 2004).

Whereas there is an enormous amount of evidence that dopamine trains the actor, there is
relatively little evidence that dopamine trains the critic (teaches the brain to predict reward
value). Below I discuss experimental evidence against dopamine's proposed role in learning to
predict reward. I then suggest that the reward prediction error of dopamine neurons is not well
suited for this function.

A well-established effect of reward prediction, and the one that is essential to dopamine-
based reinforcement learning models, involves the computation of the dopamine reward prediction error itself. Once an animal has learned to predict a reward, the prediction cancels the
excitation of dopamine neurons by the reward. When reward value is less than expected, there is

a suppression of the firing rate of dopamine neurons below their spontaneous background rate of about three impulses per second (Hollerman and Schultz, 1998; Tobler et al., 2005).

Reinforcement-learning models propose that dopamine itself drives the neural plasticity by which the system learns to predict reward. Brown et al. (1999) proposed a detailed circuit model of how neurons in striatal striosomes could use the dopamine error signal and spectral timing in order to learn to predict and cancel the reward excitation of dopamine neurons. After dopamine-dependent learning, onset of a conditioned stimulus or action initiates a process in these striatal neurons that results in an appropriately timed inhibitory signal being sent directly to dopamine neurons, thereby cancelling their excitation by reward. One means of testing dopamine's role in this learning process would be to substitute an artificial dopamine signal in place of a natural reward and to test whether we still observe the inhibitory effect of reward prediction on dopamine neurons.

Artificial dopamine signals can be elicited by electrical stimulation. Wightman and colleagues have shown that electrical stimulation in the dopamine cell body region in the ventral midbrain of rats evokes dopamine release in the striatum and nucleus accumbens (as measured with high temporal resolution by fast-scan cyclic voltammetry) (e.g. Cheer et al., 2005). Since this electrical stimulation has behavioural reward value, it is an example of 'brain stimulation reward', or BSR. Cheer et al. (2005) observed the same amount of dopamine release, regardless of whether BSR was well predicted by an action of the animal or delivered unpredictably by the experimenter.

If the electrical stimulation in this study evoked dopamine release by direct activation of the axons of dopamine neurons, then the amount of dopamine release would not be sensitive to any inhibition of the soma or dendrites that might accompany reward prediction. However, it is unlikely that substantial numbers of dopamine neurons were directly activated in the study of Cheer et al. (2005), despite electrical stimulation in the dopamine cell body region. My own unpublished observations in rat brain slices indicated that local electrical stimulation evoked action potentials in the vast majority of dopamine neurons by eliciting excitatory post-synaptic potentials. Substantially higher current intensities were needed to directly evoke action potentials. This is likely to be because axons of dopamine neurons are small and unmyelinated and therefore have higher stimulation thresholds than the larger, myelinated axons of excitatory afferents. Likewise, although the rat medial forebrain bundle contains dopamine axons, its stimulation in BSR does not directly activate substantial numbers of dopamine neurons (reviewed by Shizgal, 1997). Thus it seems likely that the excitation of dopamine neurons in the study of Cheer et al. (2005) was monosynaptic. This excitation could potentially have been predicted, and at least partially cancelled, if dopamine were involved in learning to predict and inhibit the excitation of dopamine neurons. The failure of Cheer et al. (2005) to observe any effect of reward predictability on BSR-evoked dopamine release casts doubt on the hypothesis that dopamine is important in learning to predict reward value.

However, there is evidence that the direct inhibition of dopamine neurons may play a relatively minor role in cancelling the excitation of dopamine neurons by predicted reward (Fiorillo et al., 2008). Rather, the prediction error could be substantially computed upstream of dopamine neurons. In the latter case, the monosynaptic excitation of dopamine neurons that was likely studied by Cheer et al. (2005) would be only weakly sensitive to the effects of reward prediction. If the excitation of dopamine neurons were elicited by BSR evoked further upstream from dopamine neurons (polysynaptic excitation), then there would be a greater chance to observe an effect of reward prediction on the dopamine response to BSR. In other words, the effect of monosynaptic excitation may be difficult to predict and cancel, but polysynaptic excitation of dopamine neurons (as occurs with natural reward) provides multiple sites at which neural plasticity might act to predict and counteract the excitatory effect of reward on dopamine neurons.

With this in mind, I have studied BSR evoked from the mediodorsal thalamus, a brain region that is not thought to have any direct projections to the ventral midbrain (although it is innervated by dopamine neurons of the ventral tegmental area). One hypothesis was that if electrical stimulation of mediodorsal thalamus has reward value, then it may also activate dopamine neurons. In the one macaque monkey studied, BSR in mediodorsal thalamus activated dopamine neurons with a latency and duration that was very similar to the activation observed with natural reward stimuli (latency of ~70ms, duration of ~150ms) (Fiorillo and Newsome, 2006). The latency indicates that the excitation of dopamine neurons was polysynaptic. The reward value of this BSR (measured in a choice task) was similar to a typical drop of juice (0.1mL), and likewise the increase in firing rate evoked by BSR was similar to that evoked by juice. However, unlike the case of natural reward, the activation by BSR was not diminished once BSR became predictable. Thus, despite the fact that the dopamine response to BSR was very similar in its time course and magnitude to a natural reward response, it was not able to train the circuitry to predict and cancel the activation of dopamine neurons by BSR.

Although the two experiments previously described with BSR are not conclusive, and additional work is needed, they suggest that dopamine may not be critical for learning to predict and cancel the excitation of dopamine neurons by reward stimuli. If dopamine is not critical in learning this aspect of reward prediction, which is so important to the regulation of dopamine neurons themselves, then dopamine may not be critical for learning to predict reward in general. Independent of the experimental evidence previously described, the dopamine error signal does not appear to be appropriate for learning to predict reward, as discussed next.

Dopamine is thought to drive learning by strengthening synapses that are active when dopamine levels are high (through a three-term Hebbian learning rule, in which synaptic plasticity depends on dopamine as well as pre-and post-synaptic activity), and it may also weaken synapses that are active when dopamine levels are suppressed (Reynolds and Wickens, 2002; Izhikevich, 2007). Such a rule reinforces synapses and actions associated with reward, and weakens synapses and actions that are associated with no reward (or aversive outcomes). However, in learning to predict reward value, one should not ignore 'bad news'. Thus, synapses in which activity is associated with either positive or negative reward prediction errors contain useful information and should be strengthened. A prediction error that signals the absolute value of the error would be more appropriate in learning to predict reward value, rather than the error signal of dopamine neurons, in which firing rate is modulated in opposite directions by positive and negative errors.

One possibility is that the increase in dopamine transmission that accompanies positive errors is involved in learning to predict reward value, but the relatively small decrease in dopamine that accompanies negative errors is not involved. Another group of neurons, signalling negative reward prediction errors, would then be needed in order to learn about negative reward predictors. Some neurons are indeed strongly activated by negative reward prediction errors (Matsumoto and Hikosaka, 2007).

Although an appropriate form of reward prediction error could be useful in learning to predict reward, it would be advantageous to have a system that does not depend entirely on reward prediction error in order to learn to predict reward. This is because reward prediction errors can only identify reward predictors that are temporally paired with reward. However, a stimulus event could be useful in predicting reward even though it has never before been paired with reward, as illustrated by the phenomenon of sensory preconditioning. In a sensory preconditioning experiment, two neutral stimuli are paired, such that the animal learns that stimulus A predicts stimulus B. Later, in a second phase of training, the animal learns that stimulus B predicts reward. In a subsequent test, it is found that presentation of stimulus A causes the animal to predict the occurrence of reward (as indicated by the animal's behaviour), despite the fact that stimulus A has never immediately preceded reward. It is clear from such experiments that animals learn the predictive relationship between two neutral stimuli (including the temporal relationship), and use this information to predict reward (reviewed by Arcediano and Miller, 2002). In general, dopamine neurons are only weakly activated by neutral stimuli (depending on their predictability and physical salience; unpublished observations). Thus it appears that neither dopamine nor reward prediction error is necessary for acquiring reward-predictive information. Unfortunately, it is not known whether information acquired through sensory preconditioning is used by dopamine neurons in computing reward prediction error.

It would be advantageous for dopamine neurons to have access to as much relevant information as possible for predicting reward. Recordings of dopamine neurons in behaving animals indicate that dopamine neurons can indeed make use of diverse sorts of information in predicting reward, and the experiments to date are at least consistent with the possibility that dopamine neurons have access to all the relevant information in the brain. In predicting reward, it would be useful to have access to higher-level 'cognitive' information that cannot be acquired through use of reward prediction error signals, as in the case of sensory preconditioning. Thus, in predicting reward, dopamine neurons may access information from a large portion of the brain that is devoted to making predictions in general. In this view, dopamine is not necessary for learning to make predictions in general, nor is it necessary for acquiring all of the information that contributes to the prediction of reward value, even the prediction utilized by dopamine neurons themselves. The experimental evidence described earlier suggests the more extreme possibility that dopamine may in fact not be involved in learning to predict reward at all. Rather, dopamine neurons may simply make use of reward prediction in order to drive reinforcement learning.

Comparison of dopamine and selective attention

It is interesting to compare the dopamine signal with the top-down processes that mediate selective attention in the cortex. Both signals are believed to direct information processing towards behaviourally relevant parts of the world ('future reward'). I have suggested that both dopamine and selective attention may modulate Hebbian plasticity so that a neuron's information (the stimulus that a neuron predicts) is relevant to future reward, or the biological goals of the animal (Fiorillo, 2008). In order for dopamine and selective attention to select relevant information, these signals must themselves be predictive of future reward outcomes (where reward could be good or bad). However, there are several important differences. First, whereas the dopamine signal discriminates good from bad, the attentional signal could be the same whether it is directing attention to appetitive or aversive aspects of the world. Second, the dopamine signal (measured by firing rate in the cell bodies) is global in the sense that the same signal is broadcast throughout much of the brain. Thus it is non-selective, since all target neurons receive the same information. By contrast, selective attention is thought to rely on precise circuitry in which top-down projections specify which low-level neurons should be attended to and which should be ignored. In addition, the two processes are thought to work on different timescales. Attention shapes the information that a neuron receives by waxing and waning over hundreds of milliseconds. Dopamine probably has some 'unconditioned' effects that are equally rapid and transient; but the effects of dopamine in conditioning, as described by reinforcement-learning models, are thought to be slower, with dopamine altering synaptic strengths over multiple pairings of stimuli or actions with reward. These dopamine dependent changes may then last for a very long time in the absence of additional conditioning. For example, Bao et al. (2001) trained rats for several weeks by pairing certain tones with dopamine release (resulting from BSR evoked from the ventral tegmental area). They found that training led to an expanded representation of dopamine-paired tones in primary auditory cortex when tested 24 hours after the last training session. Dopamine and the signals that mediate top-down selective attention therefore appear to exemplify two very different means of ensuring that a neuron's information is behaviourally relevant (or equivalently, predictive of future reward.)

Conclusions

I have described how the plastic regulation of a neuron's non-synaptic ion channels, and particularly potassium channels, could provide a neuron with the ability to learn to make predictions based on prior temporal information (Fiorillo, 2008). The function of these ion channels within the temporal domain would be analogous in many respects to the function of synapses within the spatial domain. Experiments will be needed to test this hypothesis.

My studies of dopamine neurons in an interval-timing task suggest that the temporal uncertainty in reward prediction is high at both the neuronal and behavioural levels, and it is more sensitive to interval duration than to variability in interval duration (Fiorillo et al., 2008). I have suggested the possibility that, in contrast to a proposal of dopamine-based reinforcement learning models, dopamine may not be involved in learning to predict reward (including both its magnitude and timing). In signalling prediction error, dopamine neurons appear to have access to a great diversity of information about reward, but dopamine itself may not be critical to the acquisition of much of that information.

References

Arcediano, F. and Millier, R.R. (2002). Some constraints for models of timing: a temporal coding hypothesis perspective. *Learning and Motivation*, **33**, 105–23.

Attneave, F. (1954). Some informational aspects of visual perception. *Psychological Reviews*, **61**, 183–93.

Bao, S., Chan, V. T., and Merzenich, M. M. (2001). Cortical remodelling induced by activity of ventral tegmental dopamine neurons. *Nature*, **412**, 79–83.

Barlow, H. B. (1961). Possible principles underlying the transformation of sensory messages. In W.A. Rosenblith (Ed.) *Sensory Communication*, pp.217–34. Cambridge, MA: MIT Press.

Barto A. G. (1995). Adaptive Critics and the Basal Ganglia. In J. C. Houk, J. L. Davis, and D. G. Beiser (Eds.) *Models of Information Processing in the Basal Ganglia*, pp.215–232. Cambridge, MA: MIT Press.

Bayer, H. M. and Glimcher, P. W. (2005). Midbrain dopamine neurons encode a quantitative reward prediction error signal. *Neuron*, **47**, 129–41.

Brody, C. D., Hernandez, A., Zanos, A., and Romo, R. (2003). Timing and neural encoding of somatosensory parametric working memory in macaque prefrontal cortex. *Cerebral Cortex*, **13**, 1196–207.

Brown, J., Bullock, D., and Grossberg, S. (1999). How the basal ganglia use parallel excitatory and inhibitory learning pathways to selectively respond to unexpected rewarding cues. *Journal of Neuroscience*, **19**, 10502–11.

Buhusi, C. V. and Meck, W. H. (2005). What makes us tick? Functional and neural mechanisms of interval timing. *Nature Reviews Neuroscience*, **6**, 755–65.

Cheer, J. F., Heien, M. L. A. V., Garris, P. A., Carelli, R. M., and Wightman, R. M. (2005). Simultaneous dopamine and single-unit recordings reveal GABAergic responses: implications for intracranial self-stimulation. *Proceedings of the National Academy of Sciences USA*, **102**, 19150–5.

Contreras-Vidal, J. L. and Schultz, W. (1999). A predictive reinforcement model of dopamine neurons for learning approach behavior. *Journal of Computational Neuroscience*, **6**, 191–214.

Dickinson A (1980). *Contemporary Animal Learning Theory*. Cambridge: Cambridge University Press.

Fiorillo, C. D., Tobler, P. N., and Schultz, W. (2003). Discrete coding of reward probability and uncertainty by dopamine neurons. *Science*, **299**, 1898–902.

Fiorillo, C. D. and Newsome, W. T. (2006). 'Activation of midbrain dopamine neurons by brain stimulation reward in mediodorsal thalamus.' 36th annual meeting of the Society for Neuroscience, Atlanta, October 14–18, 2006.

Fiorillo, C. D., Newsome, W. T. and Schultz, W. (2008). The temporal precision of reward prediction in dopamine neurons. *Nature Neuroscience*, **11**, 966–73.

Fiorillo, C. D. (2008). Towards a general theory of neural computation based on prediction by single neurons. *Public Library of Science ONE*, **3**, e3298.

Ghose, G. M. and Maunsell J. H. R. (2002). Attentional modulation in visual cortex depends on task-timing. *Nature*, **419**, 616–20.

Gibbon, J., Malapani, C., Dale, C. L., and Gallistel C. R. (1997). Toward a neurobiology of temporal cognition: advances and challenges. *Current Opinion in Neurobiology*, **7**, 170–84.

Grossberg, S. and Schmajuk, N.A. (1989). Neural dynamics of adaptive timing and temporal discrimination during associative learning. *Neural Networks*, **2**, 79–102.

Hollerman, J. R. and Schultz, W. (1998). Dopamine neurons report an error in the temporal prediction of reward during learning. *Nature Neuroscience*, **1**, 304–9.

Hosoya, T., Baccus, S. A., and Meister, M. (2005). Dynamic predictive coding by the retina. *Nature*, **436**, 71–7.

Izhikevich, E. M. (2007). Solving the distal reward problem through linkage of STDP and dopamine signaling. *Cerebral Cortex*, **17**, 2443–52.

Janssen, P. and Shadlen, M. N. (2005). A representation of the hazard rate of elapsed time in macaque area LIP. *Nature Neuroscience*, **8**, 234–41.

Jaynes, E. T. (2003). *Probability Theory: The Logic of Science*. Cambridge: Cambridge University Press.

Kobayashi, S. and Schultz, W. (2008). Influence of reward delays on responses of dopamine neurons. *Journal of Neuroscience*, **28**, 7837–46.

Ludvig, E. A., Sutton, R. S., and Kehoe, E. J. (2008). Stimulus representation and the timing of reward-prediction errors in models of the dopamine system. *Neural Computation*, **20**, 3034–54.

Malinow, R. and Malenka, R. C. (2002). AMPA receptor trafficking and synaptic plasticity. *Annual Review of Neuroscience*, **25**, 103–26.

Matell, M. S. and Meck, W. H. (2004). Cortico-striatal circuits and interval timing: coincidence detection of oscillatory processes. *Cognitive Brain Research*, **21**, 139–70.

Matsumoto, M. and Hikosaka, O. (2007). Lateral habenula as a source of negative reward signals in dopamine neurons. *Nature*, **447**, 1111–15.

Morris, G., Arkadir, D., Nevet, A., Vaadia, E., and Bergman, H. (2004). Coincident but distinct messages of midbrain dopamine and striatal tonically active neurons. *Neuron*, **43**, 133–43.

Reynolds, J. N. J. and Wickens, J. R. (2002). Dopamine-dependent plasticity of corticostriatal synapses. *Neural Networks*, **15**, 507–21.

Simoncelli, E. P. and Olshausen, B. A. (2001). Natural image statistics and neural representation. *Annual Review of Neuroscience*, **24**, 1193–216.

Schultz, W., Dayan, P., and Montague, R. R (1997). A neural substrate of prediction and reward. *Science*, **275**, 1593 –9.

Shizgal, P. (1997). Neural basis of utility estimation. *Current Opinion in Neurobiology*, **7**, 198–208.

Srinivasan, M. V. Laughlin, S. B., and Dubs, A. (1982). Predictive coding: a fresh view of inhibition in the retina. *Proceedings of the Royal Society of London B*, **126**, 427–59.

Sutton, R. S. and Barto, A. G. (1981). Toward a modern theory of adaptive networks: expectation and prediction. *Psychological Review*, **88**, 135–170.

Sutton, R. S. and Barto, A. G. (1998). *Reinforcement Learning*. Cambridge MA: MIT Press.

Tobler, P. N., Fiorillo, C. D., and Schultz, W. (2005). Adaptive coding of reward value by dopamine neurons. *Science*, **307**, 1642–5.

Turrigiano, G., Abbott, L. F., and Marder, E. (1994). Activity-dependent changes in the intrinsic membrane properties of cultured neurons. *Science*, **264**, 974–7.

Wise, R. A. (2004). Dopamine, learning and motivation. *Nature Reviews Neuroscience*, **5**, 1–12.

Acknowledgements

This research was supported by WCU (World Class University) programme through the Korea Science and Engineering Foundation funded by the Ministry of Education, Science and Technology (R32-2008-000-10218-0).

Chapter 21

Foreperiod and sequential effects: theory and data

Sander A. Los

An early contribution to the field of temporal attention was Herbert Woodrow's (1914) voluminous monograph titled 'The measurement of attention'. Woodrow provided a comprehensive review of what was known at the time about the behavioural effects of the foreperiod (FP). FP is the interval between the offset of a warning stimulus (S1) and the onset of an imperative stimulus (S2) to which the participant is instructed to respond as quickly as possible. A key characteristic of the design that Woodrow considered was that S1 (typically a brief tone) merely served to signal that S2 was impending, while being uninformative of any other feature of S2, like its location, content, or task requirement. Despite the minimal information conveyed by S1, Woodrow observed that the response time (RT) with respect to S2 was highly dependent on the duration of FP. This led him to propose that attention varies systematically during FP, and that RT is shorter to the extent that the occurrence of S2 coincides with a peak in the participant's attentional state.

Woodrow (1914) also reported several new phenomena from his own experimental work. Among these new phenomena was the sequential effect of FP, which he observed in the variable-FP paradigm, where FP varies randomly across the trials of a block. Although the robustness of this effect has been established across many publications since Woodrow's seminal contribution, its theoretical importance has not been widely appreciated. In this chapter, I will describe the sequential effect of FP and explain why I think it may cast light on some fundamental properties of temporal attention.

Effects of foreperiod: attention or preparation?

Before I consider the typical data patterns observed in the variable-FP paradigm, a comment on terminology is in order. After Woodrow's (1914) contribution, it has gradually become conventional to describe FP effects on RT in terms of non-specific preparation or preparatory set rather than in terms of temporal attention (e.g. Mowrer, 1940; Bertelson, 1967; Niemi and Näätänen, 1981; Los and Schut, 2008). The notion of temporal attention has been preserved in studies relating FP to response accuracy, when the participant is asked to identify a (masked) S2 (e.g. Rolke and Hofmann, 2007) or to estimate its duration (e.g. Grondin and Rammsayer, 2003). It is unclear whether there is a valid rationale for this schism in the literature. For instance, Ivry and Hazeltine (1995) have shown that the variability of performance in a temporal judgement task is similarly related to temporal intervals as the variability of performance in a temporal production task, strongly suggesting a common underlying mechanism.

In view of this state of affairs, I will use the term preparation for no other reason than to agree with the conventional terminology in the RT literature. In particular, I use this term as a placeholder for any mechanism, whether perceptual or action-related, whether intentional or unintentional, that starts prior to the onset of S2 and that contributes to the reduction of RT. Readers more familiar with the attention literature may wish to replace my 'preparation' by 'temporal attention'.

I am aware that preparation becomes a nearly meaningless concept after stretching its meaning in the way I propose here. However, given the rudimentary state of theory in the FP literature, it seems prudent not to confine the meaning of preparation by a set of a priori convictions. As has been the case in the more developed exact sciences, concepts often obtain a well-defined meaning only after they become embedded in a strong unified theory. Similarly, a sensible definition of preparation and its relation to attention may emerge as we gain a better understanding of the mechanisms underlying the key phenomena of the FP literature.

The classical RT–FP function

To illustrate the phenomena that I will focus on, consider one of my pilot studies in which eight participants were instructed to make a speeded choice response (a left or right key press) to a visual S2 (a square appearing left or right from fixation) that was presented after a brief auditory S1 (a 50-ms beep). FP varied randomly across trials, at 0.5, 1.0, 1.5, and 2.0 seconds, according to a uniform distribution. To simplify the exposition of ideas, I will refer to possible moments of S2 occurrence relative to S1 as *critical moments*, and to the actual moment of S2 occurrence on any given trial as the *imperative moment* of that trial. Thus, in the pilot study, there were four critical moments, one of which became the imperative moment on any given trial.

Figure 21.1A shows the classical RT–FP function that I observed, exhibiting the characteristic monotonic reduction of RT as FP increases (see also Wagener and Hoffmann, Chapter 16, this volume). By far the most common explanation of this function is in terms of an increasing conditional probability of S2 occurrence as time elapses during FP (e.g. Woodrow, 1914; Elithorn and Lawrence, 1955; Näätänen, 1970; Luce, 1986; Janssen and Shaldon, 2005; Stuss et al., 2005). In the pilot study, S2 had an equal (0.25) a priori probability of occurring at each critical moment. However, as critical moments are bypassed during FP without the presentation of S2, the conditional probability that S2 will occur at one of the remaining critical moments increases, to reach unity after the penultimate critical moment has been bypassed (since then the last critical moment must be the imperative moment of that trial). On the assumption that the participant's preparatory state develops in keeping with the conditional probability of S2 occurrence, the classical RT–FP function is readily accounted for. This assumption is justified by the belief that participants experience a high state of preparation as being strenuous and difficult to maintain (Näätänen, 1970, 1971; Gottsdanker, 1975; Van der Molen and Jennings, 2005). Therefore, they will engage it only if the probability for the impending presentation of S2 is high.

Results from studies that have manipulated the FP distribution are usually taken as support for this explanation. As the FP distribution becomes more positively skewed (i.e. by increasing the proportion of short FPs in a block of trials), the RT–FP function becomes more shallow, presumably because of an increase of the conditional probability that S2 occurs at an early critical moment (e.g. Zahn and Rosenthal, 1966; Baumeister and Joubert, 1969). Indeed, in the case of an exponential ('non-ageing') FP distribution, when the conditional probability of S2 occurrence is equal for all critical moments, the RT–FP function is usually found to be flat (e.g. Näätänen, 1971; Trillenberg, et al., 2000).[1] These findings are consistent with the notion that preparation is tuned to the changing conditional probability of S2 occurrence over time.

----

[1] It is also possible to fix the conditional probability of S2 occurrence to 1 by presenting each level of FP in a separate ('pure') block of trials. In that case, RT has been found to decrease sharply as FP increases from 0 to about 300ms, and to increase slowly as FP increases further (e.g. Müller-Getmann et al., 2003). The two segments of this function are typically taken to reflect a build-up of preparation and an increase in time uncertainty, respectively. A discussion of these concepts is beyond the scope of this chapter (see Los and Schut, 2008, for a recent contribution).

A relevant question that is usually ignored within this theoretical framework is how partici-pants acquire knowledge of the FP distribution. It is unlikely that task instruction is the answer, because effects of FP and FP distribution have been observed in populations with limited ability of understanding instruction, such as young children (e.g. Elliot, 1970; Vallesi and Shallice, 2007), monkeys (e.g. Janssen and Shadlen, 2005) or rats (Narayanan, et al., 2006). Therefore, it is more likely that participants update their knowledge of the distribution while performing the task, for instance by keeping a running average across a sample of recent trials.

The sequential effect of foreperiod

In spite of its parsimony, the explanation of the classical RT–FP function in terms of the condi-tional probability of S2 occurrence has a fundamental shortcoming: It fails to account for the sequential effect of FP. As it turns out, the data points displayed in Figure 21.1A obscure a hidden but systematic source of variance stemming from the FP that occurred on the preceding trial. To observe this effect, we should categorize the RT observed on any trial $\underline{n}$ according to the FP of both trial n (FP_n) and trial $n - 1$ (FP_{n-1}). Figure 21.1B shows mean RT of the pilot study as a function of FP_n and FP_{n-1}.

A simple summary of this data pattern is that RT is longer to the extent that FP_{n-1} exceeds the duration of FP_n. Or, as Woodrow (1914) put it nearly a century ago: '...the most marked effect of order seems to be that the reaction time to any interval is shortened when preceded by an interval of nearly the same or shorter length, and that it is lengthened when preceded by a considerably longer interval'(p.46). A crucial feature of this sequential effect is its asymmetry. As Figure 21.1B shows, the effect of FP_{n-1} is very strong for the shortest FP_n, becomes gradually less pronounced as FP_n increases, and disappears at the longest FP_n.

Despite its early discovery and proven robustness (for a recent overview, see Steinborn et al., 2008), the sequential effect of FP has been ignored in many publications on variable-FP effects,

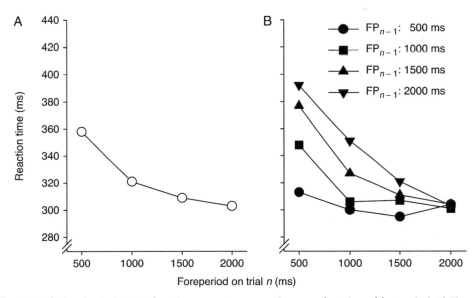

Fig. 21.1 A) The classical RT–FP function: mean response time as a function of foreperiod. B) The asymmetric sequential effect: same data as (A), with the foreperiod on the preceding trial (FP_{n-1}) as additional parameter. Pilot data by the author.

while being treated as a nuisance in others. Occasionally, an explanation has been proposed in peaceful coexistence with an explanation for the classical RT–FP function. However, this practice misinterprets the very nature of variable-FP effects. The point is that the classical RT–FP function and the asymmetric sequential effect are not independent: the stronger the asymmetry of the sequential effect, the steeper the slope of the RT–FP function.[2] Therefore, the asymmetric sequential effect of FP (Figure 21.1B) is the basic data pattern in need for explanation, rather than the classical RT–FP function (Figure 21.1A). Any explanation for this effect also explains the classical RT–FP function, but not vice versa.

Realizing this reveals the problem for the classical account of the RT–FP function in terms of the conditional probability of S2 occurrence: It fails to account for the more fundamental sequential effect of FP. This is particularly so if one assumes that the participant's subjective knowledge of the FP distribution corresponds one-to-one to the objective FP distribution. In that case, RT should be completely independent of FP_{n-1}. If instead one allows that the participant's subjective knowledge of the FP distribution emerges from a running average of a sample of past trials, it is possible to introduce some influence of trial $n - 1$. However, this influence is clearly insufficient to account for the powerful asymmetry of the sequential effect. Let me emphasize: after even a single trial with the shortest FP on trial $n - 1$, the effect of FP on trial n is dwarfed (Figure 21.1B). Therefore, an account based on preparation in keeping with the conditional probability of S2 occurrence, by itself, fails as a general account of FP effects in the variable-FP paradigm. I hasten to add that this conclusion does not necessarily disqualify conditional probability of S2 occurrence as a useful concept. As becomes clear later, it may still be important as a component within a more encompassing theoretical framework.

Accounting for the sequential effect of foreperiod

In the literature, several general ideas have been proposed to account for the sequential effect of FP, but here I will consider only those proposals that have been developed into a consistent, testable mechanism. A discussion and critique of some other ideas can be found in Niemi and Näätänen's (1981) review.

The strategic view

According to the strategic view (e.g. Alegria and Delhaye-Rebaux, 1975; Niemi and Näätänen, 1981; Requin, et al., 1991; see also Vallesi, Chapter 22, this volume), participants aim on each trial n for peak preparation at a specific critical moment. It is assumed that participants initially select the imperative moment of trial $n - 1$ for this purpose. However, if this critical moment is bypassed during FP on trial n without occurrence of S2, a high level of preparation can either be extended over time ('maintaining preparation') or shifted toward a later critical moment ('re-preparation'). As a result, the strategic view predicts relatively slow responding only when the imperative moment occurs earlier than on trial $n - 1$, when S2 catches the participant in an unprepared state. In all other conditions S2 falls within a time window of high preparation, and responding should be relatively fast, consistent with the data pattern of the asymmetric sequential effect (Figure 21.1B).

---

[2] Note that the description of the RT–FP function and the asymmetric pattern of sequential effects is more inclusive than the main effect of FP_n and the $FP_n \times FP_{n-1}$ interaction effect, respectively. Within the General Linear Model, the latter effects are of course independent.

A key feature of this view is the strategic nature of preparation. That is, participants are flexible in selecting a moment for peak preparation, an ability that Nobre and colleagues have called temporal orienting (Coull and Nobre, 1998; Nobre, 2001; Nobre et al., 2007; Correa, Chapter 26; Nobre, Chapter 27; Coull, Chapter 31, this volume). Several studies have shown that participants are capable of temporal orienting when presented with a symbolic cue at the start of the trial that specifies with high or perfect validity which one out of several critical moments will be the imperative moment of that trial. In particular, after a valid temporal cue a strong reduction has been reported for both the slope of the RT–FP function (Zahn, 1970; Mo and Kersey, 1980; Nobre, 2001) and the sequential effect (Los and Van den Heuvel, 2001; Los and Heslenfeld, 2005).

The trace-conditioning view

Trace conditioning is the quintessential theoretical framework of understanding timing processes in animals. It is a variant of classical or operant conditioning defined by a blank interval (the trace) intervening the offset of a conditioned stimulus (CS; e.g. a buzzer) and the onset of an unconditioned stimulus (US; e.g. food). As has been shown in myriads of studies since Pavlov's (1927) groundbreaking work, after only a few presentations of the CS–US pair, an animal reveals a heightened state of preparation (in terms of the conditioned response) as the moment of US presentation draws near (e.g. Machado, 1997; Gallistel and Gibbon, 2000; see also Fiorillo, Chapter 20, this volume). The relevance of this work for present purposes becomes obvious when we replace CS by S1 and US by S2: the trace-conditioning paradigm becomes equivalent to the (variable) FP paradigm.

In contrast with the strategic view, an explanation of the sequential effect of FP in terms of trace conditioning denies that participants aim their preparation at any one critical moment in particular. Instead, preparation is conceived as a time-based function, whose peaks and troughs are shaped by reinforcement and extinction. These processes are assumed to proceed autonomously, provided that S2, in the capacity of a US, has motivational significance. This is the case when the participant adopts an intentional stance to respond quickly to the occurrence of S2 (though regardless of when S2 occurs).

In its simplest form, the trace-conditioning model proposed by Los and colleagues (e.g. Los and Van den Heuvel, 2001; Los and Heslenfeld, 2005; see Bosse et al., 2007 and Los, et al., 2001, for more comprehensive formalized versions) assumes that each critical moment is associated with a conditioned strength. The higher the conditioned strength associated with a critical moment, the shorter RT will be if S2 occurs at that moment. At the same time, the conditioned strength is adjusted during FP on a trial-by-trial basis in accordance with three learning rules. First, the conditioned strength associated with any critical moment decreases as that critical moment is bypassed during FP (extinction). Second, the conditioned strength associated with the imperative moment increases when S2 is presented and responded to (reinforcement). Third, the conditioned strength associated with a critical moment that occurs later than the imperative moment remains unchanged (persistence). The rationale that extinction only applies to critical moments bypassed during FP and not to later critical moments is that the participant, in his or her striving for a fast response to S2, must suppress a disposition to respond during FP. After the response to S2, this suppression is released, thus sparing critical moments beyond the imperative moment from extinction.

To illustrate the dynamics of this model, suppose that at the start of a given trial the conditioned strength associated with each of four critical moments is equal (Figure 21.2A). Also, suppose that on this trial the third critical moment is about to become the imperative moment. As the first two critical moments are bypassed during FP without presentation of S2 their associated conditioned strength decreases (extinction; Figure 21.2B). At the third critical moment, the response to S2 causes an increase of the associated conditioned strength (reinforcement; Figure 21.2C). Finally, the fourth critical moment is neither bypassed during FP nor used for the presentation of S2, so its associated conditioned strength remains unchanged (persistence). The resulting state of conditioning after the trial (Figure 21.2D) will yield the asymmetric sequential effect, because on the next trial responding will be relatively slow when S2 occurs at a critical moment bypassed during FP_{n-1}.

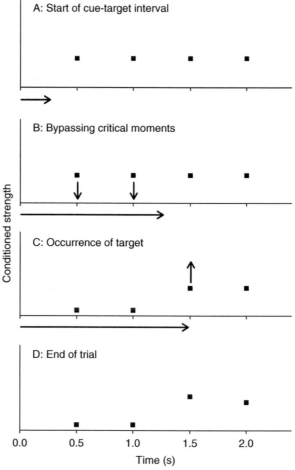

Fig. 21.2 Within-trial dynamics of the trace-conditioning model of the asymmetric sequential effect. Each critical moment (i.e. possible moment of target occurrence) is associated with a conditioned strength. A) Hypothetical equal conditioned strength associated with each of four critical moments at the start of a given trial. B) Upon bypassing a critical moment during the foreperiod, the associated conditioned strength is subject to extinction. C) The conditioned strength associated with the critical moment of target occurrence is reinforced. D) The resulting state of conditioning after the trial, which carries over to the next trial. Adapted from Los, S. A. (2004). Inhibition of return and nonspecific preparation: separable inhibitory control mechanisms in space and time. *Perception & Psychophysics*, **66**, 119–30, with permission from Psychonomic Society Publications.

The dual-process view

According to Vallesi, Shallice, and colleagues (Vallesi and Shallice, 2007; Vallesi et al., 2007a,b; Vallesi, Chapter 22, this volume), the state of preparation at each critical moment is a joint function of two influences: an influence based on the conditional probability of S2 occurrence, which develops during FP on trial n, and 'arousal modulation' stemming from trial $n-1$. The former influence is assumed to be intentional (or strategic) in nature, and it operates as described earlier. That is, during FP on trial n, the preparatory state increases with the conditional probability of S2 occurrence. Arousal modulation is conceived as an automatic consequence of the duration of the preparatory state adopted during trial $n-1$. In particular, the shorter the FP_{n-1}, the greater the participant's level of arousal on trial n, regardless of the duration of FP_n.

An important issue in this dual-process view is how intentional and automatic contributions combine to influence behaviour. Vallesi and Shallice (2007) were not very specific on this point, but they assumed that a strong intentional influence compensates for a low state of preparation due to a long FP_{n-1}. Figure 21.3 provides a simple illustration of this idea. The broken horizontal lines show the predicted RTs as a function of FP_{n-1}, if the state of preparation were fully determined by arousal modulation: the longer the FP_{n-1}, the longer the RT on trial n, regardless of FP_n. The arrows represent the growing influence of the intentional component during FP on trial n, according to the conditional probability of S2 presentation. The symbols represent the predicted joint effect. In particular, if the first critical moment turns out to be the imperative moment on trial n, arousal modulation strongly determines RT in view of the low contribution of the intentional component. During FP, the growing influence of the intentional component increasingly compensates for low arousal, resulting in a decreasing influence of FP_{n-1} on RT. As a result, the asymmetric sequential effect (Figure 21.1B) emerges.

This illustration reveals an important point of the dual-process view. Whereas the sequential effect originates from the automatic component, its asymmetry is caused by the compensating influence of the intentional component.

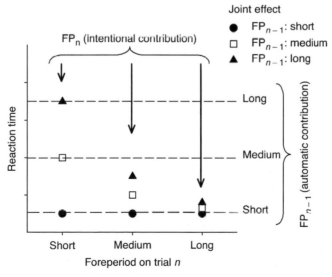

Fig. 21.3 The dual-process view of the asymmetric sequential effect. Performance (symbols) is a joint function of an automatic influence stemming from the foreperiod on trial $n-1$ (broken horizontal lines) and an intentional influence that develops during the foreperiod on trial n (arrows).

Lines of evidence

The ideas outlined in the previous section have motivated some recent studies on the nature of preparation in the variable-FP paradigm. The present section gives a brief overview of this work.

Origin of the sequential effect

According to the strategic view, the sequential effect of FP reflects the strategy of the participant to orient initially to the critical moment that was the imperative moment of the last trial, and re-prepare (or maintain preparation) if necessary. This strategy is suboptimal when FP_n is shorter than FP_{n-1}. In that case, a valid cue concerning the duration of the impending FP should help the participant optimize his or her strategy of temporal orienting. Consistent with this corollary, cue-ing studies have shown that the sequential effect of FP is strongly reduced if participants receive valid information at the start of a trial about the duration of the impending FP (Los and Van den Heuvel, 2001; Los and Heslenfeld, 2005). However, this finding does not falsify a view that attributes the sequential effect to sources other than temporal orienting. It is still possible that the sequential effect originates from conditioning or arousal modulation, but that this contribution is dominated and obscured by temporal orienting when a valid cue informs the participant of the impending imperative moment.

To test this possibility, Los and Heslenfeld (2005) used the contingent negative variation (CNV; Kornhuber and Deeke, 1965) as a covert measure of preparation at critical moments that are bypassed during FP. The CNV is a negative going brain potential during FP, which is generally believed to reflect the participant's state of preparation for S2 (e.g. Rohrbaugh and Gaillard, 1983; Van Boxtel and Brunia, 1994; see also Praamstra, Chapter 24; Pouthas and Pfeuty, Chapter 30, this volume). In conditions without a cue, Los and Heslenfeld observed that, at frontal and central brain sites, the CNV was more negative (higher preparation) throughout FP_n as FP_{n-1} was shorter. Crucially, this sequential effect was barely reduced in a condition in which all trials started with a valid cue. In particular, even on those trials where the participant knew for sure that S2 would occur at the latest critical moment, and therefore most likely abstained from temporal orienting to earlier critical moments, the earlier critical moments still exhibited a covert sequen-tial effect on the CNV. That is, the sequential effect of FP can be observed at an early critical moment when temporal orienting is deflected to a later critical moment, which strongly suggests that the sequential effect has a non-strategic origin (see Los and Van den Heuvel, 2001 for com-plementary behavioural evidence). This challenges the basic premise of the strategic view, whereas it is consistent with the conditioning and dual-process view.

Inhibition

According to the conditioning view, extinction plays a crucial role in the origin of the sequential effect as well as in its asymmetry. A straightforward extension of this view is that extinction is implemented by an inhibitory process that serves to prevent participants from premature responding during FP. This entails the paradoxical hypothesis that maintaining a state of high preparation during FP involves a continuous application of inhibition.

This hypothesis has recently received strong support from animal research focusing on bilateral dorsomedial prefrontal cortex (DMPFC). This region has been associated with several functions, including motor preparation. In one study, Narayanan and colleagues (2006) trained rats to respond quickly to an auditory S2 in the variable-FP paradigm. After training, infusion of the GABA-A agonist muscimol caused bilateral DMPFC inactivation in the experimental condi-tion, whereas saline infusion left DMPFC unaffected in the control condition. The results showed that rats responded prematurely, during the FP, more frequently in the experimental condition.

Also, in the control condition, the distribution of premature responses peaked in the vicinity of the imperative moment, whereas in the experimental condition it was relatively diffuse across FP. These findings are readily explained by assuming that, when inactivated by muscimol, DMPFC ceases to inhibit the response system during FP, which leads to responding at inappropriate moments (see Narayanan and Laubach, 2006, for converging evidence).

Whereas inhibitory control during FP seems firmly established by these findings, its role as the driving force behind the sequential effect remains to be demonstrated. One additional finding by Narayanan and colleagues (2006) is interesting in this respect. They observed that for regular responses to S2, the RT–FP function was flatter in the experimental condition (DMPFC inactivation) than in the control condition. They explained this finding by assuming that the response system is kept under inhibition until an internally set deadline approaches. This mechanism would impede responding especially on trials with short FPs (well before reaching the deadline) in the control condition (where inhibition functions normally). The alternative explanation suggested by the conditioning model attributes this finding to inhibition on the preceding trial. In particular, the inhibition (extinction) exerted in bypassing early critical moments during a long FP_{n-1} is weaker in the experimental condition than in the control condition, which ultimately leads to a flatter average RT–FP function. To test this hypothesis, future research may examine whether DMPFC inactivation reduces the sequential effect.

Demonstrating a key role for inhibition in the origin of the sequential effect would clearly be consistent with the premises of the conditioning view, while being difficult to accommodate by the strategic view. The implications for the dual-process view would be less clear. As it stands, a connection between arousal modulation and inhibition does not make sense intuitively. However, by casting the automatic component in terms of inhibition, it should be possible to revise the dual-process view without affecting its fundamental dual-process assumption.

Foreperiod-distribution effects

In my first outline of the trace-conditioning model (Los, 1996, p.178 ff), I envisaged a broad division between phenomena driven by subjective strategy (temporal orienting) and those driven by conditioning. I conjectured that conditioning was the fundamental mechanism explaining FP phenomena in absence of a temporal cue, while temporal orienting would come into play in designs that involved a temporal cue.

A corollary of this division is that the highly robust effect of FP distribution on the RT–FP function reflects conditioning rather than temporal orienting. Recall that the RT–FP function becomes flatter as the FP distribution becomes more positively skewed, which suggests a key role for temporal orienting guided by the conditional probability of S2 occurrence. However, this finding can also be explained in terms of conditioning, because changing the FP distribution necessarily involves changing the ratio of specific intertrial transitions of FPs. In particular, as the distribution becomes more positively skewed, early critical moments are increasingly more often repeated and less often bypassed during FP. According to the trace-conditioning model, this implies that the conditioned strength associated with early critical moments receives more reinforcement and less extinction, which ultimately will lead to a flatter average RT–FP function.

A similar ambiguity applies to the finding that the inclusion of catch trials (i.e. trials without S2) in the variable-FP paradigm increases RT most strongly for the longest FP (Drazin, 1961; Correa, et al., 2004, 2005; Los, 2004; Los and Agter, 2005). One explanation of this finding is that an increase in the proportion of catch trials most tangibly reduces the conditional probability of S2 occurrence at the latest critical moment, which may discourage temporal orienting at the latest critical moment. Alternatively, one may conceive of a catch trial as a trial with a very long FP, extending beyond the latest critical moment. Then, according to the trace-conditioning model, the conditioned strength associated with the latest critical moment is subject to extinction when this moment is bypassed during FP on a catch trial. Therefore, RT for the longest FP should be longer after a catch trial than after any other FP_{n-1}—a prediction that has been confirmed (Correa et al., 2004; Los, 2004; Los and Agter, 2005).

To disentangle possible influences of temporal orienting and conditioning, Los and Agter (2005) devised a procedure that allowed them to compare the RT–FP functions of different FP distributions uncontaminated by the differential contribution of specific intertrial transitions of FP (see also Drazin, 1961; Zahn and Rosenthal, 1966; Baumeister and Joubert, 1969; Alegria and Delhaye-Rembaux, 1975; Possamaï, et al., 1975). This procedure involved reweighting mean RT for each specific intertrial transition of FPs observed under one RT distribution (e.g. uniform) in accordance with the probability of occurrence of that transition under another RT distribution (e.g. exponential). If the effect of RT distribution solely reflects a changing ratio of specific inter-trial transitions, the RT–FP functions of two different distributions should become identical after reweighting.

When applying this procedure to each pair of three different FP-distributions (uniform, exponential, and peaked), Los and Agter estimated that at most 30% of the effect of RT distribution could be attributed to the sequential effect of FP. This finding clearly shows that distribution effects cannot be explained by the principles of conditioning alone. Los and Agter (2005) proposed that when the FP distribution deviates from uniform, temporal orienting is invoked as an additional process and tuned to the most frequent imperative moment of the distribution, thereby compensating possible negative consequences of conditioning. This view implies that a pure manifestation of the influence of conditioning is limited to the uniform FP distribution.

Process dissociations

With the introduction of the dual-process view, Vallesi and Shallice (2007; see also Vallesi et al., 2007a,b) challenged the trace-conditioning view even under a uniform FP distribution. According to the dual-process view, the asymmetric sequential effect always reflects the influence of two contributions: automatic arousal modulation, causing the sequential effect, and intentional preparation based on the conditional probability of S2 occurrence, causing the asymmetry of the sequential effect.

The dual-process view makes the principled prediction that the sequential effect should become symmetric after elimination of its intentional component. In particular, because of the cessation of a compensatory intentional influence, all FP_ns should come to reveal a sequential effect of the same magnitude as that of the shortest FP_n (cf. the horizontal lines in Figure 21.3). By contrast, according to the conditioning view, the sequential effect should always be asymmetric. This is because the extinction process applies only to critical moments bypassed during FP and not to critical moments beyond the imperative moment. If the extinction process is eliminated, the sequential effect should disappear altogether (assuming that reinforcement drives the conditioned strength associated with each critical moment to ceiling).

The empirical program of Vallesi, Shallice and colleagues (Stuss et al., 2005; Vallesi and Shallice, 2007; Vallesi et al., 2007a,b; Vallesi, Chapter 22, this volume) hinges on the assumption that intentional preparation based on the conditional probability of S2 occurrence is driven by the right dorsolateral prefrontal cortex (rDLPFC) (see also Coull, Chapter 31, this volume). Therefore, reducing rDLPFC functioning during FP should lead to a flatter RT–FP function and more symmetrical sequential effects. Reasoning that the prefrontal cortex matures relatively late during childhood, Vallesi and Shallice (2007) tested these predictions by comparing children of various age groups in the variable-FP paradigm. They observed that across the age range of 4–11 years, responding became considerably faster, and the RT–FP function gradually steeper. Crucially, the sizable sequential effect was symmetric for the youngest age group (4–5 years) and became gradually more asymmetric across subsequent age groups (but see Elliot, 1970, for a deviant finding). This finding is consistent with the dual-process view, but not with the conditioning view.

In another study, Vallesi, Shallice, and Walsh (2007b) manipulated rDLPFC integrity experimentally. They compared FP effects before and after a 20-minute session during which the application of transcranial magnetic stimulation (TMS) temporarily reduced normal functioning of rDLPFC. As compared to the pre-TMS control, they observed a flatter RT–FP function as well as a more symmetrical sequential effect after TMS application to rDLPFC (though not after TMS application to left DLPFC). Vallesi and colleagues took these findings as evidence for the dual-process view and against the conditioning view. Yet, on close examination, their findings do not fully agree with the pattern predicted by the dual-process view. The flattening of the RT–FP function involved not only an increase of the RT at the longest FP, but at least as much a decrease of RT at the shortest FP. In addition, TMS application caused at least as much a reduction of the sequential effect for the shortest FP, as an increase of the sequential effect for the longest FP. These findings suggest decreased extinction during FP, consistent with the conditioning view.

Capitalizing on this idea, Van Lambalgen and Los (2008) suggested that rDLPFC may fulfil an inhibitory function during FP, similar to DMPFC discussed earlier (Narayanan, et al., 2006). To test this idea, Van Lambalgen and Los used a dual task, in which participants saw a central stream of visual digits (one per 800ms) while they were performing a two-choice RT task in the variable-FP paradigm. In the experimental condition, participants were instructed to count the number of digit repetitions in the stream (i.e. a 1-back task) in addition to performing the RT task; in the control condition, they were instructed to ignore the digits. A 1-back task is a loading task, which makes a high demand on DLPFC functioning (Jonides et al., 1997; Mitchell, et al., 2002). Therefore, according to the dual-process view, it should influence the RT–FP function via the intentional component. In particular, it should flatten the RT–FP function and boost the sequential effect for the longer FPs. By contrast, according to the conditioning view, the 1-back task may influence the RT–FP function via extinction. If so, it should flatten the RT–FP function by shrinking the sequential effect for the shortest FPs.

The results showed that, while a concurrent 1-back task strongly increased RT in the variable-FP paradigm, it did not influence the slope of the RT–FP function. Furthermore, while it did somewhat reduce the sequential effect of FP, it left its asymmetry unaffected. That is, the sequential effect was neither boosted for the long FPs, as predicted by the dual-process view, nor shrunk for the short FPs, as predicted by the conditioning view. Yet, the fact that the sequential effect was sensitive to memory load while the slope of the RT–FP function was not, seems to pose a greater challenge to the dual-process view.

Conclusions

The simplicity of the classical RT–FP function is deceptive. It conceals a highly robust source of variance embodied by the asymmetric sequential effect of FP, which solicits an explanation within a learning-theoretical context. Recent studies have started to cast some light on the processes underlying the sequential effect. Of the views considered here, the strategic view seems to fare least well, whereas both the trace-conditioning view and the dual-process view provide good starting points for future research.

One way to distinguish between the latter views is to collect more data on the relation between the classical RT–FP function and the asymmetric sequential effect. Demonstrations of dissociations between these effects, similar to those reported by Vallesi and Shallice (2007), would further challenge the conditioning view. To enhance the bearing of such findings for the dual-process view, it will be important to specify the combination rule by which the postulated intentional and automatic processes contribute to preparation. Another issue worth exploring is the role of inhibition in the origin and asymmetry of the sequential effect. Confirming this role would further establish the connection between trace conditioning and preparation. Finally, I think it is pertinent to come to a more comprehensive assessment of the popular idea that preparation grows as the conditional probability of S2 occurrence increases. As I have emphasized in this chapter, this assessment should not occur without consideration of the sequential effect of FP.

References

Alegria, J. and Delhaye-Rembaux, M. (1975). Sequential effects of foreperiod duration and conditional probability of the signal in a choice reaction time task. *Acta Psychologica*, **39**, 321–8.

Baumeister, A. and Joubert, C. (1969). Interactive effects on reaction time of preparatory interval length and preparatory interval frequency. *Journal of Experimental Psychology*, **82**, 393–5.

Bertelson, P. (1967). The time course of preparation. *Quarterly Journal of Experimental Psychology*, **19**, 272–9.

Bosse, T., Jonker, C. M., Los, S. A., Torre, L. V. D., and Treur, J. (2007). Formal analysis of trace conditioning. *Cognitive Systems Research*, **8**, 36–47.

Correa, A., Lupiáñez, J., Milliken, B., and Tudela, P. (2004). Endogenous temporal orienting of attention in detection and discrimination tasks. *Perception & Psychophysics*, **66**, 264–78.

Correa, A., Lupiáñez, J., and Tudela, P. (2005). Attentional preparation based on temporal expectancy modulates processing at the perceptual level. *Psychonomic Bulletin & Review*, **12**, 328–34.

Coull, J. T. and Nobre, A. C. (1998). Where and when to pay attention: The neural systems for directing attention to spatial locations and to time intervals as revealed by both PET and fMRI. *Journal of Neuroscience*, **18**, 7426–35.

Drazin, D. (1961). Effects of foreperiod, foreperiod variability and probability of stimulus occurrence on simple reaction time. *Journal of Experimental Psychology*, **62**, 43–50.

Elithorn, A. and Lawrence, C. (1955). Central inhibition – some refractory observations. *Quarterly Journal of Experimental Psychology*, **7**, 116–27.

Elliott, R. (1970). Simple reaction time: effects associated with age, preparatory interval, incentive-shift, and mode of presentation. *Journal of Experimental Child Psychology*, **9**, 86–107.

Gallistel, C. R. and Gibbon, J. (2000). Time, rate and conditioning. *Psychological Review*, **107**, 289–344.

Gottsdanker, R. (1975). The attaining and maintaining of preparation. In Rabbitt, P. M. A. and Dornic, S. (Eds.) *Attention and Performance V*. London, Academic Press.

Grondin, S. and Rammsayer, T. H. (2003). Variable foreperiods and temporal discrimination. *Quarterly Journal of Experimental Psychology*, **56A**, 731–65.

Ivry, R. B. and Hazeltine, R. E. (1995). Perception and production of temporal intervals across a range of durations: evidence for a common timing mechanism. *Journal of Experimental Psychology: Human Perception and Peformance*, **21**, 3–18.

Janssen, P. and Shaldon, M. N. (2005). A representation of the hazard rate of elapsed time in macaque area LIP. *Nature Neuroscience*, **8**, 234–41.

Jennings, J. R. and Van Der Molen, M. W. (2005). Preparation for speeded action as a psychophysiological concept. *Psychological Bulletin*, **131**, 434–59.

Jonides, J., Schumacher, E. H., Smith, E. E., Lauber, E. J., Awh, E., Minoshima, S., and Koeppe, R. A. (1997). Verbal working memory load affects regional brain activation as measured by PET. *Journal of Cognitive Neuroscience*, **9**, 462–75.

Los, S. A. (1996). On the origin of mixing costs: Exploring information processing in pure and mixed blocks of trials. *Acta Psychologica*, **94**, 145–188.

Los, S. A. (2004). Inhibition of return and nonspecific preparation: separable inhibitory control mechanisms in space and time. *Perception & Psychophysics*, **66**, 119–30.

Los, S. A. and Agter, F. (2005). Reweighting sequential effects across different distributions of foreperiods: Segregating elementary contributions to nonspecific preparation. *Perception & Psychophysics*, **67**, 1161–70.

Los, S. A. and Heslenfeld, D. J. (2005). Intentional and unintentional contributions to nonspecific preparation: Electrophysiological evidence. *Journal of Experimental Psychology: General*, **134**, 52–72.

Los, S. A., Knol, D. L., and Boers, R. M. (2001). The foreperiod effect revisited: Conditioning as a basis for nonspecific preparation. *Acta Psychologica*, **106**, 121–45.

Los, S. A. and Schut, M. L. J. (2008). The effective time course of preparation. *Cognitive Psychology*, **57**, 20–55.

Los, S. A. and Van Den Heuvel, C. E. (2001). Intentional and unintentional contributions to nonspecific preparation during reaction time foreperiods. *Journal of Experimental Psychology: Human Perception and Performance*, **27**, 370–86.

Luce, R. D. (1986). *Response Times*. New York, Oxford University Press.

Machado, A. (1997). Learning the temporal dynamics of behavior. *Psychological Review*, **104**, 241–65.

Mitchell, J. P., Macrae, C. N., and Gilchrist, I. D. (2002). Working memory and the suppression of reflexive saccades. *Journal of Cognitive Neuroscience*, **14**, 95–103.

Mo, S. S. and Kersey, R. (1980). Foreperiod effects on time estimation and simple reaction time in schizophrenia. *Journal of Clinical Psychology*, **36**, 94–9.

Mowrer, O. H. (1940). Preparatory set (expectancy): some methods of measurement. *Psychological Monographs*, **52**.

Müller-Gethmann, H., Ulrich, R., and Rinkenauer, G. (2003). Locus of the effect of temporal preparation: evidence from the lateralized readiness potential. *Psychophysiology*, **40**, 597–611.

Näätänen, R. (1970). The diminishing time-uncertainty with the lapse of time after the warning signal in reaction-time experiments with varying fore-periods. *Acta Psychologica*, **34**, 399–419.

Näätänen, R. (1971). Nonaging foreperiod and simple reaction time. *Acta Psychologica*, **35**, 316–27.

Narayanan, N. S. and Laubach, M. (2006). Top-down control of motor cortex ensembles by dorsomedial prefrontal cortex. *Neuron*, **52**, 921–31.

Narayanan, N. S., Horst, N. K., and Laubach, M. (2006). Reversible inactivations of rat medial prefrontal cortex impair the ability to wait for a stimulus. *Neuroscience*, **139**, 865–76.

Niemi, P. and Näätänen, R. (1981). Foreperiod and simple reaction time. *Psychological Bulletin*, **89**, 133–62.

Nobre, A. C. (2001). Orienting attention to instants in time. *Neuropsychologia*, **39**, 1317–28.

Nobre, A. C., Correa, A., and Coull, J. T. (2007). The hazards of time. *Current Opinion in Neurobiology*, **17**, 465–70.

Pavlov, I. P. (1927). *Conditioned Reflexes*. London: Oxford University Press.

Possamaï, C. A., Granjon, M., Reynard, G., and Requin, J. (1975). High order sequential effects and the negative gradient of the relationship between simple reaction time and foreperiod duration. *Acta Psychologica*, **39**, 263–70.

Requin, J., Brener, J., and Ring, C. (1991). Preparation for action. In Jennings, J. R. and Coles, M. G. H. (Eds.) *Handbook of Cognitive Psychophysiology: Central and Automatic Nervous System Approaches*. New York: Wiley.

Rohrbaugh, J. W. and Gaillard, A. W. K. (1983). Sensory and motor aspects of the contingent negative variation. In Gaillard, A. W. K. and Ritter, W. (Eds.) *Tutorials in ERP Research: Endogenous Components*. Amsterdam: North-Holland.

Rolke, B. and Hofmann, P. (2007). Temporal uncertainty degrades perceptual processing. *Psychonomic Bulletin & Review*, **14**, 522–6.

Steinborn, M. B., Rolke, B., Bratzke, D., and Ulrich, R. (2008). Sequential effects within a short foreperiod context: Evidence for the conditioning account of temporal preparation. *Acta Psychologica*, **129**, 297–307.

Stuss, D. T., Alexander, M. P., Shallice, T., Picton, T. W., Binns, M. A., MacDonald, R., et al. (2005). Multiple frontal systems controlling response speed. *Neuropsychologia*, **43**, 396–417.

Trillenberg, P., Verleger, R., Wascher, E., Wauschkuhn, B., and Wessel, K. (2000). CNV and temporal uncertainty with 'ageing ' and 'nonageing' S1-S2 intervals. *Clinical Neurophysiology*, **111**, 1216–26.

Vallesi, A. and Shallice, T. (2007). Developmental dissociations of preparation over time: deconstructing the variable foreperiod phenomena. *Journal of Experimental Psychology: Human Perception and Performance*, 33, 1377–88.

Vallesi, A., Mussoni, A., Mondani, M., Budai, R., Skrap, M., and Shallice, T. (2007a). The neural basis of temporal preparation: Insights from brain tumor patients. *Neuropsychologia*, **45**, 2755–63.

Vallesi, A., Shallice, T. and Walsh, V. (2007b). Role of the prefrontal cortex in the foreperiod effect: TMS evidence for dual mechanisms in temporal preparation. *Cerebral Cortex*, **17**, 466–74.

Van Boxtel, G. J. M. and Brunia, C. H. M. (1994). Motor and non-motor aspects of slow brain potentials. *Biological Psychology*, **38**, 37–51.

Van Lambalgen, R. M., and Los, S. A. (2008). The role of attention in nonspecific preparation. In B. C. Love, K. McRae, and V. M. Sloutsky (Eds.), *Proceedings of the 30th Annual Conference of the Cognitive Science Society*. Austin, TX: Cognitive Science Society, 1525–30.

Woodrow, H. (1914). The measurement of attention. *Psychological Monographs*, **17**, 1–158.

Zahn, T. P. (1970). Effects of reductions in uncertainty on reaction time in schizophrenic and normal subjects. *Journal of Experimental Research in Personality*, **4**, 135–43.

Zahn, T. P. and Rosenthal, D. (1966). simple reaction time as a function of the relative frequency of the preparatory interval. *Journal of Experimental Psychology*, **72**, 15–19.

Acknowledgement

I would like to thank Chris Olivers for helpful comments on an earlier draft of this article.

Chapter 22

Neuroanatomical substrates of foreperiod effects

Antonino Vallesi

Preparation usually implies the ability to anticipate future events by reducing uncertainty about them. Preparation over time, in particular, involves reduction of uncertainty about 'when' (rather than what or where) an event will occur (Requin et al., 1991). The need for this capacity is ubiquitous in everyday life. For example, temporal preparation plays an important role in music (e.g. resuming play after a pause), in driving (e.g. waiting for the traffic light to turn green), or in sport, when athletes have to anticipate the timing of critical events, such as the start signal in a 100-meter sprint or the penalty kick in football.

Temporal preparation can be achieved explicitly or implicitly. Explicit mechanisms of temporal preparation are required, for example, when an external precue announces the timing of the next critical event. Many studies have demonstrated that attention can be effectively oriented to a certain point in time under these conditions (e.g. Coull and Nobre, 1998; Nobre, 2001). In contrast, implicit temporal preparation occurs when individuals prepare to perform a task without advance information about how much time will elapse before they have to execute the task. Yet, time has a dramatic effect on behaviour in these situations, suggesting that temporal information also affects cognitive processing when it is not task-relevant.

Although implicit temporal preparation has been studied by cognitive psychologists for a long time (Woodrow, 1914), consensus has not yet been achieved regarding the cognitive processes involved. Moreover, the neural bases of these phenomena have only recently begun to be investigated. In this chapter, behavioural effects of implicit temporal preparation and the hypothetical cognitive processes underlying these effects will be briefly introduced. Recent studies of the neuroanatomical substrates of temporal preparation will be then selectively reviewed and their impact on cognitive theories will be discussed.

The foreperiod phenomena

Experimentally, implicit temporal preparation has been extensively investigated in studies using the foreperiod paradigm (Woodrow, 1914). In this paradigm, the foreperiod is the time gap between a non-informative warning stimulus and a target stimulus that requires a response. If the foreperiod is kept constant across trials in a block, responses to the target are typically faster for short intervals than for long ones (fixed-foreperiod effect; e.g. Mattes and Ulrich, 1997).

However, behavioural effects change radically if the foreperiod is varied from trial to trial rather than between blocks. In the classic variable-foreperiod paradigm, a range of different foreperiods randomly occurs across trials, each foreperiod having the same a priori probability. Participants are instructed to respond to the target as quickly as possible. A typical finding in this paradigm is that responses are slower after short foreperiods than after long ones, a pattern that is referred to as the variable- foreperiod effect (see Niemi and Näätänen, 1981, for a review). A second phenomenon concerns sequential effects: for a given foreperiod on the current trial, subjects are slower when a longer foreperiod, rather than when an equal or shorter foreperiod, occurred on the preceding trial (Karlin, 1959). Sequential effects are strongest on trials with shortest foreperiods (Los, Chapter 21, this volume).

The foreperiod phenomena are extremely robust. They have been replicated for different foreperiod averages and ranges, at least within certain upper and lower boundaries (Niemi and Näätänen, 1981), using both simple and choice response-time (RT) tasks (Karlin, 1959; Bertelson and Boons, 1960), with warning stimuli presented in different modalities (Los and van den Heuvel 2001; Vallesi et al., 2007a), and even without warnings (Stuss et al., 2005). However, despite the robustness of the behavioural effects, there is so far no agreement about the underlying cognitive processes and neural mechanisms.

Cognitive accounts of foreperiod effects

Increased temporal uncertainty and reduced accuracy in time estimation with long time intervals (Gibbon et al., 1984) have been frequently used to explain slowed responding in fixed-foreperiod tasks with long foreperiods (e.g. Gottsdanker 1970; Requin et al., 1991). In turn, better time estimation and better motor tuning mechanisms for short time ranges (e.g. Hasbroucq et al., 1997; see later) have been suggested to explain the RT advantage for relatively short fixed foreperiods.

Different kinds of explanations have been proposed for the variable-foreperiod effect, that is shorter RTs for longer foreperiods when foreperiods vary from trial to trial. Traditionally, this effect has been attributed to strategic processes (Niemi and Näätänen, 1981). In variable-foreperiod paradigms, the passage of time provides information about when the next stimulus will occur even when the a priori probability of stimulus presentation is equal across the various foreperiods (Elithorn and Lawrence, 1955). Indeed, as time passes during a given foreperiod without the target stimulus occurring, the conditional probability of its occurrence increases in the next possible foreperiod. The cognitive system presumably learns this changing conditional probability early in the experimental session and exploits it to increase response preparation (e.g. Näätänen, 1970). However, this account does not explain sequential effects (e.g. Karlin, 1959).

More recently, Los and colleagues (Los et al., 2001; Los and van den Heuvel 2001; Los, Chapter 21, this volume) proposed an alternative account based on conditioning mechanisms. This model explains both the foreperiod and sequential effects within a single theoretical model. According to this model, the occurrence of a given foreperiod reinforces the strength of preparation associated with this foreperiod, so that if it occurs again, participants' readiness to respond will be enhanced. Moreover, on any trial, the preparation strength for a foreperiod is extinguished if a longer foreperiod occurs. The rationale for this assumption is that during shorter foreperiods it is necessary to prevent premature responding when short foreperiods pass without the target being presented. Withholding a response is effortful and aversive (Näätänen, 1971) and therefore provokes extinction. Moreover, the longest foreperiods benefit from reinforcement without ever being extinguished because foreperiods that are even longer cannot occur. It follows that the conditioned strength of preparation for the longest foreperiods can never decrease. The model thus explains the asymmetric sequential effects for short and long foreperiods. According to this single-process view, the foreperiod effect is a direct consequence of sequential effects, because the response speed on a given trial is a function of the conditioning influences produced on previous trials.

Los and van den Heuvel (2001) also provided evidence against alternative strategic accounts of sequential effects (cf. Karlin 1959). In this study, a temporal cue at the beginning of each trial indicated which foreperiod would occur. Timing information provided by the cue could be valid, neutral or invalid. Subjects were able to prepare efficiently during validly cued foreperiods, as indicated by faster responses after valid cues than after invalid ones. Importantly, pronounced sequential effects were observed for infrequent invalid temporal cues, when strategic attention to foreperiod sequences was unlikely to occur because attention was diverted to invalidly cued foreperiods. This work demonstrates a dissociation between intentional processes (cue-related effects) and unintentional ones (sequential effects) in temporal preparation (see also Correa et al., 2006b).

In the absence of explicit temporal cues that enable intentional preparation, the single-process model (Los et al., 2001) would posit that conditioning processes alone can explain foreperiod and sequential effects. This leads to the prediction that the neural substrates of foreperiod and sequential effects should overlap because both effects are manifestations of the same core mechanism. However, to presage the following discussion, recent empirical evidence seems to support a more nuanced account.

Neural substrates of the fixed-foreperiod effect

Besides a better time estimation for shorter time ranges (Gibbon et al., 1984), motor mechanisms have also been used to explain the RT advantage for short foreperiods in fixed-foreperiod paradigms. Transcranial magnetic stimulation (TMS; see Box 22.1) has been used to examine these putative motor mechanisms. TMS can be applied to the motor cortex to assess corticospinal excitability by recording motor-evoked potentials (MEP) in peripheral nerves of the responding hand. Corticospinal excitability has been reported to decrease gradually with increasing temporal proximity to the target, resulting in reduced MEP amplitude (Hasbroucq et al., 1999; Burle et al., Chapter 18, this volume). This effect is generally interpreted as resulting from peripheral inhibition, an adaptive mechanism that enhances the sensitivity of the motoneurons responding to supraspinal commands during preparation (Requin et al., 1991). Importantly, the decrease in MEP amplitude has been observed during a fixed foreperiod of 500ms but not during a longer foreperiod of 2500ms (Hasbroucq et al., 1997).

Another index of preparation is the contingent negative variation (CNV), a slow negative-going event-related potential (ERP; see Box 22.1) that increases during the foreperiod (Walter et al., 1964). Source analysis has suggested that the generators of CNV are more spread out across the cortex than the mechanism involved in the generation of MEPs, and possibly include, besides the motor cortex, other associative areas like for instance pre-supplementary and supplementary motor areas (e.g. Hamano et al., 1997; Nobre, 2001). A testable hypothesis would be that, during temporal preparation, the neural circuitry generating the CNV sends inhibitory projections to motoneurons in the primary motor cortex in order to hold the motor system in check (Hasbroucq et al., 1999). This mechanism seems to be more effective for short time intervals.

In a recent neuropsychological (see Box 22.1) study, Stuss and colleagues (2005) tested patients with brain lesions, divided into four subgroups according to which prefrontal region was affected by the lesion: right lateral, left lateral, superior medial, and inferior medial. Patients performed fixed- and variable-foreperiod tasks. In the fixed-foreperiod task, a visual warning signal occurred either 1 or 3 seconds prior to the target, constantly in each block. Participants were required to perform a shape discrimination task on the target. All four patient groups and controls showed the fixed-foreperiod effect, that is, slower responses for longer foreperiods. However, patients with lesions in superior medial prefrontal regions showed exaggerated response slowing

---

Box 22.1 Cognitive neuroscience methodologies

Transcranial magnetic stimulation (TMS) is a technique that transitorily perturbs the ongoing processing of a small cortical area by inducing, through a stimulation coil, a magnetic field that penetrates the scalp. A single pulse has a short-lived effect (a few milliseconds), and can be used to understand 'when' a brain area is essential for behaviour. With frequent repetitive TMS pulses, the interfering effects can last several minutes after stimulation.

Event-related potentials (ERP) are scalp voltage fluctuations resulting from the electrical activity of cortical neural populations involved in the processing of sensory, cognitive or motor events. Given their high temporal resolution, ERPs are useful for tracking ongoing cognitive processes.

Neuropsychology is the study of cognitive processes in patients with discrete brain lesions. A main assumption of neuropsychology is that if a brain area is critical for the processes underlying a given behavioural effect, a lesion to that area will impair that behavioural effect.

Functional magnetic resonance imaging (fMRI) measures changes in blood oxygenation over time. Since neural activity in a brain area requires consumption of glucose and oxygen carried in the blood, it yields an increase in local blood flow. However, the increase in blood flow exceeds oxygen extraction, thus resulting in a local increase in blood oxygenation levels. Therefore, fMRI is useful for inferring the localization of brain activity associated with different cognitive processes. Block and event-related fMRI designs allow measurement of brain activity involved in tasks performed over a relatively long time-period (half a minute or more), or in a single-event trial, respectively. To isolate areas involved in the process of interest, a subtraction (*contrast*) may be performed between brain activity in two tasks, one of which supposedly involves all the processes involved in the other task plus the process of interest.

---

for longer foreperiods. These results were interpreted in terms of an energization deficit (Stuss et al., 1995), a time-dependent decline in the ability to energize the neural systems involved in response preparation.

Neural substrates of the variable-foreperiod effect

The role of right lateral prefrontal cortex: neuropsychological and TMS evidence

The study by Stuss and colleagues (2005) also investigated effects of frontal lesions on the variable-foreperiod effect. Subjects performed simple and choice RT tasks in which the target stimulus appeared randomly after one of five foreperiods (range: 3–7 seconds). Only patients with lesions in right lateral prefrontal cortex failed to show the typical variable-foreperiod effect of shorter RTs for longer foreperiods, suggesting a deficit in monitoring the conditional probability of stimulus occurrence (Elithorn and Lawrence, 1955). However, sequential effects were not analysed in that study.

The investigation of the anatomical bases of the foreperiod phenomena continued with a subsequent study (Vallesi et al., 2007b). One goal of this study was to test whether the neuropsychological results (Stuss et al., 2005) could be reproduced in healthy adults by means of transient inhibition of the right dorsolateral prefrontal cortex (DLPFC) with TMS (see Box 22.1; Figure 22.1A). The left DLPFC was also inhibited as a control site, since lesions in this area had no influence on the foreperiod effect (Stuss et al., 2005). The study also assessed the role of the right

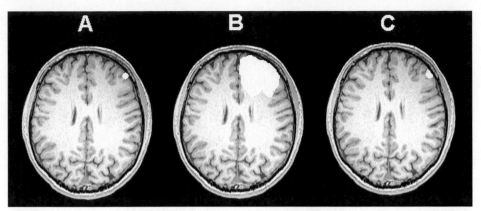

Fig. 22.1 (See also Plate 6) Approximate locations (in white) of the right lateral prefrontal region involved in the variable-foreperiod effect in three different studies. A) The right dorsolateral prefrontal area stimulated by TMS in Vallesi et al. 2007b (coordinates were taken from the fMRI study by Lewis and Miall, 2003); B) Pre-surgical tumour location in the group of right lateral prefrontal patients tested in Vallesi et al. 2007a; C) Cluster in the right dorsolateral prefrontal cortex activated in the variable versus fixed foreperiod contrast in the fMRI study by Vallesi et al. (2009). To allow comparison across studies, the regions are superimposed to the same axial slice (MNI z: 26) of an individual subject's standardized brain.

angular gyrus (AG), an area often associated with temporal processing (Lewis and Miall, 2003; Harrington et al., 1998; Janssen and Shadlen, 2005). Besides the variable-foreperiod effect, sequential effects were also investigated. The rationale was that, if a common mechanism underlies both foreperiod and sequential effects (e.g. Los et al., 2001), TMS on right DLPFC should affect these two measures simultaneously. By contrast, if different processes are involved in these two effects, TMS on this area should modulate the foreperiod effect but not necessarily the sequential effects.

Two experiments were designed with simple and choice RT tasks, respectively, using a variable-foreperiod paradigm. The relatively long foreperiod range used in Stuss and colleagues' (2005) study (i.e. 3–7 seconds) may suggest vigilance-related impairment in right prefrontal patients, rather than a deficit in monitoring stimulus presentation over time. For this reason, a shorter foreperiod range was used (0.5–1.5 seconds). Participants were tested on three different days. In each session, participants first performed a baseline variable-foreperiod task, then received inhibitory TMS on one of the three areas, and finally again performed the foreperiod task while the inhibitory effects of TMS were still active. In the second experiment, two task blocks were performed after TMS instead of one. Pilot studies had indicated that the influence of learning effects across blocks was negligible (Vallesi, 2007).

Results from both experiments showed no TMS effect over the left DLPFC and right angular gyrus. TMS over the right DLPFC significantly reduced the foreperiod effect with respect to a pre-TMS baseline block, confirming findings from the neuropsychological study (Stuss et al., 2005). On the other hand, sequential effects were not significantly reduced. Importantly, in the second block post-TMS in experiment 2, the RT lengthening after a long foreperiod on trial n − 1 was present even for long foreperiods on trial n (symmetric sequential effects). The second block was administered for 7–14 minutes after TMS on right DLPFC, namely the time-window when the inhibitory effect of the TMS used in that study was expected to be at its strongest (Huang et al., 2005). The implications of this result will be discussed in a later section.

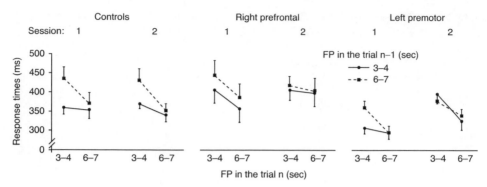

Fig. 22.2 Response times of three of the patient groups tested in Vallesi et al. (2007a). FP = foreperiod. Error bars: standard error of the mean.

An issue left open by the two previous studies (Stuss et al., 2005; Vallesi et al., 2007b) is the neural locus of sequential effects. Investigation of the neural bases of the foreperiod phenomena was therefore, in another study, extended to lesions outside the prefrontal regions (Vallesi et al., 2007a). In that study, 58 right-handed tumor patients were assigned to six groups according to tumor location: right or left lateral prefrontal, right or left premotor, and right or left parietal cortex. Patients were tested in a variable-foreperiod paradigm similar to the simple-RT task employed by Stuss and colleagues (2005). They underwent testing in two sessions, which took place 1–3 days before and 2–6 days after surgical resection of the tumor, respectively. Twelve hospitalized orthopedic patients were also tested with a similar time schedule as a control group.

RT data from three selected groups are presented in Figure 22.2. Results showed no difference between any tumor patient group and controls in the baseline session, demonstrating no effects of the tumor per se on the foreperiod phenomena. Confirming previous findings, a significant reduction of the foreperiod effect from the pre- to the post-surgery session was selectively observed in patients with right lateral prefrontal lesions only (Figure 22.1b), whereas the sequential effects disappeared after left premotor tumor excision (see Figure 22.1c and later section).

In summary, lesions or inhibitory TMS on the right DLPFC reduce the foreperiod effect while the size of sequential effects remains unaffected (Vallesi et al., 2007b), although their shape may change as discussed in a later section. On the other hand, sequential effects disappear after surgical removal of left premotor cortex despite an intact foreperiod effect (Vallesi et al., 2007a). These findings suggest that the mechanisms underlying the foreperiod and the sequential effects are functionally and anatomically dissociable.

The role of different prefrontal regions: brain imaging evidence

A subsequent study (Vallesi et al., 2009) investigated the neural bases of the foreperiod phenomena at the whole-brain level using fMRI (see Box 22.1). A blocked fMRI experiment was administered to 14 healthy participants. Foreperiod length (1 versus 3 seconds) and paradigm type (fixed versus variable) were manipulated within-subject. Subjects were required to make a choice response to a target shape (a square or a triangle).

Fixed short- and long-foreperiod paradigms were used as baseline tasks for the variable-foreperiod paradigm. Fixed and random timing conditions share the same basic perceptual and motor demands. However, if the foreperiod is kept constant, the conditional probability of

stimulus occurrence also remains constant across trials, and monitoring this conditional probability cannot be used for temporal preparation. In the variable paradigm, in contrast, the foreperiod varies randomly, allowing the monitoring process thought to underlie the variable-foreperiod
effect to play a role (e.g. Elithorn and Lawrence, 1955). On the basis of the previously reviewed
neuropsychological and TMS evidence (Stuss et al., 2005; Vallesi et al., 2007a,b), right DLPFC
activation was expected to be greater for the variable-foreperiod paradigm compared with the
fixed one. Results confirmed this prediction (Figure 22.1C). Moreover, across subjects, the degree
of right DLPFC activation predicted the size of the behavioural foreperiod effect. The only other
activated area showing a positive correlation with the foreperiod effect was left precuneus (see
the next section). None of the areas activated in the variable- versus fixed-foreperiod contrast
correlated with sequential effects.

Other areas were also more activated in the variable- versus fixed-foreperiod contrast,
including left DLPFC. Since this area did not show a causal role on the foreperiod phenomena in
previous studies (Stuss et al., 2005; Vallesi et al., 2007a,b), it is probably not as critical as the right
DLPFC. However, another fMRI study also showed involvement of left DLPFC in irregular timing (Dreher et al., 2002). In that study, a hybrid paradigm was used, orthogonally manipulating
task-switching demands (switch versus no switch) and time regularity (regular versus irregular
foreperiods). As results showed, activation of left DLPFC (and of its right hemisphere homologue) during the variable-foreperiod paradigm interacted with task-switching demands. This
finding fits with the hypothesis that left DLPFC is mostly involved in setting the relevant task
criteria (Derfuss et al., 2004; Stuss and Alexander, 2007). This role may be especially important
when the target onset is unpredictable and task-relevant processes need to be continuously
re-established.

In contrast to Vallesi and colleagues (2009), Dreher and colleagues (2002) did not observe
right DLPFC activation as a main effect in the variable- versus fixed-foreperiod contrast. It should
be noted that the reduction of RTs with longer foreperiods was a non-significant trend in Dreher
and colleagues' study (p = 0.09). Participants may not have used strategic processes efficiently to
optimize preparation with longer foreperiods in that study, probably due to the complex task
demands. This may explain the absence of right DLPFC differential activation in the variable-
foreperiod task. In line with this account, Vallesi et al.'s data (2009) also showed that only subjects
with a significant variable-foreperiod effect activated the right DLPFC.

Anterior cingulate and superior medial frontal cortex also showed differential activation in
the variable- versus fixed-foreperiod contrast (Vallesi et al., 2009). This finding was interpreted in
terms of an energization account (e.g. Stuss et al., 1995): whenever the response conditions are
non-optimal (e.g. due to temporal uncertainty), a superior medial prefrontal system energizes
lower-level systems that sustain task-relevant processes. This energization account was also supported by the finding that the anterior cingulate was more strongly activated in the last two runs
than in the first two runs of the variable-foreperiod task, probably to provide additional energization to counter fatigue.[1] A final result of note in Vallesi et al.'s study (2009) was the absence
of regions showing stronger activation for the fixed- than for the variable-foreperiod paradigm.

---

[1] A role of superior medial prefrontal regions in energization would also have been supported by Vallesi
et al.'s fMRI study (2009) if a greater involvement of this region for the long versus short fixed-foreperiod
contrast could be shown. Patients with lesions to this region, indeed, had an exaggerated RT lengthening
for long fixed foreperiods (Stuss et al., 2005). This contrast failed to show differential activation in this
region. However, statistical power was probably not optimal, considering that there was only one run per
fixed foreperiod.

This suggests that fixed-foreperiod tasks do not involve brain areas outside of a subset of those also required to perform the variable-foreperiod task.

In summary, the fMRI evidence provided by Vallesi et al. (2009) confirms the role of right DLPFC in modulating temporal preparation during variable-foreperiod tasks. The findings also extend the previous literature (Stuss et al., 2005; Vallesi et al., 2007a) by showing that other brain regions, ranging from primary sensory areas to prefrontal regions, may also be involved in temporal preparation.

The role of sensory areas

The involvement of perceptual processes in temporal preparation has been a subject of controversy. Some authors initially argued that early perceptual processes were not influenced by temporal preparation, since perceptual degradation did not interact with foreperiod effects (e.g. Sanders 1980). However, more recent psychophysical studies have found interactions between perceptual manipulations (e.g. target luminance) and foreperiod effects, at least in the fixed-foreperiod paradigm (e.g. Los and Schut, 2008). In support of these findings, attention to time has been shown to increase perceptual sensitivity in visual discrimination tasks (Correa et al., 2005; Rolke and Hofmann, 2007).

This controversy extends to electrophysiological findings. Some studies reported that ERP components marking visual perceptual analysis are insensitive to foreperiod duration in visual detection tasks (e.g. Miniussi et al., 1999; Rudell and Hu, 2001). However, these negative results may be task-specific because, when finer perceptual analysis is required, temporal preparation enhances visual and auditory evoked potentials (Griffin et al., 2002; Lange et Al., 2003; Correa et al., 2006a; Lange and Röder, Chapter 28, this volume).

Involvement of areas responsible for perceptual processing specifically in variable-foreperiod tasks was found in the fMRI results reported earlier (Vallesi et al., 2009). Visual cortex (left precuneus) was not only more strongly activated during the variable- (compared to the fixed-) foreperiod paradigm, but its activation was also positively correlated with the size of the variable-foreperiod effect. This suggests that preparation in variable-foreperiod paradigms may involve top-down modulation of perceptual processes.

The role of motor regions

Some fMRI studies have shown that left premotor cortex is selectively more involved in temporal orienting of attention than in spatial attention (Coull and Nobre, 1998; Coull et al., 2000; Coull, Chapter 31, this volume). Premotor areas also appear to be important for sequential effects in the variable-foreperiod paradigm. After lesions to left premotor regions (Vallesi et al., 2007a), no RT reduction was observed when a short foreperiod in the trial n −1 preceded a short foreperiod in the trial n (Figure 22.2C). This finding suggests a premotor/motor locus of facilitation following short-foreperiod trials. Since paretic patients were excluded, explanations related to purely motor deficits can be discarded. Nevertheless, the tumor patient study (Vallesi et al., 2007a) allowed no strong conclusions to be drawn about the anatomical locus of sequential effects. Indeed, although left premotor patients did not show significant sequential effects post-surgery, in contrast to their pre-surgery baseline and to control subjects, their sequential effects were not statistically different from those of other patients with surgical lesions in the frontal lobes (anterior to the central sulcus). The left premotor involvement in sequential effects thus deserves further investigation.

Indirect evidence of a possible premotor locus of sequential effects comes from an ERP study by Van der Lubbe and colleagues (2004; see also Los and Heslenfeld 2005). These authors investigated effects of the preceding foreperiod on the CNV, an ERP index of preparation. They found that around the possible occurrence of the shortest foreperiod in trial n, CNV was more pronounced when short foreperiods had occurred in trial n −1 than long ones. This suggests that preparation was maximal after short foreperiods and low after long foreperiods in the preceding trial. Similar trends were also observed for longer current foreperiods. CNV is partially generated in premotor and motor areas (Hamano et al., 1997). Therefore, these data are compatible with an involvement of premotor regions in sequential effects.

Developmental evidence

The evidence reviewed in earlier sections (e.g. Vallesi et al., 2007b) strongly suggests that foreperiod and sequential effects are due to different processes and depend on two neural systems. A prediction can thus be made about the developmental trajectories followed by the two effects. Since the foreperiod effect depends upon the functioning of the right DLPFC, it might be expected to follow the neurodevelopmental curve of the prefrontal cortex, which matures at a slower pace than the rest of the brain (Huttenlocher and Dabholkar, 1997) and shows exponential maturation between ages 4–7 years (e.g. Delalle et al., 1997). Many frontally-based tasks, indeed, begin to be performed well at this age (Zelazo et al., 1996). On the other hand, a different developmental curve is expected for the emergence of sequential effects, given the data suggesting that these effects are independent of the right DLPFC (Vallesi et al., 2007b) and may instead involve premotor regions (Vallesi et al., 2007a).

These predictions were tested in a recent developmental study (Vallesi and Shallice 2007). In a first experiment, children (4–11 years of age) and adults (19–30 years) were tested in a variable-foreperiod paradigm with foreperiods of 1, 3, and 5 seconds occurring equiprobably and randomly. The results showed a dissociation in the developmental trajectories followed by the two foreperiod phenomena. Sequential effects were already present at ages 4-5, whereas the foreperiod effect appeared gradually around ages 6–7. These results were replicated longitudinally in a subgroup of 4–5-year-old children tested 14 months later, and in a subsequent experiment (foreperiods: 1, 2, and 3 seconds) carried out with a new cohort of 4–6-year-old children. The presence of sequential effects, in the absence of a foreperiod effect, in the youngest children tested suggests that they have at least partially different neuroanatomical and functional origins (cf. Los et al., 2001).

Another interesting finding was that sequential effects changed shape as a function of age: they were symmetrically present across all three current foreperiods in 4-year-old children, but decreased for the longest current foreperiod in 5- and 6-year-old children, as is normally observed in adults. Although previous studies also reported a smaller foreperiod effect in children than in adults (e.g. Adams and Lambos, 1986), no study showed age-related differences in sequential effects (Elliott, 1970; Czudner and Rourke, 1972). However, children tested in the previous studies were older than the critical age (i.e. more than 4 years old).

A tentative dual-process account

A dual-process account of the foreperiod phenomena has been recently proposed to explain the developmental dissociations described earlier (Vallesi and Shallice, 2007). The symmetrical sequential effects found in 4-year-old children were explained by a mechanism of readiness regulation. Readiness to respond is believed to be facilitated following short foreperiods, and to decrease following long foreperiods, regardless of the current foreperiod. This refractory-like effect may derive from the fact that maintaining temporal preparation requires cognitive resources (cf., Näätänen 1971). It is possible that these resources are exhausted after long foreperiods, and require time to recover. This hypothesis receives support from accuracy data in the study by

Vallesi and Shallice (2007). In their second experiment, children (especially 4- and 5-year-old ones) were more likely to give a very slow response (>1500ms), or to fail to respond, as the preceding foreperiod increased. This pattern suggests a refractory-like effect of long preceding foreperiods on preparation level during the current trial. Moreover, all children in this experiment (4–6 years old) were more likely to give premature responses after short preceding foreperiods, suggesting a facilitation of their preparation level. A similar tendency was observed in the accuracy data of children aged 4–5 (and some older children) in the previous experiment. Ceiling effects due to low task difficulty may explain why accuracy effects are not usually found for older children and adults.

According to the dual-process account (Vallesi and Shallice, 2007), the pattern of asymmetric sequential effects usually observed in older children and adults' RTs reflects the compensatory influence of an additional process of endogenous preparation (Niemi and Näätänen, 1981). This process checks the increasing conditional probability of target occurrence across time in order to enhance preparation. This monitoring process would partially offset the process of sustained readiness modulation that produces sequential effects at longer foreperiods. If the monitoring process is impaired, sequential effects can also occur for long foreperiods, even in adults (Vallesi et al., 2007b).

Electrophysiology is more sensitive for tracking readiness regulation in adults, than purely behavioural measures. Los and Heslenfeld (2005) showed that, in adults, temporal cue validity and preceding foreperiod independently affected the CNV, an ERP measure of readiness. Importantly, CNV amplitude was larger throughout the current foreperiod with a short than with a long preceding foreperiod, irrespective of the current foreperiod length. That is, sequential effects on the CNV were similar for short and long current foreperiods (mirroring the symmetrical sequential effects on RTs in 4-year-old children).

During development, processes pertaining to lower level cognitive systems are acquired before processes belonging to higher-level systems (Zelazo et al., 1996; Shallice, 2004). The latter are localized mainly in the prefrontal cortex, a structure that matures more slowly than other brain regions (e.g. Delalle et al., 1997). In this context, the fact that the developmental onset of the foreperiod effect was delayed relative to the onset of sequential effects suggests that the former depends more heavily on prefrontal cortex than the latter. As reviewed in earlier sections, other findings point to a critical role of right DLPFC in the foreperiod effect. Unlike sequential effects, the foreperiod effect is significantly attenuated when right DLPFC is permanently damaged, transitorily inhibited, or not yet mature (Stuss et al., 2005; Vallesi and Shallice, 2007; Vallesi et al., 2007a,b). That multiple processes may underlie temporal preparation is also suggested by the fact that different psychophysiological indices of preparation poorly correlate with each other (Jennings and van der Molen, 2005), possibly because each index marks partially distinct preparation processes.

Future directions

Future research should further investigate the neural bases of the less strategic, but equally relevant, processes underlying the fixed-foreperiod effect and sequential effects. An fMRI design with more than only one run per fixed foreperiod (cf. Vallesi et al., 2009) would be useful for identifying areas differentially involved in foreperiods of various lengths within the fixed foreperiod paradigm. Event-related fMRI or neuropsychological studies with higher lesion specificity (cf. Vallesi et al., 2007a) could help unveil the neural network involved in sequential effects.

Dopaminergic agonists and antagonists can respectively improve or impair performance in explicit temporal processing tasks (Meck, 1996). Some studies have suggested that dopamine might also be important in the foreperiod effect. Patients with schizophrenia who suffer from dopaminergic up-regulation (Kapur, 2003) show an enhanced variable-foreperiod effect (Zahn et al., 1963). In contrast, Parkinson's patients who suffer from dopaminergic down-regulation (e.g. Rakshi et al., 1999) may exhibit a reduction of this effect (Jurkowski et al., 2005). The role of different neurotransmitters in producing foreperiod phenomena should also be investigated.

Although studies to date have mainly focused on the role of cortical structures, it is plausible that input from subcortical areas (basal ganglia, thalamus) and cerebellum also plays a role in temporal preparation during foreperiod paradigms (e.g. Brunia and van Boxtel, 2001; Vallesi et al., 2008).

Conclusions

Temporal preparation involves anticipation of the timing of future events. The data reviewed here suggest that several processes underlie this cognitive ability. Some of these processes, such as those underlying the variable-foreperiod effect, are probably strategic and flexible but are capacity-limited and develop later. These strategic processes optimize the activity in brain structures involved in perception, information processing, and action. Which of these stages receive greater optimization may depend on specific task demands. Other processes contributing to temporal preparation, such as those underlying sequential effects, seem to be more robust, but are less flexible than the strategic processes.

To conclude, the evidence to date supports the view that preparation is a multi-componential cognitive capacity, consisting of supervisory processes on the one hand, and more automatic factors on the other. Although these processes and underlying brain regions normally interact, they can be also dissociated. Preparation is not a unitary phenomenon.

References

Adams, R.J. and Lambos, W.A. (1986). Developmental changes in response preparation to visual stimuli. *Percept Mot Skills*, **62**, 519–22.

Bertelson, P. and Boons, J.P. (1960). Time uncertainty and choice reaction time. *Nature*, **187**, 531–2.

Brunia, C.H. and van Boxtel, G.J. (2001). Wait and see. *Int J Psychophysiol*, **43**, 59–75.

Correa, A., Lupiáñez, J., and Tudela, P. (2005). Attentional preparation based on temporal expectancy modulates processing at the perceptual level. *Psychon Bull Rev*, **12**, 328–34.

Correa, A., Lupiáñez, J., Madrid, E., and Tudela, P. (2006a). Temporal attention enhances early visual processing: a review and new evidence from event-related potentials. *Brain Res*, **1076**, 116–28.

Correa, A., Lupiáñez, J., and Tudela, P. (2006b). The attentional mechanism of temporal orienting: determinants and attributes. *Exp Brain Res*, **169**, 58–68.

Coull, J. T. and Nobre, A. C. (1998). Where and when to pay attention: the neural systems for directing attention to spatial locations and to time intervals as revealed by both PET and fMRI. *J Neurosci*, **18**, 7426–35.

Coull, J. T., Frith, C. D., Buchel, C., and Nobre, A. C. (2000). Orienting attention in time: behavioural and neuroanatomical distinction between exogenous and endogenous shifts. *Neuropsychologia*, **38**, 808–19.

Czudner, G. and Rourke, B. P. (1972). Age differences in visual reaction time of 'brain-damaged' and normal children under regular and irregular preparatory interval conditions. *J Exp Child Psychol*, **13**, 516–26.

Delalle, I., Evers, P., Kostovic, I., and Uylings, H. B. (1997). Laminar distribution of neuropeptide Y-immunoreactive neurons in human prefrontal cortex during development. *J Comp Neurol*, **379**, 515–22.

Derfuss, J., Brass, M., and Von Cramon, D. Y. (2004). Cognitive control in the posterior frontolateral cortex: evidence from common activations in task coordination, interference control, and working memory. *NeuroImage*, **23**, 604–12.

Dreher, J. C., Koechlin, E., Ali, S. O., and Grafman, J. (2002). The roles of timing and task order during task switching. *NeuroImage*, **17**, 95–109.

Elithorn, A. and Lawrence, C. (1955). Central inhibition: some refractory observations. *Q J Exp Psychol*, **11**, 211–20.

Elliott, R. (1970). Simple reaction time: effects associated with age, preparatory interval, incentive-shift, and mode of presentation. *J Exp Child Psychol*, **9**, 86–107.

Gibbon, J., Church, R.M., and Meck, W.H. (1984). Scalar timing in memory. *Ann N Y Acad Sci*, **423**, 52–77.

Gottsdanker, R. (1970). Uncertainty, time keeping and simple reaction time. *J Motor Behav*, **2**, 245–60.

Griffin, I. C., Miniussi, C., and Nobre, A. C. (2002). Multiple mechanisms of selective attention: differential modulation of stimulus processing by attention to space or time. *Neuropsychologia*, **40**, 2325–40.

Hamano, T., Luders, H. O., Ikeda, A., Collura, T. F., Comair, Y. G., and Shibasaki, H. (1997). The cortical generators of the contingent negative variation in humans: a study with subdural electrodes. *Electroencephalogr Clin Neurophysiol*, **104**, 257–68.

Harrington, D. L., Haaland, K. Y., and Knight, R. T. (1998). Cortical networks underlying mechanisms of time perception. *J Neurosci*, **18**, 1085–95.

Hasbroucq, T., Kaneko, H., Akamatsu, M., and Possamai, C. A. (1997). Preparatory inhibition of cortico-spinal excitability: a transcranial magnetic stimulation study in man. *Brain Res Cogn Brain Res*, **5**, 185–92.

Hasbroucq, T., Kaneko, H., Akamatsu, M., and Possamai, C. A. (1999). The time-course of preparatory spinal and cortico-spinal inhibition: an H-reflex and transcranial magnetic stimulation study in man. *Exp Brain Res*, **124**, 33–41.

Huang, Y. Z., Edwards, M. J., Rounis, E., Bhatia, K. P., and Rothwell, J. C. (2005). Theta burst stimulation of the human motor cortex. *Neuron*, **45**, 201–6.

Huttenlocher, P. R. and Dabholkar, A. S. (1997). Regional differences in synaptogenesis in human cerebral cortex. *J Comp Neurol*, **387**, 167–78.

Janssen, P. and Shadlen, M. N. (2005). A representation of the hazard rate of elapsed time in macaque area LIP. *Nat Neurosci*, **8**, 234–41.

Jennings, J. R. and van der Molen, M. W. (2005). Preparation for speeded action as a psychophysiological concept. *Psychol Bull*, **131**, 434–59.

Jurkowski, A. J., Stepp, E., and Hackley, S. A. (2005). Variable foreperiod deficits in Parkinson's disease: dissociation across reflexive and voluntary behaviors. *Brain Cogn*, **58**, 49–61.

Kapur, S. (2003). Psychosis as a state of aberrant salience: a framework linking biology, phenomenology, and pharmacology in schizophrenia. *Am J Psychiatry*, **160**, 13–23.

Karlin, L. (1959). Reaction time as a function of foreperiod duration and variability. *J Exp Psychol*, **58**, 185–91.

Lange, K., Rosler, F., and Roder, B. (2003). Early processing stages are modulated when auditory stimuli are presented at an attended moment in time: an event-related potential study. *Psychophysiology*, **40**, 806–17.

Lewis, P. A. and Miall, R. C. (2003). Brain activation patterns during measurement of sub- and supra-second intervals. *Neuropsychologia*, **41**, 1583–92.

Los, S. A. and Heslenfeld, D. J. (2005). Intentional and unintentional contributions to nonspecific preparation: electrophysiological evidence. *J Exp Psychol Gen*, **134**, 52–72.

Los, S. A. and Schut, M. L. (2008). The effective time course of preparation. *Cognit Psychol*, **57**, 20–55.

Los, S. A. and van den Heuvel, C. E. (2001). Intentional and unintentional contributions to nonspecific preparation during reaction time foreperiods. *J Exp Psychol Hum Percept Perform*, **27**, 370–86.

Los, S. A., Knol, D. L., and Boers, R. M. (2001). The foreperiod effect revisited: conditioning as a basis for nonspecific preparation. *Acta Psychol*, **106**, 121–45.

Mattes, S. and Ulrich, R. (1997). Response force is sensitive to the temporal uncertainty of response stimuli. *Percept Psychophys*, **59**, 1089–97.

Meck, W. H. (1996). Neuropharmacology of timing and time perception. *Brain Res Cogn Brain Res*, **3**, 227–42.

Miniussi, C., Wilding, E. L., Coull, J. T., and Nobre, A. C. (1999). Orienting attention in time. Modulation of brain potentials. *Brain*, **122**, 1507–18.

Näätänen, R. (1970). The diminishing time-uncertainty with the lapse of time after the warning signal in reaction-time experiments with varying foreperiods. *Acta Psychologica*, **34**, 399–419.

Näätänen, R. (1971). Nonaging foreperiod and simple reaction time. *Acta Psychologica*, **35**, 316–27.

Niemi, P. and Näätänen, R. (1981). Foreperiod and simple reaction time. *Psychol Bull*, **89**, 133–62.

Nobre, A. C. (2001). Orienting attention to instants in time. *Neuropsychologia*, **39**, 1317–28.

Rakshi, J. S., Uema, T., Ito, K., Bailey, D. L., Morrish, P. K., Ashburner, J., et al. (1999). Frontal, midbrain and striatal dopaminergic function in early and advanced Parkinson's disease A 3D [(18)F]dopa-PET study. *Brain*, **122**, 1637–50.

Requin, J., Brener, J., and Ring, C. (1991). Preparation for action. In J. R. Jennings and M. G. H. Coles (Eds.) *Handbook of Cognitive Psychophysiology: Central and Autonomic Nervous System Approaches*, pp.357–448. New York: Wiley.

Rolke, B. and Hofmann, P. (2007). Temporal uncertainty degrades perceptual processing. *Psychon Bull Rev*, **14**, 522–6.

Rudell, A. P. and Hu, B. (2001). Does a warning signal accelerate the processing of sensory information? Evidence from recognition potential responses to high and low frequency words. *Int J Psychophysiol*, **41**, 31–42.

Sanders, A. F. (1980). Stage analysis of reaction processes. In G. G. Stelmach and J. Requin (Eds.) *Tutorials in Motor Behavior*, pp.331–54. Amsterdam: North-Holland Publishing Company.

Shallice, T. (2004). The fractionation of supervisory control. In M.S.Gazzaniga (Ed.) *The Cognitive Neurosciences III*, pp.943–56. Cambridge, MA: MIT Press.

Stuss, D. T. and Alexander, M. P. (2007). Is there a dysexecutive syndrome? *Philos Trans R Soc Lond B Biol Sci*, **362**, 901–15.

Stuss, D. T., Alexander, M. P., Shallice, T., Picton, T. W., Binns, M. A., Macdonald, R., et al. (2005). Multiple frontal systems controlling response speed. *Neuropsychologia*, **43**, 396–417.

Stuss, D.T., Shallice, T., Alexander, M.P., and Picton, T.W. (1995). A multidisciplinary approach to anterior attentional functions. *Ann N Y Acad Sci*, **769**, 191–211.

Vallesi, A. (2007). 'The monitoring role of right lateral prefrontal cortex: evidence from variable foreperiod and source memory tasks.' PhD Dissertation. Trieste: SISSA.

Vallesi, A. and Shallice, T. (2007). Developmental dissociations of preparation over time: deconstructing the variable foreperiod phenomena. *J Exp Psychol Hum Percept Perform*, **33**, 1377–88.

Vallesi, A., Mussoni, A., Mondani, M., Budai, R., Skrap, M., and Shallice, T. (2007a). The neural basis of temporal preparation: insights from brain tumor patients. *Neuropsychologia*, **45**, 2755–63.

Vallesi, A., Shallice, T., and Walsh, V. (2007b). Role of the prefrontal cortex in the foreperiod effect: TMS evidence for dual mechanisms in temporal preparation. *Cereb Cortex*, **17**, 466–74.

Vallesi, A., McIntosh A. R., Stuss D. T. (2008). Role of the cerebellum in temporal preparation: an fMRI study. Abstract presented at the Twenty-sixth European Workshop on Cognitive Neuropsychology, Bressanone, Italy. January 2008.

Vallesi, A., McIntosh, A. R., Shallice, T., and Stuss, D. T. (2009). When time shapes behaviour: fMRI evidence of brain correlates of strategic preparation over time. *J Cog Neurosci* **21**(6), 1116–26.

Van der Lubbe, R. H., Los, S. A., Jaskowski, P., and Verleger, R. (2004). Being prepared on time: on the importance of the previous foreperiod to current preparation, as reflected in speed, force and preparation-related brain potentials. *Acta Psychol (Amst)*, **116**, 245–62.

Walter, W. G., Cooper, R., Aldridge, V. J., McCallum, W. C., and Winter, A. L. (1964). Contingent negative variation: an electric sign of sensorimotor association and expectancy in the human brain. *Nature*, **203**, 380–4.

Woodrow. (1914). The measurement of attention. *Psychol Monogr* **5**(76), 1–158.

Zahn, T. P., Rosenthal, D., and Shakow, D. (1963). Effects of irregular preparatory intervals on reaction time in schizophrenia. *J Abnorm Soc Psychol*, **67**, 44–52.

Zelazo, P., Carter, S., Resnick, K., and Frye, C. (1996). The development of executive functions in children. *Rev Gen Psychol*, **1**, 198–226.

Acknowledgments

The preparation of this chapter was in part supported by a postdoctoral fellowship award from the Canadian Institute of Health Research (CIHR, MFE-87658) to the author. The author thanks all the collaborators contributing to his articles reviewed here and Julia Spaniol for proofreading the chapter.

Chapter 23

Attending to sound patterns and the role of entrainment

Mari Riess Jones

Isolated sounds often serve an alerting function; we re-orient to an unanticipated sound. But, when sounds collectively form sequences arising from animate creatures, they typically serve a communicative function, eliciting various anticipatory behaviours in listeners. This chapter is about how humans react, in-the-moment, to sound patterns created by others. One feature of this behaviour is that listeners seem to 'keep time' effortlessly with the common patterns of speech and music, an observation which suggests the presence of an effective tracking mechanism. I have suggested that entrainment is a good candidate for such a mechanism (Jones, 1976). The idea is that temporal regularities within extended events induce a low-level attending activity with resulting temporal expectancies that figure into a listener's dynamic tracking of such events.

This chapter focuses upon attending to sounds, although clearly temporal regularities characterize light as well as sound patterns. In the first section, I review tasks requiring judgements about time in the context of sound (monotonic) sequences and provide evidence for listeners' sensitivities to temporal regularities in these events. A second section addresses theoretical issues involving attention and timing through the lens of entrainment and dynamic attending theory (DAT). A final section considers the impact of implicit rhythmic timing on listeners' ability to judge the pitch component of non-monotonic (melodic) sequences.

Temporal expectancies: anticipating the 'when' of events

Expectancies are inherently temporal by virtue of their reference to time. Expected 'moments' are scaled future time regions (minutes, days, etc.); the 'when' of a happening distinguishes an expectancy (future time) from a memory (past time). Although temporal expectancies can be probabilistically elicited by discrete cues (cf. Nobre, 2001; Correa, Chapter 26; Nobre, Chapter 27, this volume), they also arise from structural relations within a prevailing temporal context. On various time scales, expectancies can manifest themselves as extrapolations of attending into the future. I propose that context, supplied by a pattern's rate and/or rhythm (visual or auditory), shapes such extrapolations.

To understand the role of attending in this process, my colleagues and I have examined the influence of temporal aspects of stimulus contexts. This focus upon stimulus structure does not preclude roles for more conventional, voluntary, aspects of attending. Rather, it suggests that dynamic aspects of our surroundings contribute to how we focus attending in time. For instance, conversations entail turn-taking wherein listeners tacitly monitor utterances of interlocutors, anticipating future phrase endings (Boltz, 2005; Wilson and Wilson, 2005). Similarly, when listeners track a melodic theme, they typically anticipate 'when' critical tones will arrive (Klein and Jones, 1996). These examples suggest that attending in dynamic contexts is aimed to coincide *in time* with upcoming elements. In other words, synchrony is an implicit goal. Indeed, a hall-mark of attending is that some internal process must co-occur with an external (target) stimulus. Achieving synchrony in dynamic environments is more challenging than in static environments because elements comprising unfolding events appear and disappear in time (Jones, 2001). Attending must 'keep pace': heightening to anticipate successive sounds (*anticipatory attending*) and, failing this, re-orienting following an unanticipated sound (*reactive attending*).

The temporal component of attending

I begin by describing some effects of sequential context in *explicit* timing tasks where listeners judge time itself. Two illustrative tasks involve, respectively, categorical judgements and dis-criminative time judgements. Our general strategy embeds a pair of to-be-judged time intervals in a patterned context with the aim of examining effects of context rate/ rhythm on listeners' responses to time.

Time-judgement tasks

Time-judgement tasks were designed to determine how well listeners judged the durations of expected, versus unexpected, time spans. Listeners were to categorize durations of comparison intervals, relative to a preceding standard interval. A standard/comparison pair followed a monot-onic induction sequence having a fixed rate (Large and Jones, 1999; Barnes and Jones, 2000; McAuley and Jones, 2003). The induction sequence usually comprised a series of brief (60-ms) sine tones (all middle C), presented in an isochronous rhythm (identical inter-onset-intervals, IOIs). In one study, sequence rate was determined by IOIs of 600ms. Our primary independent variable was the duration of a standard time interval (S), which followed the sequence; equally often S ended 'early' (S = 524, 579ms), 'on time' (S = 600ms), or 'late' (S = 621, 676ms). A com-parison, yoked to the standard, followed (comparison intervals were identical to the standard, S, or differed by 12%, a suprathreshold amount). Subjects were explicitly told to '*focus upon stand-ard (S) and comparison (C) intervals*' and to '*ignore the induction sequence*'. They reported whether a comparison interval was the same duration, longer, or shorter than its standard.

Figure 23.1A shows proportion of correct categorization responses as a function of standard duration. This inverted U-shaped accuracy profile conforms to a *theoretical expectancy profile*, indicating best performance with the expected standard and worst with very unexpected ones. Similar profiles emerged for induction sequences of other rates (McAuley and Kidd, 1998; Barnes and Jones, 2000). Furthermore, we found that the value of a comparison, judged to be subjec-tively equal to a standard (i.e. a point of subjective equality), revealed that participants systemati-cally distorted durations of standards ending unexpectedly early or late. That is, regardless of the standard presented, listeners' judgements tended to be based on a standard value that approxi-mated the induction IOI, not the veridical value of the particular standard; this favoured performance with the expected standard. This reliance on an induced pace even persists to affect judgements about delayed standard/comparison pairs that occur following a silence of two IOIs (McAuley and Jones, 2003).

Apparently a rhythmically coherent induction sequence is sufficiently compelling that listeners tend to disregard instructions to ignore it, as evidenced by the fact that induction rate leads to systematic distortions in judgements of unexpected standards. We hypothesized that sequence rate activates a persisting periodic attending activity which, in turn, subtly biases listeners to expect certain forthcoming time intervals. A full explanation requires a process that is: 1) periodic; 2) context sensitive; and 3) sustainable. In the next section, I outline an entrainment model with these properties that predicts findings of Figure 23.1A.

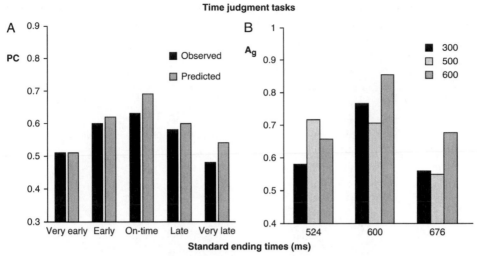

Fig. 23.1 Performance for categorical time judgment experiments. A) Inverted-U profiles of proportion correct (PC) judgments (observed, predicted) are shown for duration judgments of comparisons that followed one of five different standards (abscissa), given an isochronous induction rate of 600ms. Predicted PCs (light bars) are based on task-specific applications of Box 1 equations (Large and Jones, 1999). B) In a similar task, A_g, indexes accuracy (chance A_g = 0.50; perfect performance A_g = 1.00) is shown for duration judgements of three standards (abscissa) that follow different (isochronous) induction rates (IOIs of 300ms, 500ms, 600ms). Reproduced from Barnes, R. and Jones, M. R. (2000). Expectancy, attention, and time. *Cognitive Psychology*, **41**, 254–311.

Barnes and Jones (2000) addressed the proposal that attending is periodic. Three groups of participants listened to monotonic induction sequences of different rates (IOIs = 300ms, 500ms, or 600ms). As in the preceding experiment, following an isochronous rhythm, listeners judged yoked standard-comparison durations. But in this experiment, all groups received the same three standard (S) values where S = 524ms, 600ms, or 676ms. We used a two-choice (same, different) task to calculate a non-parametric measure of differentiation based on signal detection theory, namely A_g. We expected best performance for standards ending after 600ms in listeners receiving the 600ms induction rate. But, if a periodic process is elicited by each induction rate, then listeners receiving the 300-ms induction rate should show an inverted U-shaped A_g profile similar to that of the 600-ms rate group. That is, periodic attending, if sensitive to context rate, implies that the harmonic ratio (1:2) between 300ms and 600ms rates will render these conditions similar. Furthermore, if this periodicity is sustained, then attending to the 300-ms rate will 'beat through' a 600-ms standard interval to correctly anticipate its ending time. By contrast, listeners receiving the non-harmonic, 500ms, rate should show a linear A_g profile with best performance at S = 524ms.

It is possible, of course, that attending is not periodic. A contrary view holds that psychological time is registered on an interval, not a harmonic, scale (Church, 2003). This view maintains that performance of the 300-ms and 600-ms rate groups will be maximally different (i.e. by 300ms); indeed, on an interval scale the 300-ms rate group is closer to the 500-ms (a 200-ms difference). Thus, an interval time hypothesis predicts that performance of listeners receiving the 300-ms rate should resemble that of listeners in the 500-ms condition, not that of listeners receiving 600-ms induction rates.

Results, in Figure 23.1B, favour a periodic attending interpretation. Induction groups with harmonically related rates (300ms, 600ms) both revealed best performance for the harmonically congruent standard interval of 600ms. They showed statistically comparable inverted-U profiles of A_g, which differed significantly from a linear profile of the 500-ms rate group. These findings were replicated by McAuley and Jones (2003).

In sum, tasks involving duration judgements show that an isochronous context rhythm of a given rate: 1) increases judgement accuracy of expected time intervals, while decreasing estimation accuracy of unexpected intervals; 2) induces temporal expectancies based on periodic attending; 3) elicits a sustained periodicity. More generally, although temporal expectancies are often linked to speeded motor responses, a purely motor explanation of expectancy does not readily apply to temporal categorization data.

Time-discrimination tasks

Time-discrimination tasks ask 'What is the smallest detectable difference between two time intervals?' A temporal *just noticeable difference* (JND) is determined by presenting a standard interval of duration, S, and comparison intervals, C, which differ from S in small amounts (C = S + Δt). Over trials, the relative magnitude of the time change (Δt/S) is varied, and participants report if they detect a difference between S and C. The JND is a temporal acuity threshold that is statistically determined from detection accuracy scores for all time changes. Note that this task differs from the categorical judgement task because here the comparison time interval (which assumes some subthreshold values) is now the relevant independent variable. It is useful to note that the typical discrimination task presents listeners with only two time intervals, S and C. This two-interval psychophysical design yields a common finding: the average temporal JND corresponds to ratio, Δt/S, near 0.06 (Allan, 1979).

We asked 'Does temporal acuity change in dynamic contexts?' In tackling this question, Large and I (Large and Jones, 1999) adapted psychophysical designs to incorporate various temporal contexts. We embedded two short isochronous '*test*' regions distinguished by higher pitched tones in longer auditory sequences. Test regions alternated with context regions of lower pitched tones: context, *test*, context, *test*, context. Although test regions were isochronous, context regions could be temporally variable, containing several different IOIs. Overall, mean IOI, denoted T, was identical for context and test regions, T = 600ms. Adapting conventional terminology, in this design a standard becomes the mean IOI of the sequence (i.e. S = T), and a comparison interval (in a test region) becomes: C = T + Δt. Whereas in the preceding task, the standard duration varied, here it is constant (T). Instead, the comparison varies as function |Δt|; three values[1] of C were determined by Δt/T of 0.035, 0.065, 0.095. Equally often a single deviant comparison occurred in each test region, and listeners identified which region contained this anisochrony. A second important variable involved temporal variability of context regions. Contextual irregularity varied as a function the standard deviation (SD) of context IOIs, from low (SD = 21ms) to high (SD = 75ms).

We reasoned that detection of an anisochrony should depend upon a listener's sensitivity to an expectancy violation elicited by a deviant time-change. One prediction is that detection performance will increase with the magnitude of an expectancy violation based on |Δ|/T. In addition, because temporally regular contexts (low IOI variability) induce strong temporal expectancies, which should continue into isochronous test regions, a second prediction is that regular contexts

---

[1] Psychophysical convention averages data over comparisons smaller (−Δt) and larger (+Δt) than the standard, S (Figure 23.2). By contrast, plots of detection PCs that distinguish signed deviations (i.e. smaller and larger than S) are U-shaped accuracy profiles with lowest PC for smallest |Δt| value.

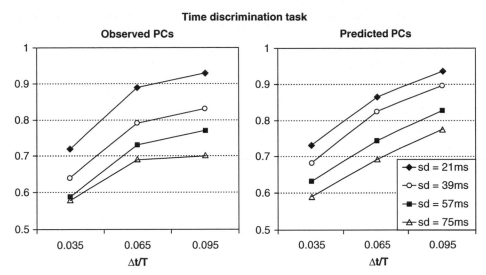

Fig. 23.2 Left panel shows proportion correct (PC) detections of time-changes |Δt| in a comparison IOI (relative to a standard, T = 600ms), as a function of relative magnitude: |Δt|/T. Using long sequences, the comparison time-change appeared randomly in one of two isochronous test regions that alternated with rhythmically variable context regions (see text). Best detections occurred with the largest time-deviation (data are collapsed over positive and negative time-changes, see footnote 1). Accuracy declined as context variability (i.e., standard deviation, SD, of context IOIs) increased from low (SD = 21ms) to high (SD =75ms). Right panel shows task-specific entrainment model predictions derived from Box 23.1 equations (Large and Jones, 1999).

will heighten the detectability of any time-change, leading to good performance. By contrast, temporally irregular contexts (high IOI variability) yield weak expectancies, hence poor detection performance.

Figure 23.2 (left panel) shows that both predictions are supported. Accuracy (proportion correct, PC) increased with Δt/T and decreased with context variability. In addition, calculations of temporal acuity thresholds, i.e. JNDs, revealed that temporal resolution was extremely good (JND = 0.023) in isochronous control conditions (not shown in Figure 23.2), but worsened as rhythmic regularity declined, and was quite poor (JND = 0.10) with very irregular rhythmic contexts. Relative to conventional estimates in two-interval designs (JND = 0.06), it seems that, depending upon rhythmic regularity, dynamic contexts either enhance or degrade temporal acuity.

In summary, listeners' ability to detect small deviations from isochrony is estimated using a new paradigm that incorporates dynamic contexts. Listeners appear to detect time changes (Δt/T) as violations from temporal expectancies that are induced by a surrounding rhythmic context. Performance improves with rhythmically regular contexts. We conclude that attentional monitoring: 1) is context sensitive; 2) persists over time; and 3) can be 'attuned' or 'thrown off-track', respectively, by regular or irregular temporal contexts.

Attention and perceiving time: theoretical implications

How might we formalize expectancy and expectancy violations? To answer this, I outline a theoretical framework which clarifies anticipatory attending, and hence expectancies, as well as reactive attending, hence expectancy violations.

First I consider common reactions to this general approach, which raise these questions: Is this *really* attention? Isn't this time perception? Such queries imply: 1) attention is not involved in time perception; and 2) 'real' attention is insensitive to contextual timing. Yet, opinions differ widely on what constitutes attention. In what follows, I address both points. First, in this section, I show that contrasting definitions of attention figure, respectively, in two different approaches to time perception: scalar expectancy theory (SET) and dynamic attending theory (DAT). Second, to address the claim that attention is insensitive to temporal contexts, in the final section, I describe research that adapts conventional attention tasks to assess the implicit influence of temporal structure (of sound patterns) on judgements of pitch and timbre.

Scalar expectancy theory (SET)

SET is an influential theory, which for many, is the accepted explanation of time perception (Gibbon et al., 1984; Church, 2003). According to SET, attention is defined in terms of a switch that starts and stops a counter. An attentional switch is closed at the onset of a to-be-judged time interval, allowing ticks from a 'pacemaker' clock (which emits a stochastic stream of ticks) to flow to an accumulator/counter; conversely, attention opens the switch at an interval's offset, ceasing tick accumulation. Next, a time interval is coded as a numerical count of accumulated ticks, scaled, then stored in memory. A temporal expectancy reflects retrieval of a likely interval time code. Pairwise time judgements involve relating a comparison time code (in working memory) to an expected standard (in reference memory). In sum, SET assumes that time judgements involve comparing interval (numerical) codes of two (standard/comparison) durations that are discretely delimited by attention.

Dynamic attending theory (DAT)

A contrasting definition of attention emerges in DAT. Unlike SET, in DAT attending does not control an on/off switch. Instead, it is defined as a contextually driven, synchronized, series of energy pulses. The main theoretical mechanism is *entrainment*. Because DAT links attention to entrainment, McAuley and Jones (2003) have shown that it may be better suited than SET to address time perception and attention in dynamic environments.

Assumptions central to DAT entrainment models:

1) *Driving rhythms*: sequential patterns can function as driving *rhythms*. Typically, a stimulus driving rhythm is formalized as series of sound onsets specified by timed *intensity changes* (i.e. $t_1, t_2 .... t_n, t_{n+1} ...$) where an IOI = $(t_{n+1} - t_n)$. For any rate (i.e. T, the mean IOI), a driving rhythm describes a stimulus context which affords some temporal regularity, where greater regularity yields more effective driving rhythms.

2) *Driven rhythms*: biological oscillations of various sorts exist. Either singly, or in temporally organized groups, brain oscillations exhibit amplitude (energy) periodicities. Most are *limit-cycle oscillators;* a limit cycle is a closed trajectory reflecting traversal through states in a state space, defined by state variables (e.g. phase, period). Many trajectories in this space converge to this closed trajectory when it is *stable* (Strogatz, 1994). Stability explains an oscillator's 'bounce back' potential, namely its ability to recover from perturbations (e.g. a temporally deviant tone onset). Such resilience means that a stable limit-cycle oscillation can: 1) exhibit a periodicity; 2) sustain this periodicity; 3) respond to perturbations, yet restore its periodicity. In short, a stable limit cycle functions as a periodic attractor, with self-sustaining properties (here, limit cycle means stable limit cycle). Cycle time specifies an oscillator's intrinsic (resonant) period, P_0.

3) *Entrainment*: in living things, a non-linear dynamical system can describe a pairing of a *driving rhythm with a driven, biological, rhythm* which corresponds to entrainment. As outlined in Box 23.1, entrainment reflects shifts in phase (Equation 1) and period (Equation 2) of a neural oscillation in response to a driving rhythm (see also Kilavik and Riehle, Chapter 19; Praamstra, Chapter 24, this volume). An entraining oscillator is adaptive: changes in phase and manifest period, P, move a *driving-plus-driven system* toward attractor states (phase synchrony, period matching). Entrainment is most evident when a driving rhythm is regular, with a rate approximating the intrinsic period of a driven oscillation.

Historically, entrainment theories have focused on circadian rhythms where driven oscillations of long intrinsic periods (ca. 24 hours) adapt to driving rhythms marked by light changes (dawn, dusk). Few have considered entrainments at smaller time scales or those marked by sound changes (but see Jones, 1976). Yet the human species has greatly refined communication via sound patterns. Musical patterns are prime examples of events that offer well-structured driving rhythms. Although artful and complex, music exploits powerful temporal regularities that allow examination of universal features of dynamic attending (e.g. synchrony, context sensitivity). I maintain that significant, untapped, explanatory potential for understanding con-specific communication resides in small-scale entrainments to such patterns. Undoubtedly, developing this potential presents mathematical challenges because the field of nonlinear dynamics is daunting. Nevertheless, recent mathematical advances in neurobiology (Izhikevich, 2007) as well as empirical evidence for entraining neuronal oscillations (Snyder and Large, 2005; Zanto et al., 2006; Will and Berg, 2007; Lakatos et al., 2008), suggest that it is not far-fetched to imagine neural oscillations that entrain to relatively small time spans.

DAT entrainment models

Entrainment is a consistent feature of DAT (Jones, 1976; Jones and Boltz, 1989). Recently, attentional entrainment been formalized in nonlinear dynamic models which appeal to joint, interactive, activities of multiple attending oscillations (Large, 1994; McAuley, 1995; Large and Jones, 1999; Jones, 2008). The simplest model, developed by Large, involves one oscillator. As shown in Box 23.1, it features three basic properties: oscillator phase; oscillator period; and an attentional pulse (Large, 1994; Large and Kolen, 1995; Large and Jones, 1999).

Box 23.1 DAT entrainment terms and equations

Three components of a one-oscillator model (Large and Jones model, 1999):

1. *Relative phase*, φ: phase difference between expected time and that of observed tone onset.

2. *Oscillator period*, P_0: intrinsic (asymptotic) duration of an oscillator's limit cycle; P, manifest period, is the adapted period.

3. *Attentional pulse*: burst of concentrated, high frequency, energy at an expected phase point.

Equation 1: $\varphi_{n+1} = \varphi_n + [t_{n+1} - t_n / P] + \eta_N F(\varphi_n)$ (mod −0.5, 0.5, 1),

Equation 2: $P_{n+1} = P_n + P_0 \eta_p F(\varphi_n)$

where $F(\varphi_n) = -\frac{1}{2}\pi\sin 2\pi\varphi$

Control parameters: η_N, η_p

Oscillator phase is expressed through a critical model variable, relative phase, φ. Relative phase refers to the period-normalized time difference between expected and observed time points in an oscillator's cycle. An expected phase, $\varphi = 0$, receives heightened (peak) attentional energy. By contrast, less energy is allocated to a sound onset at an unexpected phase, $\varphi \neq 0$. Within limits, a driving rhythm can force phase changes (when $\varphi \neq 0$) that move the system through various states in phase space toward the attractor state of synchrony ($\varphi = 0$). Corrective, phase changes, described by a sine-circle mapping (Equation 1, Box 23.1) reflect a phase change from φ_n, at time t_n, to φ_{n+1} at t_{n+1}. Phase corrections are often swift and transient (depending on φ_n). Although gross irregularities in a driving (stimulus) rhythm context disrupt entrainment, fairly regular driving rhythms can lead to synchrony between an oscillatory pulse and tone onsets.

The intrinsic period (P_0) of an oscillator is critical to entrainment. If P_0 differs greatly from the average rate, T, of a regular stimulus rhythm, then phase synchrony fails. Conversely, if T is within *entrainment region limits* ($P_0 \sim T$) of an internal oscillation, then synchrony is possible (Jones, 2004; McAuley et al., 2006). Equation 2 of Large's model specifies changes in manifest period, P, of a driven oscillator as it gradually adapts to T and sustains this rate. Period adjustments explain rate tracking, but they often transpire more slowly than phase corrections.

Entrainment describes how listeners 'tune into' an event. Synchrony and temporal expectancies become more precise as a regular driving rhythm unfolds. This results from adaptive updating of phase and period of an attending oscillation, as suggested in Figure 23.3A. Is this attunement largely implicit, as it appears to be? Or can entrainment be brought under voluntary

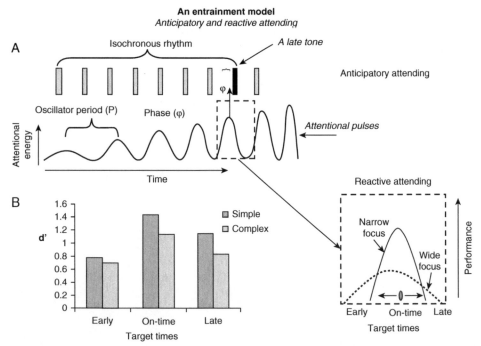

An entrainment model
Anticipatory and reactive attending

Fig. 23.3 Schematic of entrainment, where oscillator period, P, and phase, φ, adapt to a regular driving rhythm. *Anticipatory attending* periodically paces the attentional pulse. Insert shows *reactive attending* as attempted adaptive reactions to ill-timed targets. B) Accuracy, measured by d', is shown for pitch judgements of early, on time, or late tones embedded in different melodies: simple (smooth pitch motion) or complex (jagged pitch motion) (Jones, et al. 2006).

control by, for example, explicit instructions? In this respect, control parameters may play an unheralded role. The parameter, η_N, of Equation 1 controls phase correction speed, whereas η_p of Equation 2 controls period adaptability. Values of control parameters determine a system's behaviour, including the speed of adjusting phase and period to event timing. Conventionally, such parameters reflect the force of a driving rhythm (e.g. tone intensity) and neural responsiveness to force levels; but, broader interpretations of control parameters remain possible. Future theories may enlist control parameters to explain listeners' voluntary responsiveness to event timing as a function of instructions and task demands.

Finally, the attentional pulse is the third component of Large's model. It represents a 'tunable,' symmetrical, attentional *focus in time* (Large and Jones, 1999). Perhaps burst oscillators are involved (Izhikevich, 2007). Thus, a pulse corresponds to a burst of energy (e.g. beta, gamma band frequencies), localized symmetrically about an expected phase point carried by a slower periodicity (e.g. delta frequency) (e.g. Snyder and Large, 2005). In addition to the phase of a pulse at a focal point within a cycle, the width of a symmetrical pulse (about $\varphi = 0$) is important. Pulse width corresponds to phase variance. Thus, pulse width gauges precision of focal attending: as pulse narrows, the concentration of attending energy about an expected time point increases. Theoretically, irregular driving rhythms will increase phase variability, thereby widening the attentional pulse. As with other parameters, pulse parameters may be sensitive to factors other than stimulus timing, such as instructions.

In sum, entrainment models describe a tacit dance between driving rhythms and attending oscillations. Important aspects of this dance involve oscillator phase, period, and pulse. And, because a driving rhythm partners in this dance, entrainment theory gives new meaning to the term 'stimulus driven' attending. Does DAT, then, preclude roles for task demands and voluntary control of attending? No. Different task-sensitive strategies (future oriented versus analytic attending; selective versus divided attending) also play a role (Jones and Boltz, 1989; Jones et al., 1995). It is more accurate to conclude that the structure of a driving rhythm can facilitate or inhibit the execution of a task-induced attentional set. A complete account will involve, among other things, broader interpretations of control parameters.

Task-specific entrainment models

To assess DAT, we applied two task-specific entrainment models to the categorical and discrimination tasks, described earlier. These models adapt Box 23.1 equations in respectively different ways to reflect task demands. Each model considers the potential impact of relevant independent variables on certain components of the driving-plus-driven system. The trick is to account for interactions among model components (phase, period, pulse; control parameters) that change over time. Accordingly, task-specific DAT models express hypotheses about the collective state of a system, *at the moment of responding*; this state is summarized by a *collective variable*. For entrainment models, the collective variable is relative phase, φ (i.e. mean and/or variance of φ), which reflects the time difference between expected and observed sound onsets.

To illustrate, DAT implies that attending synchronizes with a rhythmic sequence as it unfolds, i.e. as a listener 'tunes into' the pattern. Consider a hypothetical experiment where participants overtly predict ending times of isochronous sequences. Let the independent variable be sequence length: short versus long. The collective variable, φ, reflects a momentary difference between expected and observed phase points throughout sequence monitoring. But, at the time of a response (i.e. sequence ending), the value of φ should be smaller for long than short sequences, due to more phase correction opportunities in longer sequences. This predicts greater accuracy in predicting ending times of the longer sequences (cf. McAuley and Miller, 2007). The following paragraphs develop similar hypotheses for categorization and discrimination tasks with other independent variables.

In revisiting the time-judgement task, recall that listeners who categorized comparison (C) intervals that followed one of several standard durations (S), erred primarily with comparisons yoked to unexpected standards (Figure 23.1A). Here a task-specific model (from Box 23.1) focuses upon the impact of the independent variable, standard duration, upon an entrained oscillator period and resulting temporal expectancies at the time of judging a comparison. According to DAT, the self-sustaining property of a limit-cycle oscillator induces periodic attending, leading to judgement errors in this task. Due to a sustained oscillation, listeners *fail to period adapt* to an unexpected standard (i.e. η_p of Equation 2 is low). An induced oscillator's period persists, *changing only minimally*, following a single unexpected standard. In other words, a limit cycle property is responsible for the inverted U accuracy profile of Figure 23.1. At the moment of responding to a yoked comparison, the collective variable, φ, reflects the degree to which a listener relies upon a distorted standard. Larger φ values are predicted for unexpected standards than expected ones, meaning poorer judgements of comparisons yoked to unexpected standards. Conversely, best performance is predicted for comparisons yoked to expected standards because here φ approximates zero. This reasoning generated a good fit to the inverted U profile in Figure 23.1a (Large and Jones, 1999). In brief, this task features a primary role for a persisting temporal expectancy (oscillator period), hence *final φ values negatively correlate with accuracy*: more deviant standard durations (larger φ values) create greater time distortions, hence poorer categorical judgements.

By contrast, the time-discrimination task, described earlier, features a role for expectancy violations. That is, listeners must detect a rhythmic anisochrony within isochronous test regions embedded in longer sequences. Whereas in the preceding experiment the independent variable was standard duration, in this discrimination task, the important independent variable is the magnitude of a to-be-detected comparison interval. We assume that sequence context elicits a periodic expectancy (period, P), based upon average sequence rate, T (i.e. $P \sim T$); expectancy violations, elicited by a deviant comparison, should increase with the magnitude of a comparison change ($\Delta t / T$). Note, the collective variable, φ, turns out to be a direct gauge of such violations: φ increases as $\Delta t / T$ increases. A task-specific DAT model (Box 23.1) predicts better time-change detection with more pronounced expectancy violations, i.e. larger mean φ values. In other words, in this task φ *correlates positively with accuracy*. A time discrimination accuracy profile is *opposite* to the inverted U predicted for a time categorization task (see footnote 1). A second prediction holds that increases in context irregularity increase φ variance; entrainment weakens, the attentional pulse widens and performance declines. The right panel of Figure 23.2 indicates support for both predictions (Large and Jones, 1999; McAuley and Jones, 2003).

In sum, categorization tasks reveal persisting effects of an induced expectancy (i.e. a limit cycle) whereas time discrimination tasks reveal the impact of an expectancy violations (i.e. relative phase). Task-specific DAT models capture these opposing effects of different independent variables and task demands using the same collective variable.

Attending to the pitch component

Curiously, in listening to sound patterns in music or speech, we are often unaware of underlying temporal expectancies: Our attention seems focused on the 'what' of forthcoming sounds, not the 'when'. Nonetheless, I suggest that we tacitly 'use' event timing to attend. In the first section, I showed that driving rhythms of monotonic sequences affect explicit judgements about time, even when people are told to ignore context rhythms. However, such tasks are open to criticisms, namely that they arguably assess time perception, not attention. Furthermore, when listeners explicitly judge time, time becomes a task-relevant dimension. Perhaps, then, listeners do not entrain, but instead voluntarily use rhythm as an explicit 'cue' to judge time. The latter begs thorny issues concerning 'cues' and how they work. Nevertheless, because DAT implies that attending 'in-the-moment' is effortlessly controlled by event timing, it suggests an implicit influence of event time on attending to non-temporal targets.

To answer the question, 'Does the time structure of a pitch pattern affect attending to non-temporal features, such a pitch?' we asked participants to judge pitch or timbre of targets embedded within rhythmic pitch sequences, i.e. melodies. Adapting conventional attention tasks, we varied attentional set (instructions, task) as well as sequence structure. One goal was to discover if rhythmic context *implicitly* affects listeners' identification of targets defined by non-temporal features, and, if so, whether such effects are modulated by attentional set.

Pitch-judgement tasks pose different demands than time-judgement tasks. Because pitch is task-relevant, listeners must focus directly upon features of time-markers themselves, e.g. tones. Moreover, pitch judgements are usually blatantly relative, involving pitch relations: 'Is this pitch higher or lower than a preceding one?' In 1976, I proposed that pitch relations are usefully conceived as distances in pitch space (in semitones). Further, melodies project a series of space-like distances over time, meaning they may be experienced as pitch motion (Jones, 1976; Hahn and Jones, 1981; Johnston and Jones, 2006). Perhaps listeners generate 'motion-like' expectancies, aimed jointly at the 'where' (in pitch space) and 'when' (in time) of forthcoming sounds. If so, listeners may have difficulty separating pitch changes from covarying time changes (Jones, 1976).

Current entrainment models do not formally incorporate pitch relations (or pitch motion). Driving rhythms are defined by changes in intensity, *not pitch*. Nevertheless, DAT offers two indirect ways of incorporating pitch. One way interprets the attentional pulse as a *general source of attentional energy*. Therefore, regular (versus irregular) rhythms elicit anticipatory attending that targets narrower, more focused, bursts of attentional energy to expected times which can facilitate assessment of *any* property of an expected tone. A second way to incorporate pitch relationships *recasts driving rhythms*. Significant pitch changes may function, along with intensity changes, as time markers, thereby modulating sequence regularity. For instance, complex melodies, with large, poorly timed, pitch changes (i.e. jagged pitch motion), can create irregular driving rhythms; indeed, in fast sequences large pitch changes phenomenally 'break-up' rhythmic percepts (Jones, 1976). Together, these interpretations raise two possibilities: 1) rhythmically regular melodies will elicit anticipatory attending, facilitating feature identification of any 'well-timed' tone; conversely, rhythmically irregular distractor tones will elicit poor anticipatory attending to distractors, thereby reducing their interference; 2) pitch irregularities in melodic contexts may lessen entrainment effectiveness of a driving rhythm.

In addressing the first possibility, Klein and I (Klein and Jones, 1996) used a sustained attending task to discover if rhythmic regularity/irregularity implicitly affects anticipatory attending. Listeners monitored long patterns of alternating pitches (high, H, low, L) to detect randomly occurring targets (timbre changes). Different groups of participants heard, respectively, one of three rhythms (binary, trinary, complex). We also manipulated attentional set by exploiting pitch distance; either listeners divided attending (to H and L tones) or they selectively attended (to H tones) where low tones functioned as distractors. In all six conditions, high tones formed an isochronous rhythm (2000ms IOIs). In the binary rhythm, low tones interleaved with high tones to create an isochronous HLHLH . . . rhythm; in the trinary rhythm, low tones formed regular three-tone groups around alternate high tones (. . . LHL . . . H . . . . LHL . . .). In the complex rhythm, similar three tone groups appeared, but timing of low tones was relatively irregular.

We predicted an interaction of rhythm with attentional set. In examining target detection with high tones, we found the predicted interaction. In divided attending conditions, listeners were worst at detecting targets in the complex rhythm and best in the binary rhythm, where overall rhythmic regularity should facilitate anticipatory attending. Conversely, in selective attending conditions, isochrony of high tones should facilitate performance *only if* listeners ignore distracting low tones. Striking evidence confirmed this hypothesis. In the complex rhythm, low tone irregularity should disrupt anticipatory attending to these distractors, thereby reducing their interference. It did. Selective attending was best in the complex rhythm (higher accuracy, faster RTs) and worst in the binary rhythm, suggesting listeners more successfully 'tuned out' distractors when selectively attending to high tones in the complex rhythm. Although attentional set clearly modulated listeners 'use' of time structure in this study, it did not override rhythmic constraints. Overall, rhythm exerted an implicit, and critical, influence on performance.

We addressed the second possibility in recent studies on implicit timing. In two pitch-judgement experiments, time was technically irrelevant (Jones et. al. 2006). We manipulated melodic as well as rhythmic structure where the latter, expressed by intensity changes, was iso-chronous except when a target tone appeared: It could be early, on time, or late. Pitch targets occurred at the penultimate serial location in recurrent nine tone melodies (Jones et al., 2006). Melodic context varied to ascertain if pitch changes affected entrainment: simple melodies had small pitch changes, leading to smooth pitch motion, whereas complex melodies contained many large pitch changes, leading to jagged pitch motion.

In the first experiment listeners were to focus upon pitch (time was not mentioned). They judged whether the target pitch in a comparison melody changed to a higher or lower pitch (by one semitone) or remained the same as in an immediately preceding, standard, melody. Results appear in Figure 23.3B. They support an implicit timing account; pitch identification was best for on-time targets, as measured by the sensitivity index, d'. Performance was also better with simple than complex melodies, suggesting effects of melodic structure on entrainment. One interpretation is that large, perturbing, pitch changes in complex melodies contribute to driving rhythm irregularities, thereby disrupting entrainment. In brief, efficient anticipatory attending, induced by regular sequence timing, elicited superior performance with on-time targets and simple melodies, whereas reactive attending was responsible for poor performance with ill-timed targets.

In a follow-up study listeners were instructed to *ignore timing of early and late targets* and focus strictly on pitch. If listeners comply with instructions, they should voluntarily ignore target timing and focus upon pitch, leading to better performance with ill-timed tones than in the preceding experiment (Figure 23.3B). This did not happen. Accuracy remained low with ill-timed tones, indicating listeners were handicapped in responding to unexpectedly timed sounds.

We infer that event structure (melody, rhythm) implicitly guides anticipatory attending to on-time tones, whereas reactive attending to ill-timed tones is resistant to voluntary control (instructions). In addition, complex melodies seem to reduce entrainment effectiveness. The latter finding converges with others in showing that large pitch changes affect listeners' sense of rhythmic regularity. Such findings suggest a need to recast driving rhythms to include pitch relationships (Jones et al., 1995, Ellis and Jones, 2009).

Finally, an unresolved issue surrounds accuracy profiles. Because current entrainment models incorporate a *symmetrical* attentional pulse, they predict equal accuracy for early and late targets. However, accuracy profiles of Figure 23.3B reveal mild asymmetry; listeners are somewhat better with late than earlier targets. More pronounced asymmetries have also been reported (Mackenzie et al., 2009). Others, using probabilistic cues and visual rhythms, also find asymmetries (Correa and Nobre, 2008). Although reasons for asymmetries are unclear (but see Nobre et al., 2007), they call for theoretical modifications to address differential phase responses to expectancy violations.

In sum, when people pay attention to pitch (timbre) in auditory patterns, sequence timing implicitly affects performance. Listeners perform best in monitoring tasks when target tones conform to a regular rhythm (see also Schubotz, Chapter 25, this volume). If people selectively monitor certain pitches, but not others (distractors), then rhythmic irregularity of the latter facilitates 'tuning them out'. Furthermore, listeners are more effective in temporally targeting attending to rhythmically expected tones within simple (versus complex) melodies, suggesting that in tracking a melody, they implicitly use event timing that emerges jointly from pitch and intensity changes.

Conclusions

Attending to sound patterns can be paced by regularities of rhythmic context. This in-the-moment attending is addressed using DAT wherein entrainment plays a featured role. Current entrainment models formalize how rhythmic stimuli (i.e. driving rhythms) shape the dynamics of listeners' attending to sound patterns (i.e. via driven rhythms, namely neural oscillations). Task-specific DAT models predict people's performance in time judgement tasks (explicit timing) and pitch judgement tasks (implicit timing) as a function of temporal context (rate, rhythm). Explicit judgements about time depend upon rhythmic contexts, but in respectively different ways for categorization and discrimination tasks. Simply put, in temporal categorization tasks, performance is better with rhythmically expected (than unexpected) sounds whereas in discrimination tasks performance is better with rhythmically unexpected (than expected) sounds. Models involving entrainment constructs (e.g. limit cycle oscillations, relative phase as a collective variable) explain such findings. In addition, DAT is applicable to tasks where listeners implicitly use rhythmic structure to attend to pitch (timbre) targets and where both attentional set and melodic structure are varied.

References

Allan, L. G. (1979). The perception of time. *Perception and Psychophysics*, **26**, 340–54.

Barnes, R. and Jones, M. R. (2000). Expectancy, attention, and time. *Cognitive Psychology*, **41**, 254–311.

Boltz, M. (2005). Temporal dimensions of conversational interactions: the role of response latencies and pauses in social impression formation. *Journal of Language and Social Psychology*, **24**, 103–38.

Church, R. M. (2003). A concise introduction to scalar timing theory. In Meck, W. H. (Ed.) *Functional and Neural Mechanisms of Interval Timing*. Boca Raton, FL: CRC Press.

Correa, A. and Nobre, A. C. (2008). Neural modulation by regularity and passage of time. *Journal of Neurophysiology*, **100**, 1649–55.

Gibbon, J., Church, R. M. and Meck, W. H. (1984). Scalar timing in memory. In Gibbon, J. and Allan, L. G. (Eds.) *Annals of the New York Academy of Sciences*. New York: New York Academy of Sciences.

Hahn, J. and Jones, M. R. (1981). Invariants in auditory frequency. *Scandinavian Journal of Psychoogyl*, **22**, 129–44.

Izhikevich, E. M. (2007). *Dynamical Systems in Neuroscience: The Geometry of Excitability and Bursting*. Cambridge, MA: MIT Press

Johnston, M. H. and Jones, M. R. (2006). Higher order pattern structure influences auditory representational momentum. *Journal of Experimental Psychology: Human Perception and Performance* **32**, 2–17.

Jones, M. R. (1976). Time, our lost dimension: toward a new theory of perception, attention, and memory. *Psychological Review*, **83**, 323–55.

Jones, M. R. (2001). Temporal expectancies, capture and timing in auditory sequences. In Gibson, C. F. B. (Ed.) *Attraction, Distraction, and Action: Multiple Perspectives on Attentional Capture*. Amsterdam: Elsevier Science, B.V.

Jones, M. R. (2008). Musical time. In Hallam, S., Cross, I., Thaut, M. (Ed.) *Oxford Handbook of Music Psychology*. Oxford: Oxford University Press.

Jones, M. R. and Boltz, M. (1989). Dynamic attending and responses to time. *Psychological Review*, **96**, 459–91.

Jones, M. R., Jagacinski, R. J., Yee, W., Floyd, R. L. and Klapp, S. (1995). Tests of attentional flexibility in listening to polyrhythmic patterns. *Journal of Experimental Psychology: Human Perception & Performance*, **21**, 293–307.

Klein, J. M. and Jones, M. R. (1996). Effects of attentional set and rhythmic complexity on attending. *Perception & Psychophysics*, **58**, 34–46.

Lakatos, P., Karmos, G., Mehta, A. D., Ulbert, I. and Schroeder, C. E. (2008). Entrainment of neuronal oscillations as a mechanism of attentional selection. *Science*, **320**, 110–13.

Large, E. W. (1994). Dynamic representation of musical structure. *Psychology*. Ohio State University, Columbus, OH.

Large, E. W. and Jones, M. R. (1999). The dynamics of attending: how people track time-varying events. *Psychological Review*, **106**, 119–59.

Large, E. W. and Kolen, J. (1995). Resonance and the perception of musical meter. *Connection Science*, **6**, 177–208.

Mackenzie, N., Ellis, R. J. and Jones, M. R. (2009). Anticipatory and reactive attending to auditory events. *Music Perception*, under review.

McAuley, J. D. (1995). 'Perception of time phase: Toward an adaptive oscillator model of rhythmic pattern processing.' Unpublished PhD. Bloomington, Indiana University.

McAuley, J. D. and Miller, N. S. (2007). Picking up the pace: Effects of global temporal context on sensitivity to the tempo of auditory sequences. *Perception & Psychophysics*, **69**, 709–18.

McAuley, J. D. and Jones, M. R. (2003). Modeling effects of rhythmic context on perceived duration: a comparison of interval and entrainment approaches to short-interval timing. *Journal of Experimental Psychology: Human Perception & Performance*, **29**, 1102–25.

McAuley, J. D. and Kidd, G. R. (1998). Effect of deviations from temporal expectations on tempo discrimination of isochronous tone sequences. *Journal of Experimental Psychology: Human Perception & Performance*, **24**, 1786–800.

Nobre, A. C. (2001). Orienting attention to instants in time. *Neuropsychologia*, **39**, 1317–28.

Nobre, A. C., Correa, A. and Coull, J. T. (2007). The hazards of time. *Current Opinion in Neurobiology*, **17**, 465–70.

Snyder, J. S. and Large, E. W. (2005). Gamma-band activity reflects the metric structure of rhythmic tone sequences. *Cognitive Brain Research*, **24**, 117–26.

Strogatz, S. H. (1994). *Nonlinear Dynamics and Chaos*. Cambridge, MA: Perseus Books Publishing, LLC.

Will, U. and Berg, E. (2007). Brain wave synchronization and entrainment to periodic acoustic stimuli. *Neuroscience Letters*, **424**, 55–60.

Wilson, M. and Wilson, T. (2005). An oscillator model of the timing of turn-taking. *Psychonomic Bulletin and Review*, **12**, 957–68.

Zanto, T. P., Snyder, J. S. and Large, E. W. (2006). Neural correlates of rhythmic expectancy. *Advances in Cognitive Psychology*, **2**, 221–31.

Acknowledgements

Research reported in this chapter was supported by grants from the National Science Foundation (1981–2006). I am grateful to Robert Ellis for comments on earlier versions of this chapter.

Chapter 24

Electrophysiological markers of foreperiod effects

Peter Praamstra

In the long history of studies on foreperiod effects and reaction time, it has been asked whether reaction time constitutes a valid index of covert cognitive processes if this measure is subject to timing variables related to the foreperiod duration (Niemi and Näätänen, 1981). The predominant interest, however, has always been the exploitation of foreperiod effects as an experimental window on preparatory processes mediated by temporal expectations. Relevant physiological measures for the investigation of temporal preparation, used in conjunction with reaction times, include not only measures of brain activity, but also measures such as heart rate and pupillary dilation (eg. Jennings et al., 1998). This chapter will focus on the electroencephalographic (EEG) markers of brain activity used to investigate the brain-based timing mechanisms that presumably underlie temporal preparation as manifested in foreperiod effects. Several different types of marker can be distinguished. One is the slow preparatory brain potential called the contingent negative variation (CNV), and a second type is the modulation of sensory-evoked potentials. The CNV is often regarded as closely related to the timing processes under study, while sensory-evoked potentials index the changes in sensory processing resulting from anticipatory timing. An increasingly important third type is represented by event-related changes in power and phase-relations across different EEG frequency components.

Electrophysiological measures have been used predominantly in explicit timing tasks (Pouthas and Pfeuty, Chapter 30, this volume), i.e. tasks that require participants to judge interval durations (time perception), to produce intervals of a certain duration (time production), or to attend selectively to sensory stimuli occurring in a certain time window (temporal orienting). However, there is a small body of work that has used EEG measures in tasks where timing is manipulated by means of the foreperiod duration, and is incidental to the performance of the task. The chapter is divided into separate sections dealing with implicit timing effects on the CNV, on sensory-evoked potentials, and on oscillatory activity. These are followed by a section on the basal ganglia and timing, and a final section that attempts to relate the electrophysiological findings to models of timing and the neural representation of timing processes.

The CNV as a marker of temporal preparation

Foreperiod effects on reaction time and CNV

In their seminal report on the CNV, Walter and colleagues (1964) described the now well-known features of a sustained potential of negative polarity developing in the interval between a conditional and an imperative stimulus. The paper examined the dependence of the CNV on the contingency of the association between the two stimuli, including an observation that the events that start and terminate the CNV need not be external stimuli, but can be represented by a purely mental judgement of a time interval. This observation established the CNV as a potential marker of timing processes.

The experimental paradigm for eliciting the CNV lends itself in a straightforward way to electrophysiological exploration of foreperiod effects on reaction time. Thus, McAdam and colleagues (1969) addressed the reaction-time effects observed when blocks of trials with a constant foreperiod are compared with other blocks of trials with a different fixed foreperiod. Across blocks of increasing foreperiod duration, reaction times increase, which has been attributed to decreasing accuracy of predicting the time of stimulus presentation. Comparing constant foreperiods of 800ms, 1600ms, and 4800ms, McAdam and co-workers confirmed this reaction-time increase and established a concurrent decrease of CNV amplitude.

When foreperiods vary from trial to trial, instead of between blocks or sessions, the subjective probability of stimulus delivery at any time point will be determined by the probability distribution of different foreperiod durations. Thus, with a rectangular distribution of foreperiod durations, the longest foreperiods yield the fastest response times because the conditional probability of stimulus occurrence, given that it has not yet occurred, increases (Los, Chapter 21; Vallesi, Chapter 22, this volume). In such a variable foreperiod paradigm, with five equiprobable foreperiod durations ranging from 500–900ms (100-ms steps), CNV amplitude was found to increase with foreperiod duration alongside decreases in reaction time (Loveless, 1973). Given that the variable foreperiod effect on reaction time is dependent on the probability distribution of different foreperiod durations, both reaction time and CNV findings should show a different pattern when foreperiod durations have a different probability distribution. Trillenberg and colleagues (2000) compared an aging probability distribution with a non-aging and a Gaussian distribution. Their findings *confirmed* those of Loveless (1973) in that the aging probability distribution (with equiprobable foreperiod durations) produced steadily increasing CNV amplitudes. Their findings *extended* those of Loveless in that CNV amplitude remained constant across foreperiod durations in a non-aging distribution, and reached its highest amplitude with the most frequent foreperiod duration in the Gaussian distribution.

The interpretation of these studies on foreperiod effects and the CNV depends on what is measured by the CNV. While the observations of Walter and colleagues (1964) indicated that the CNV can be elicited without an overt motor response as the terminating event, the CNV has always been considered to be closely associated with the preparation of movement, given the resemblance of the terminal CNV with the readiness potential preceding voluntary movements (Rohrbaugh et al., 1976). From this point of view, the previously discussed studies confirm a relation between reaction times and response readiness (represented by CNV amplitude), demonstrated by the foreperiod effects on reaction time. However, the studies do not substantially contribute to the interpretation that foreperiod effects are produced by temporal expectations. While the Trillenberg and colleagues (2000) study, using different foreperiod distributions, could have contributed to this perspective, its relevance is diminished by the fact that the time-course variations of the CNV, related to different foreperiod distributions, were mediated not by internal timing but by continuous timing information available to the subjects. It is therefore relevant to turn to explicit timing studies for evidence that the CNV can convey information about timing processes in ways that do not rely on response readiness or an inverse relationship between CNV amplitude and reaction time.

CNV in explicit timing tasks

The CNV has been exploited in a variety of different timing tasks, with some of the studies providing clear evidence for timing processes being reflected in the CNV. For instance, Macar and colleagues (1999) showed that in a time-production task where subjects were asked to estimate a target duration of 2.5 seconds by means of two button presses, CNV amplitude correlated with the duration of the produced interval. In a time-discrimination task performed by the same subjects, probe durations judged to be shorter than the target duration led to a smaller CNV amplitude than (equally long) probe durations that were judged too long. These results reveal a relationship between CNV amplitude and perceived or produced time intervals.

Subsequent work began to examine the influence of a memorized duration on the time-course of the CNV elicited by a probe duration that subjects had to compare against the memorized (standard) duration (Macar and Vidal, 2003; Pfeuty et al., 2003; Pouthas and Pfeuty, Chapter 30, this volume). Two sets of results are important for the work on implicit timing to be discussed later. The first concerns the strong impact that a memorized standard exerts on the CNV that accompanies a probe stimulus. As illustrated in Figure 24.1, during the presentation of the probe stimulus, the CNV continues to rise for the duration of the memorized standard, but demonstrates a change in slope when that duration has elapsed, even when the probe stimulus continues (Macar and Vidal 2003; Pfeuty et al., 2003). This result is interpreted as reflecting a comparison process between the memory trace of the standard duration and the probe duration that is actually being presented. This process unfolds until the memorized duration has elapsed and causes the CNV to peak at that time point; during the remaining portion of a longer probe the CNV drops in amplitude as the signal no longer needs to be timed (Macar and Vidal, 2003).

The second set of results also relates to the comparison between a probe and a memorized standard duration. Pfeuty and colleagues (2005; Pouthas and Pfeuty, Chapter 30, this volume) investigated whether the behaviour of the CNV is consistent with predictions of a timing model based on 'climbing neuronal activity'. In this model, neural activity encodes intervals of different

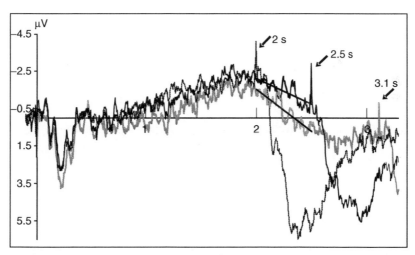

Fig. 24.1 The figure shows the CNV recorded during the presentation of three probe durations (2, 2.5, and 3.1 seconds), which participants compared to a previously presented 2-second duration standard. The figure shows that the CNV continues to rise for the approximate duration of the memorized standard, but then changes in slope even when the probe stimulus is not yet extinguished. Traces are measured from the medial centro-parietal area (electrode CPz) and represent grand averages across 10 subjects. The end of each probe duration, indicated by arrows, is detectable due to a brief artefact. Reproduced with permission from Macar, F. and Vidal, F. (2003). The CNV peak: an index of decision making and temporal memory. *Psychophysiology*, **40**, 950–4.

duration by means of adjustments in the slope of firing rate increases (Durstewitz 2003; Reutimann et al., 2004). Thus, neural activity patterns encoding a short and a longer duration differ in that the slope of firing rate increase is steeper for the short interval, while they peak at the same firing rate. By comparing a range of different test durations against two different standards, Pfeuty and colleagues (2005) established that the CNV peak amplitude at the end of the memorized standard duration was identical for short and long standards.

Both sets of results highlight effects of timing processes on the CNV that are *independent* of motor preparation. The properties of the CNV established in these explicit timing tasks have been exploited in implicit timing tasks, based on manipulation of foreperiod duration, to readdress whether foreperiod effects on reaction time are mediated by temporal expectations.

CNV and implicit timing

In order to demonstrate and investigate the operation of interval timing mechanisms in reaction-time tasks, Praamstra and colleagues (2006) examined whether the timing properties of the CNV also come to the fore when subjects perform an ordinary choice-reaction task with no other requirements than to respond quickly and accurately to each stimulus. To this end, the traditional warned reaction-time task with a foreperiod between warning and reaction stimulus was abandoned. Instead, reaction stimuli, requiring a choice response, were presented at regular intervals and the CNV was measured between successive reaction stimuli. Two manipulations were key to the experiment. First, by varying the interval between reaction stimuli (SOA: stimulus-onset-asynchrony) across different trial series, the design allowed an evaluation of adjustments in slope of the CNV. Second, by introducing a deviant SOA at the end of each trial series, the design allowed an evaluation of the effects of previous 'standard' intervals on the resolution of the CNV in the perturbed interval (see Figure 24.2A). This created a situation similar to the comparison of a probe duration against a memorized standard (cf. Macar and Vidal 2003; Pfeuty et al., 2003, 2005), except that in this case implicit timing effects are measured, as subjects are not required to make an explicit temporal judgement.

If CNV-like slow preparatory brain potentials between successive reaction stimuli are influenced by an implicit timing mechanism, then their slope and time-course should be different for short and long SOA conditions such that the amplitude reached before the next stimulus is the same for short and long SOA conditions. By contrast, if they are not under the control of such a timing mechanism, then the amplitude should be higher for long SOAs than for short SOAs, as the CNV has more time to build up. The results (see Figure 24.2B) show that the CNV between successive stimuli reached a fixed amplitude just before the anticipated termination of the entrained interval. This amplitude was independent of the duration of the interval, since the slope of the CNV was adjusted to the interval after repeated exposure. These results thus resemble the findings reported by Pfeuty and colleagues (2005) in an explicit timing task, showing that CNV activity peaks at the end of a memorized duration, and that its slope varies inversely with the length of this duration.

Note that one could still interpret the development of CNVs with identical amplitude in short and long SOA conditions as merely reflecting the build-up of a non-specific state of motor readiness. However, this interpretation can be rejected on the basis of the behaviour of the CNV during the deviant SOAs. During deviant SOAs that were longer than the preceding standard, the CNV reached its peak around the time of the expected stimulus arrival, and then dropped in amplitude before the delayed stimulus arrived (see Figure 24.2C). This behaviour is similar to that observed when a test duration is judged against a memorized standard of shorter duration (Macar and Vidal, 2003; Pfeuty et al., 2003, 2005), demonstrating that the CNV, in these experimental

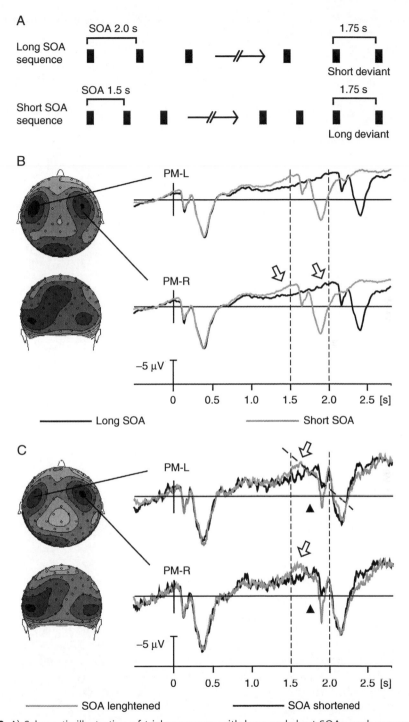

Fig. 24.2 A) Schematic illustration of trial sequences with long and short SOAs, each sequence ending with a final deviant SOA that was longer or shorter than the preceding standard SOA. B) Scalp topography and CNV waveforms in short and long SOA conditions. The waveforms demonstrate an adjustment in slope according to the length of the SOA such that the CNV reaches

Fig. 24.2 (*continued*) the same fixed amplitude (see open arrows) just before the anticipated arrival of the next stimulus, whether the SOA is short or long. Waveforms represent averaged activity of four electrodes overlying the left (PM-L) and right (PM-R) pre-motor cortex activation maxima. Line spacing in the scalp maps is 0.5μV. The dashed lines indicate the 1500-ms and 2000-ms standard SOA durations. C) Effect of the sequence-final timing perturbation on slow brain potentials. The topography of the CNV in the long deviant condition (plotted for the interval 1400–1500ms) is similar to that seen with the standard SOA. The CNV over left and right pre-motor areas peaks around 1600ms (see open arrows), i.e. shortly after the expected time of stimulus arrival, and drops in amplitude before stimulus presentation at 1750ms (indicated by black arrow head). The dashed lines indicate the standard 1500-ms and 2000-ms SOA durations. In the top traces, a regression line is fitted to the downgoing slope of the CNV in the long deviant condition. Line spacing in the scalp maps is 0.5μV. Figure adapted with permission from Praamstra, P., Kourtis, D., Kwok, H. F., and Oostenveld, R. (2006). Neurophysiology of implicit timing in serial choice reaction-time performance. *Journal of Neuroscience*, **26**, 5448–55.

conditions, does not just reflect motor readiness, but expresses the duration of a stored standard interval. As shown here, the standard duration does not need to be learned by explicit memorization of a given time interval, but can consist of a duration learned through repeated presentation of stimuli and/or repeated actions, i.e. through conditioning.

Modulation of sensory-evoked responses by temporal expectancy

The conclusion of the previous section on the CNV is that this slow brain potential is not only a marker of interval timing mechanisms probed in explicit timing tasks; it can also be regarded as a marker of interval timing in tasks where temporal parameters are manipulated in an implicit fashion. These timing processes influence reaction times, as demonstrated by foreperiod effects. A further question is whether, in addition to optimizing the timing of motor responses, it is also the case that processes of interval timing create a window of temporal attention that facilitates sensory processing. This question is answered in the affirmative by work with temporal orienting paradigms (e.g. Lange et al., 2003; Rolke and Ulrich, Chapter 17; Correa, Chapter 26; Lange and Röder, Chapter 28, this volume). Behavioural results with subliminal visual stimulation suggest that implicitly shaped temporal expectations can also influence perceptual processing. For example, Naccache and colleagues (2002) found that priming effects of masked stimuli, which were not consciously recognized, depended on the regular timing of stimulus presentation.

Foreperiod effects on sensory ERP components were not evaluated in early CNV studies discussed earlier, nor in a more recent study (Müller-Gethmann et al., 2003). However, temporal expectation effects on early ERP components were investigated in an elegant study using a naturalistic approach by Doherty and colleagues (2005). Their task created spatial and temporal expectations on the basis of the trajectory and speed of motion of a moving stimulus (Nobre, Chapter 27, this volume). Following temporary disappearance of the stimulus under an occlusion zone on the computer display, evaluation for the presence of a specific visual feature was facilitated when the previous trajectory enabled spatial, temporal, or spatial-temporal prediction of the location and timing of reappearance. In terms of detection speed, effects of temporal and spatial expectation were additive. However, the early P1 visual component revealed a synergistic effect of temporal attention on the spatial attentional modulation of the P1, thus supporting that exogenously driven temporal expectations do influence perceptual processing.

Correa and Nobre (2008) extended this approach to address further questions related to temporal expectation driven by exogenous rhythmic stimulation (Coull, Chapter 31; Nobre, Chapter 27, this volume). As Doherty and colleagues (2005), they induced temporal expectancy by means of regular time steps at which a visual stimulus moved across the display. Reappearance of the stimulus after occlusion was manipulated to be in-step (valid temporal orienting) or out-of-step (invalid temporal orienting) with the established rhythm. Variation of the regular time step between trials (range 200–900ms), in combination with the validity manipulation, created a range of occlusion times split into short, medium, and long categories. It was found that on invalid, but not valid trials, the duration of the occlusion affected the visual N1 amplitude. Specifically, in the 'long' category of occlusion times (where the stimulus predominantly occurred later than expected) the N1 was attenuated relative to the N1 in the 'short' category. This resembles a result of Praamstra and colleagues (2006) who reported an attenuation of the N1 when the eliciting stimulus occurred later than expected on the basis of an entrained rhythm. These data thus provide further confirmation for an effect of temporal expectancy on perceptual processes.

Oscillatory correlates of foreperiod preparation

EEG phenomena linked to movement preparation are not confined to slow brain potentials, but also comprise changes in ongoing oscillatory activity especially in the beta frequency range (see also Kilavik and Riehle, Chapter 19, this volume). Task-related modulations of beta activity consist of a preparatory reduction in power and a post-movement increase, labelled as event-related desynchronization and synchronization, respectively. Beta synchronization and desynchronization are localized to the sensorimotor cortex (Jurkiewicz et al., 2006).

The modulation of beta-range activity during different foreperiod manipulations is largely consistent with effects observed for the CNV, reported in previous sections. Thus, preparatory beta desynchronization, in a task where subjects had to respond with a simple hand movement to a response signal, occurs only when the response signal is presented at regular intervals, allowing temporal prediction. It is not observed when the stimulus occurs at variable intervals (Alegre et al., 2003). This conforms to the presence/absence of the CNV before predictable/unpredictable response signals (Cunnington et al., 1995). When the predictable interval between response signals is varied between conditions, the time-course of both beta desynchronization and the CNV are adjusted to the foreperiod (Praamstra et al., 2006; Praamstra and Pope 2007). In a warned reaction-time task with randomly intermixed foreperiod durations of 1.5, 3, and 4.5 seconds, Alegre et al. (2006) observed a sustained beta desynchronization of growing amplitude with increasing foreperiod duration. This, likewise, is congruent with the CNV amplitude that increases with foreperiod duration, and is assumed to reflect increasing response readiness when the conditional probability of response signal occurrence grows (Loveless 1973; Trillenberg et al., 2000).

It should be noted that the reduction of beta power associated with increasing response readiness is observed not only when reaction signals have an aging probability distribution, i.e. a distribution in which the occurrence becomes gradually more likely if the signal has not yet been presented. Schoffelen and colleagues (2005) contrasted such a distribution (i.e. increasing hazard rate) with a decreasing hazard rate distribution and found that beta power remained inversely related to response readiness. This behaviour of beta activity was exactly opposite to the modulation of gamma activity in the 40–70Hz range, which was found to increase with response readiness. Hazard functions in relation to action are treated more extensively in Chapter 19 by Kilavik and Riehle in this volume.

Whereas modulation of the sensorimotor beta rhythm during foreperiod manipulations has not provided information beyond what is known on the basis of the CNV, this is not the case for the modulation of alpha activity. In spatial attention tasks, the lateral distribution and power of alpha activity over occipital scalp regions has been found to vary with the direction of spatial attention. When spatial attention is cued for the occurrence of a stimulus in one visual hemifield, alpha activity increases over the ipsilateral occipital cortex in order to reduce the sensitivity to input from the non-attended hemifield (Worden et al., 2000), while alpha activity is reduced over the contralateral occipital cortex in order to facilitate input from the attended field (Kelly et al., 2006). As for temporal attention, there is evidence that temporal expectancies based on foreperiod duration can also affect occipital alpha power and influence the processing of visual input. In the implicit-timing task described earlier (see Figure 24.2A), Praamstra and colleagues (2006) found a modulation of occipital alpha activity during perturbations of the standard foreperiod duration. Specifically, alpha activity diverged in amplitude between conditions where the foreperiod was shortened and where it was lengthened. In the latter case, alpha activity showed a sharp drop in amplitude at the expected time of occurrence of the reaction signal. At the same time, the visual-evoked N1 response to the delayed reaction signal was attenuated, indicating that perturbed timing of the reaction signal affected its perceptual processing. The drop in alpha-band amplitude, combined with the reduction of the visual-evoked response amplitude, could suggest that the reduction of alpha activity *terminates* a state of heightened sensitivity around the time of expected stimulation. However, reduction of alpha activity is usually considered to facilitate active information processing (eg. Fries et al., 2001; Klimesch et al., 2007), and to be beneficial to visual detection and discrimination performance. It is therefore also possible that the observed reduction of alpha *initiated* a window in which temporal attention facilitated sensory processing. This reduction would normally (when an expected stimulus is not delayed) go unnoticed due to stimulus-related effects on alpha amplitude.

The modulation of occipital alpha activity by temporal attention was not observed in a similar study with older subjects and patients with Parkinson's disease (Praamstra and Pope 2007), possibly indicating a sensitivity to age. There are, however, related observations of anticipatory phase adjustments of alpha activity (Barry et al., 2004). Importantly, these instances of a modulation of occipital alpha activity by temporal expectation underline that temporal preparation is not exclusive to the motor domain.

Timing and the basal ganglia: electrophysiological markers of foreperiod effects in Parkinson's disease

Foreperiod effects demonstrate that performance in behavioural tasks is influenced by temporal expectations that are shaped by the temporal structure of the task. As seen in previous sections, such implicit temporal preparation is reflected in slow brain potentials, in sensory-evoked potentials, and in EEG oscillations. This preparation is attributed to interval timing mechanisms that are widely regarded as dependent on intact basal ganglia function. It is, therefore, of interest to evaluate temporal preparation and associated electrophysiological indices in Parkinson's disease, which is caused by basal ganglia dysfunction related to degeneration of dopamine producing cells in the substantia nigra.

A role for the basal ganglia in the processing of temporal information is supported by animal models of striatal dysfunction and neuropharmacological experiments (MacDonald and Meck 2004; Buhusi and Meck 2005) and by human functional neuroimaging (Rao et al., 2001; Coull et al., 2004; Jahanshahi et al., 2006). Consistent with a timing function of the basal ganglia, patients with Parkinson's disease display abnormal performance in motor and perceptual timing tasks (eg. Pastor et al., 1992; O'Boyle et al., 1996) although normal timing performance has also been reported (Schnider et al., 1995; Spencer and Ivry, 2005). As for temporal expectancies underlying foreperiod effects, there is evidence suggesting that these partly rely on the same substrate as interval timing mechanisms (MacDonald and Meck 2004), thus predicting that foreperiod effects and associated electrophysiological markers are altered in Parkinson's disease.

Cunnington and colleagues (1995) examined preparatory slow brain potentials in Parkinson's disease patients in a task that contrasted predictably timed versus variably timed reaction signals. Control subjects demonstrated preparatory slow brain potentials preceding predictably timed reaction signals. However, such activity was absent in Parkinson's patients, although they did show preparatory activity when they produced the movements without timing cues. The authors concluded that patients are deficient in anticipatory temporal control of movements, a function they assumed relies on the supplementary motor area. In contrast to the results of Cunnington and co-workers, Jahanshahi et al. (1995) did not find differences in pre-movement slow brain potentials between Parkinson's patients and controls when they made externally cued movements in response to a predictably timed response signal occurring at ~3-second intervals.

Praamstra and Pope (2007) investigated implicit temporal expectations in Parkinson's disease, applying the same implicit timing paradigm as Praamstra and colleagues (2006), illustrated in Figure 24.2A. In elderly control subjects, adjustments in task timing manifested themselves in the slope and rise time of the CNV, as they had done in younger subjects performing the same task (Praamstra et al, 2006) (see Figure 24.2B). By contrast, in Parkinson's patients there was no CNV as such, a result similar to that reported by Cunnington and colleagues (1995) for EEG activity preceding predictably timed reaction signals. This result suggests that Parkinson's patients did not engage in temporal preparation, although it does not imply that this was due to impaired interval timing related to their basal ganglia dysfunction. Indeed, during perturbations of the standard inter-stimulus interval, patients, as well as controls, showed an abrupt drop in CNV amplitude at the time of expected stimulus arrival when the inter-stimulus interval had actually been lengthened. This suggests that, even in the absence of CNV indices of temporal preparation, patients built up a representation of the inter-stimulus interval duration, enabling the neural detection of the deviant interval.

In the same investigation, deficient temporal preparation was also revealed in time-frequency analyses of task-related changes in alpha and beta band power. In essence, a biphasic desynchronization/synchronization pattern of alpha and beta activity modulation in control subjects was replaced by a monophasic desynchronization pattern of modulation. That is, patients showed an attenuated or absent synchronization phase and very little *anticipatory* desynchronization, but still a brisk and high amplitude desynchronization response *following* the reaction stimuli. This was particularly pronounced for alpha activity over posterior brain regions. The lack of anticipatory desynchronization indicates that task-relevant neural populations were released from background oscillatory activity to engage in visual and motor processes in a largely stimulus-driven fashion, rather than in a predictive mode. Likewise, the reduced (beta band) or absent (alpha band) synchronization indicates that the recruitment back into ensemble oscillatory activity was clearly abnormal (Praamstra and Pope, 2007).

Together, these abnormal foreperiod effects show that patients with Parkinson's disease do not spontaneously engage in temporal preparation in a context in which temporal regularity would strongly encourage such preparation. However, this seems to be due not to compromised interval timing per se but rather to a failure to exploit temporal information. Such a dissociation might be explained in terms of abnormal implicit learning and habit formation related to basal ganglia dysfunction (Graybiel, 1995; Knowlton et al., 1996).

How do electrophysiological results inform psychological and neural models of timing?

Early studies using the CNV to investigate foreperiod effects interpreted amplitude variations of this component in terms of 'preparatory set' (Loveless, 1973) or 'level of expectancy' (McAdam et al., 1969). Later studies using the CNV in explicit timing tasks exploited information derived from its scalp distribution to argue for a major contribution of the supplementary motor area (SMA) to generation of the CNV (e.g. Macar et al., 1999). Strengthened by neuroimaging evidence that the SMA subserves timing functions (for review see Macar et al., 2002), this suggested a direct link between the CNV and timing functions. This relation has been framed in terms of a pacemaker-accumulator model of interval timing, which posits an internal clock or pacemaker that emits regular pulses that are stored in an accumulator for comparison with a reference memory (cf. Buhusi and Meck 2005). Specifically, the SMA has been proposed to represent the accumulator, storing the pulse units and acting as working memory for temporal information (Macar et al., 2002; see also Pfeuty et al., 2005). In this view, the basal ganglia represent the internal clock, projecting to the SMA via basal ganglia-thalamocortical pathways. Similarly, Cunnington et al. (1995) regarded basal ganglia-thalamocortical loops through the SMA as vital for temporal prediction in sequential motor tasks and the SMA as the main generator for the associated pre-movement EEG activity.

According to current standards of EEG source reconstruction, the previously discussed studies do not provide very strong evidence for the claim that the SMA accounted for timing-related modulations of the CNV. Perhaps the more important question, however, is whether the CNV data support the existence of a specialized neural module or system for interval timing. Relevant to this question is the observation that implicit timing effects on the time course of the CNV (Praamstra et al., 2006; Praamstra and Pope 2007) replicated similar effects found in explicit timing tasks (Macar et al., 1999; Pfeuty et al., 2005). However, unlike in explicit timing tasks, these effects originated in lateral premotor structures instead of the SMA, as established on the basis of high-resolution EEG methods. The involvement of lateral premotor structures is in keeping with data from primate neurophysiology (Mauritz and Wise 1986) and human functional neuroimaging on event predictability (Schubotz et al., 2000; Schubotz and Von Cramon 2001; Schubotz, Chapter 25; Coull, Chapter 31, this volume). The divergence suggests that distinct cortical substrates implement similar timing mechanisms for different behaviours. This is still compatible with a specialized timing system if these different cortical substrates show the same effects by virtue of their participation in basal ganglia-thalamocortical circuits that implement a flexible, general-purpose timing function (Buhusi and Meck, 2005), with parts of the basal ganglia acting as a 'core timer' (Meck et al., 2008).

While existing CNV data are certainly compatible with a distributed specialized timing system, they do not exclude the possibility that temporal information is processed in a local task-dependent manner. As previously observed by Pfeuty and colleagues (2005), the temporal processing exhibited in the CNV resembles the anticipatory behaviour of delay period sustained activity recorded in neurons from frontal (Niki and Watanabe, 1979; Akkal et al., 2004), parietal (Leon and Shadlen, 2003), and thalamic neurons (Komura et al., 2001). Both demonstrate a temporal profile characterized by climbing neuronal activity (Durstewitz, 2003; Reutimann et al., 2004). Like the CNV, the slope of climbing activity changes as the typical interval between relevant events changes. Moreover, both the CNV and climbing activity suddenly drop when an anticipated stimulus (or predicted reward) does not occur at the expected time (Komura et al., 2001; Durstewitz, 2003). These similarities between the CNV and delay period activity across different neural structures may be interpreted as an argument in favour of local task-dependent computation of temporal information.

Conclusions: an oscillatory perspective

In the preceding sections of this review, slow brain potentials, sensory-evoked responses, and task-related modulations of oscillatory activity were dealt with as distinct neurophysiological phenomena. However, recent work on the generation of evoked responses has assigned an important role to phase-resetting of spontaneously occurring oscillations as a possible generator mechanism (e.g. Makeig et al., 2002). Lakatos and colleagues (2008) have proposed that this account might be extended to include the generation of the CNV. Their work further proposes that entrainment of oscillations acts as a mechanism for attentional selection (Schroeder and Lakatos, 2009). Since this potentially provides a more unified perspective on electrophysiological implicit timing phenomena related to foreperiod effects, this chapter ends with a brief discussion of this recent work.

Recording local field potentials and multiunit activity in the macaque primary auditory cortex, Lakatos and co-workers (2005) provided evidence for what they refer to as the 'oscillatory hierarchy hypothesis'. According to this hypothesis, the amplitude of oscillations at different frequencies is modulated by the phase of a local, lower frequency oscillation. This nested structure of oscillations holds for delta waves up to gamma range frequencies. Given that oscillatory activity reflects cyclical change in neural excitability, an entrainment of the oscillatory hierarchy to rhythmic stimulus components in the environment may optimize stimulus processing. Lakatos and co-workers confirmed the hierarchical structure of EEG oscillations and the entrainment of ongoing slow delta activity to the timing of stimulus presentation. Moreover, they confirmed that nested higher frequency oscillations are associated with changes in excitability and concomitant changes in responsiveness to stimulation. In subsequent work, Lakatos and colleagues (2008) showed that selective attention can shift entrainment of the oscillatory hierarchy between different concurrent rhythmic event streams so that high-excitability phases will coincide with events in the attended stimulus stream.

Lakatos and colleagues (2008) speculated that the warning signal in an explicit temporal orienting task resets frontal slow wave activity, thus generating the CNV. It is clear from the preceding sections in this chapter that existing CNV data already provide support for this proposal. In particular, CNV data from implicit timing tasks (Praamstra et al., 2006; Praamstra and Pope, 2007) and from sequential motor tasks with predictable stimuli (Cunnington et al., 1995) might be viewed as instances of entrainment of slow oscillations to rhythmic events. Resetting and entrainment effects on slow oscillations might also play a role in the sequential influence (Los, Chapter 21, this volume) that one foreperiod duration can exert on temporal expectations operating during a subsequent foreperiod of a different duration. Moreover, hierarchical cross-frequency coupling (Lakatos et al., 2005) provides a basis for the explanation of temporal attention effects on sensory-evoked responses, both in explicit temporal orienting tasks (e.g. Lange et al., 2003) and implicit timing tasks (Doherty et al., 2005; Praamstra et al., 2006; Correa and Nobre 2008).

The entrainment effects on slow EEG rhythms observed by Lakatos and co-workers were recorded in the auditory and visual cortex, i.e. areas that are not regarded as important to the generation of the CNV. However, there is a notion that the distribution of the CNV is influenced by the sensory modality of the warning and imperative signal. In the implicit timing task of Praamstra and colleagues (2006), in which visual stimuli were presented at regular inter-stimulus intervals, the scalp distribution of the CNV was characterized not only by bilateral frontal maxima, but also contained discrete maxima over the lateral occipital cortex (see Figure 24.2). This distribution is obviously in line with entrainment to the visual reaction stimulus and leads one to expect a different distribution for reaction stimuli in another modality.

Overall, the work reviewed in this chapter demonstrates that the investigation of temporal preparation is still influenced by early reaction time studies of foreperiod effects. At the same time, neurophysiological investigations of the timing mechanisms underlying such effects have evolved beyond the classical foreperiod paradigm. The results of these investigations not only underline the importance of temporal preparation; they also begin to be relevant to questions such as whether the processing of temporal information is organized in a localized or a distributed manner, and whether timing is under the control of a specialized system or is task-dependent. Scalp-recorded EEG methods provide the means to study the neurophysiology of timing processes in humans and show promise for making a significant contribution to further investigations of the role of entrainment and phase resetting of spontaneous EEG oscillations in timing and temporal attention.

References

Akkal, D., Escola, L., Bioulac, B., and Burbaud, P. (2004). Time predictability modulates pre-supplementary motor area neuronal activity. *Neuroreport*, **15**, 1283–6.

Alegre, M., Gurtubay, I. G., Labarga, A., Iriarte, J., Malanda, A., and Artieda, J. (2003). Alpha and beta oscillatory changes during stimulus-induced movement paradigms: effect of stimulus predictability. *Neuroreport*, **14**, 381–5.

Alegre, M., Imirizaldu, L., Valencia, M., Iriarte, J., Arcocha, J., and Artieda, J. (2006). Alpha and beta changes in cortical oscillatory activity in a go/no go randomly-delayed-response choice reaction time paradigm. *Clinical Neurophysiology*, **117**, 16–25.

Barry, R. J., Rushby, J. A., Johnstone, S. J., Clarke, A. R., Croft, R. J., and Lawrence, C. A. (2004). Event-related potentials in the auditory oddball as a function of EEG alpha phase at stimulus onset. *Clinical Neurophysiology*, **115**, 2593–601.

Buhusi, C. V. and Meck, W. H. (2005). What makes us tick? Functional and neural mechanisms if interval timing. *Nature Reviews Neuroscience*, **6**, 755–65.

Correa, A. and Nobre, A. C. (2008). Neural modulation by regularity and passage of time. *Journal of Neurophysiology*, **100**, 1649–55.

Coull, J. T., Vidal, F., Nazarian, B., and Macar, F. (2004). Functional anatomy of the attentional modulation of time estimation. *Science*, **303**, 1506–8.

Cunnington, R., Iansek, R., Bradshaw, J. L., and Phillips, J. G. (1995). Movement-related potentials in Parkinson's disease. Presence and predictability of temporal and spatial cues. *Brain*, **118**, 935–50.

Doherty, J. R., Rao, A., Mesulam, M. M., and Nobre, A. C. (2005). Synergistic effect of combined temporal and spatial expectations on visual attention. *Journal of Neuroscience*, **25**, 8259–66.

Durstewitz, D. (2003). Self-organizing neural integrator predicts interval times through climbing activity. *Journal of Neuroscience*, **23**, 5342–53.

Fries, P., Reynolds, J. H., Rorie, A. E., and Desimone, R. (2001). Modulation of oscillatory neuronal synchronization by selective visual attention. *Science*, **291**, 1560–3.

Graybiel, A. M. (1995). Building action repertoires: memory and learning functions of the basal ganglia. *Current Opinion in Neurobiology*, **5**, 733–41.

Jahanshahi, M., Jenkins, I. H., Brown, R. G., Marsden, C. D., Passingham, R. E., and Brooks, D. J. (1995). Self-initiated versus externally triggered movements. I. An investigation using measurement of regional cerebral blood flow with PET and movement-related potentials in normal and Parkinson's disease subjects. *Brain*, **118**, 913–33.

Jahanshahi, M., Jones, C. R., Dirnberger, G., and Frith, C. D. (2006).The substantia nigra pars compacta and temporal processing. *Journal of Neuroscience*, **26**, 12266–73.

Jennings, J. R., van der Molen, M. W., S and teinhauer, S. R. (1998). Preparing the heart, eye, and brain: foreperiod length effects in a nonaging paradigm. *Psychophysiology*, **35**, 90–8.

Jurkiewicz, M. T., Gaetz, W. C., Bostan, A. C., and Cheyne, D. (2006). Post-movement beta rebound is generated in motor cortex: evidence from neuromagnetic recordings. *Neuroimage*, **32**, 1281–9.

Kelly, S. P., Lalor, E. C., Reilly, R. B., and Foxe, J. J. (2006). Increases in alpha oscillatory power reflect an active retinotopic mechanism for distracter suppression during sustained visuospatial attention. *Journal of Neurophysiology*, **95**, 3844–51.

Klimesch, W., Sauseng, P., and Hanslmayr, S. (2007). EEG alpha oscillations: The inhibition-timing hypothesis. *Brain Research Brain Research Reviews*, **53**, 63–88.

Knowlton, B. J., Mangels, J. A., and Squire, L. R. (1996). A neostriatal habit learning system in humans. *Science*, **273**, 1399–402.

Komura, Y., Tamura, R., Uwano, T., Nishijo, H., Kaga, K., and Ono, T. (2001). Retrospective and prospective coding for predicted reward in the sensory thalamus. *Nature*, **412**, 546–9.

Lakatos, P., Shah, A. S., Knuth, K. H., Ulbert, I., Karmos, G., and Schroeder, C. E. (2005). An oscillatory hierarchy controlling neuronal excitability and stimulus processing in the auditory cortex. *Journal of Neurophysiology*, **94**, 1904–11.

Lakatos, P., Karmos, G., Mehta, A. D., Ulbert, I., and Schroeder, C. E. (2008). Entrainment of neuronal oscillations as a mechanism of attentional selection. *Science*, **320**, 110–13.

Lange, K., Rösler, F., and Röder, B. (2003). Early processing stages are modulated when auditory stimuli are presented at an attended moment in time: an event-related potential study. *Psychophysiology*, **40**, 806–17.

Leon, M. I. and Shadlen, M. N. (2003). Representation of time by neurons in the posterior parietal cortex of the macaque. *Neuron*, **38**, 317–27.

Loveless, N. E. (1973). The contingent negative variation related to preparatory set in a reaction time situation with variable foreperiod. *Electroencephalography and Clinical Neurophysiology*, **35**, 369–74.

Macar, F. and Vidal, F. (2003). The CNV peak: an index of decision making and temporal memory. *Psychophysiology*, **40**, 950–4.

Macar, F., Vidal, F., and Casini, L. (1999). The supplementary motor area in motor and sensory timing: evidence from slow brain potential changes. *Experimental Brain Research*, **125**, 271–80.

Macar, F., Lejeune, H., Bonnet, M., Ferrara, A., Pouthas, V., Vidal, F., and Maquet, P. (2002). Activation of the supplementary motor area and of attentional networks during temporal processing. *Experimental Brain Research*, **142**, 475–85.

McAdam, D. W., Knott, J. R., and Rebert, C. S. (1969). Cortical slow potential changes in man related to interstimulus intevval and to pre-trial prediction of interstimulus interval. *Psychophysiology*, **5**, 349–58.

MacDonald, C. J. and Meck, W. H. (2004). Systems-level integration of interval timing and reaction time. *Neuroscience and Biobehavioral Reviews*, **28**, 747–69.

Makeig, S., Westerfield, M., Jung, T.P., Enghoff, S., Townsend, J., Courchesne, E., et al. (2002). Dynamic brain sources of visual evoked responses. *Science*, **295**, 690–4.

Mauritz, K. H. and Wise, S. P. (1986). Premotor cortex of the rhesus monkey: neuronal activity in anticipation of predictable environmental events. *Experimental Brain Research*, **61**, 229–44.

Müller-Gethmann, H., Ulrich, R., and Rinkenauer, G. (2003). Locus of the effect of temporal preparation: evidence from the lateralized readiness potential. *Psychophysiology*, **40**, 597–611.

Naccache, L., Blandin, E., and Dehaene, S. (2002). Unconscious masked priming depends on temporal attention. *Psychological Science*, **13**, 416–24.

Niemi, P. and Näätänen, R. (1981). Foreperiod and simple reaction time. *Psychological Bulletin*, **89**, 133–62.

Niki, H. and Watanabe, M. (1979). Prefrontal and cingulate unit activity during timing behavior in the monkey. *Brain Research*, **171**, 213–24.

O'Boyle, D. J., Freeman, J. S., and Cody, F. W. (1996). The accuracy and precision of timing of self-paced, repetitive movements in subjects with Parkinson's disease. *Brain*, **119**, 51–70.

Pastor, M. A., Artieda, J., Jahanshahi, M., and Obeso, J. A. (1992). Time estimation and reproduction is abnormal in Parkinson's disease. *Brain*, **115**, 211–25.

Pfeuty, M., Ragot, R., and Pouthas, V. (2003). When time is up: CNV time course differentiates the roles of the hemispheres in the discrimination of short tone durations. *Experimental Brain Research*, **151**, 372–9.

Pfeuty, M., Ragot, R., and Pouthas, V. (2005). Relationship between CNV and timing of an upcoming event. *Neuroscience Letters*, **382**, 106–11.

Praamstra, P. and Pope, P. (2007). Slow brain potential and oscillatory EEG manifestations of impaired temporal preparation in Parkinson's disease. *Journal of Neurophysiology*, **98**, 2848–57.

Praamstra, P., Kourtis, D., Kwok, H. F., and Oostenveld, R. (2006). Neurophysiology of implicit timing in serial choice reaction-time performance. *Journal of Neuroscience*, **26**, 5448–55.

Reutimann, J., Yakovlev, V., Fusi, S., and Senn, W. (2004). Climbing neuronal activity as an event-based cortical representation of time. *Journal of Neuroscience*, **24**, 3295–303.

Rao, S. M., Mayer, A. R., and Harrington, D. L. (2001). The evolution of brain activation during temporal processing. *Nature Neuroscience*, **4**, 317–23.

Rohrbaugh, J. W., Syndulko, K., and Lindsley, D. B. (1976). Brain wave components of the contingent negative variation in humans. *Science*, **191**, 1055–7.

Schnider, A., Gutbrod, K., and Hess, C. W. (1995). Motion imagery in Parkinson's disease. *Brain*, **118**, 485–93.

Schoffelen, J. M., Oostenveld, R., and Fries, P. (2005). Neuronal coherence as a mechanism of effective corticospinal interaction. *Science*, **308**, 111–13.

Schroeder, C. E. and Lakatos, P. (2009). Low frequency neuronal oscillations as instruments of sensory selection. *Trends in Neuroscience*, **32**, 9–18.

Schubotz, R. I. and von Cramon, D. Y. (2001). Interval and ordinal properties of sequences are associated with distinct premotor areas. *Cerebral Cortex*, **11**, 210–22.

Schubotz, R. I., Friederici, A. D., and von Cramon, D. Y. (2000). Time perception and motor timing: a common cortical and subcortical basis revealed by fMRI. *Neuroimage*, **11**, 1–12.

Spencer, R. M. and Ivry, R. B. (2005). Comparison of patients with Parkinson's disease or cerebellar lesions in the production of periodic movements involving event-based or emergent timing. *Brain and Cognition*, **58**, 84–93.

Trillenberg, P., Verleger, R., Wascher, E., Wauschkuhn, B., and Wessel, K. (2000). CNV and temporal uncertainty with aging and non-aging S1-S2 intervals. *Clinical Neurophysiology*, **111**, 1216–26.

Walter, W. G., Cooper, R., Aldridge, V. J., McCallum, W. C., and Winter, A. L. (1964). Contingent negative variation: an electric sign of sensorimotor association and expectancy in the human brain. *Nature*, **203**, 380–4.

Worden, M. S., Foxe, J. J., Wang, N., and Simpson, G.V. (2000). Anticipatory biasing of visuospatial attention indexed by retinotopically specific alpha-band electroencephalography increases over occipital cortex. *Journal of Neuroscience*, **20**, RC63.

Chapter 25

Neural bases of rhythm prediction

Ricarda I. Schubotz

When we perceive a rhythm we are often able to anticipate upcoming temporal structure on the basis of the temporal structure given by the first few seconds heard or observed (see also Jones, Chapter 23, this volume). The ability to predict a rhythm becomes especially manifest when we synchronize our movements to it, for instance by tapping or nodding. In everyday life, we display more or less accurate rhythm prediction for tuning-in behaviour in many situations: we dance to music, enter escalators, adapt to the flow of the traffic when crossing a street, and walk side by side with a friend. Rhythmic information is inherent to so many situations in our daily routines that we are mostly unaware of the fact that we engage in the prediction of external rhythms or adapt our movements and actions to them. It is obvious that we could not plan our actions or even survive in a continuously changing environment if we did not engage in rhythm prediction and timing.

What renders rhythm prediction a particularly exciting topic for brain research is that it seems to span diametrically opposed sides of so many processes: it seems very closely related to basic motor functions but, at the same time, can be flexibly applied to many situations including cultural behaviours such as dance or music. It is most often applied without our particular notice or even our awareness but it can call for all of our attentional resources, and then can be as exhausting as it is pleasurable.

From an information-processing perspective, rhythms can be conceptualized as combining interval and ordinal information, i.e. they instantiate serial orders of (empty or filled) temporal intervals. From an ontological point of view, rhythms are classified as events (as opposed to, for example, objects or facts), which means that they behave like processes and are temporally extended and structured. These two perspectives represent different approaches for investigating rhythm prediction as a cognitive function: on the one hand, rhythm prediction can be considered a special case of *sequential* prediction, and on the other hand, rhythm prediction can be seen as akin to the prediction of dynamics and actions, i.e. another exemplification of inanimate or animate *events*.

From either perspective, it is evident that prediction of rhythm pertains to cognitive functions that are suggestive of an 'internal model' (also 'simulation' or 'emulation') framework. The application of internal models across a wide range of motor and non-motor cognitive functions was put forward by Wolpert and Flanagan (2001) and furthered by a discussion in *Behavioral and Brain Sciences* initiated by the philosopher Rick Grush (2004). Originally developed in applied mathematics and cybernetics to describe the behaviour of dynamic systems, internal models have since been proposed to guide anticipatory computations that make us faster and more efficient in many cognitive and behavioural domains. The core architecture, in which an internal forward model (or predictor) is embedded, comprises a controller that sends efferent copies to the predictor, which converts them to mock (i.e. hypothesized or modelled) re-afferents that are then sent to a comparator module; there, mock re-afferents are matched on-line to real afferent input from the environment. Depending on the current learning stage, mismatches between mock and real afferents are interpreted to signal that either the subject's own expectations (forward models) are still deficient, or that the environment has changed unexpectedly.

Conceiving of rhythm perception as a kind of anticipatory computation such as event prediction, action planning, or serial learning, implies common roots for these functions with respect to their cerebral implementation. In the last decade, we have conducted several studies using functional magnetic resonance imaging (fMRI) to understand the neural basis for rhythm prediction. The paradigm that was used, in various versions, is called the Serial Prediction Task (SPT, Schubotz 1999). A sequence of visual or auditory stimuli is presented, with presentation durations of stimuli typically ranging from about 200–1800ms. Sequences are usually structured in a predictable manner, comprising either repetitive (1–2–3–1–2–3 . . .) or monotonous (1–2–3–4–5 . . . or 1–1–1 . . .) subsequences, or hybrids thereof. Subjects are asked to attend to the order of stimuli and to try to predict upcoming stimuli on that basis. In order to control subjects' engagement in the prediction process, a forced-choice task is implemented at the end of each trial where subjects have to indicate by button press whether or not the sequence developed or ended as predicted. Target detection tasks or serial match-to-sample tasks are used as control conditions that place equal demands on perception, alertness, and response selection, but have no requirement in terms of prediction. That is, the temporal relationship between consecutive stimuli is task-irrelevant in the control condition.

Depending on the study and question at hand, brain activation was analysed for two phases of interest: the phase in which subjects tried to predict upcoming stimuli, and the moment of sequential deviance, i.e. the violation of expectation (occurring in half of the trials). In computational terms, the former task phase reflects slow but flexible unsupervised learning (cf. Doya, 1999) of sequential information, whereas the latter relates to a mismatch in the 'comparator'. While we have recently started to investigate the latter question (Bubic et al., 2008), the bulk of our fMRI studies focused on the prediction interval. One of our major aims was to find out which influence the property (such as its duration, its colour, or its position) of the stimulus (based on which prediction is made) has on the haemodynamic activity pattern. To this end, we investigated prediction on the basis of spatial, object, and pitch information as well as prediction of rhythm information, using abstract (i.e. not meaningful or natural) stimuli in the visual or auditory domains. The following will mainly focus on the specificity of rhythm prediction (as opposed to other kinds of prediction).

Rhythm prediction was found to correlate with an over-proportional increase of metabolism in the inferior portion of the lateral ventral premotor cortex (Schubotz et al., 2000, 2003; Schubotz and von Cramon, 2001a; Wolfensteller et al., 2007; see also Coull, Chapter 31, this volume). Activation encompassed parts of Brodmann area (BA) 6 (i.e. the inferior precentral sulcus extending up to the crown of the precentral gyrus while excluding the central sulcus) as well as BA 44 (ventral portions of the pars opercularis of the inferior frontal gyrus). Activation was always bilateral and it was absolutely robust across all studies related to rhythm prediction. Further activations were found in the supplementary motor area (SMA), the striatum, and the lateral cerebellum (cf. O'Reilly et al., 2008), but with larger variance across studies and with stepwise decreasing effect size.

Considering fMRI studies on rhythm prediction in more detail, one of the first findings was that corresponding brain activity was largely independent of input modality and, perhaps even more interesting, that activation patterns suggested rhythm prediction to be a special case of (event) prediction in general (Schubotz and von Cramon, 2001a; Schubotz et al., 2003). Thus, when comparing rhythm prediction to object-based or spatial prediction, we showed that the entire lateral premotor cortex was engaged in each of these tasks but with a significant variation in the local maximum of the activity. Specifically, we found the inferior ventral premotor cortex,

Rhythm > position, object

Z > 3.09

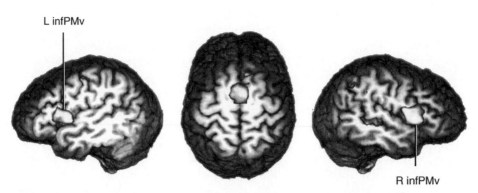

Fig. 25.1 Rhythm prediction (contrasted with object-based and spatial prediction) reveals significant engagement of the inferior ventral premotor cortex (infPMv), an area related to vocal and articulatory control. Concurrent activation is most often seen in the supplementary motor area (SMA), striatum, and cerebellar cortex. L = left, R = right. Adapted with permission from Wolfensteller, U., Schubotz, R. I., and von Cramon, D. Y. (2007). Understanding non-biological dynamics with your own premotor system. *Neuroimage*, **36**(Suppl 2), T33–43.

superior ventral premotor cortex, and dorsal premotor cortex to be most engaged in rhythm-based, object-based, and space-based prediction, respectively (Figure 25.1).

A further difference between rhythm prediction and other kinds of prediction is that duration is an *intrinsically* dynamic stimulus property and hence attention to rhythm is probably predictive by nature. This concept was substantiated in a recent fMRI study in which the effect of predictability of stimulus sequences was investigated without explicitly instructing the subjects to make predictions (Schubotz and von Cramon, 2005). We presented sequences of pictures that were either ordered (repetitions or alternations) or random with regard to their object properties, spatial properties, or rhythmic properties. We asked subjects to respond to each picture immediately in a forced-choice response mode. In the rhythm task, they were asked to judge whether a picture was 'long' (400ms) or 'short' (100ms). In the object task, they had to indicate whether the picture was a 'square' or a 'circle'; and finally, in the position task, 'horizontal' versus 'vertical' arrangements of shapes were to be indicated. It should be noted that, in contrast to the serial prediction tasks, sequential order of stimuli was task-irrelevant. As a result, only the timing task was found to trigger activation in the premotor cortex (namely its inferior ventral part, in line with previous findings). Interestingly, this activation was found for both predictable (regular) and non-predictable (random) rhythms. These findings show that merely focusing attention on temporal duration is sufficient to trigger premotor activation, which is indistinguishable from premotor activation during rhythm prediction. It is important to note that premotor activation vanished for the object-based and spatial tasks, corroborating by analogy a predictive account for timing tasks.

How can we make sense of fMRI findings on rhythm prediction? The most robustly activated area in rhythm prediction, the inferior ventral premotor area, is known to function in the representation of vocal configurations (Tonkonogy and Goodglass, 1981; Dronkers, 1996; Fox et al., 1996; R. J. Wise et al., 1999; Fadiga et al., 2002). The extension from BA 6 inferiorly into the frontal opercular cortex, and adjacent to the anterior insula, is called the precentral operculum (Peters and Jones, 1985) and contains a face representation. In combination with the inferior ventrolateral premotor cortex, it is taken to be implicated in the organization of complex behaviours related to the face, mouth, and fingers. In humans, activations in this region were reported for rhythmic pattern production in singing (Perry et al., 1999; Riecker et al., 2000; Ozdemir et al., 2006; Kleber et al., 2007), as well as for rhythmic pattern rehearsal in speech (Riecker et al., 2002).

Thus, obviously, a *motor-related network* is engaged during rhythm prediction, including cortical and subcortical structures that are typically found for the performance, observation, and imagery of articulation and vocalization (for references, see Schubotz and von Cramon, 2003).[1] The same applies to object-based and spatial prediction, with the difference that the motor functions of these areas are related to grasping and manipulation in the former case and to reaching in the latter. In order to interpret these differences (and similarities) between rhythm, object-based, and spatial prediction, macaque studies can be considered. They show that the premotor cortex contains a variety of differently tuned sensorimotor neurons (Fadiga et al., 2000); their regional prevalence points to spatially tuned neurons prevailing in dorsal premotor sites (e.g. Lebedev and Wise, 2001) and object-tuned neurons in ventral premotor sites (e.g. Rizzolatti et al., 2002). However, while spatial and object-based prediction thus match the regional functional tuning in macaque premotor cortex, no experimental evidence exists for rhythm-tuned neurons in macaque inferior ventral premotor cortex. Unfortunately, there are no brain studies on macaques' rhythm perception (although it has been behaviourally demonstrated that, for example, New World monkeys use rhythmic cues in perception; Ramus et al., 2000; Tincoff et al., 2005).

Moreover, as recently discussed (Schubotz et al., 2008), most single-cell and anatomical-connection studies on premotor areas, neglect the inferior-most part of the postarcuate region. Therefore, it is very difficult to estimate whether the inferior ventral premotor cortex that is typically activated during rhythm and pitch prediction in humans is comparable to monkey area 6V or rather to a dysgranular area that has been referred to as 6bβ (Vogt and Vogt, 1919) or as the precentral operculum (as mentioned earlier) (Roberts and Akert, 1963; Preuss and Goldman-Rakic, 1989). A further potential barrier we face when trying to benefit from comparative models arises from the fact that macaque monkeys have not evolved the capacity of language; yet language and speech evolution in humans are likely to have called for further development, and even quantitative increase of audiomotor neurons in the premotor area controlling speech and articulation. This difference clearly limits the cross-species comparability of man and macaque.

From a conceptual perspective, a plausible explanation for finding 'motor areas' being engaged by rhythm prediction is that forward models are exploited not only for dynamics that we control (i.e. our action) but also for those that we don"t (e.g. the actions of others, or the rhythm of external sources, such as music or escalators). This view generalizes a predictive account from action to event perception (HAPEM framework, Schubotz, 2007). With regard to the inferior ventral premotor cortex, it is postulated that this region houses sensorimotor neurons that are tuned to transformations in the domain of temporal duration (i.e. acceleration and deceleration) and transformations in the domain of pitch (i.e. rising and falling). These sensorimotor premotor neurons code for exteroceptive as well as for interoceptive change (re-afference) that is triggered particularly in the case of vocal and articulatory production, since this kind of change is largely defined by timing and pitch properties (Figure 25.2).

---

[1] More tentatively, we could say that both rhythm prediction and vocal or articulatory production overlap in a cerebral network, though it may well be that neuronal populations covered in these overlapping voxels differ with regard to their functional tuning.

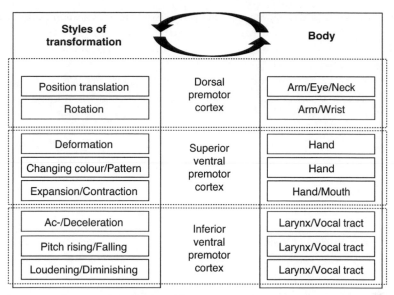

Styles of transformation		Body
Position translation	Dorsal premotor cortex	Arm/Eye/Neck
Rotation		Arm/Wrist
Deformation	Superior ventral premotor cortex	Hand
Changing colour/Pattern		Hand
Expansion/Contraction		Hand/Mouth
Ac-/Deceleration	Inferior ventral premotor cortex	Larynx/Vocal tract
Pitch rising/Falling		Larynx/Vocal tract
Loudening/Diminishing		Larynx/Vocal tract

Fig. 25.2 The HAPEM framework holds that different styles of transformation in action and perception are supported by different portions of the lateral premotor cortex and its associated projection sites. Accordingly, prediction of rhythm engages the inferior ventral premotor cortex because this region is the one which is best adapted to specify its motor output in terms of rhythm (in addition to pitch). However, rhythm prediction does not amount to vocal or articulatory imagery, but to an audiomotor and/or visuomotor fraction of action only (cf. Schubotz, 2007, for a detailed theoretical account). Adapted with permission from Schubotz, R. I. (2007). Prediction of external events with our motor system: towards a new framework. *Trends Cog Sci*, **11**(5), 211–18.

The account outlined here is based on the assumption that computations in the inferior ventral premotor areas are not principally different from computations in the superior ventral and dorsal premotor areas. As mentioned previously, macaque premotor neurons in superior ventral and dorsal areas exhibit tuning to object-based and spatial transformations during grasping and reaching actions that can be activated not only internally (by action) but also externally (by perception and attention) (Fadiga et al., 2000). The same could hold for sensorimotor neurons in the inferior ventral premotor area that are tuned not only for rhythmic and pitch-related transformations during articulation and vocalization, but also during perception of externally generated rhythms.

A major issue in this line of reasoning is, of course, what kind of attended external stimulus is appropriate (sufficient) to trigger this premotor activation. This point has been specifically addressed in the outline of the HAPEM framework (Schubotz, 2007). The core problem this account has to cope with is how it could be possible for the motor system to emulate dynamics (e.g. environmental rhythms) of whose production we are incapable. That is, we may well be able to *predict* the emergence of the next step on an escalator, but we certainly cannot *move* like an escalator. We can *predict* the flow of traffic but we cannot *move* like cars. This problem also relates to the notorious observation that performance teaches us to predict, but prediction does not teach us to perform (for example, somebody may know exactly how Glenn Gould played the first tones of Bach's Goldberg Variation No. 11 in the 1981 recordings, but unfortunately (s)he cannot play it like him). As to an empirical observation supporting this notion, we found superior ventral premotor activation for the prediction of a rapidly presented sequence of colour transitions filling the entire presentation screen, for which it seems impossible to identify some kind of action of which those stimuli could be reminiscent (Schubotz and von Cramon, 2002). Hence, we seem capable of predicting a stimulus sequence that we cannot reproduce ourselves, and the premotor cortex becomes engaged when doing so.

The solution that has been put forward by the HAPEM framework is related to the fact that sensorimotor neurons in the premotor cortex of the macaque code for, so to speak, *fractions* of actions. That is, they are either tuned to vision (and a body part), or to touch (and a body part), or to audition (and a body part), or to mixtures thereof (Fadiga et al., 2000). That means we can imagine audiomotor neurons that establish a representation of the rhythmic and pitch-related changes that define a melody, without therewith establishing a full-blown 'motor' representation with all of its interoceptive and exteroceptive re-afferents. Rhythm prediction thus does not amount to latent vocalization or articulation but only to a fraction of it.

Empirical evidence for this claim comes from a comparison between brain activity during motor imagery and serial prediction: one would expect overlap in the premotor cortex but activation of distinct networks otherwise, indicating full-blown action representation in the case of motor imagery but not for serial prediction. In a recent fMRI study, we focused particularly on the similarities of a vocal imagery task and a rhythmic prediction task (Wolfensteller et al., 2004). However, when considering potential dissimilarities, a direct contrast showed clear differences between vocal imagery and rhythm prediction: vocal imagery elicited higher responses than rhythm prediction particularly in the posterior supplementary motor area and in primary motor, as well as primary and secondary somatosensory, areas; the reverse contrast revealed higher activation in the intraparietal sulci, dorsal and superior ventral premotor cortex[2], thalamus and the fusiform gyrus. Another fMRI study has shown that monitoring a stimulus sequence, with the intention of subsequently reproducing it, differs from monitoring a stimulus sequence with the intention of predicting further sequence repetitions with regard to brain activation in the supplementary motor area, the primary motor cortex, and the cerebellar cortex, but not with regard to activation in premotor (or parietal) sites (Schubotz and von Cramon, 2001b).

Conclusions

Many questions remain as yet unresolved. This chapter has focused on the inferior ventral premotor cortex in rhythm prediction, but, of course, this area functions in close collaboration with many others, e.g. the supplementary motor area, the striatum, the cerebellar cortex and the parietal projection sites. The characteristic neuronal tuning in the ventral premotor cortex may merely result from the position of this area in a specific network. Thus, with the same justification, the chapter could have focused on one of these other areas in the motor system. One of the many challenging but unsettled issues in this regard is the relative functional contribution of the closely related areas BA 44 (called Broca's area in the left brain) and the adjacent BA 6, which is implicated in numerous functional domains, especially that of action and language (cf. Schubotz and Fiebach, 2006 and further papers in the same special issue). Therefore an interesting question here would be whether BA 6 and BA 44 contribute in different ways to rhythm prediction. A comparison of activation maxima across six fMRI studies we conducted shows maxima for rhythm prediction in BA 6 and those for pitch prediction in BA 44 (Figure 25.3). The inferior

---

[2] Note that the entire lateral premotor cortex is typically engaged for serial prediction, with maximum activation being determined by the property that prediction is based on. Accordingly, while vocal imgery and rhythm prediction both draw particularly on the inferior ventral premotor cortex, the direct contrast reveals additional activation spreading all over the lateral premotor belt for rhythm prediction.

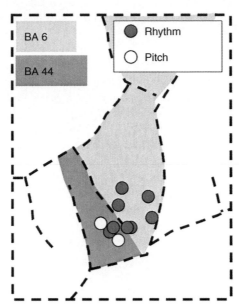

Fig. 25.3 A plot of local maxima of fMRI activation generated during rhythm and pitch prediction in the inferior ventral premotor cortex (BA 6, light grey, and BA 44, dark grey; dashed lines indicate sulci in an individual brain). Activations in the right brain were mirrored in the left brain. The abscissa corresponds to the y-axis and the ordinate to the z-axis of Talairach space (the x-axis was levelled).

precentral sulcus can be used as a fairly reliable macroanatomical landmark separating BA 44 and BA 6 (Keller et al., 2009). This finding corresponds well with the pronounced auditory projections into the ventral prefrontal area adjacent to BA 6 in the macaque (Deacon, 1992). However, activation of either task (rhythm and pitch) usually extends across both cortical fields. Moreover, none of the studies involved in this analysis investigated both rhythm and pitch prediction within one and the same session and group. Even so, the moderate difference in local maxima for rhythm and pitch prediction could motivate a systematic experimental investigation.

Finally, some limitations of fMRI evidence on rhythm perception and its brain correlates should be addressed. Imaging studies sometimes report not only inferior ventral, but also superior ventral and even dorsal premotor activation for rhythm perception tasks. FMRI findings thus seem to sink into arbitrariness: rhythm induces some motor activity, sometimes here, sometimes there—the gain in insight is limited. In the last part of this chapter, I wish to refute this nihilistic view.

First, when considering brain correlates of rhythm prediction or perception, it is crucial to eliminate or control as far as possible motor components of the paradigm employed in order to disentangle attentional from motor contributions of the motor system. When trying to identify in the experimental literature a formal definition of what renders a function 'motor', one realizes that a large body of research makes use of a fairly intuitive notion (as opposed to knowing all precise semantic rules when playing the language-game in a Wittgensteinian sense). For instance, is a cognitive application of an internal forward model (cf. Grush, 2004) by definition a 'motor function' if it exploits the efference copy architecture? Approaching this issue from the safe side, motor paradigms typically employ finger tapping as a means of generating (and measuring the effects of) synchronization with (or 'tuning into') an externally provided rhythm. Thus, not surprisingly, these studies report dorsal premotor cortex in addition to ventral premotor activity (Lewis et al., 2004; Jantzen et al., 2005; Chen et al., 2006; Karabanov et al., 2009), since two representations of the digits are found in the premotor cortex, one dorsal and one ventral (Dum and Strick, 2005).

Even when investigating 'passive listening', which has no motor task requirements, the involvement of motor areas due to micro-movements and motor imagery is a potential, and even probable, source of brain activation that has to be carefully controlled. It is easy to see that our eyes, heads, and fingers tend to tune into the beat of musical rhythms we perceive (this effect could be even greater in a scanner environment where subjects are forced to merely listen, deprived of other sources of information and trying *not* to move). Thus, 'silence' or 'empty trials' do not provide a sufficient contrast for rhythm perception, even during passive listening. In this case, the primary motor areas for vocal and articulatory production, as well as the frontal eye fields, would be expected to become active, and thus possibly be reflected in the data (e.g. Chen et al., 2008). The same restriction applies to the usage of 'resting baselines' when investigating effector-independent motor timing, as eye movements may be systematically related to rhythm but random during rest (e.g. Bengtsson et al., 2005). Thus, even carefully and intelligently designed fMRI paradigms run the risk of motor confounds when drawing on resting state conditions for contrast against rhythmic ones. Methods such as transcranial magnetic stimulation that can assess a lowering of the motor threshold, or studies in patients who suffer from upper motoneuron degeneration, should be used to complement imaging findings so as to rule out influences of motor strategies or 'subliminal' motor activity definitively. Even then, however, it remains largely unclear where and how we draw the border between metabolic signs of 'cognitive' and those of 'motor' processes, and whether this border can be drawn at some procedural or anatomical level in the brain at all.

Second, it may be particularly irritating to insist on disentangling rhythm perception from rhythmic production on the one hand, and to postulate a particularly tight link between rhythm and voice-related brain areas on the other. Obviously we produce rhythms not only with our voice but with many body parts. This issue relates to the fact that the premotor cortex is engaged in arbitrary (or 'non-standard') sensorimotor mappings (Wise et al., 1996). This function allows us to adapt flexibly to highly developed cultural cues, for instance when a car driver learns to press the brake pedal with the right foot when approaching a red traffic light. In a recent fMRI study, we found that, surprisingly, the premotor cortex codes neither for the body part involved in such a mapping (e.g. the right foot) nor for the stimulus (the red light), but for the *transformation* that we associate with the stimulus (push the pedal down) (Wolfensteller et al., 2004). This finding also shows that the standard premotor map for transformation styles in action and perception, as postulated in the HAPEM framework (Schubotz, 2007), is clearly modifiable by experience. However, as long as we do not assign specific movements to rhythm due to acquired arbitrary sensorimotor mappings (such as, for example, piano players do with their finger movements), maximal brain activity will be located at inferior ventral premotor sites, i.e. the premotor vocal/ articulatory areas.

Finally, and perhaps most importantly, the entire premotor cortex is activated by predictive tasks, and it was argued earlier that timing tasks may be predictive by nature (i.e. duration is intrinsically event-like). The property-specific effects in the premotor cortex are only relative differences that are found by directly contrasting one prediction condition with another. Does this mean that there is almost no functional specialization in the premotor cortex with regard to prediction tasks? This view seems to be supported by the observation that motor representations show considerable (but functionally meaningful, cf. Schieber, 2001) overlap in the premotor cortex; however, it is a proposal that is definitely to be rejected. Predicting rhythm will always activate the entire premotor cortex, because whenever an event is attended to (e.g. a melody, a rhythm, a ball trajectory), this event has, by definition, spatial, temporal, and object properties. Even if we draw the subject's attention to one out of these different sources of information, it is probable that perception cannot perfectly filter (i.e. entirely suppress) all task-irrelevant stimulus properties. But we cannot present our subjects with a 'purely temporal' stimulus (a pure rhythm) or a 'purely spatial' stimulus (a pure place in space). This means that only by controlling all these concurrent sources of information we will be able to elucidate the specific functional contribution of each premotor subarea to predictive attention.

References

Bengtsson, S. L., Ehrsson, H. H., Forssberg, H., and Ullén, F. (2005). Effector-independent voluntary timing: behavioural and neuroimaging evidence. *Eur J Neurosci*, **22**(12), 3255–65.

Bubic, A., von Cramon, D. Y., Jacobsen, T., Schröger, E., and Schubotz, R. I. (2008). Violation of expectation: neural correlates reflect bases of prediction. *J Cogn Neurosci*, **21**(1), 155–68.

Chen, J. L., Zatorre, R. J., and Penhune, V. B. (2006). Interactions between auditory and dorsal premotor cortex during synchronization to musical rhythms, *NeuroImage*, **32**, 1771–81.

Chen, J. L., Penhune, V. B., and Zatorre, R. J. (2008). Listening to musical rhythms recruits motor regions of the brain. *Cereb Cortex*, **18**(12), 2844–54.

Deacon, T. W. (1992). Cortical connections of the inferior arcuate sulcus cortex in the macaque brain. *Brain Res*, **573**, 8–26.

Doya, K. (1999). What are the computations of the cerebellum, the basal ganglia and the cerebral cortex? *Neural Netw*, **12**, 961–74.

Dronkers, F. E. (1996). A new brain region for coordinating speech articulation. *Nature*, **384**, 159–61.

Dum, R. P. and Strick, P. L. (2005). Frontal lobe inputs to the digit representations of the motor areas on the lateral surface of the hemisphere. *J Neurosci*, **25**(6), 1375 –86.

Fadiga, L., Fogassi, L., Gallese, V., and Rizzolatti, G. (2000). Visuomotor neurons: ambiguity of the discharge or 'motor' perception? *Int J Psychophysiol*, **35**(2–3), 165–77.

Fadiga, L., Craighero, L., Buccino, G., and Rizzolatti, G. (2002). Speech listening specifically modulates the excitability of tongue muscles: a TMS study. *Eur J Neurosci*, **15**, 399–402.

Fox, P. T., Ingham, R. J., Ingham, J. C., Hirsch, T. B., Downs, J. H., Martin, C., et al. (1996). A PET study of the neural systems of stuttering. *Nature*, **382**, 158–61.

Grush, R. (2004). The emulation theory of representation: motor control, imagery, and perception. *Behav Brain Sci*, **27**, 377–442.

Jantzen, K. J., Steinberg, F. L., and Kelso, J. A. (2004). Brain networks underlying human timing behavior are influenced by prior context. *Proc Natl Acad Sci USA*, **101**, 6815–20.

Karabanov, A., Blom, O., Forsman, L., and Ullén, F. (2009). The dorsal auditory pathway is involved in performance of both visual and auditory rhythms. *NeuroImage*, **44**(2), 480–8.

Keller, S. S., Crow, T., Foundas, A., Amunts, K., and Roberts, N. (2009). Broca's area: nomenclature, anatomy, typology and asymmetry. *Brain Lang*, **109**(1), 29–48.

Kleber, B., Birbaumer, N., Veit, R., Trevorrow, T., and Lotze, M. (2007). Overt and imagined singing of an Italian aria. *NeuroImage*, **36**, 889–900.

Lebedev, M. A. and Wise, S. P. (2001). Tuning for the orientation of spatial attention in dorsal premotor cortex. *Eur J Neurosci*, **13**(5), 1002–8.

Lewis, P. A., Wing, A. M., Pope, P. A., Praamstra, P., and Miall, R. C. (2004). Brain activity correlates differentially with increasing temporal complexity of rhythms during initialisation, synchronisation, and continuationphases of paced finger tapping. *Neuropsychologia*, **42**, 1301–12.

O'Reilly, J. X., Mesulam, M. M., and Nobre, A. C. (2008). The cerebellum predicts the timing of perceptual events. *J Neurosci*, **28**(9), 2252–60.

Ozdemir E, Norton A, and Schlaug G (2006). Shared and distinct neural correlates of singing and speaking. *NeuroImage*, **33**, 628-635.

Perry, D. W., Zatorre, R. J., Petrides, M., Alivisatos, B., Meyer, E., and Evans, A. C., (1999). Localization of cerebral activity during simple singing. *Neuroreport*, **10**, 3979–84.

Peters, A. and Jones, E. G., (1985). *Cerebral Cortex, Vol. 4, Association and Auditory Cortices*. New York: Plenum.

Preuss, T. M. and Goldman-Rakic, P. S. (1989). Connections of the ventral granular frontal cortex of macaques with perisylvian premotor and somatosensory areas: anatomical evidence for somatic representation in primate frontal association cortex. *J Comp Neurol*, **282**, 293–316.

Ramus, F., Hauser, M. D., Miller, C., Morris, D., and Mehler, J. (2000). Language discrimination by human newborns and by cotton-top tamarin monkeys. *Science*, **288**(5464), 349–51.

Riecker, A., Ackermann, H., Wildgruber, D., Dogil, G., and Grodd, W. (2000). Opposite hemispheric lateralization effects during speaking and singing at motor cortex, insula and cerebellum. *Neuroreport*, **11**, 1997–2000.

Riecker, A., Wildgruber, D., Dogil, G., Grodd, W., and Ackermann, H. (2002). Hemispheric lateralization effects of rhythm implementation during syllable repetitions: an fMRI study. *NeuroImage*, **16**, 169–176.

Rizzolatti, G., Fogassi, L., and Gallese, V. (2002). Motor and cognitive functions of the ventral premotor cortex. *Curr Opin Neurobiol*, **12**(2):149–54.

Roberts, T. S. and Akert, K. (1963). Insular and opercular cortex and its thalamic projection in *Macaca mulatta*. *Schweizer Archiv für Neurologie, Neurochirurgie und Psychiatrie*, **92**, 1–43.

Schieber, M. H. (2001). Constraints on somatotopic organization in the primary motor cortex. *J Neurophysiol*, **86**(5), 2125–43.

Schubotz, R. I. (1999). Instruction differentiates the processing of temporal and spatial sequential patterns: Evidence from slow wave activity in humans. *Neurosci Lett*, **265**, 1–4.

Schubotz, R. I. (2007). Prediction of external events with our motor system: towards a new framework. *Trends Cog Sci*, **11**(5), 211–18.

Schubotz, R. I. and Fiebach, C. (2006). Integrative models of Broca's area and the ventral premotor cortex. *Cortex*, **42**(4), 461–3.

Schubotz, R. I. and von Cramon, D. Y. (2001a) Functional organization of the lateral premotor cortex: fMRI reveals different regions activated by anticipation of object properties, location and speed. *Cog Brain Res*, **11**, 97–112.

Schubotz, R. I . and von Cramon, D. Y. (2001b). Interval and ordinal properties of sequences are associated with distinct premotor areas. *Cereb Cortex*, **11**(3), 210–22.

Schubotz, R. I . and von Cramon, D. Y. (2002). Dynamic patterns make the premotor cortex interested in objects: influence of stimulus and task revealed by fMRI. *Brain Res Cogn Brain Res*, **14**(3), 357–69.

Schubotz, R. I . and von Cramon, D. Y. (2003). Functional-anatomical concepts of human premotor cortex: evidence from fMRI and PET studies. *NeuroImage*, **20**(Suppl 1), S120–31.

Schubotz, R. I. and von Cramon, D. Y. (2005). Premotor activation in fMRI: duration and order in abstract stimulus sequences [German]. *Klinische Neurophysiologie*, **36**, 29–35.

Schubotz, R. I., Friederici, A. D. and von Cramon, D. Y. (2000). Time perception and motor timing: a common cortical and subcortical basis revealed by event-related fMRI. *NeuroImage*, **11**, 1–12.

Schubotz, R. I., von Cramon, D. Y. and Lohmann, G. (2003). Auditory what, where, and when: A sensory somatotopy in lateral premotor cortex. *NeuroImage*, **20**, 173–185.

Schubotz, R. I., Kalinich, C., and von Cramon, D. Y. (2008). How anticipation recruits our motor system: the habitual pragmatic body map revisited. In P. Haggard, Y. Rossetti, and M. Kawato (Eds.) *Sensorimotor Foundations of Higher Cognition. Attention and Performance XXII*, pp.141–62. Oxford: Oxford University Press.

Tincoff, R., Hauser, M., Tsao, F., Spaepen, G., Ramus, F., and Mehler, J. (2005). The role of speech rhythm in language discrimination: further tests with a non-human primate. *Dev Sci*, **8**(1), 26–35.

Tonkonogy, J. and Goodglass, H., (1981). Language function, foot of the third frontal gyrus, and rolandic operculum. *Arch. Neurol,* **38**, 468–90.

Vogt, C. and Vogt, O. (1919). Allgemeine Ergebnisse unserer Hirnforschung [German; General results of our brain research]. *J Psychologie Neurologie,* **25**, 279–462.

Wise, R. J., Greene, J., Büchel, C., and Scott, S.K., (1999). Brain regions involved in articulation. *Lancet,* **353**, 1057–61.

Wise, S. P., di Pellegrino, G., and Boussaoud, D. (1996). The premotor cortex and nonstandard sensorimotor mapping. *Can J Physiol Pharmacol,* **74**(4), 469–82.

Wolfensteller, U., Schubotz, R. I., and von Cramon, D. Y. (2004). "What" becoming "where": functional magnetic resonance imaging evidence for pragmatic relevance driving premotor cortex. *J Neurosci,* **24**(46), 10431–9.

Wolfensteller, U., Schubotz, R. I., and von Cramon, D. Y. (2007). Understanding non-biological dynamics with your own premotor system. *Neuroimage,* **36**(Suppl 2), T33–43.

Wolpert, D.M. and Flanagan, J.R. (2001). Motor prediction. *Curr Biol,* **11**, R729–R732.

Section 3b

Temporal predictions guided by endogenous cues

Chapter 26

Enhancing behavioural performance by visual temporal orienting

Ángel Correa

Tempus omnia revelat
(Latin proverb: time will reveal all things)

Temporal orienting of attention belongs to the general field of research on 'temporal expectations'. Temporal expectation involves a prediction about when a forthcoming event will occur. As defined by Coull and Nobre (1998), temporal orienting concerns 'how information about time intervals can be used to direct attention to a point in time when a relevant event is expected, to optimise behaviour' (p.7426). This chapter will focus on studies of temporal orienting, in which expectations are induced by cues providing explicit and predictive information about the temporal onset of a task-relevant stimulus ('target'). I will describe the behavioural consequences of temporal orienting through a variety of tasks demanding specific aspects of cognitive processing, such as perception, action, language, and executive control. The main message of these sections is that temporal orienting facilitates the processing of task-relevant stimulus representations flexibly, through a broad spectrum of cognitive processes. Finally, temporal orienting is discussed in a broader context, in relation to other types of temporal expectations that guide attention. The picture here reveals rich interrelations between attentional preparation and different types of temporal information.

A brief history of temporal orienting

The origins of temporal orienting can be traced back to the first studies about attentional preparation, in the early days of Experimental Psychology as a scientific discipline (Wundt, 1887). Early scholars observed the essential role of time in attentional preparation by manipulating the duration of the preparatory interval, the so-called 'foreperiod'. They showed that preparation develops over time and relies on temporal certainty about the target onset (Woodrow, 1914).

The closest antecedent to investigations of temporal orienting is probably the study by Zahn and Rosenthal (1966). In this study, two foreperiods of different durations (1 and 3 seconds) were randomly intermixed during the experiment. The key manipulation concerned the distribution or relative proportion of these foreperiods, which could be either biased to the short duration (high probability of 1-second foreperiods), biased to the long duration (high probability of 3-second foreperiods), or unbiased (equal probability of 1-second and 3-second foreperiods). Reaction times (RTs) to detect a target were collected and then plotted as a function of foreperiod duration ('RT-foreperiod functions') for each condition of foreperiod distribution. Although participants received no information about the duration and distribution of foreperiods, the three RT-foreperiod functions clearly revealed differential temporal-expectation profiles.

The critical finding was that the distribution biased toward short intervals strongly decreased RTs at the short foreperiod, as if a high proportion of short foreperiods induced an early expectation, which tuned temporal preparation optimally to the short interval.

Could participants voluntarily use these temporal expectations if they were based on explicit information about when a target would appear? This question gave birth to the formal study of the temporal orienting of attention. A decade ago, Coull and Nobre (1998) conducted a neuroimaging study with positron emission tomography (PET) and functional magnetic resonance imaging (fMRI) to address this question. In an analogous manner to what had happened in the general field of time perception (see Macar et al., 2002, for a review), the neural approach followed by Nobre and her colleagues contributed to the renaissance of the classical field of temporal preparation in the contemporary context of Cognitive Neuroscience. Since that initial study (Coull and Nobre, 1998) the number of publications on temporal orienting has grown continually and exponentially.

Box 26.1 Temporal expectations outside the laboratory: three everyday examples

Example 1: little David got sick and his mum took him to the nursery. David was very anxious, as he knew he would be given an injection. However, the experienced nurse played the following trick. She started counting: 'One, two, and . . .' and suddenly, she gave the injection; '. . . and three?' asked David with surprise and relief, as he felt much less pain than he had anticipated. Why did the nurse give him the injection earlier than expected? She was applying one principle of temporal orienting: perception (in this case, the perception of pain) is impaired for stimuli occurring at unexpected times. The nurse induced in David a late expectancy about the occurrence of the painful injection, but she 'delivered' the pain before that moment. Distracting attention away from the actual moment of the delivery of pain served to attenuate the perception of pain.

Example 2: 'Ready . . .'—the athletes were perfectly lined up behind the starting line. 'Steady . . .' the expectation dramatically increased millisecond by millisecond in the stadium, the athletes increased their readiness to the maximum: muscles taut, attention highly focused, awaiting the auditory go signal . . . 'Bang!'—Carl Lewis was the first athlete who started running. He reacted just 250 milliseconds after hearing the gunshot, and most importantly, 50 milliseconds earlier than the second runner. What was the secret of his temporal advantage? Carl was very good at orienting his attention to the exact moment at which the gun fired. With his attention temporally tuned, he was the fastest participant to perceive the sound, and the fastest one to trigger the motor activity of his leg muscles. That crucial advantage helped Carl win that race.

Example 3: one day, there was general confusion in the office about the onset of a meeting. Immanuel believed it would start at 10:30. Helen said the right meeting time was 11:00, whereas Rose expected the meeting to happen at 11:30. There was nobody at the office when Immanuel arrived. He was prepared to start at 10:30, but had to delay that moment for at least half an hour. During that time interval, Immanuel thought: 'sooner or later the meeting will take place today, so I am going to rehearse my speech one more time'—thus, he became fully prepared for the meeting even though its onset did not confirm his initial temporal expectation. The boss arrived at 11:00 and the meeting started. Helen appeared on

---

Box 26.1 Temporal expectations outside the laboratory: three everyday examples *(continued)*

time, she was prepared and her speech was hence excellent. Immanuel also did a good job when his turn began since he was also prepared—well, strictly speaking, he was re-prepared. Poor Rose received a phone call from her boss at 11:15. 'Damn! I needed those fifteen minutes for the final rehearsal of my speech!'—Rose arrived late and unprepared for the meeting, which was evident from her speech. 'If only I could go back in time' she lamented. As she realized that people can only prepare for the future, not for the past, she decided to follow the same strategy as Immanuel. For the next meeting, Rose would be ready on time, and in fact, a bit earlier!

Temporal orienting speeds up motor responses

Can attention be oriented to specific moments in time, analogously to the orienting of attention in the spatial domain? Coull and Nobre (1998) developed a temporal version of the Cost and Benefits procedure, introduced by Posner (1980) to study how attention could be oriented covertly to different locations in space (see also Coull, Chapter 31; Nobre, Chapter 27, this volume). In a temporal-orienting procedure (see Figure 26.1), a temporal cue explicitly indicates that the task-relevant stimulus ('target') will appear either after a short interval ('early') or after a long interval ('late'). Temporal cues are predictive, since in most trials the early cue is validly associated with target onsets at the short interval, whereas the late cue is related to target onsets at the long interval. When the target appears (e.g. the 'X' stimulus), participants have to respond as quickly as possible by pressing a key. That is, they perform a speeded simple-RT detection task.

The results typically show that the early cue produces the fastest RTs at the short interval, whereas the late cue produces the fastest RTs at the long interval. These opposite temporal-expectation profiles can be attributed to the predictive temporal information explicitly provided by the cues. 'Temporal orienting effects' are generally indexed by comparing early versus late cue conditions at the short interval only. In Figure 26.1, temporal orienting effects refer to faster RTs to detect expected targets at the short interval as compared to RT to detect earlier-than-expected targets also appearing at the short interval. At the long interval, however, temporal orienting effects are diminished or absent because they are masked by another form of temporal expectation, foreperiod effects (see Los, Chapter 21; Vallesi, Chapter 22, this volume). Following our example, the target could occur either at the short or at the long interval with similar a priori probability ($p = 0.5$). However, the *conditional probability* of target occurrence increases with time, such that the target always appears at the long interval ($p = 1$) if it has not yet appeared at the short interval. Obviously, explicit temporal cues are more effective when they serve to predict uncertain rather than certain target onsets (i.e. in short-interval rather than long-interval conditions; see 'Temporal orienting in relation to other forms of temporal expectation' section for further details). To summarize, we can conclude that temporal orienting optimizes behaviour by speeding up performance in detection tasks (Coull and Nobre, 1998).

But what was the nature of this behavioural enhancement? Was it due to faster perception or to faster responses to the target stimulus? The answer was clear according to the initial evidence based on fMRI and event-related potentials (ERPs): temporal orienting speeds up behaviour by enhancing the preparation of motor responses (Coull and Nobre, 1998; Miniussi et al., 1999; Coull et al., 2000; Nobre, Chapter 27, this volume). The implication was that the effects of temporal orienting were constrained to modulating the preparation of motor processing. However, this interpretation did not fit with the general view of attention as a mechanism that selects information flexibly, not only at late response stages, but also at early perceptual stages of

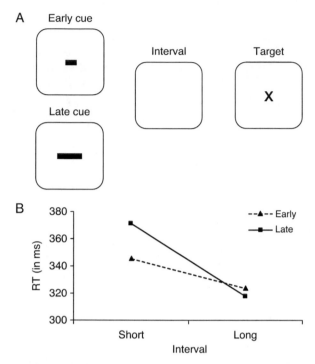

Fig. 26.1 A) How to study temporal orienting. A standard temporal-orienting experiment is composed of a set of trials. Each trial includes a sequence of a temporal cue, interval, and target, which can be visually presented to the participants via computer screen. The temporal cue provides explicit and predictive information about the time interval after which the target will appear. The short bar in the figure indicates that the target will appear after 400ms with a probability of 0.75, whereas the long bar indicates that the target will appear after 1400ms with the same probability. On each trial, only one temporal cue is presented, which is followed by a blank interval. The duration of this interval can be either short (400ms) or long (1400ms) with equal probability. In 'valid' trials, the target appears at the cued interval (early cue—short interval and late cue—long interval conditions). In 'invalid' trials, the target appears either earlier than expected (late cue—short interval) or later than expected (early cue—long interval) according to the temporal cue. The participants' task is to detect the letter 'X' (i.e. target) and press a key as quickly as possible (simple-RT detection task). B) Typical results in temporal orienting experiments. Mean reaction times (RTs) averaged across participants are plotted as a function of temporal cue (early, late) and interval (short: 400ms; long: 1400ms). Note that RTs are faster for long, as compared to short, intervals; this is the 'foreperiod effect'. Most importantly, the early expectation induced by the temporal cue attenuates the slope of the foreperiod effect. As a result, RTs at the short interval are faster for early cues rather than for late cues; this is the 'temporal orienting effect' (or validity effect). In contrast, RTs at the long interval are generally similar for both early and late cues, which reflect the interaction between temporal orienting and foreperiod effects. The facilitation in task performance at cued intervals is ascribed to the orienting of attention to the interval specified by the temporal cue. Procedure and data are taken from Correa, Á., Lupiáñez, J., Milliken, B., and Tudela, P. (2004). Endogenous temporal orienting of attention in detection and discrimination tasks. *Perception and Psychophysics,* **66**(2), 264–78.

stimulus processing. In fact, the possibility that temporal orienting could also influence early perceptual analysis had been acknowledged in the first two review articles that Nobre and colleagues published about temporal orienting (Griffin, Miniussi, and Nobre, 2001; Nobre, 2001). However, empirical evidence was still needed to support this hypothesis. The search for evidence of temporal orienting effects upon perceptual processing had just begun.

Temporal orienting improves stimulus perception

Why did the initial studies fail to observe perceptual enhancement by temporal orienting? An answer to this intriguing question could be found in research showing that spatial orienting enhances stimulus perception through the visual system (see Mangun, 1995, for a review). The visual system is rich in spatial rather than temporal information, as it is spatially organized following retinotopic maps. Given that all temporal orienting studies had so far been conducted in the visual modality only, it was possible that the tasks were not sensitive enough to show perceptual modulation. Perhaps, temporal orienting effects would be most clearly observed if a temporally rich modality, such as audition, was involved. Following this logic, Lange and her colleagues found that temporal orienting enhanced the auditory N1, an ERP component linked to early perceptual analysis of auditory information (Lange, Rösler, and Röder, 2003; Lange and Röder, Chapter 28, this volume).

At that time, my colleagues and I realized that the evidence restricting the effects of temporal orienting to motor preparation in the visual modality was exclusively based on simple-RT detection tasks. These tasks emphasize the execution of a speeded response, but do not require a detailed perceptual analysis of the visual features of the target. This circumstance could have favoured the effect of attention upon response rather than perceptual levels of processing. The use of tasks imposing stronger demands on perceptual analysis might instead strengthen the beneficial effects of attention on stimulus perception.

For example, choice-RT discrimination tasks require that participants respond selectively to target stimuli that differ along a particular perceptual feature, such as shape. In a shape discrimination task, participants should make one response if they see 'X', and a different response if they see 'O'. Indeed, the behavioural findings in visual discrimination tasks suggested that temporal orienting might enhance the perceptual analysis of visual stimuli (Griffin et al., 2001; Los and Van den Heuvel, 2001; Milliken et al., 2003; Correa et al., 2004). However, these findings relied on RT measures, in which it is difficult to isolate the contribution of perceptual versus motor factors to the attentional benefits that were observed. Thus, faster RT performance for attended versus unattended targets in a discrimination task could be due to faster stimulus perception (perceptual preparation), faster responses (motor preparation), or both. Behavioural indices other than RT were therefore necessary to investigate temporal orienting effects on perceptual preparation. To that end, an appropriate index should be a measure of perceptual processing that is collected free from time pressure during participants' responses.

The use of psychophysical methods can provide behavioural indices of perceptual accuracy, such as d' (Green and Swets, 1966). In a first study (Correa, Lupiáñez, and Tudela, 2005), we used rapid serial visual presentation (RSVP), in which the target (the 'X' letter) was embedded within a stream of distractors (other letters). The participants' task was to decide (without time pressure) whether the target had been presented in the stream. This task was perceptually challenging, as stimuli were successively presented so fast (14ms per item) that they masked one another. We explicitly cued participants to attend to the specific points in time at which the target could appear, and tested whether d' improved as a consequence of these temporal expectations. The results showed that visual perception, as indexed by d', was most accurate for targets appearing at the cued temporal interval (Correa et al., 2005). This finding provided the first behavioural evidence that temporal orienting improves visual perception (see also Rolke and Ulrich, Chapter 17, this volume).

In a later study we used another measure of perceptual accuracy uncontaminated by response time pressures to gain convergent evidence that temporal orienting improves visual perception (Correa et al., 2006a). Participants performed a 'temporal order judgment' task, in which they had to judge (without time pressure) the order of occurrence of two peripheral flashes presented very close in time (ranging from 10–110-ms separation). The dependent variable of interest was the 'just noticeable difference (JND)'—the minimum temporal separation between the onsets of the two stimuli allowing correct report of their order of occurrence with 75% accuracy. Therefore, a smaller JND indicated better temporal resolution. We instructed participants to attend selectively to the interval indicated by the cue, and tested whether the JND decreased with valid temporal expectations. The results showed that the JND was smaller for targets appearing at the expected interval (JND = 41ms) as compared to the unexpected interval (JND = 46ms). In other words, temporal orienting improved the temporal resolution to perceive the order of two visual events that occurred almost simultaneously.

Supporting these findings, there is growing evidence from electrophysiological studies demonstrating facilitation of perceptual-related ERPs by temporal orienting (Doherty et al., 2005; Correa et al., 2006b, 2007; Lange, Krämer, and Röder, 2006; Sanders and Astheimer, 2008; Lange, 2009). A key feature that emerges after reviewing these studies is the common use of tasks involving strong demands on perceptual processing (see Correa et al., 2006b, for a review). This set of studies was important to temporal-orienting research, not only because they proved the flexible nature of the underlying attentional mechanism, but also because they enriched the range of cognitive tasks used to study temporal orienting. The initial simple-RT tasks were replaced by increasingly sophisticated tasks to address complex phenomena in human cognition. This idea is illustrated in the following section, which describes research on the effects of temporal orienting upon linguistic processing and executive control.

Temporal orienting beyond perception and action: effects on semantic processing and executive control

Does the flexibility of temporal orienting go beyond the modulation of simple perceptual and motor representations? The studies described in this section show that temporal orienting also influences high-level central cognition, such as linguistic processing of semantic categories and the executive control needed to perform complex selection of competing stimuli and responses.

Semantic processing can be studied by measuring priming effects produced by a stimulus (prime) upon the processing of a subsequent stimulus (target), with which it shares a semantic category. A study by Naccache and colleagues (Naccache, Blandin, and Dehaene, 2002) found that temporal orienting can facilitate semantic categorization, as indexed by unconscious semantic priming effects. Semantic priming was measured at the unconscious level by embedding primes and targets within a RSVP of visual masks. Specifically, semantic priming was only observed when the prime and target occurred within the attended time window, which suggests that temporal orienting facilitates semantic processing. Another study using RSVP found that temporal orienting also facilitated the conscious identification of target letters presented within a stream of distractor digits (Martens and Johnson, 2005). Furthermore, the main result of that study was that temporal cuing reduced the attentional blink (Raymond, Shapiro, and Arnell, 1992; Shapiro and Raymond, Chapter 3; Olivers, Chapter 4, this volume). This interesting finding suggests that temporal orienting can optimize the deployment of attentional resources at critical time intervals, in order to overcome the temporal limitations of working memory.

In most studies mentioned so far, the attentional selection of cognitive representations was relatively simple, that is, it did not involve controlled selection of mutually competing representations. Competing or incompatible representations produce conflict during information processing, which can be resolved by executive control according to internal goals (Atkinson and Shiffrin, 1968; Norman and Shallice, 1986). For example, executive control is engaged during the resolution of response conflict in the flanker task (Eriksen and Eriksen, 1974). In the arrows-version of this task, participants have to respond according to whether the direction of a central arrow (target) points left or right. Response conflict arises in the incongruent condition, in which a set of arrows flanking the target points in the opposite direction (e.g. '> > < > >'). Controlled selection is then needed to inhibit the response associated with the incompatible flankers and/or to activate the response associated with the target. In contrast, the congruent condition does not involve response conflict because target and flankers call for the same response (e.g. '< < < < <'). When task performance is compared for congruent and incongruent conditions (i.e. the *conflict effect* index), it becomes clear that controlled selection is difficult and time-consuming (i.e. errors are more frequent and RTs are slower on incongruent as compared to congruent conditions).

We have recently started investigating the effects of temporal orienting upon executive control processes required to resolve between conflicting representations during task performance. The results of the first study showed temporal orienting to have different effects depending on whether the task involves conflicting representations at the perceptual-selection or motor-selection levels (Correa et al., in press). Temporal orienting *facilitated* executive control when the task involved the resolution of conflict at *perceptual* rather than response levels, such as in the spatial Stroop task. In the incongruent condition of the spatial Stroop task, perceptual conflict arises from a mismatch between two stimulus dimensions, target location and orientation (e.g. a target arrow is presented at the top of the display—meaning 'up', whereas the arrow is pointing downwards—meaning 'down').

However, temporal orienting *disrupted* rather than facilitated the resolution of *response conflict* as indexed by flanker and Simon (Simon and Small, 1969) tasks. In the incongruent condition of the Simon task, response conflict arises from a mismatch between the location at which a stimulus is presented and the side of the motor response specifically associated with that stimulus according to task instructions (e.g., a target is presented in the left visual field, whereas the participant has to use the right hand to respond correctly to that target). In this particular condition, participants committed many more errors when the conflicting target appeared at the *attended* rather than the unattended moment. Do these puzzling findings imply that temporal orienting impairs executive control? They at least suggest that the enhancement of response readiness conferred by temporal orienting is only beneficial when simple response selection is required (e.g. in simple-RT detection tasks; Coull and Nobre, 1998), but not when the controlled selection of competing response tendencies is involved. Research on temporal orienting effects upon executive control is still in the initial phase; forthcoming studies should explore temporal orienting with other types of executive-control tasks.

The preceding sections have addressed the question of the locus of temporal orienting effects. We have concluded that this locus is flexible, and mainly depends on the cognitive demands of the task at hand. Another important question that has emerged in the field concerns the relationship between temporal orienting and other time-related attentional processes. The following section will focus on the interrelationship between temporal orienting and other forms of temporal expectation.

Temporal orienting in relation to other forms of temporal expectation

Temporal expectation is a broad concept that includes multiple types of attentional preparation in time. Temporal expectations can rely on many different sources to provide the relevant temporal information, such as explicit predictive cues (temporal orienting), temporal regularity (rhythmic expectations), probabilistic information associated with the passage of time (hazard functions and foreperiod effects), and inter-trial sequences of repetitions/alternations of foreperiod durations (sequential effects). However, the interrelationship between different types of temporal expectations has been considered only recently (see Nobre, Correa, and Coull, 2007; Coull and Nobre, 2008, for reviews). Foreperiod effects refer to the finding of faster RTs at long as compared to short foreperiods (i.e. preparatory intervals) in variable foreperiod procedures, in which short and long foreperiods are intermixed within a block of trials (Los, Chapter 21; Vallesi, Chapter 22, this volume). Sequential effects refer to the finding that RTs are faster when the current short foreperiod is a repetition of a previously short foreperiod rather than a switch from a previously long foreperiod (Woodrow, 1914; see also Los, Chapter 21, this volume). Rhythmic expectations refer to the finding that optimal task performance occurs at time intervals coinciding with a regular rhythm (Jones et al., 2002; see also, Olson and Chun, 2001; Jones, Chapter 23; Praamstra, Chapter 24; Schubotz, Chapter 25, this volume).

The diversity of these phenomena included under the concept of temporal expectations naturally calls for a taxonomy. One possible criterion to divide them considers the implicit versus explicit nature of the source of temporal prediction. Explicit temporal expectations are produced by temporal orienting, whereas implicit temporal expectations are produced by foreperiod effects, sequential effects, and rhythmic expectations, since they occur naturally regardless of the participant's explicit knowledge about underlying temporal contingencies. Alternatively, temporal expectations can be classified as a function of the automatic versus controlled nature of the processing underlying the behavioural effects (Los and Van den Heuvel, 2001; Capizzi, Sanabria, and Correa, 2009).

Capizzi and colleagues recently tested the automaticity of different types of temporal expectations by asking participants to perform a temporal preparation task, similar to the task shown in Figure 26.1, under both single-task and dual-task conditions. In the latter condition, we found that the addition of a concurrent working memory task interfered selectively with temporal orienting and foreperiod effects; in contrast, sequential effects survived the dual-task interference (Capizzi, Sanabria, and Correa, 2009). This result supports the idea that temporal orienting and foreperiod effects involve controlled temporal expectations since they both: 1) are influenced by a working memory task that competes for limited resources of controlled processing (Posner and Snyder, 1975); 2) rely on the strategic computation of conditional probabilities over time (Correa and Nobre, 2008); and 3) engage prefrontal brain areas linked to attentional control (Coull and Nobre, 1998; Coull et al., 2000; Stuss et al., 2005; Vallesi, Shallice, and Walsh, 2007; Vallesi et al., 2007, 2009) (see also Vallesi, Chapter 22; Coull, Chapter 31, this volume).

On the other hand, sequential effects and rhythmic expectations involve automatic temporal expectations, as they can guide temporal expectation in a bottom-up manner solely on the basis of non-predictive stimuli (Los and Van den Heuvel, 2001; Jones et al., 2002; Steinborn et al., 2008). Moreover, automatic sequential effects are immune to a competing working memory task (Capizzi, Sanabria, and Correa, 2009), and they probably involve brain structures: 1) that follow an earlier development in life than the prefrontal cortex (Vallesi and Shallice, 2007; Vallesi, Chapter 22, this volume) and 2) that might be involved in processes of trace conditioning (Los and Van den Heuvel, 2001; Los, Chapter 21, this volume).

As can be observed, the two suggested taxonomies are highly overlapping, such that sequential effects and rhythmic expectations are considered to involve implicit and automatic processing, whereas temporal orienting involves explicit and controlled processing. More research in this area should improve this taxonomy and clarify the relationships between different types of temporal expectations. In this context, some studies have already revealed that temporal orienting and sequential effects exert dissociable consequences on behaviour (Correa et al., 2004; Los and Van den Heuvel, 2001; Los and Agter, 2005; Los and Heslenfeld, 2005; Correa, Lupiáñez, and Tudela, 2006).

The dissociation between temporal orienting and sequential effects has been further observed at the neural level in lesion studies (Vallesi, Shallice et al., 2007; Vallesi et al., 2007; Vallesi, Chapter 22, this volume). Instead, other studies find strong interactions rather than dissociations between different forms of temporal expectation, namely, between temporal orienting and foreperiod effects (Correa, Lupiáñez, and Tudela, 2006, see also Figure 26.1), and between rhythmic expectations and foreperiod effects (Correa and Nobre, 2008).

Recently, we have developed a simple experimental task that can be administered to neuropsychological patients in order to evaluate functioning of three types of temporal expectations (temporal orienting, foreperiod and sequential effects), and to study the interaction between them (Triviño et al., in press). The task consists of an adaptation of the task shown in Figure 26.1. The preliminary results obtained with this task seem promising: patients with frontal lesions presenting frontal symptoms in neuropsychological testing were impaired on temporal orienting and foreperiod effects, whereas sequential effects remained intact. This finding hence confirms the association between temporal orienting and foreperiod effects (suggesting a common mechanism), and the dissociation between temporal orienting/foreperiod effects versus sequential effects. This neurological dissociation also fits well with the taxonomy in which sequential effects reflect automatic processing, whereas temporal orienting and foreperiod effects reflect controlled processing dependent upon the prefrontal cortex. Taking into account the interaction between temporal orienting and foreperiod effects, temporal orienting can be understood as the explicit and controlled modulation of the foreperiod effect.

Conclusions

The main conclusion to be drawn from this chapter is that temporal orienting is a mechanism that selects information with a high degree of *flexibility*. Temporal orienting can prioritize both perceptual and motor processing, depending on the types of representations that are particularly task-relevant within a specific context. The benefits of temporal orienting upon behavioural performance seem *widespread*, as they are evident across a variety of behavioural tasks involving low- as well as high-level cognitive demands. These attributes of temporal orienting fit perfectly with the notion of selective attention, with the particularity that the selection of information is controlled by explicit predictions about the temporal onset of events.

References

Atkinson, R. and Shiffrin, R. (1968). Human memory: a proposed system and its control processes. In K. Spence and J. Spence (Eds.) *The Psychology of Learning and Motivation: Advances in Research and Theory*, Vol. 2, pp.742–75. New York: Academic Press.

Capizzi, M., Sanabria, D., and Correa, A. (2009). 'Dual-task evidence for automatic and controlled mechanisms in temporal preparation.' Paper presented at the XVI Conference of the European Society for Cognitive Psychology, Krakov (Poland). 2–5 September, 2009.

Correa, Á. and Nobre, A. C. (2008). Neural modulation by regularity and passage of time. *Journal of Neurophysiology,* **100**(3), 1649–55.

Correa, Á., Lupiáñez, J., and Tudela, P. (2005). Attentional preparation based on temporal expectancy modulates processing at the perceptual-level. *Psychonomic Bulletin and Review,* **12**(2), 328–34.

Correa, Á., Lupiáñez, J., and Tudela, P. (2006). The attentional mechanism of temporal orienting: Determinants and attributes. *Experimental Brain Research,* **169**(1), 58–68.

Correa, Á., Lupiáñez, J., Milliken, B., and Tudela, P. (2004). Endogenous temporal orienting of attention in detection and discrimination tasks. *Perception & Psychophysics,* **66**(2), 264–78.

Correa, Á., Lupiáñez, J., Madrid, E., and Tudela, P. (2006). Temporal attention enhances early visual processing: A review and new evidence from event-related potentials. *Brain Research,* **1076**(1), 116–28.

Correa, Á., Sanabria, D., Spence, C., Tudela, P., and Lupiáñez, J. (2006a). Selective temporal attention enhances the temporal resolution of visual perception: Evidence from a temporal order judgment task. *Brain Research,* **1070**(1), 202–5.

Correa, Á., Kane, R., Lupiáñez, J., and Nobre, A. C. (2007). 'Temporal orienting facilitates perception: Electrophysiological evidence based on steady-state visual evoked potentials.' Paper presented at the XV Conference of the European Society for Cognitive Psychology, Marseille (France). 29 August–1 September, 2007.

Correa, Á., Cappucci, P., Nobre, A. C., and Lupiáñez, J. (in press). The two sides of temporal orienting: facilitating perceptual selection, disrupting response selection. *Experimental Psychology.*

Coull, J. T. and Nobre, A. C. (1998). Where and when to pay attention: the neural systems for directing attention to spatial locations and to time intervals as revealed by both PET and fMRI. *Journal of Neuroscience,* **18**(18), 7426–35.

Coull, J. T. and Nobre, A. (2008). Dissociating explicit timing from temporal expectation with fMRI. *Current Opinion in Neurobiology,* **18**, 1–8.

Coull, J. T., Frith, C. D., Buchel, C., and Nobre, A. C. (2000). Orienting attention in time: behavioural and neuroanatomical distinction between exogenous and endogenous shifts. *Neuropsychologia,* **38**(6), 808–19.

Doherty, J. R., Rao, A., Mesulam, M. M., and Nobre, A. C. (2005). Synergistic effect of combined temporal and spatial expectations on visual attention. *Journal of Neuroscience,* **25**, 8259–66.

Eriksen, B. A. and Eriksen, C. W. (1974). Effects of noise letters upon the identification of a target letter in a nonsearch task. *Perception & Psychophysics,* **16**, 143–9.

Green, D. M. and Swets, J. A. (1966). *Signal Detection Theory and Psychophysics.* New York: Wiley.

Griffin, I. C., Miniussi, C., and Nobre, A. C. (2001). Orienting attention in time. *Frontiers in Bioscience,* **6**, 660–71.

Jones, M. R., Moynihan, H., MacKenzie, N., and Puente, J. (2002). Temporal aspects of stimulus-driven attending in dynamic arrays. *Psychological Science,* **13**(4), 313–19.

Lange, K. (2009). Brain correlates of early auditory processing are attenuated by expectations for time and pitch. *Brain and Cognition,* **69**(1), 127–37.

Lange, K., Krämer, U. R., and Röder, B. (2006). Attending points in time and space. *Experimental Brain Research,* **173**(1), 130–40.

Lange, K., Rösler, F., and Röder, B. (2003). Early processing stages are modulated when auditory stimuli are presented at an attended moment in time: an event-related potential study. *Psychophysiology,* **40**, 806–17.

Los, S. A. and Agter, F. (2005). Reweighting sequential effects across different distributions of foreperiods: Segregating elementary contributions to nonspecific preparation. *Perception & Psychophysics,* **67**(7), 1161–70.

Los, S. A. and Heslenfeld, D. J. (2005). Intentional and unintentional contributions to nonspecific preparation: Electrophysiological evidence. *Journal of Experimental Psychology: General,* **134**, 52–72.

Los, S. A. and Van den Heuvel, C. E. (2001). Intentional and unintentional contributions to nonspecific preparation during reaction time foreperiods. *Journal of Experimental Psychology: Human Perception and Performance,* **27**, 370–86.

Macar, F., Lejeune, H., Bonnet, M., Ferrara, A., Pouthas, V., Vidal, F., et al. (2002). Activation of the supplementary motor area and of attentional networks during temporal processing. *Experimental Brain Research,* **142**, 475–85.

Mangun, G. R. (1995). Neural mechanisms of visual selective attention. *Psychophysiology,* **32**, 4–18.

Martens, S. and Johnson, A. (2005). Timing attention: cuing target onset interval attenuates the attentional blink. *Memory and Cognition,* **33**(2), 234–40.

Milliken, B., Lupiáñez, J., Roberts, M., and Stevanovski, B. (2003). Orienting in space and time: Joint contributions to exogenous spatial cuing effects. *Psychonomic Bulletin and Review,* **10**(4), 877–83.

Miniussi, C., Wilding, E. L., Coull, J. T., and Nobre, A. C. (1999). Orienting attention in time: modulation of brain potentials. *Brain,* **122**, 1507–18.

Naccache, L., Blandin, E., and Dehaene, S. (2002). Unconscious masked priming depends on temporal attention. *Psychological Science,* **13**(5), 416–24.

Niemi, P. and Näätänen, R. (1981). Foreperiod and simple reaction time. *Psychological Bulletin,* **89**, 133–62.

Nobre, A. C. (2001). Orienting attention to instants in time. *Neuropsychologia,* **39**, 1317–28.

Nobre, A. C., Correa, A., and Coull, J. T. (2007). The hazards of time. *Current Opinion in Neurobiology,* **17**, 1–6.

Norman, D. A. and Shallice, T. (1986). Attention to action: willed and automatic control of behaviour. In R. J. Davidson, G. E. Schwartz, and D. Shapiro (Eds.), *Consciousness and Self-Regulation: Advances in Research and Theory* (pp.1–18). New York: Plenum Press.

Olson, I. R., and Chun, M. M. (2001). Temporal contextual cuing of visual attention. *Journal of Experimental Psychology: Learning, Memory and Cognition,* **27**(5), 1299–313.

Posner, M. I. (1980). Orienting of attention. *Quarterly Journal of Experimental Psychology,* **32**, 3–25.

Posner, M. I., and Snyder, C. R. R. (1975). Attention and cognitive control. In R. Solso (Ed.), *Information processing and cognition: The Loyola Symposium,* pp.55–85. Hillsdale, NJ: Lawrence Erlbaum.

Raymond, J. E., Shapiro, K. L., and Arnell, K. M. (1992). Temporary suppression of visual processing in an RSVP task: An attentional blink? *Journal of Experimental Psychology: Human Perception and Performance,* **18**(3), 849–60.

Sanders, L. D. and Astheimer, L. B. (2008). Temporally selective attention modulates early perceptual processing: event-related potential evidence. *Perception & Psychophysics,* **70**(4), 732–42.

Simon, J. R. and Small, A. J. (1969). Processing auditory information: interference from an irrelevant cue. *Journal of Applied Psychology,* **53**(5), 433–5.

Steinborn, M. B., Rolke, B., Bratzke, D., and Ulrich, R. (2008). Sequential effects within a short foreperiod context: Evidence for the conditioning account of temporal preparation. *Acta Psychologica,* **129**(2), 297–307.

Stuss, D. T., Alexander, M. P., Shallice, T., Picton, T. W., Binns, M. A., Macdonald, R., et al. (2005). Multiple frontal systems controlling response speed. *Neuropsychologia,* **43**(3), 396–417.

Triviño, M., Correa, Á., Arnedo, M., & Lupiáñez, J. (in press) Temporal orienting deficit after prefrontal damage. *Brain.*

Vallesi, A., and Shallice, T. (2007). Developmental dissociations of preparation over time: deconstructing the variable foreperiod phenomena. *Journal of Experimental Psychology: Human Perception and Performance,* **33**(6), 1377–88.

Vallesi, A., Shallice, T., and Walsh, V. (2007). Role of the prefrontal cortex in the foreperiod effect: TMS evidence for dual mechanisms in temporal preparation. *Cerebral Cortex,* **17**(2), 466–74.

Vallesi, A., Mussoni, A., Mondani, M., Budai, R., Skrap, M., and Shallice, T. (2007). The neural basis of temporal preparation: insights from brain tumor patients. *Neuropsychologia,* **45**(12), 2755–63.

Vallesi, A., McIntosh, A. R., Shallice, T., and Stuss, D. T. (2009). When time shapes behaviour: fMRI evidence of brain correlates of strategic preparation over time. *Journal of Cognitive Neuroscience* **21**(6), 1116–26.

Woodrow, H. (1914). The measurement of attention. *Psychological Monographs,* **17**, 1–158.

Wundt, W. (1887). *Grundzüge der Physiologischen Psychologie.* Leipzig: Engelmann.

Zahn, T. P., and Rosenthal, D. (1966). Simple reaction time as a function of the relative frequency of the preparatory interval. *Journal of Experimental Psychology,* **72**, 15–19.

Acknowledgements

The writing of this chapter was supported by grants from the RYC-2007-00296 Ramón y Cajal programme, SEJ2007-63646 and SEJ2007-63247 (Spanish Ministerio de Ciencia e Innovación), and the CSD2008-00048 CONSOLIDER INGENIO (Dirección General de Investigación).

Chapter 27

How can temporal expectations bias perception and action?

Anna C. Nobre

Over its brief history, experimental psychology has taught us to accept the counterintuitive notion that our perception is highly biased. Perceptual functions do not build a veridical copy of external reality for our musings. Instead, perception is adapted flexibly, moment-to-moment, to deliver the events that are relevant to our current behavioural goals. 'Selective attention' is the set of functions that prioritizes and filters information-processing in order to determine the contents of our awareness and guide our actions. At its core is the ability to integrate experience over various time-scales in order to extract regularities and build predictions about selective attributes of forthcoming relevant events.

To date, 'attention' research has been primarily concerned with how predictions about the location, identity, or simple features of relevant events can influence neural processing. Tremendous strides have been made in understanding the neural systems and cellular mechanisms of attention (Kastner and Ungerleider, 2000; Nobre, 2001b; Reynolds and Chelazzi, 2004; Serences and Yantis 2006), enabling the development of increasingly sophisticated theoretical and computational models (Desimone and Duncan, 1995; Maunsell and Treue 2006; Lee and Maunsell 2009; Reynolds and Heeger 2009).

According to prevailing accounts, neural coding of task goals in executive control areas leads to top-down feedback signals which 'bias' the competitive interactions among neurons in sensory areas to prioritize the coding of stimulus features that are relevant to task goals (Desimone and Duncan, 1995; see also Maunsell and Treue 2006). Most of the research has been carried out in the visual system. Here, attention-related modulation has been observed across several cortical and subcortical areas, suggesting the flexibility to influence processing at several stages, possibly according to the types of attributes that are relevant or expected, or the actions that are to be performed (Kastner and Pinsk 2004; Nobre, 2004). Top-down biasing is achieved through a combination of cellular mechanisms. Single-unit recordings from non-human primates have shown that selective attention optimizes perceptual analysis by increasing the tonic firing rate of neurons coding relevant locations, objects, or features (Chelazzi et al., 1993, 1998; Luck et al., 1997; Treue and Martínez Trujillo, 1999); changing the effective size of receptive fields to filter out signals from irrelevant locations or objects (Moran and Desimone, 1985; Chelazzi et al., 1993, 1998, 2001; Reynolds et al., 1999); and increasing synchronization of high-frequency oscillatory activity among neurons coding relevant locations to maximize the impact of their outputs in downstream areas (Fries et al., 2001; 2008; Womelsdorf et al., 2006). Additional mechanisms may yet be revealed, but an underlying commonality to these mechanisms is that they capitalize on the receptive-field properties of visual neurons, using the spatial and feature-configuration tuning of neurons to highlight relevant items and remove distractions.

Missing from the mainstream theories and models of attention, however, is an essential dimension for organizing our perceptual experience—time (Kant, 1781/1999). Because the environment and our experience within it are not static, it is often not sufficient to select the identity and locations of relevant events, but also necessary to consider when these will occur and how to time our actions toward them. Think of the simple problem of intercepting the ball in a football game.

In principle, it should be possible to extract temporal predictions from the dynamic properties of stimuli or recurring temporal associations between events to bias perception and action toward the relevant moments of relevant events. Indeed, the psychological and neuroscientific literatures are filled with examples, often incidental, of how temporal regularities and expectations modulate behavioural performance and neural activity (Nobre et al., 2007). Yet, these lines of evidence did not influence research into selective attention until relatively recently.[1]

Some years ago, Coull and I set out to redress the omission of temporal factors in the cognitive neuroscience literature on attention (Coull and Nobre 1998; Coull, Chapter 31, this volume). We developed an experimental paradigm in which it was possible to manipulate temporal expectations for task-relevant target stimuli in an analogous way to how spatial expectations are typically manipulated (Posner, 1980). Our goals were to reveal the brain areas involved in controlling the orienting of attention to relevant moments in time, testing whether these were co-extensive with brain areas involved in the control of spatial orienting; and to reveal the mechanisms through which temporal expectations could bias perception or action. Predictably, but unforeseen, the path ahead was much more difficult than it appeared on the surface.

In hindsight, the daunting nature of the enterprise should have been obvious. In the case of other types of attention, our basic understanding about the neural organization of perceptual and motor systems has provided valuable guidance. As mentioned briefly earlier, the spatial layout and functional tuning of receptive fields for features and feature-configurations provide a clear substrate for top-down feedback signals to bias neuronal processing in order to select task-relevant locations and objects. Likewise, frontoparietal sensorimotor circuits organized in terms of spatially directed action goals, and especially the oculomotor circuit, provide a logical source for the attentional biasing signals (Nobre 2001b; Moore and Armstrong, 2003; Moore and Fallah, 2004; Taylor et al., 2007; Ruff et al., 2009).

Sources of temporal expectations

When it comes to how temporal expectations are coded and how they can influence information processing, intuitions from basic neuroscience are sorely lacking. Knowledge about how the brain codes temporal intervals on the scale that is relevant to organize cognition[2] would be instrumental in guiding hypotheses about putative control system(s) for temporal orienting of attention.

But, very little is known, and even less is agreed upon. The existence of a dedicated *timing* system in the brain is hotly debated. Some propose that temporal intervals are computed by a

---

[1] Scholars have considered for a long time how the length and the certainty of temporal intervals between events (foreperiod) can influence performance variables (see Niemi and Näätänen, 1981). However, little consideration was given to the possibility that foreperiod effects could come under flexible endogenous or exogenous control, according to task goals and changing predictions. With a few notable exceptions (see Posner and Petersen, 1990; Jones, 2004), the foreperiod effects in particular or the temporal dimension in general were also not taken into consideration in the mainstream research on selective attention.

[2] Of primary interest is the neural coding of intervals on the order of hundreds of milliseconds, within the upper limits of 'interval timing'.

centralized neural system, possibly organized around thalamo-cortical-striatal motor circuits (Matell and Meck, 2000; Coull et al., 2004), the cerebellum (Ivry, 1996; Ivry and Schlerf, 2008) or their combination (O'Reilly et al., 2008). Others propose that the computation of temporal parameters occurs in a distributed fashion, across many or all neural systems (Mauk and Buonomano, 2004; Nobre and O'Reilly 2004; Karmarkar and Buonomano, 2007). Within distributed models, temporal estimations have often been linked to circuits involved in processing spatial representations and spatially guided actions (Leon and Shadlen, 2003; Burr, Tozzi, Morrone, 2007; Morrone and Burr, Chapter 13, this volume). Given this state of affairs, there is no clear theoretically motivated favourite starting point for identifying the system(s) that control the orienting of attention to relevant temporal intervals.

As a first step, Coull and I used non-invasive brain imaging to compare directly, in the same participants and tasks, brain areas that were activated when attention was oriented to spatial locations versus temporal intervals (Coull and Nobre, 1998; see also Coull, Chapter 31, this volume). We found that activity in the dorsal frontoparietal circuit, which is well known to control spatial attention (Kastner and Ungerleider, 2000; Nobre 2001b; Corbetta and Shulman, 2002), was also modulated by temporal orienting. In addition, we found that a network of areas related to manual action preparation was selectively engaged by temporal orienting, including: left posterior parietal and left inferior premotor cortex. Involvement of these areas in temporal orienting, and especially of the left parietal cortex, proved reliable over subsequent experiments of ours (Coull et al., 2000, 2001) and is compatible with findings using tasks that have manipulated temporal expectations in different ways (Sakai et al., 2000; Schubotz and von Cramon, 2001; Assmus et al., 2003; Schubotz et al., 2003; Coull et al., 2008).

The working hypothesis derived from these imaging findings is that sensorimotor circuits specialized for manual action selection and preparation may contribute to the control of the temporal allocation of attention in a way that is analogous to how the oculomotor system participates in the spatial allocation of attention (Nobre 2001a, 2004). Timing is of exquisite importance for the preparation and execution of limb movements, suggesting these multisensory sensorimotor circuits may represent with a high level of precision the temporal dynamics of relevant stimuli as well as the temporal orchestration of complex goal-directed actions. Recently, a role has also been proposed for the cerebellum to influence this circuitry, by providing a temporal forward model that can be used for predicting the timing of sensory events as well as actions (O'Reilly et al., 2008; see also Miall et al., 1993; Ivry et al., 2002; Ramnani, 2006).

However, the case for these limb-related sensorimotor circuits to serve as a control system for temporal orienting of attention, possibly in combination with the oculomotor circuit, is not yet sealed. It remains unclear whether the areas identified comprise a general control network or a set of regions whose activity is modulated by temporal expectations in the tasks. Imaging studies so far have not separated brain activity related to temporal expectations triggered by the cues and the subsequent modulation of imperative target events.[3] Therefore modulation of activity in sensorimotor areas may be related to resultant biases in decision-making or response preparation upon target presentation. The problem is compounded by the fact that many tasks so far have required speeded manual responses to target stimuli.

Additional investigations, testing the role of action preparation in general, and of specific sensorimotor demands of tasks in particular, will be essential to determine whether there exists a

---

[3] This is a particularly problematic aspect of temporal orienting studies, since manipulating temporal expectations often requires imposing temporal correlations between events, which in turn makes separating their haemodynamic responses impossible.

network for the control of temporal orienting, which can be dissociated from any intrinsic task-related sensorimotor networks. Recently, studies have begun testing the involvement of brain areas in coding temporal expectations and predictions in the absence of speeded action requirements (Coull et al., 2008; O'Reilly et al., 2008), though these experiments may not have been able to rule out completely the contribution of implicit decisions or motor preparation. Current investigations are also underway to test whether and how the types of action required by a task (i.e. manual responses or saccades) influence the brain areas that participate in temporal orienting (Cotti et al., 2009). To test the generality of any candidate temporal orienting control network, it will also be necessary to test its involvement in tasks using non-visual and cross-modal stimuli. Finally, the causal involvement of brain areas identified by imaging will need to be confirmed by interference-based methods, using lesion or transcranial magnetic stimulation (TMS) studies (Vallesi, Chapter 22, this volume).

If action-related sensorimotor circuits turn out to play a critical role in the control of temporal orienting, it may be difficult to tell whether time-keeping is intrinsic in these circuits or whether the relevant intervals are provided by a separate, dedicated clock mechanism (Nobre et al., 2007; Coull and Nobre, 2008). If a separate, dedicated clock mechanism does exist, it may prove difficult for brain-imaging methods to reveal it. For example, reliable timekeeping may require activity in critical brain areas to remain relatively unaffected by ongoing task demands (Nobre and O'Reilly, 2004). In such a scheme, top-down control signals related to temporal predictions would arise from the interaction of dedicated time-keeping mechanisms and action-related sensorimotor systems.

As I see it, the two competing views about the sources of temporal expectations are still very much still in the running. Temporal expectations may be mediated by a general 'control' network, related to action preparation, regardless of the specific stimulus parameters or task goals. Under this first possibility, temporal predictions may be generated internally within this system or may arise from the interaction of this system with a dedicated neural clock mechanism. Alternatively, temporal expectations may emerge within the brain areas that specifically participate in the task, according to stimulus parameters and task goals. Under this second possibility, task-related multisensory sensorimotor circuits may play a prominent role, since these provide a plausible substrate for organizing and translating sensory experience into behavioural output. While these two alternatives are fundamentally different at the conceptual level, their implications for predicted patterns of neural activity may be much more subtle, especially for investigations in the human brain where the imaging methods are relatively blunt.

Biasing perception by temporal expectations

Even more puzzling than considering the sources of temporal predictions is to reflect upon how these may come to influence perception. There is no clear intuition about the units for temporal selection. In the case of feature-based or object-based attention, it is possible to augment the baseline activity or excitability in neurons coding the features or feature-configurations of relevant objects (Chelazzi et al., 1993; Treue and Martínez Trujillo, 1999; Stokes et al., 2009). In the case of case of spatial attention, it is possible to enhance activity or excitability of neurons with receptive fields that overlap with relevant locations (Moran and Desimone, 1985; Luck et al., 1997; Fries et al., 2001). But what would serve as the neural substrate for selective biasing by a temporal prediction? As far as we know, there is no explicit coding of temporal intervals in the receptive fields of sensory areas. It would not be possible, therefore, to enhance selectively the activity in neurons that code relevant moments in time. One option would be to enhance activity across all sensory neurons, as in a phasic alerting signal, but such a mechanism would be highly metabolically taxing and would lack the selectivity to enhance target items relative to simultaneously present distractor items.

Despite the puzzle of how this might come about, behavioural work does suggest the ability of temporal expectations to influence perceptual functions (Rolke and Ulrich, Chapter 17; Jones, Chapter 23; Schubotz, Chapter 25; Correa, Chapter 26; Lange and Röder, Chapter 28, this volume). Though it is often difficult to pinpoint the stage of processing that is modulated by behavioural performance measures alone, some findings suggest early influences. For example, the degree of temporal certainty between events can modulate perceptual thresholds for luminance, orientation and stereoscopic discriminations (Lasley and Cohn, 1981; Westheimer and Ley, 1996) and can increase perceptual discriminability of visual stimuli (Correa et al., 2005; Rolke and Hofmann, 2007).

Cued temporal expectations of visual stimuli

To investigate directly whether, when, and how perceptual functions were modulated by temporal expectations, my colleagues and I recorded event-related potentials during performance of a cued visual temporal orienting task (Miniussi et al., 1999). These voltage fluctuations measured at the scalp, which vary systematically with stimulus events in a task, serve as a rich dependent variable with which to track ongoing brain activity directly and in real-time, albeit with poor spatial resolution.[4]

In the first study, a foveal version of the temporal orienting task was used (see Figure 27.1A). Central cues whose appearance was counterbalanced across participants predicted the appearance of a central target stimulus after a short or long stimulus-onset asynchrony (600ms or 1400ms) (Miniussi et al., 1999). The task required simple speeded detection of the target stimulus, and cues were valid on 80% of trials (10% invalid trials and 10% catch trials). Modulation of behavioural performance and neural activity by temporal orienting cues was restricted to targets appearing at the first, short interval. After passage of an empty short interval, it became highly predictable that the target would occur at the longer interval, enabling participants to re-orient their attention to this next relevant time point (also see Coull, Chapter 31, this volume), an effect that is also compatible with improved performance at the longer foreperiods in variable-foreperiod tasks (Wagener and Hoffman, Chapter 16; Los, Chapter 21; Vallesi, Chapter 22, this volume). Given the demands of the task, behavioural effects were expressed as improvements in the reaction times to detect targets appearing at the short interval after valid versus invalid temporal cues.

Event-related potentials elicited by cues and targets revealed how neural activity was modulated during anticipation and processing of the targets respectively. After cues, there was a pronounced difference in a slow negative potential linked to the anticipation of stimuli or responses, known as the 'contingent negative variation' (Walter et al., 1964), which is thought to be generated in brain areas related to motor preparation (Vidal et al., 1995; Rektor, 2002; Praamstra et al., 2006). The potential was significantly steeper after cues predicting short target intervals, suggesting the ability of temporal expectations to act through sensorimotor circuits to tune motor preparation for detecting target stimuli. Our observation is in line with several others,

----

[4] Event-related potentials provide a read-out of extracellular voltage signals associated with synchronized synaptic activity across large populations of well aligned neurons (mainly pyramidal cortical neurons) (Allison et al., 1986; Hämäläinen and Hari, 2002). Because of spatial summation across all simultaneously active synaptic fields across the folds of cortex, locating the brain areas generating the voltage fields measured over the scalp is intractable (Helmholtz, 1853).

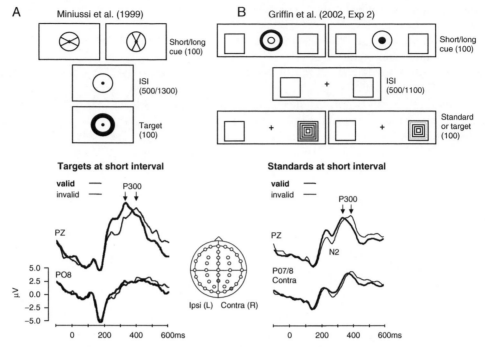

Fig. 27.1 ERP results from two experiments manipulating temporal expectation by endogenous temporal cues. A) Task schematic and grand-averaged ERPs elicited by target stimuli appearing at the short interval in the study by Miniussi et al. (1999): participants viewed a brief (100-ms) cue followed by a central target stimulus (100) at either 600ms or 1400ms after cue onset. The cue consisted of a narrow or wide cross (30° or 60°, counterbalanced) and predicted the interval (600ms, 1400ms) at which the target would appear (80% validity.) The target consisted of the brightening of the central circle (1.7°), and required a simple detection response. Grand-averaged waveforms elicited by central target stimuli appearing at the short interval when participants expected targets at the short interval (valid trials, thick line) or the long interval (invalid trials, thin line). Results showed significant attenuation of the N2 by temporal expectation and a significant anticipation of the P3 latency by valid temporal expectation. B) Task schematic and grand-averaged ERPs elicited by standard stimuli appearing at the short interval in the study by Griffin et al. (2002): participants (N = 12) viewed a brief (100-ms) cue followed by a unilateral stimulus (100ms, centred at 7.5° horizontal eccentricity and 1.5° below the vertical meridian) at either 600s or 1200ms after cue onset. The cue consisted of the brightening of either the inner or outer circle, and indicated which interval (600ms, 1200ms) was relevant for target discrimination. Participants responded only to occasional targets (19% of trials) appearing at the cued interval. Standard and target stimuli consisted of a pattern of concentric squares. Targets were defined by one of the inner squares being fainter. Grand-averaged waveforms in the temporal orienting condition elicited by unilateral standard peripheral stimuli when subjects were attending the short (thick line) and long (thin line) intervals. Results showed a marginally significant attenuation of the N2 by temporal expectation and a significant anticipation of the P3 latency by valid temporal expectation.

showing that this potential ramps up gradually and peaks at the anticipated time of the relevant target or response (Macar and Vidal, 2004; Pfeuty et al., 2005), and is strongly influenced by changes in the ongoing temporal predictability of events either by the temporal pattern of events inherent to the task or by explicit temporal cues (Trillenberg et al., 2000; Los and Heslenfeld, 2005; Praamstra et al., 2006; Los, Chapter 21; Pouthas and Pfeuty, Chapter 30; Praamstra, Chapter 24, this volume).

Event-related potentials triggered by target stimuli at the short interval showed clear modulation of later potentials associated with post-perceptual processes.[5] Most notably, the prominent late positive potential was brought forward in time as well as enhanced in magnitude. Taking into account the preceding modulation of cue-related potentials, we speculated that predictive information about temporal intervals may be used to prepare or synchronize processes linked to decisions or responses. Many subsequent studies have also shown the acceleration of potentials linked to preparation and execution of responses by controlled temporal expectations in orienting paradigms (Griffin et al., 2002; Lange et al., 2003; Doherty et al., 2005; Correa et al., 2006; Correa and Nobre, 2008) as well as by automatic temporal expectations in foreperiod paradigms (Muller-Gethmann, et al., 2003; Los and Helensfeld 2005; Hackley et al., 2007; Burle et al., Chapter 18, this volume). Together, these results complement findings from single-unit recordings in motor and premotor areas in demonstrating the strong effects of temporal expectations upon the level and synchronizationon of neuronal activity in response-related areas (Heinen and Liu 1997; Riehle et al., 1997; Luchetti and Bon, 2001; Renoult et al., 2006; Kilavik and Riehle, Chapter 19, this volume).

Disappointingly, however, no early modulation of perceptual processes was observed in target-related potentials in our task (Figure 27.1A) (Miniussi et al., 1999). Several possibilities for this null finding were considered and ruled out. The perceptual demands of the task might have been too low, so that it was sufficient to tune motor functions without modulating perceptual analysis of the target stimuli. Miniussi and I tested this possibility with a version of the task in which difficulty was titrated on an ongoing basis by a staircase procedure that maintained performance between 70% and 80% accuracy. Rather than simply detecting a circular target, participants had to discriminate a small break in the outline of the target, which could appear in any part of the circumference. The potentials elicited by targets in this perceptually demanding task still showed no evidence of early perceptual modulation. Given the null-effects nature of the findings and the ferocity of the publications game, we never submitted a manuscript based on this experiment, but it is described in Miniussi's doctoral thesis (Miniussi, 1999). Next, it was considered whether the foveal location of the targets may have jeopardized the ability to observe attentional modulations, since perceptual analysis may already be naturally enhanced and optimized by foveation. To test this, Miniussi conducted a spatial attention experiment using foveal target stimuli, but in this case clear modulation of the visual potentials of foveal stimuli was

---

5 It is important to note that the temporal correlations required by most modulations of temporal expectations also pose difficulties for investigating their modulation of neural processing with event-related potentials. It is important to rule out contamination of target-related waveforms by late potentials that are time-locked to preceding cue stimuli. Overlap between potentials from preceding and current stimuli can lead to erroneous interpretations (Woldorff, 1993). For example, an effect that looks like early modulation of target-related activity could really signal modulation of a late potential from the preceding stimulus. It is important, therefore, to ensure that baseline activity preceding target-related potentials is well equated and to plot the distribution of target-related effects to ensure that it differs significantly from any lingering cue-related effects. Replicating findings across different ranges of intervals would also provide greater confidence for interpreting target-related results.

observed (Miniussi et al., 2002). Finally, we tested whether temporal expectations could modulate perceptual analysis of peripheral stimuli requiring difficult perceptual discriminations (Griffin et al., 2002). Two experiments were carried out, manipulating either the probability of targets appearing at a given interval (Experiment 1) or the task-relevance of targets appearing at a given interval (Experiment 2). In neither case was the earlier visual potential (P1) modulated by temporal expectations (Figure 27.1B). In Experiment 1, a small but significant enhancement of the later N1 potential was observed bilaterally. This effect, however, has not proven reliable across visual temporal orienting tasks, and it is also possible that post-perceptual variables related to sensori-motor integration or motor preparation contribute to this stage of analysis (e.g. Doherty et al., 2005). Without additional supporting evidence, it may be imprudent to attach too much weight to this finding of 'visual' modulation by temporal expectations.

One experiment by Correa et al. (2006) stands as an exception in the visual temporal orienting literature. In this case, a blocked manipulation of the predicted intervals between temporal cues and subsequent targets in a shape-discrimination task using foveal stimuli did result in modulation of the visual P1 potential. In their experiment, the extent to which late cue-related activity over posterior electrodes contributed to the early P1 effects, which peaked unusually late (>150ms), is not clear. It will be important to resolve the matter by replicating the findings using different temporal intervals and showing that the early modulation shares the same underlying distribution as the visual P1 potential. If reliable modulation of visual processing is confirmed, it would suggest that the stronger manipulation of temporal expectations achieved using a blocked design, combined with high perceptual demands, is sufficient to drive early perceptual modulation. In this case, however, it may be difficult to tell whether the effects result from voluntary orienting of temporal attention based on cues, or automatic associations that develop across the consistent temporal pairing of intervals between stimuli across trials (Los and Van den Heuvel, 2001; Los and Helensfeld 2005; Los, Chapter 21, this volume). Blocked manipulations may also lead to contributions of state-dependent variables, such as increased alertness or error-monitoring in difficult blocks.

Rhythmic temporal expectations of visual stimuli

Isolated temporal expectations

More recently, we have developed an experimental task to investigate the effects of temporal expectations under more naturalistic conditions (Doherty et al., 2005). Though symbolic cues that explicitly predict the attributes or timing of upcoming events are experimentally convenient, they have few counterparts in the real world. Instead, expectations about perceptual events typically develop by observing their dynamic qualities, such as their speed and spatial trajectory. These can be used, for example, to anticipate the reappearance of transiently occluded objects (Wertheimer, 1961; Michotte et al., 1964; Assad and Maunsell, 1995). Furthermore, whereas it is experimentally meaningful to manipulate temporal expectations in isolation, in the real world temporal expectations tend to be linked to specific events and are thus bound to the other predictable stimulus attributes. Think again about intercepting the ball in a football game.

In the task we developed, an object—a ball—appears at the side of a display monitor and moves across to the other side of the monitor in discrete steps, passing 'under' an occluding band along its way (Figure 27.2A). The participants' goal was to monitor the moving ball covertly, and to discriminate a small shape embedded within the ball upon its reappearance after occlusion. There were no explicit predictive cues, but temporal and/or spatial expectations could be derived from the inherent dynamics with which the ball moved across the screen. In different conditions, the ball appeared at regular intervals (550ms, temporal expectation) or at

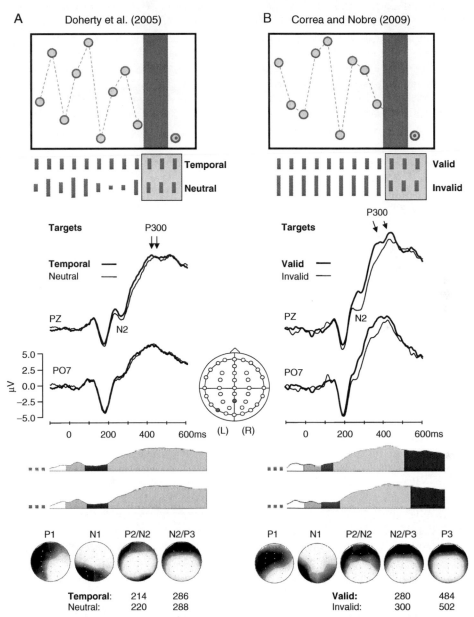

Fig. 27.2 ERP results from two experiments manipulating temporal expectation by the regularity versus irregularity of discrete motion steps of an object passing 'under an occluding band'.
A) *Top panel:* task schematic in the study by Doherty et al. (2005): a red ball appeared at the left side of a black screen and moved in discrete steps and disappeared underneath an occluding band (11.4–14.7° eccentricity) for two steps. Only one ball was ever present on the screen. The schematic, however, shows the entire sequence of steps. The dashed lines illustrate the apparent trajectory. The small bars underneath the display schematic illustrate graphically the duration of each motion step, which could be regular (equal size) or irregular (different sizes). Participants were required to respond only if the ball contained a black dot upon its reappearance (go/no-go,

Fig. 27.2 (*continued*) 50% probability). The task manipulated spatial and temporal expectations factorially. Shown here are two conditions without spatial expectation. In the Temporal condition, the ball moved in regular steps (550 ms), which generated a focused temporal expectation about when the ball would reappear. In the Neutral condition, the ball moved in irregular steps (200–900 ms), which did not generate a focused temporal expectation. *Middle panel:* grand-averaged ERPs for the temporal and neutral conditions (N = 24 participants) showed no modulation of early visual P1 (see lateral posterior electrode contralateral to ball, PO7). Instead significant modulations were observed over later N2 and P300 potentials (see midline parietal electrode PZ). The N2 was significantly attenuated by temporal expectation, and the P300 was larger and earlier in the temporal condition in the case of go (but not no-go) targets. *Bottom panel:* a new topographical analysis of the data using Cartool (D. Brunet, Functional Brain Mapping Laboratory, Geneva, Switzerland). Topographies of grand-averaged ERPs referenced to the average of all scalp electrodes and normalized by the global field power were subjected to a spatiotemporal clustering algorithm to determine the number, nature, and timings of topographies that best explained topographical variance across conditions (Atomize & Agglomerate Hierarchical Clustering; minimum segment duration 20 ms, topographies with >95% correlation were collapsed). The results showed equivalent stable topographical in the two conditions, but a shift in the timing of the later neural states, so that late potentials started earlier in the temporal condition relative to the neutral condition. The global field power waveforms are shown starting from 100ms (P1 potential), with different shades of grey indicating different topographical states. The corresponding topographical maps are shown just below from a bird's-eye perspective (top corresponds to front of head, left to left), with white indicating positive values and black negative values. Onsets of the final two topographical states are indicated for the two conditions (in ms). B) *Top panel:* task schematic in the study by Correa and Nobre (2009): a yellow ball appeared at the left side of a grey screen and moved in discrete steps and disappeared underneath an occluding band (11.7–14.3° eccentricity) for two steps. Participants were required to respond only if the ball contained a black dot upon its reappearance (go/no-go, 80% probability). The task manipulated temporal expectations in the absence of spatial expectations. In the Valid temporal condition, the ball moved in regular steps (200–900ms, fixed within trial), and reappeared at the predicted moment from 'under' the occluding band. In the Invalid temporal condition, the ball reappeared either at least 200ms before or at least 200ms after the predicted moment. *Middle panel:* grand-averaged ERPs for the valid and invalid short-occlusion conditions (N = 16 participants) showed no modulation of early visual P1 (see lateral posterior electrode contralateral to ball, PO7). Later, the N2 was attenuated and the P300 was anticipated for valid versus invalid targets appearing after short occlusion periods (see midline parietal electrode PZ). *Bottom panel:* topographical analysis using the same procedures and parameters as in panel (A). The results showed equivalent stable topographical in the two conditions, but a shift in the timing of the later neural states, so that late potentials started earlier in the valid condition relative to the invalid condition.

irregular intervals (200–900ms, no temporal expectation), and following a linear spatial trajectory (spatial expectation) or erratic spatial trajectory (no spatial expectation).[6] The ball remained occluded for two motion steps (1100ms). Temporal and spatial expectations were manipulated in a factorial fashion, to yield four possible types of expectation about when and/or where the

---

[6] Discrete motion steps were used instead of continuous motion so that it was possible to manipulate temporal versus spatial predictions factorially within the same task. It would not have been possible to equate speeds of motion across conditions where a ball moves in a spatially predictable linear trajectory and in a spatially unpredictable erratic trajectory.

ball would reappear. In the condition of combined temporal and spatial expectations (TS), participants could predict the exact moment and location for the re-appearance of the ball after occlusion. In the condition of isolated temporal expectation (T), the participants could anticipate the exact moment but could not anticipate where along the vertical occlusion band the target would reappear. In the condition of isolated spatial expectation (S) the participants could antici-pate the exact location but could not anticipate when the target would reappear after occlusion. In the no-expectation condition (N), the participants could anticipate neither the exact moment nor location for target reappearance.

The behavioural results confirmed the ability of both temporal and spatial expectations derived from the motion properties of the ball to speed reaction times (additive main effects) (Figure 27.2A). Again, we used event-related potentials to chart the time course and nature of neural modulation by isolated and combined temporal and spatial expectations. When temporal or spatial expectations occurred in isolation, the pattern of effects was remarkably similar to the results from previous studies using endogenous predictive cues. In the case of isolated spatial expectation, the characteristic amplitude enhancement of the contralateral visual P1 was observed (reviewed in Mangun, 1995; Eimer, 1998; Hillyard et al., 1998). In the case of isolated temporal expectation there was no modulation of the early visual P1 potential, but again later post-perceptual potentials showed the characteristic effects including the earlier latency of the late positive potential. The inclusion of a go/no-go manipulation in this task also enabled us to prove the hypothesized dependency of the effects of temporal expectation on motor variables (Miniussi et al., 1999), including at the level of the late 'visual' N1 potential, which was diminished for targets appearing at expected moments, but only if these required responses.

A new topographical segmentation of the data from this experiment (Doherty et al., 2005) provides a graphical visualization of one of the main ways through which temporal expectations influence post-perceptual analysis. Analysis of stimuli occurring at expected and unexpected temporal moments proceeds through an equivalent series of distinct neural stages, but valid temporal expectations makes processing more efficient so that processing reaches successive stages progressively earlier (Figure 27.2A).

Correa and I recently replicated this pattern of modulation by isolated temporal expectations in a similar, but more flexible occlusion task (Correa and Nobre, 2008) (Figure 27.2B). In the new task, the regular intervals used to drive temporal expectations, as well as the occlusion periods, varied on a trial-by-trial basis, providing important validation about the generality of the effects. In addition, by varying the intervals, it was possible to observe the interaction between the effects of temporal predictability driven by the regularity of temporal rhythms and the length of the occlusion interval (foreperiod). Applying topographical segmentation to data from this experi-ment also showed the progressive speeding of information processing through successive stages of analysis by temporal expectations (Figure 27.2B).

Synergies between temporal and spatial expectations

The most sensible conclusion from the results of experiments in my laboratory is that isolated temporal expectations enhance information processing of visual stimuli primarily by optimizing post-perceptual stages of analysis. Early visual stages of analysis remain largely unaffected. Of course, it is not possible to rule out the ability of temporal expectations to influence perceptual functions under different, as yet untested experimental conditions. In addition, some perceptual effects may occur that cannot be measured by the method of event-related potentials.

However, the experiment by Doherty revealed that the impact of temporal expectations on early visual processing changes dramatically when these are combined with spatial expecta-tions. In this case, a striking synergy occurs. Whereas temporal expectations in isolation exerted no effect upon the early visual P1 potential, when temporal expectation was combined with spatial expectation, it greatly boosted the effect of spatial expectation in enhancing the P1 (Figure 27.3A). Rohenkohl and I have now replicated this intriguing effect in a new version of the occlusion task (Rohenkohl and Nobre, 2009) (Figure 27.3B). Modulation of early visual potentials has also been observed by Praamstra and colleagues (2006; Praamstra, Chapter 24, this volume) in a task where foveal target stimuli appeared synchronously with or deviated slightly from a regular rhythm set up by a preceding train of visual stimuli. Here too, temporal expectations set up by rhythmic stimulation occurred in the context of spatial expectations.

These new findings suggest a sensible and ecologically valid way in which temporal expectations can selectively bias visual perceptual functions. Temporal expectations rarely, if ever, occur in isolation. Time is, by nature, anchored to events and their interrelations. Therefore temporal expectations may serve mainly to organize other types of expectations about unfolding events. A logical prediction is that temporal expectation for visual stimuli exerts the strongest effects when coupled with predictions about other features that can be clearly mapped onto neuronal receptive-field properties. In the absence of explicit coding of timing in visual cortex, temporal expectations may nevertheless tune activity in neurons coding relevant stimulus locations or features. So far, we have only demonstrated interaction between temporal and spatial expectations (Doherty et al., 2005; Rohenkohl and Nobre 2009), but we are currently testing the ability of temporal expectations to interact with other predicted receptive-field properties (e.g. object colour or shape). In addition, the consistent and strong effects on motor-related processing show that temporal expectations also help select and prepare specific responses required in a task to optimize performance. Motor-related activity can be optimized even in the absence of other predicted target attributes or of visual modulation, suggesting multiple possible sites for biasing signals to influence information processing according to temporal expectations.

Our findings and interpretations of synergistic effects of temporal and spatial expectations are compatible with single-unit studies showing modulation of spatial-attention effects by the evolving temporal probability of target appearance in areas V4 (Ghose and Maunsell, 2002) and LIP (Janssen and Shadlen, 2005).

Temporal expectations in other sensory modalities

Although it is intuitively appealing to suppose that temporal expectations tune sensory processing across sensory modalities though analogous mechanisms, this appears not to be the case. In contrast to the findings using visual stimuli, perceptual modulation is routinely reported in auditory studies of temporal orienting (Lange et al., 2006; Lange and Röder 2006; Lange and Heil, 2008; Sanders and Astheimer 2008). The enhancement of the auditory N1 potential for stimuli occurring at the relevant moment is a consistent finding across these studies (Lange and Röder, Chapter 28, this volume). It would be interesting to test whether perceptual modulation can occur at even earlier stages, influencing the mid-latency potentials which reflect the initial stages of cortical processing (see Woldorff et al., 1987).

Studies comparing the stages of modulation of visual versus auditory processing using well equated stimuli and task conditions are still missing, but a descriptive comparison of results between the visual and auditory modalities points to heterogeneity in how temporal expectation optimizes information-processing across the sensory modalities. Vision and audition are complementary in their levels of sensitivity to spatial and temporal parameters, and attentional modulations may be guided accordingly. In audition—a sense characterized by its high temporal acuity and sensitivity—the extensive subcortical processing and the coding of temporal parameters from the earliest stages may provide the necessary substrate for temporal biases, which is absent

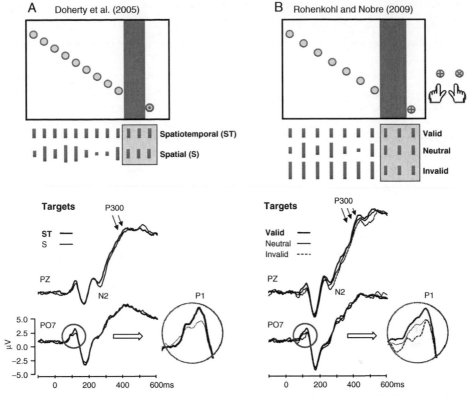

Fig. 27.3 ERP results from two experiments manipulating temporal expectation by the regularity versus irregularity of discrete motion steps in the presence of spatial expectation (see Figure 27.2 for further details). A) *Top panel:* SpatioTemporal (ST) and Spatial (S) conditions in the study by Doherty et al. (2005). In the SpatioTemporal condition, the ball moved in regular steps (550ms) and followed a linear spatial trajectory, which generated focused temporal and spatial expectations about when and where the ball would reappear. In the Spatial condition, the ball moved in irregular steps (200–900 ms) but followed a linear spatial trajectory, which generated focused spatial expectation in the absence of temporal expectation. *Bottom panel:* grand-averaged ERPs for the spatiotemporal and spatial conditions (N = 24 participants) showed significant enhancement of the visual P1 potential. This was functionally equivalent to the augmentation of the P1 enhancement by spatial expectation (S) relative to neutral trials (not shown). In addition, the N2 was attenuated and the P300 was anticipated by temporal expectation. B) *Top panel:* task schematic in the study by Rohenkohl and Nobre (2009): A white ball appeared at the top or bottom of the left side of a grey screen and moved in temporally regular (200-ms ball duration; 200-ms or 600-ms interval, fixed) or irregular (200-ms ball duration; 100–700-ms interval, randomized) discrete steps along a diagonal spatial trajectory, disappearing underneath an occluding band (11.4–14.7° eccentricity) for one step. Participants were required to make a forced-choice discrimination as to whether the ball contained an upright or tilted cross upon its reappearance (50% probability). The occlusion period was either short (600ms) or long (1400ms). Data were analysed for balls reappearing after the short interval. In valid trials (44%), the occlusion interval was correctly predicted according to the regular speed of the ball during the pre-occlusion period. In Neutral trials (44%), the speed of the ball was irregular during the pre-occlusion period. In Invalid trials (12%), the ball appeared earlier than predicted by the regular slow speed of the ball during the pre-occlusion period. *Bottom panel:* grand-averaged ERPs for Valid, Neutral, and Invalid conditions (N = 20 participants) showed significant and systematic enhancement of the P1 potential as a function of temporal validity; as well as attenuation of the N2 and anticipation of the P300.

in vision (Viemeister and Plack, 1993; Poeppel, 2003; Thompson et al., 2006; King and Nelken, 2009).

However, before it is possible to draw strong conclusions about the degree of similarity or difference in how temporal attentional biases operate in vision and audition, it is necessary to rule out other possible explanations for the divergent findings. For example, auditory experiments of cued temporal orienting have tended to use blocked manipulations of relevant temporal intervals (Lange et al., 2003, 2006; Lange and Röder, 2006; Sanders and Astheimer, 2008) whereas visual experiments have tended to use trial-by-trial manipulations. The one exception in the visual domain is the study in which early visual modulations were reported (Correa et al., 2006). An important next step, therefore, is to design appropriate tasks to compare and contrast directly modulation of visual and auditory processing by temporal expectations. Additional studies investigating the effects of temporal expectations in other sensory modalities, as well as across modalities (Lange and Röder, 2006), will also be essential for deriving the underlying principles governing how temporal expectations operate upon perceptual functions.

Cellular mechanisms of perceptual biases by temporal expectations

Within the vast literature dealing with the mechanisms of attention at the cellular level, only a handful of studies have considered the role of temporal biases (Ghose and Maunsell, 2002; Janssen and Shadlen, 2005; Lakatos et al., 2007, 2008; Anderson and Sheinberg, 2008). This disappointing situation is bound to change soon. Facing the fundamental importance of the temporal factor for the organization of perception is simply inevitable.

As mentioned earlier, the lack of any direct mapping of time in the receptive-field properties of sensory neurons means that the mechanisms for biasing sensory signalling by temporal expectations cannot be isomorphic with the mechanisms available for spatial or feature-based biasing. It is not possible, for example, to change the baseline level of activity or to synchronize the activity only in neurons coding the predicted relevant interval. On the other hand, it might be possible to time the activity in neurons coding relevant task stimuli or to select neurons that are in a particular dynamic state (Karmarkar and Buonomano, 2007), mechanisms that are not available when only spatial or feature-based expectations are present. The studies so far are too few in number to provide a comprehensive view of the cellular mechanisms of temporal biases, but they already provide some tantalizing clues.

Two studies have demonstrated that temporal predictions can make use of the spatial coding of task-relevant events to modulate the timing of neuronal activity in a spatially selective way. Ghose and Maunsell (2002) showed temporal tuning of spatial attention effects in visual area V4 according to evolving temporal expectations. Monkeys had to detect a change in the orientation of a Gabor patch in one location, while ignoring changes at another location. The differential rate of firing in neurons coding the spatially relevant versus irrelevant location fluctuated according to the temporal conditional probability function for the orientation change to occur. Janssen and Shadlen (2005) observed a similar effect in a delayed-saccade task, where modulation of neuronal firing in parietal area LIP by spatial attention and/or saccade planning varied according to the subjective temporal probability for the occurrence of the response signal. In both cases, temporal expectations were able to sharpen the attentional biases selectively by making use of the spatial properties of neuronal receptive fields. These findings at the single-unit level are compatible with the findings and interpretations from our observations using event-related potentials with visual tasks (Doherty et al., 2005; Rohenkohl and Nobre, 2009).

The most direct investigation of temporal expectations upon cellular activity to date has been conducted by Anderson and Sheinberg (2008; Anderson and Sheinberg, Chapter 29, this volume). In their task, two stimuli occurred successively in spatially predictable locations, and the second, target stimulus required a pre-learned categorization response. Monkeys had also learned that, at the beginning of a trial, particular images of objects predicted the interval at which the target image would appear. Temporal expectations were therefore manipulated by endogenous cues on a trial-by-trial basis. Two intervals were used, and, in line with the increasing predictability of events at the later interval, the effects of temporal expectation were more pronounced for the targets occurring at the short interval. At these intervals, valid temporal expectations enhanced the spiking rates and field potentials triggered by the target image, and increased the degree of coherence between the spikes and the field potentials in the beta-gamma frequency range. These effects appear more striking than the effects in cued visual temporal orienting studies using event-related potentials in humans, in which visual modulation tends to be absent (Miniussi et al., 1999; Griffin et al., 2002). However, it is difficult to know the contribution of visual area IT to scalp-recorded potentials. This initial study stimulates several interesting questions. In order to understand whether and how the effects observed are selective across neuronal populations, it would be important to know whether the effect would also occur in conditions of spatial uncertainty, and whether the modulation differentially affects the processing of images that are effective versus ineffective at driving neuronal activity. Taking this one step further, it would be critical to test whether temporal expectations can influence the selection of a relevant target item when another task-irrelevant item is also present in the receptive field of the neuron. It would also be very informative to verify the extent to which the effects observed in the monkeys depend on long-term learning of the temporal prediction of the stimuli.

Recently, additional mechanisms for changing neuronal excitability have been revealed in situations involving rhythmic stimulation. Using field-potential recordings in visual and auditory cortices, Lakatos, Schroeder, and colleagues have shown that oscillatory activity in neuronal ensembles become entrained to the timing of task-relevant rhythmic stimuli according to their modality and location (Lakatos et al., 2005, 2007, 2008, 2009). They propose that alignment of low-frequency oscillations (in the theta range) to the timing of rhythmic or regular events provides a central mechanism for regulating cortical excitability by temporal expectations. These slow oscillatory rhythms in turn entrain higher-frequency oscillations (in the beta and gamma ranges), so that the state of cortical excitability is optimized for processing relevant events occurring at predicted moments (Canolty et al., 2006; Schroeder et al., 2008; Schroeder and Lakatos, 2009). These authors also propose that the slow contingent-negative-variation potential may reflect the underlying low-frequency carrier oscillations, whose amplitude and time-course has clearly been linked to temporal expectations (Lakatos et al., 2008; Schroeder and Lakatos, 2009; see also Pouthas and Pfeuty, Chapter 30, this volume). This simple yet thought-provoking proposal deserves concerted investigation. Initial findings by Praamstra and colleagues using scalp-recorded EEG in human participants are promising, showing modulation of oscillatory activity induced by visual stimuli occurring in- or off-phase relative to a preceding regular train of stimuli (Praamstra et al., 2006; Praamstra and Pope, 2007; Praamstra, Chapter 24, this volume).

Conclusions

In its proactive interface with reality, the brain continuously generates predictions about expected relevant events to guide perception and action. These predictions also incorporate the temporal dimension to anticipate the timing of events. Though effects of temporal expectations are conspicuous throughout the psychology and neuroscience literatures (Griffin and Nobre, 2005; Nobre et al., 2007), the neural systems and mechanisms by which temporal expectations bias perception and action are only beginning to be investigated. In these pages I have summarized my personal view of the current state of affairs, highlighting the many fundamental lacunae in our current understanding. Further research will confirm or challenge the budding notion that temporal expectations are mediated via networks closely associated with spatial and motor control; will chart the levels and types of neural activity that can be biased; and will reveal how neuronal activity and computation is modulated by this elusive dynamic dimension. The research tempo is picking up. As the rhythms carry us to our destination, we will witness major break-throughs in our understanding of the neural dynamics that shape our experience.

References

Allison, T., Wood, C. C., and McCarthy, G. (1986). The central nervous system. In M.G.H. Coles, E. Donchin, and S.W. Porges (Eds.) *Psychophysiology: Systems, Processes, and Applications*, pp.5–25. New York: Guilford Press.

Anderson, B. and Sheinberg, D. L. (2008). Effects of temporal context and temporal expectancy on neural activity in inferior temporal cortex. *Neuropsychologia*, **46**, 947–57.

Assad, J. A. and Maunsell, J. H. (1995). Neuronal correlates of inferred motion in primate posterior parietal cortex. *Nature*, **373**, 518–21.

Assmus, A., Marshall, J. C., Ritzl, A., Noth, J., Zilles, K., and Fink, G. R. (2003). Left inferior parietal cortex integrates time and space during collision judgments. *Neuroimage*, **20**(Suppl 1), S82–8.

Burr, D., Tozzi, A., and Morrone, M. C. (2007). Neural mechanisms for timing visual events are spatially selective in real-world coordinates. *Nat Neurosci*, **10**, 423–5.

Canolty, R. T., Edwards, E., Dalal, S. S., Soltani, M., Nagarajan, S. S., Kirsch, H. E., et al. (2006). High gamma power is phase-locked to theta oscillations in human neocortex. *Science*, **313**, 1626–8.

Chelazzi, L., Miller, E. K., Duncan, J., and Desimone, R (1993). A neural basis for visual search in inferior temporal cortex. *Nature*, **363**, 345–7.

Chelazzi, L., Duncan, J., Miller, E. K., and Desimone, R. (1998). Responses of neurons in inferior temporal cortex during memory-guided visual search. *J Neurophysiol*, **80**, 2918–40.

Chelazzi, L., Miller, E. K., Duncan, J., and Desimone, R. (2001). Responses of neurons in macaque area V4 during memory-guided visual search. *Cereb Cortex*, **11**, 761–72.

Corbetta, M. and Shulman, G. L. (2002). Control of goal-directed and stimulus-driven attention in the brain. *Nat Rev Neurosci*, **3**, 201–15.

Correa, Á. and Nobre, A. C. (2008). Neural modulation by regularity and passage of time. *J Neurophysiol*, **100**, 1649–55.

Correa, Á., Lupiáñez, J., Milliken, B., and Tudela, P. (2004). Endogenous temporal orienting of attention in detection and discrimination tasks. *Percept Psychophys*, **66**, 264–78.

Correa, Á., Lupiáñez, J., and Tudela, P. (2005). Attentional preparation based on temporal expectancy modulates processing at the perceptual level. *Psychon Bull Rev*, **12**, 328–34.

Correa, Á., Lupiáñez, J., Madrid, E., and Tudela, P. (2006). Temporal attention enhances early visual processing: a review and new evidence from event-related potentials. *Brain Res*, **1076**, 116–28.

Cotti, J., Rohenkohl, G., Stokes, M., Nobre, A. C., and Coull, J. (2009). Functional and neural dissociation of temporal versus motor expectations. *NeuroImage*, **47**(S1), S42.

Coull, J. T. and Nobre, A. C. (1998). Where and when to pay attention: the neural systems for directing atten-tion to spatial locations and to time intervals as revealed by both PET and fMRI. *J Neurosci*, **18**, 7426–35.

Coull, J. and Nobre, A. (2008). Dissociating explicit timing from temporal expectation with fMRI. *Curr Opin Neurobiol*, **18**, 137–44.

Coull, J. T., Frith, C. D., Buchel, C., and Nobre, A. C. (2000). Orienting attention in time: behavioural and neuroanatomical distinction between exogenous and endogenous shifts. *Neuropsychologia*, **38**, 808–19.

Coull, J. T., Nobre, A. C., and Frith, C. D. (2001). The noradrenergic alpha2 agonist clonidine modulates behavioural and neuroanatomical correlates of human attentional orienting and alerting. *Cereb Cortex*, **11**, 73–84.

Coull, J. T., Vidal, F., Nazarian, B., and Macar, F. (2004). Functional anatomy of the attentional modulation of time estimation. *Science*, **303**, 1506–8.

Coull, J. T., Vidal, F., Goulon, C., Nazarian, B., and Craig, C. (2008). Using time-to-contact information to assess potential collision modulates both visual and temporal prediction networks. *Front Hum Neurosci*, **2**, 10.

Desimone, R. and Duncan, J. (1995). Neural mechanisms of selective visual attention. *Annu Rev Neurosci*, **18**, 193–222.

Doherty, J. R., Rao, A., Mesulam, M. M., and Nobre, A. C. (2005). Synergistic effect of combined temporal and spatial expectations on visual attention. *J Neurosci*, **25**, 8259–66.

Eimer, M. (1998). Mechanisms of visuospatial attention: evidence from event-related brain potentials. *Vis Cogn*, **5**, 257–86.

Fries, P., Reynolds, J. H., Rorie, A. E., and Desimone, R. (2001). Modulation of oscillatory neuronal synchronization by selective visual attention. *Science*, **291**, 1560–3.

Fries, P., Womelsdorf, T., Oostenveld, R., and Desimone, R. (2008). The effects of visual stimulation and selective visual attention on rhythmic neuronal synchronization in macaque area V4. *J Neurosci*, **28**, 4823–35.

Ghose, G. M. and Maunsell, J. H. (2002). Attentional modulation in visual cortex depends on task timing. *Nature*, **419**, 616–20.

Griffin, I. C. and Nobre, A. C. (2005). Temporal orienting of attention. In Itti L, Rees G, Tsotsos J (Eds.) *Neurobiology of Attention*, pp.257–63. San Diego, CA: Elsevier.

Griffin, I. C., Miniussi, C., and Nobre, A. C. (2001). Orienting attention in time. *Front Biosci*, **6**, D660–71.

Griffin, I. C., Miniussi, C., and Nobre, A. C. (2002). Multiple mechanisms of selective attention: differential modulation of stimulus processing by attention to space or time. *Neuropsychologia*, **40**, 2325–40.

Hackley SA, Schankin A, Wohlschlaeger A, and Wascher E (2007). Localization of temporal preparation effects via trisected reaction time. *Psychophysiology*, **44**, 334–8.

Hämäläinen, M. and Hari, R. (2002). Magnetoencephalographic characterization of dynamic brain activation: Basic principles and methods of data collection and source analysis. In A.W. Toga and J.C. Mazziotta (Eds.) *Brain Mapping: The Methods* (2nd edition), pp.227–53. San Diego, CA: Academic Press.

Heinen, S. J. and Liu, M. (1997). Single-neuron activity in the dorsomedial frontal cortex during smooth-pursuit eye movements to predictable target motion. *Vis Neurosci*, **14**, 853–65.

Helmholtz, H. L. F. (1853). Ueber einige Gesetze der Vertheilung elektrischer Ströme in körperlichen Leitern mit Anwendung auf die thierisch-elektrischen Versuche. *Annalen der Physik und Chemie*, **89**, 211–233, 353–77.

Hillyard, S. A. and Vogel, E. K., and Luck, S. J. (1998). Sensory gain control (amplification) as a mechanism of selective attention: electrophysiological and neuroimaging evidence. *Philos Trans R Soc Lond B Biol Sci*, **353**, 1257–70.

Ivry, R. B. (1996). The representation of temporal information in perception and motor control. *Curr Opin Neurobiol*, **6**, 851–7.

Ivry, R. B. and Schlerf, J. E. (2008). Dedicated and intrinsic models of time perception. *Trends Cogn Sci*, **12**, 273–80.

Ivry RB, Spencer RM, Zelaznik HN, and Diedrichsen J (2002). The cerebellum and event timing. *Ann N Y Acad Sci*, **978**, 302–17.

Janssen, P. and Shadlen, M. N. (2005). A representation of the hazard rate of elapsed time in macaque area LIP. *Nat Neurosci*, **8**, 234–41.

Jones, M. R. (2004). Attention and timing. In Neuhoff, J. (Ed) *Ecological Psychoacoustics*. San Diego, CA: Elsevier Academic Press.

Kant, I. (1781/1999). *Critique of Pure Reason*. Cambridge: Cambridge University Press.

Karmarkar, U. R. and Buonomano, D. V. (2007). Timing in the absence of clocks: encoding time in neural network states. *Neuron*, **53**, 427–38.

Kastner, S. and Pinsk, M. A. (2004). Visual attention as a multilevel selection process. *Cogn Affect Behav Neurosci* **4**, 483–500.

Kastner, S. and Ungerleider, L. G. (2000). Mechanisms of visual attention in the human cortex. *Annu Rev Neurosci,* **23**, 315–41.

King, A. J. and Nelken, I. (2009). Unraveling the principles of auditory cortical processing: can we learn from the visual system? *Nat Neurosci,* **12**, 698–701.

Lakatos, P., Chen, C. M., O'Connell, M. N., Mills, A., and Schroeder, C. E. (2007). Neuronal oscillations and multisensory interaction in primary auditory cortex. *Neuron,* **53**, 279–92.

Lakatos, P., Karmos, G., Mehta, A. D., Ulbert, I., and Schroeder, C. E. (2008). Entrainment of neuronal oscillations as a mechanism of attentional selection. *Science,* **320**, 110–13.

Lakatos, P., O'Connell, M.N., Barczak, A., Mills, A., Javitt, D.C., and Schroeder, C.E. (2009). The leading sense: supramodal control of neurophysiological context by attention. *Neuron,* **64**: 419–30.

Lakatos, P., Shah, A. S., Knuth, K. H., Ulbert, I., Karmos, G., and Schroeder, C. E. (2005). An oscillatory hierarchy controlling neuronal excitability and stimulus processing in the auditory cortex. *J Neurophysiol,* **94**, 1904–11.

Lange, K. and Heil, M. (2008). Temporal attention in the processing of short melodies: Evidence from event-related potentials. *Musicae Scientiae* **12**, 27–48.

Lange, K., Kramer, U. M., and Röder, B. (2006). Attending points in time and space. *Exp Brain Res* **173**, 130–40.

Lange, K. and Röder, B. (2006). Orienting attention to points in time improves stimulus processing both within and across modalities. *J Cogn Neurosci* **18**, 715–29.

Lange, K., Rosler, F., and Röder, B. (2003). Early processing stages are modulated when auditory stimuli are presented at an attended moment in time: an event-related potential study. *Psychophysiology* **40**, 806–17.

Lasley, D. J. and Cohn, T. E. (1981). Detection of luminance increment: effect of temporal uncertainty. *J Opt Soc Am* **71**, 845–50.

Lee, J. and Maunsell, J. H. (2009). A normalization model of attentional modulation of single unit responses. *PLoS ONE,* **4**, e4651.

Leon, M. I. and Shadlen, M. N. (2003). Representation of time by neurons in the posterior parietal cortex of the macaque. *Neuron,* **38**, 317–27.

Los, S. A. and Heslenfeld, D. J. (2005). Intentional and unintentional contributions to nonspecific preparation: electrophysiological evidence. *J Exp Psychol Gen,* **134**, 52–72.

Los, S. A. and Van den Heuvel, C. E. (2001). Intentional and unintentional contributions to nonspecific preparation during reaction time foreperiods. *J Exp Psychol: Hum Percep Perform,* **27**, 370–86.

Lucchetti, C. and Bon, L. (2001). Time-modulated neuronal activity in the premotor cortex of macaque monkeys. *Exp Brain Res* **141**, 254–60.

Luck, S. J., Chelazzi, L., Hillyard, S. A., and Desimone, R. (1997). Neural mechanisms of spatial selective attention in areas V1, V2, and V4 of macaque visual cortex. *J Neurophysiol* **77**, 24–42.

Macar, F. and Vidal, F. (2004). Event-related potentials as indices of time processing: a review. *J Psychophysiol* **18**, 89–104.

Mangun, G. R. (1995). Neural mechanisms of visual selective attention. *Psychophysiology* **32**, 4–18.

Matell, M. S. and Meck, W. II. (2000). Neuropsychological mechanisms of interval timing behavior. *Bioessays* **22**, 94–103.

Mauk, M. D. and Buonomano, D. V. (2004). The neural basis of temporal processing. *Annu Rev Neurosci* **27**, 307–40.

Maunsell, J. H. and Treue, S. (2006). Feature-based attention in visual cortex. *Trends Neurosci* **29**, 317–22.

Miall, R. C., Weir, D. J., Wolpert, D. M., and Stein, J. F. (1993). Is the cerebellum a Smith predictor? *J Mot Behav* **25**, 203–16.

Michotte, A., Thines, G., and Crabbe, G. (1964). *Amodal completion and perceptual organization* (Tr.). Louvein: Studia Psychologica.

Miniussi, C. (1999). 'Orienting attention in the temporal domain.' Doctoral thesis from the University of Verona, Faculty of Medicine, Verona, Italy.

Miniussi, C., Rao, A., and Nobre, A. C. (2002). Watching where you look: modulation of visual processing of foveal stimuli by spatial attention. *Neuropsychologia* **40**, 2448–60.

Miniussi, C., Wilding, E. L., Coull, J. T., and Nobre, A. C. (1999). Orienting attention in time. Modulation of brain potentials. *Brain* **122**(Pt 8), 1507–18.

Moore, T. and Armstrong, K. M. (2003). Selective gating of visual signals by microstimulation of frontal cortex. *Nature* **421**, 370–3.

Moore ,T. and Fallah, M. (2004). Microstimulation of the frontal eye field and its effects on covert spatial attention. *J Neurophysiol* **91**, 152–62.

Moran, J. and Desimone, R. (1985). Selective attention gates visual processing in the extrastriate cortex. *Science* **229**, 782–4.

Muller-Gethmann, H., Ulrich, R., and Rinkenauer, G. (2003). Locus of the effect of temporal preparation: evidence from the lateralized readiness potential. *Psychophysiology* **40**, 597–611.

Niemi, P. and Näätänen, R. (1981). Foreperiod and simple reaction time. *Psychol Bulletin* **89**, 133–62.

Nobre, A. C. (2001a). Orienting attention to instants in time. *Neuropsychologia* **39**, 1317–28.

Nobre, A. C. (2001b). The attentive homunculus: now you see it, now you don't. *Neurosci Biobehav Rev* **25**, 477–96.

Nobre, A. C. (2004). Probing the flexibility of attentional orienting in human brain. In: Posner MI (Ed), *Cognitive Neuroscience of Attention*, pp.157–79. Guilford Press.

Nobre, A. C. and O'Reilly, J. (2004). Time is of the essence. *Trends Cogn Sci* **8**, 387–9.O'Reilly, J. X., Mesulam, M. M., and Nobre, A. C. (2008). The cerebellum predicts the timing of perceptual events. *J Neurosci* **28**, 2252–60.

Nobre, A., Correa, A., and Coull, J. (2007). The hazards of time. *Curr Opin Neurobiol* **17**, 465–70.

Pfeuty, M., Ragot, R., and Pouthas, V. (2005). Relationship between CNV and timing of an upcoming event. *Neurosci Lett* **382**, 106–11.

Poeppel, D. (2003). The analysis of speech in different temporal integration windows: cerebral lateralization as 'asymmetric sampling in time'. *Speech Communication* **41**, 245–55.

Posner, M. I. (1980). Orienting of attention. *Q J Exp Psychol*, **32**, 3–25.

Posner, M. I. and Petersen, S. E. (1990). The attention systems of the human brain. *Annu Rev Neurosci*, **13**, 25–42.

Praamstra, P., Kourtis, D., Kwok, H. F., and Oostenveld, R. (2006). Neurophysiology of implicit timing in serial choice reaction-time performance. *J Neurosci* **26**, 5448–55.

Praamstra, P. and Pope, P. (2007). Slow brain potential and oscillatory EEG manifestations of impaired temporal preparation in Parkinson's disease. *J Neurophysiol* **98**, 2848–57.

Ramnani, N. (2006). The primate cortico-cerebellar system: anatomy and function. *Nat Rev Neurosci* **7**, 511–22.

Rektor, I. (2002). Scalp-recorded Bereitschaftspotential is the result of the activity of cortical and subcortical generators—a hypothesis. *Clin Neurophysiol* **113**, 1998–2005.

Renoult, L., Roux, .S, and Riehle, A. (2006). Time is a rubberband: neuronal activity in monkey motor cortex in relation to time estimation. *Eur J Neurosci* **23**, 3098–108.

Reynolds, J. H. and Chelazzi, L. (2004). Attentional modulation of visual processing. *Annu Rev Neurosci* **27**, 611–47.

Reynolds, J. H. and Heeger, D. J. (2009). The normalization model of attention. *Neuron* **61**, 168–85.

Reynolds, J. H., Chelazzi, L., and Desimone, R. (1999). Competitive mechanisms subserve attention in macaque areas V2 and V4. *J Neurosci* **19**, 1736–53.

Riehle, A., Grun, S., Diesmann, M., and Aertsen, A. (1997). Spike synchronization and rate modulation differentially involved in motor cortical function. *Science* **278**, 1950–3.

Rohenkohl, G. and Nobre, A. C. (2009). 'Neural modulation by rhythm-induced temporal expectations.' In 16th Annual Meeting of the Cognitive Neuroscience Society (Society CN, ed), p.45. San Francisco, CA.

Rolke, B. and Hofmann, P. (2007). Temporal uncertainty degrades perceptual processing. *Psychon Bull Rev* **14**, 522–6.

Ruff ,C. C., Driver, J., and Bestmann, S. (2009). Combining TMS and fMRI: from 'virtual lesions' to functional-network accounts of cognition. *Cortex* **45**, 1043–9.

Sakai, K., Hikosaka, O., Takino, R., Miyauchi, S., Nielsen, M., and Tamada, T. (2000). What and when: parallel and convergent processing in motor control. *J Neurosci* **20**, 2691–700.

Sanders, L. D. and Astheimer, L. B. (2008). Temporally selective attention modulates early perceptual processing: event-related potential evidence. *Percept Psychophys* **70**, 732–42.

Schroeder, C. E. and Lakatos, P. (2009). Low-frequency neuronal oscillations as instruments of sensory selection. *Trends Neurosci* **32**, 9–18.

Schroeder, C. E., Lakatos, P., Kajikawa, Y., Partan, S., and Puce, A. (2008). Neuronal oscillations and visual amplification of speech. *Trends Cogn Sci* **12**, 106–13.

Schubotz, R. I . and von Cramon, D. Y. (2001). Interval and ordinal properties of sequences are associated with distinct premotor areas. *Cereb Cortex* **11**, 210–22.

Schubotz, R. I., von Cramon, D. Y., and Lohmann, G. (2003). Auditory what, where, and when: a sensory somatotopy in lateral premotor cortex. *Neuroimage* **20**, 173–85.

Serences, J. T. and Yantis, S. Selective visual attention and perceptual coherence (2005). *Trends Cogn Sci* **10**, 38–45.

Stokes, M., Thompson, R., Nobre, A.C., and Duncan, J. (2009). Shape-specific preparatory activity mediates attention to targets in human visual cortex. *Proceedings of the National Academy of Sciences, USA*. In Press.

Taylor, P. C., Nobre, A. C., and Rushworth, M. F. (2007). FEF TMS affects visual cortical activity. *Cereb Cortex* **17**, 391–9.

Thompson, S. K., von Kriegstein, K., Deane-Pratt , A., Marquardt, T., Deichmann, R., Griffiths, T. D., et al. (2006). Representation of interaural time delay in the human auditory midbrain. *Nat Neurosci* **9**, 1096–8.

Treue, S. and Martínez Trujillo, J. C. (1999). Feature-based attention influences motion processing gain in macaque visual cortex. *Nature* **399**, 575–9.

Trillenberg, P., Verleger, R., Wascher, E., Wauschkuhn, B., and Wessel, K. (2000). CNV and temporal uncertainty with 'ageing' and 'non-ageing' S1–S2 intervals. *Clin Neurophysiol* **111**, 1216–26.

Viemeister, N. F. and Plack, C. J. (1993). Time analysis. In Yost, W. A., Popper, A. N., and Fay, R. R. (Eds.) *Springer Handbook of Auditory Research*, pp.116–54. New York: Springer.

Vidal, F., Bonnet, M., and Macar, F. (1995). Programming the duration of a motor sequence: role of the primary and supplementary motor areas in man. *Exp Brain Res* **106**, 339–50.

Walter, W. G., Cooper, R., Aldridge, V. J., McCallum, W. C., and Winter, A. L. (1964). Contingent negative variation: an electrical sign of sensorimotor association and expectancy in the human brain. *Nature* **203**, 380–4.

Westheimer, G. and Ley, E. (1996). Temporal uncertainty effects on orientation discrimination and stereoscopic thresholds. *J Opt Soc Am* **13**, 884–6.

Woldorff, M. G. (1993). Distortion of ERP averages due to overlap from temporally adjacent ERPs: analysis and correction. *Psychophysiology* **30**, 98–119.

Woldorff, M., Hansen, J. C., and Hillyard, S. A. (1987). Evidence for effects of selective attention in the mid-latency range of the human auditory event-related potential. *Electroencephalogr Clin Neurophysiol Suppl.* **40**, 146–54.

Womelsdorf, T., Fries, P., Mitra, P. P., and Desimone, R. (2006). Gamma-band synchronization in visual cortex predicts speed of change detection. *Nature* **439**, 733–6.

Acknowledgements

Most of this work has been funded by The Wellcome Trust (project grant to A.C.N). Other sources of funding have come from the NIH (collaborative projects with Marsel Mesulam), Medical Research Council (studentship to Ivan Griffin), Programme AlBan (studentship to Gustavo Rohenkohl), Spanish Ministerio de Educación y Cultura (postdoctoral fellowship to Angel Correa).

Chapter 28

Temporal orienting in audition, touch, and across modalities

Kathrin Lange and Brigitte Röder

The ability to orient attention voluntarily in space has been studied extensively. By contrast, voluntary shifts of attention in time has received more interest only recently (Coull and Nobre, 1998; for reviews see Nobre, 2001, 2004). The first studies on 'temporal orienting' were conducted in the visual modality using a temporal variant of the classical Posner cuing paradigm (Posner, 1980). A symbolic cue indicated the duration of the cue–target interval (short, e.g. 600ms, or long, e.g. 1400ms, e.g. Miniussi et al., 1999). The target appeared with a higher probability after the indicated interval (valid trials) than after the other interval (invalid trials). As in spatial cueing tasks, a reaction-time benefit for validly cued targets compared to invalidly cued targets was consistently observed (Coull and Nobre, 1998; Miniussi et al., 1999; Coull et al., 2000, 2001; Griffin et al., 2001; Coull, Chapter 31; Nobre, Chapter 27, this volume). Moreover, temporal orienting has been found to lead to more accurate responding (Correa et al., 2005; Correa, Chapter 26, this volume). Thus, explicit temporal orienting results in behavioural benefits similar to those observed for spatial orienting.

For spatial attention, it has been investigated intensively whether behavioural attention effects arise from a modulation of early, sensory processing stages or of later, decision or response-related processing stages. A useful method for identifying the processing stage affected by an experimental manipulation is to analyse when this manipulation has an effect on event-related potentials (ERPs). ERPs are voltage fluctuations, which are time-locked to an external or internal event. ERPs are derived from the electroencephalogram by averaging equivalent recording epochs (e.g. Coles and Rugg, 1995; Fabiani et al., 2000). An ERP consists of a systematic sequence of positive and negative deflections, which are considered to be related to the various neural stages of stimulus processing. It is reasonable to assume that the earlier a deflection occurs, the more it is related to perceptual processing. Deflections associated with perception include e.g. the auditory P1 and N1 (latencies approximately 50ms and 100ms) and the visual P1 and N1 (latencies approximately 100ms and 180ms). Later deflections (>200ms; e.g. the N200 and the P300) are typically regarded as depending more on decision- or response-related processes.

Modulations of visual temporal orienting have most often been observed on the N2 and the P3 of the visual ERP, suggesting that temporal attention modulates predominantly decision- or response-related processing stages (Miniussi et al., 1999; Griffin et al., 2002; Nobre, Chapter 27, this volume). By contrast, ERP correlates of early visual processing stages (visual ERPs with latencies <200ms) have not consistently been observed to be affected by temporal orienting: Whereas Correa et al. (2006) reported an enhancement of the visual P1, Miniussi et al. (1999) did not observe early ERP effects of temporal orienting. Griffin et al. (2002, Experiment 1) found an enhancement of the visual N1 by temporal orienting. However, this effect had a broad rather than a focal scalp topography, as observed for spatial attention in the same participants, and it was not replicated in Experiment 2 of the same study. These authors concluded that visual temporal orienting mainly affects later, decision- or response-related processing. Consistent with this interpretation, functional magnetic resonance imaging studies of temporal orienting have shown activations of brain areas usually associated with motor planning or motor control (e.g. the inferior ventrolateral premotor cortex; Coull and Nobre, 1998; Coull et al., 2000, 2001; Coull, Chapter 31, this volume). The results for visual temporal orienting contrast with findings obtained for visual spatial orienting. Here, modulations of the visually evoked P1 and N1 have been taken as evidence that spatial orienting exerts an influence on stimulus processing by modulating early, perceptual stages (e.g. Van Voorhis and Hillyard, 1977; Eason, 1981; see also Mangun, 1995).

In sum, temporal orienting speeds up responding to stimuli presented at an attended compared to an unattended time point. Moreover, initial data imply that response accuracy can also be enhanced by temporal orienting. These behavioural effects appear to result from qualitatively different mechanisms than effects of visual *spatial* orienting: visual *spatial* orienting seems to rely on an enhanced processing at perceptual stages, whereas visual *temporal* orienting most likely improves processing at later, decision- or response-related stages (see also Nobre, Chapter 27, this volume).

Nevertheless, spatial attention studies have not always observed early ERP effects: a facilitation of early, perceptual processing stages depends on experimental conditions. These conditions were identified by Hillyard et al. (1973), who were the first to show a clear enhancement of the auditory N1 by selective attention. These authors presented 800-Hz and 1500-Hz tone pips randomly to the left and right ear. In one block, participants were instructed to attend to the left ear and to respond only when they heard an infrequent deviant tone in their left ear. In another block, participants were asked to attend to the right ear and to respond only to deviant tones in the right ear. To assess effects of selective attention on stimulus processing, physically identical stimuli were compared as a function of whether they belonged to the attended spatial channel. For example, ERPs to left standard stimuli (i.e. stimuli that did not require a response) were compared between conditions when the left side versus the right side was attended. The main finding was an enhancement of the auditory N1 potential to standards presented to a particular ear while this ear was attended versus unattended.

Hillyard et al. (1973) identified three properties that distinguished their study from earlier work, in which a modulation of the N1 was not reported (e.g. Smith et al., 1970), and suggested that these characteristics favour the modulation of perceptual processing stages (see also Hillyard and Picton 1987). First, attended and unattended stimuli could be easily distinguished (they differed with respect to location and pitch). Second, participants had to focus strongly on the to-be-attended channel: stimuli were presented too rapidly to allow them to process all stimuli. Moreover, unattended stimuli did not require a response and could thus be completely ignored. Note that in most probabilistic cueing experiments, stimulation rate is slower and participants have also to respond to invalidly cued targets (but see, e.g. Griffin et al., 2002). Third, a demanding within-channel discrimination task was required for stimuli of the to-be-attended channel.

A temporal variant of the 'Hillyard paradigm'

We wondered if temporal orienting could modulate early, sensory processing stages if similar task conditions were introduced as in the spatial attention paradigm used by Hillyard et al., i.e. if attended and unattended time points could be easily distinguished and if participants had to focus strongly on the attended time point (see also Correa et al., 2006). To answer this question, we employed a temporal variant of the Hillyard paradigm (Lange et al., 2003). We presented empty time intervals, which lasted 600ms (short) and 1200ms (long), in a random order (Figure 28.1A). The onset and offset of each interval were marked by auditory stimuli. Auditory stimuli were chosen, because the auditory system has a higher temporal accuracy than the visual system (Rousseau et al., 1983; Grondin et al., 1998; Westheimer, 1999; Ulrich et al., 2006). The onset stimulus was presented centrally, whereas the offset stimulus was presented either to the left or the right side. Short and long intervals were equally likely, as were presentations to the left or right side. Infrequently, 'deviant' offset stimuli were presented (deviants) that

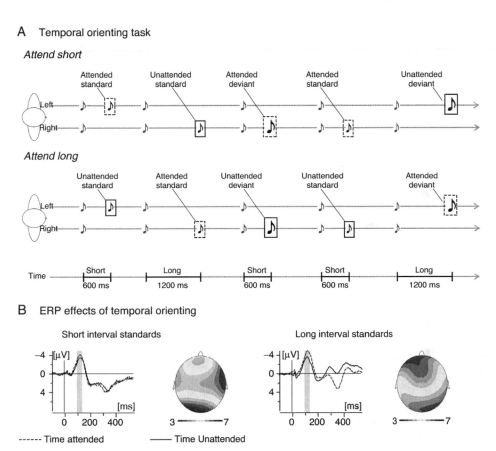

Fig. 28.1 (See also Plate 8) Schematic drawing of the temporal orienting task (A) and grand average ERPs time locked to attended and unattended standards (B). A) Musical notes represent onset (grey) and offset (black) of short and long intervals. The Attend Short condition is displayed above the Attend Long condition. Each offset marker is indicated as being either attended (dashed black marking) or unattended (black marking). The timing of the on- and offset markers and the interval durations are marked in a timeline along the bottom. B) Grand average ERPs for standards at the attended (dashed black) versus unattended (black) time. ERPs to the short interval standards (left) are shown at a representative fronto-central electrode. ERPs to the long interval standards (right) are shown at a representative frontal electrode. Next to each waveform, the normalized topography (mean = 5, SD = 2) of the N1 effect is shown (top view). Blue shadings indicate relatively more negative amplitudes for the attended than the unattended condition; red shadings indicate relatively more positive amplitudes for the attended than the unattended condition. Here, and in the following figures, the time epoch used for statistical analyses of the displayed effect is shaded grey, all traces are aligned with respect to a 100-ms pre-stimulus baseline, and Negativity is up.

differed in loudness from the frequent 'standard' offset stimuli (standards). In separate blocks, the participants were asked to attend to the time point that ended either the short or the long interval. Responses were only required to deviants at this attended time point. To assess attention effects, ERPs to standards were compared as a function of whether they appeared at a time point that was currently attended versus unattended. For example, the processing of a standard at the end of a short interval when short intervals were attended was compared to the processing of a standard at the end of a short interval when long intervals were attended (see Figure 28.1A).

There are both commonalities and differences between our temporal orienting paradigm and the original spatial attention paradigm introduced by Hillyard et al. Commonalities include the relative ease of discriminating the attended and the unattended channel, the fact that unattended stimuli could be entirely ignored, and the use of stimulus discrimination as the within-channel task. Differences are mostly related to properties inherent to the time dimension. First, attention can remain on one side for an entire block in the spatial paradigm, whereas attention has to be oriented in every trial in the temporal orienting task. Note, however, that the same time point was attended within each block in our experiment, whereas the focus of attention usually changes between trials in trial-by-trial cueing tasks (e.g. Coull and Nobre, 1998). Second, in the spatial attention paradigm participants cannot distribute their attention across two different locations, since they would hardly be able to perform the difficult within-channel discrimination. In the temporal version of the task, it is possible that participants focus their attention successively on each time point (although it is not necessary to attend to the task-irrelevant time point). This is particularly likely when no stimulus is presented after the short interval (see also Coull and Nobre 1998; Miniussi et al., 1999). Finally, in the spatial task, it is impossible to predict whether the next stimulus is a to-be-attended or a to-be-ignored one. This is essential in order to rule out alternative explanations for the attention effects, such as differences in arousal or alertness (Näätänen, 1975). In temporal orienting tasks, participants cannot predict at the onset of a trial whether a stimulus will appear after the short interval, or which stimulus will be presented. However, once the time point ending the short interval has passed without a stimulus being presented, participants know that a stimulus will occur after the long interval. In this condition it is totally predictable whether the next stimulus is an attended (in the 'attend long' condition) or an unattended stimulus (in the 'attend short' condition). Thus, when just two intervals are used, only the short interval effects can be unequivocally related to temporal orienting. To further distinguish temporal orienting from non-specific arousal, one has to show that processing is enhanced at the to-be-attended time point but not at earlier *nor* at later time points. (Recently, this has been demonstrated by Sanders and Astheimer (2008), who reported effects of temporal orienting for *three* different intervals. Consistent with the notion that temporal orienting is truly selective, the auditory N1 for their medium interval was larger when the medium interval was attended compared to when either the short or the long interval was attended.)

A modulation of the auditory N1 by temporal orienting

In our study of temporal orienting (Lange et al., 2003), we used the basic paradigm described earlier. We found an enhancement of the auditory N1 (100–140ms) in the ERPs elicited by attended compared to unattended standard stimuli. The effect observed for standards at short intervals had its maximum over fronto-temporal areas (Figure 28.1B, left); the effect observed for the long intervals had a frontal topography (Figure 28.1B, right). It has been suggested that the auditory N1 wave is generated in or near the primary auditory cortex, partly contralateral to the ear of stimulation (e.g. Woods, 1995; Picton, et al., 1999; for a review see Näätänen and Picton, 1987). The N1 has been associated with perceptual processing stages (for a review see Näätänen and Picton, 1987). Modulations of the N1 amplitude by spatial attention have been repeatedly demonstrated (e.g. Hillyard et al., 1973, Näätänen et al., 1978; Giard et al., 1988; Woldorff and Hillyard, 1991; Woods and Alain, 2001; but see Woldorff and Hillyard, 1991 for an even earlier effect). Thus, the N1 effect of temporal orienting may be regarded as evidence that temporal orienting can influence perceptual processing—at least for audition.

There are two main interpretations of N1 attention effects (for a recent review see Näätänen and Alho, 2004). Hillyard and colleagues proposed a filter- or gating-mechanism that modulates the amplitude of the N1 (Hillyard et al., 1973). By contrast, Näätänen (e.g. 1982) suggested that the enhanced N1 was actually due to the superposition of an endogenous *processing negativity*, which was assumed to reflect the comparison of the incoming stimulus with a memory representation of the to-be-attended stimulus. Thus, the crucial difference between the two approaches is whether early processing of attended and unattended stimuli differs quantitatively (Hillyard's position) or qualitatively (Näätänen's view). Whether the temporal orienting N1 is due to an enhancement of the genuine N1 wave (thus reflecting quantitative different processing) or results from different processing negativities to attended and unattended stimuli (thus reflecting qualitative different processing) has to be addressed by future research. Although temporal and spatial orienting are not necessarily based on identical neural mechanisms, the spatial domain may be used as a model when investigating mechanisms of temporal orienting.

Similar to other temporal orienting studies, the negative slow wave between the onset and the offset of the intervals was also enhanced by attention in our initial study (Lange et al., 2003). This effect has been related to expectancy or to the timing of the interval (e.g. Miniussi et al., 1999; Sanders and Astheimer, 2008). It seems unlikely, that the slow wave temporal orienting effect and the N1 effect observed in our study reflect identical processes, because their topographies differed significantly (Lange et al., 2003). Therefore, the temporal orienting N1 effect is unlikely to be an artefact of the pre-stimulus ERP difference. Additionally, to account for the pre-stimulus ERP differences, the ERPs to standard stimuli were referenced to a pre-stimulus (i.e. standard) baseline. Thus, we consider our results to be consistent with the view that—at least in audition—orienting attention to a point in time can modulate levels of stimulus processing as early as those modulated by spatial attention.

An influence of temporal orienting on later processing stages was also observed in our first study. We found a relative positivity to attended compared to unattended standards in the time range of the P3. Again, this effect was seen for standards of the short and standards of the long interval. Similar findings observed in the visual modality (Miniussi et al., 1999; Griffin et al., 2002) were interpreted as an index that temporal orienting mainly affects response-related processes. However, the P3 is also sensitive to processes not directly related to a response, e.g. the information content of the stimulus (e.g. Sutton et al., 1967; Johnson, 1986). This is consistent with the enhanced P3 to attended compared to unattended standards in our data, because events at an attended time point contain more information (whether or not to respond) than events at an unattended time point, which never required a response.

Comparing N1 effects of temporal and spatial orienting

The temporal orienting N1 effect resembled the N1 effect that has consistently been observed in auditory spatial attention tasks (for a review, see Woods, 1990). Thus, the question arises, whether these effects reflect the same neural mechanisms. To answer this question, we directly compared effects of spatial and temporal orienting within the same participants (Lange et al., 2006).

We extended the basic experimental paradigm by adding a manipulation of spatial orienting (Figure 28.2A; Lange et al., 2006). Short and long empty intervals were presented. The offset

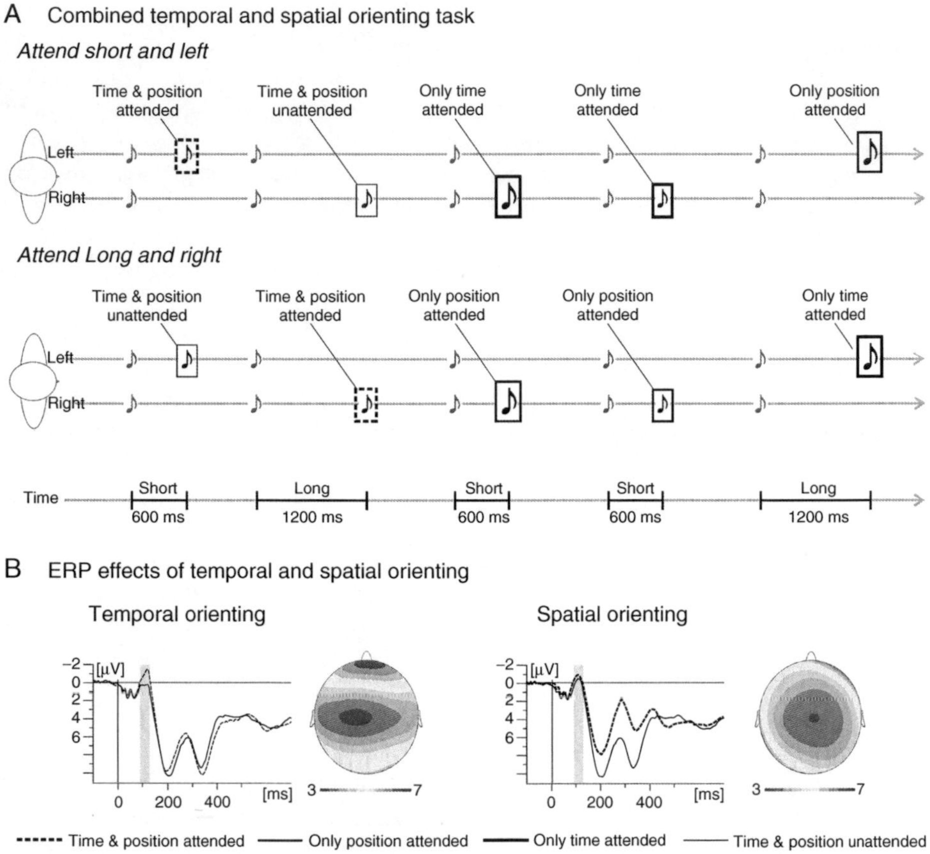

Fig. 28.2 (See also Plate 9) Schematic drawing of the combined temporal and spatial orienting task (A) and grand average ERPs time locked to attended and unattended standards (B). A) Two of the four possible conditions are shown for illustrative purposes: the Attend Short and Left condition is displayed above the Attend Long and Right condition. Each offset marker is indicated as being 'time and position attended' (bold dashed marking), 'time attended' (fine dashed marking), 'position attended' (bold black marking), or 'time and position unattended' (fine black marking). The timing of the on- and offset markers and the interval durations are marked in a timeline along the bottom. B) Grand average ERPs for standards of short intervals at an attended (dashed line) versus unattended (black line) time point for the unattended position (left) and grand average ERPs for standards of short intervals at an attended (bold line) versus unattended (fine line) location for the unattended time point (right). ERPs are shown at a contralateral central electrode cluster. Next to each waveform, the normalized topography (mean = 5, SD = 2) of the N1 effect is shown (top view). Blue shadings indicate relatively more negative amplitudes for the attended than the unattended condition; red shadings indicate relatively more positive amplitudes for the attended than the unattended condition. In the topographic maps, electrodes ipsilateral to stimulation are on the left, electrodes contralateral to stimulation are on the right.

stimulus appeared either on the left or on the right side. Participants were asked to focus on one time point (short or long interval) and one position (left or right side). The combination of the temporal and the spatial attention manipulation resulted in four conditions: 'attend short interval and left side'; 'attend short interval and right side'; 'attend long interval and left side'; and 'attend long interval and right side'. Depending on the attention condition, the stimuli were classified as: 'time and position attended'; 'time attended' (and position unattended); 'position attended' (and time unattended); or 'time and position unattended' (see also Figure 28.2A). The simultaneous manipulation of temporal and spatial orienting allows for a direct comparison of the associated ERP effects. Moreover, using this approach it is possible to investigate whether temporal and spatial information are used independently, or conjointly, for stimulus selection. If temporal and spatial information are used independently, additive attention effects in the ERPs are expected. By contrast, if temporal and spatial features interact, non-additive ERP effects are predicted.

Both temporal and spatial orienting enhanced the auditory N1 (90–130ms; Figure 28.2B). Time course and scalp topography of spatial and temporal orienting effects were similar. This result pattern suggests that spatial and temporal attention influence—at least partly— overlapping brain systems related to early auditory processing. Moreover, the spatial and temporal N1 orienting effects were not independent, suggesting that the underlying mechanisms may be related. Interestingly, the N1 effects of both temporal and spatial orienting were only reliable when the other dimension (space and time, respectively) were not attended. Possibly, an additional attended feature does not add extra benefit to stimulus processing (ceiling effect). Alternatively, the processing of stimuli lacking any attended feature may be associated with costs. Future research may implement a neutral condition in a combined temporal and spatial orienting task in order to decide between these alternatives.

While spatial and temporal orienting showed comparable influence on the N1, the ERP effects observed in later time epochs differed markedly. Spatial orienting was accompanied by a sustained, fronto-central negativity for attended compared to unattended stimuli. This sustained negativity is typically observed in auditory spatial attention tasks and has been referred to as the negative difference (Hansen and Hillyard, 1980). It may reflect further processing of stimuli that passed an initial selection mechanism (possibly indexed by the enhanced N1; Hansen and Hillyard, 1980; but see Näätänen et al., 1978; Näätänen 1982). For temporal orienting, an enhancement of the P3 was observed, just as in our earlier study (Lange et al., 2003).

Probing the hierarchy of temporal and spatial selection

In the visual system, selection by space seems to precede selection by time (Nobre 2001; Griffin et al., 2002). In the auditory domain, by contrast, the earliest effects of temporal and spatial orienting were found in the same time epoch, rendering a hierarchical selection by time and space unlikely. Rather, time and space seem to be weighted equally in audition. This may be an inherent property of the auditory system. Alternatively, a hierarchical stimulus selection may be observed when specific conditions prompt participants to rely more on one, or other, feature.

Congenitally blind individuals show superior temporal discrimination skills both in the auditory (Muchnik et al., 1991; Gougoux et al., 2004; Stevens and Weaver, 2005) and in the tactile system (Röder et al., 1996; Röder et al., 2000). They may thus favour a selection based on temporal features over a selection by space. This hypothesis was investigated in a group of congenitally blind people (Röder et al., 2007). In the blind participants, the N1 was modulated only by temporal attention but not by spatial attention, whereas in the sighted participants of Lange et al. (2006), both a temporal and a spatial orienting N1 effect were observed. A long-lasting spatial attention negativity was also observed in the blind participants. Only in the blind individuals however, was this effect was further modulated by temporal attention. Finally, the posterior positivity associated with temporal orienting was also observed in the blind group. The data of Röder et al. (2007) indicate that selection by temporal and spatial features is susceptible to long-term changes. Future studies may investigate whether stimulus selection can also be altered by short-term adaptations, e.g. when task requirements emphasize selection by one, or other, feature.

Auditory temporal orienting within and across audition and touch

The results reported so far suggest that early stages of auditory processing can be enhanced when attention is oriented to the time at which a stimulus is presented, similar to when attention is oriented to the position of a stimulus. Because spatial attention is relatively well investigated, it may be a useful approach to use spatial attention as a model when generating hypotheses about the properties and mechanisms of temporal orienting.

Spatial attention can spill over from one modality to another (for a review, see e.g. Calvert et al., 2004; Spence and Driver 2004). For example, when attention is oriented to one position for the visual modality, participants also respond more quickly to an auditory stimulus at this position (cross-modal attention effect; e.g. Spence and Driver, 1996; Spence et al., 1998; for a review see Driver and Spence, 2004). Cross-modal ERP effects of spatial attention were similar to early uni-modal ERP attention effects with respect to morphology and scalp topography (e.g. Hillyard et al., 1984; Eimer and Schröger, 1998; Eimer and Driver, 2000; Eimer, 2001; Eimer et al., 2002; Hötting et al., 2003). These findings suggest that cross-modal spatial attention affects early processing levels that have been associated with modality specific processing (for a review, see Eimer, 2004).

Because time, like space, can be coded by different modalities, we postulated that the temporal orienting of attention improves stimulus processing both in a task-relevant (attended) and in a task-irrelevant (unattended) modality. To investigate this hypothesis, we conducted a behavioural and an ERP experiment (Lange and Röder, 2006) with a multi-modal version of our temporal orienting paradigm. The offset markers of the intervals were auditory and tactile stimuli. Participants' attention was oriented to the short or the long interval for one modality only (e.g. attend short auditory). In the behavioural experiment, stimuli of one modality (the attended modality) appeared with higher probability than stimuli of the other modality. For the attended modality, stimuli appeared with higher probability after one interval (the attended interval) than after the other interval. The participants indicated for every offset stimulus whether it was continuous or had a gap. In the ERP experiment, participants were instructed to attend to one modality and one interval. They were asked to respond only when an offset stimulus of the attended interval was of the attended modality and only when it had a gap (i.e. was a deviant stimulus).

Effects of temporal orienting were assessed by comparing the processing of offset markers as a function of whether the time of their occurrence was currently attended or not. This was done separately for stimuli of the attended (uni-modal effects) and unattended modality (cross-modal effects). Participants responded more quickly to auditory and tactile stimuli at the attended compared to the unattended time point, irrespective of which modality was attended. Thus both uni-modal and cross-modal processing gains due to temporal attention were obtained. Error rates were not affected by the attention conditions, thus ruling out the possibility that the observed reaction-time benefits were due to a speed-accuracy trade-off.

To investigate which processing stages are affected by cross-modal temporal orienting, we analysed ERPs to auditory and tactile standard offset markers as a function of which time point and which modality were attended (Lange and Röder, 2006). For the auditory modality, the N1 effect of temporal orienting (e.g. Lange et al., 2003) was replicated. Most importantly, this effect was found both when audition was attended (uni-modal effect; Figure 28.3A, left side) and when touch was attended (cross-modal effect; Figure 28.3B, left side). The cross-modal N1 effect had a similar morphology as the uni-modal N1 effect. This is consistent with findings of spatial attention tasks, where attention effects for stimuli of a task-irrelevant modality have been observed in the time-range of the auditory N1 (e.g. Eimer and Schröger, 1998; Eimer et al., 2002; Hötting et al., 2003). In our temporal orienting study, the uni-modal N1 effect was larger over the hemisphere contralateral to the stimulated ear, whereas the cross-modal N1 effect was symmetrically distributed. This pattern might be achieved if the generators contributing to the N1 are differently weighted when the auditory versus another modality is attended. A cross-modal modulation of the P3 by temporal attention was not observed in the multi-modal study.

For touch, the uni-modal effect consisted of an enhancement of the somatosensory N140 (Figure 28.3A, right). The N140 is supposed to be generated in secondary somatosensory cortex (Frot et al., 1999; but see Allison et al., 1992) and it has been interpreted as a sign of sensory

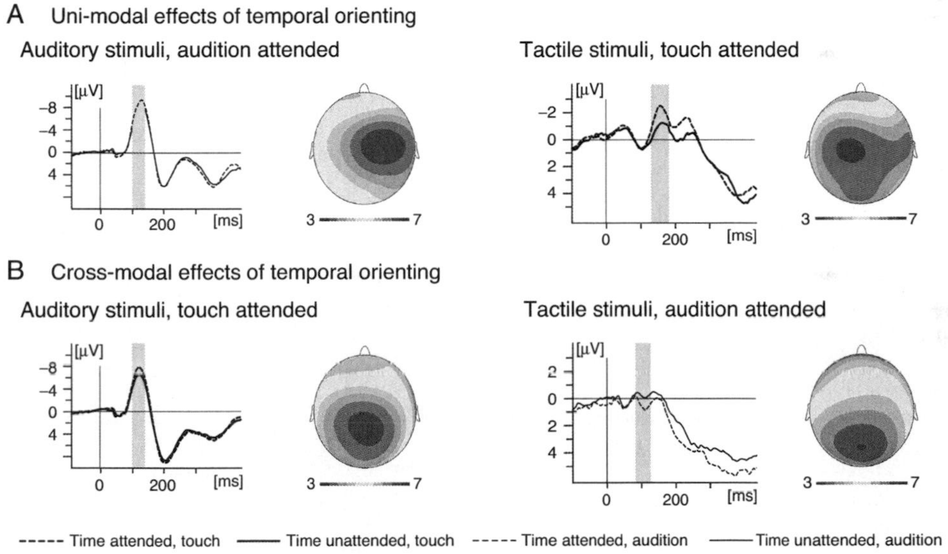

A Uni-modal effects of temporal orienting

Auditory stimuli, audition attended   Tactile stimuli, touch attended

B Cross-modal effects of temporal orienting

Auditory stimuli, touch attended   Tactile stimuli, audition attended

----- Time attended, touch   —— Time unattended, touch   ----- Time attended, audition   ——Time unattended, audition

Fig. 28.3 (See also Plate 10) Grand average ERPs to attended (dashed lines) and unattended (solid lines) standards for the uni-modal (A) and cross-modal (B) effects of temporal orienting. A) Left panel: ERPs to auditory stimuli, audition attended. Right panel: ERPs to tactile stimuli, touch attended. B) Left panel: ERPs to auditory stimuli, touch attended. Right panel: ERPs to tactile stimuli, audition attended. ERPs to auditory stimuli are shown at a contralateral central cluster. ERPs to uni-modal and cross-modal effects in the tactile modality are shown at an ipsilateral central and a contralateral parietal cluster, respectively. Next to each waveform, the normalized topography (mean = 5, SD = 2) of the depicted effect is shown (top view). Blue shadings indicate relatively more negative amplitudes for the attended than the unattended condition; red shadings indicate relatively more positive amplitudes for the attended than the unattended condition. Electrodes ipsilateral to stimulation are on the left, electrodes contralateral to stimulation are on the right.

specific processing, similar to the auditory N1 (e.g. Desmedt and Debecker, 1979). A modulation in the time range of the tactile N140 is a common finding in studies investigating the impact of spatial attention on tactile processing (Michie et al., 1987; García-Larrea et al., 1995; Eimer and Driver, 2000; Eimer et al., 2002; Hötting et al., 2003). Unlike audition, cross-modal effects in touch differed qualitatively from the uni-modal effect. Relative positivities between 80–120ms and 190–230ms were observed when a tactile stimulus was presented at a time point that was attended versus unattended for the auditory modality (Figure 28.3B, right).

To summarize the findings of our multi-modal study (Lange and Röder, 2006): we provided evidence for behavioural benefits of temporal orienting for modalities other than vision. We demonstrated enhanced perceptual processing for both the auditory and the tactile modality. We found cross-modal temporal orienting effects and thus provided evidence that time—like space— acts as a supramodal feature allowing for cross-modal binding. Since effects of temporal orienting on stimulus processing depended partly on whether the modality of the stimulus was currently attended, these data also argue against the view that effects of temporal orienting can be explained by non-specific arousal.

Conclusions

Initially, we asked whether the temporal orienting of attention modulates early perceptual processing. We have presented four studies providing evidence that explicit temporal orienting enhances early, perceptual stages of auditory processing (Lange et al., 2003; Lange et al., 2006; Lange and Röder, 2006; Röder et al., 2007). Moreover, we demonstrated that early tactile processing stages are also enhanced by temporal attention (Lange and Röder, 2006). Future research should investigate, more systematically, the preconditions for enhancement of perceptual processing steps by temporal orienting. Stimulus modality may be important, but there is evidence that crucial factors include the way attention is manipulated (Correa et al., 2006; Lange and Heil 2008; Lange, 2009) and task requirements, such as the use of a discrimination task (Correa et al., 2006). Consistent with findings observed in the visual modality, temporal orienting also influences later, decision- or response-related stages of auditory processing (Lange et al., 2003, 2006).

References

Allison, T., McCarthy, G., and Wood, C. C. (1992). The relationship between human long-latency somatosensory evoked potentials recorded from the cortical surface and from the scalp. *Electroencephalography and clinical Neurophysiology,* **84**, 301–14.

Calvert, G. A., Spence, C., and Stein, B. E. (Eds.) (2004). *The Handbook of Multisensory Processes.* Cambridge, MA: The MIT Press.

Coles, M. G. H. and Rugg, M. D. (1995). Event-related brain potentials: an introduction. In M. D. Rugg and M. G. H. Coles (Eds.) *Electrophysiology of Mind. Event-Related Brain Potentials and Cognition,* pp.1–26. Oxford: Oxford University Press.

Correa, Á., Lupiánez, J., and Tudela, P. (2005). Attentional preparation based on temporal expectancies modulates processing at the perceptual level. *Psychonomic Bulletin and Review,* **12**, 328–34.

Correa, Á., Lupiánez, J., Madrid, E., and Tudela, P. (2006). Temporal attention enhances early visual processing: A review and new evidence from event-related potentials. *Brain Research,* **1076**, 116–28.

Coull, J. T. and Nobre, A. C. (1998). Where and when to pay attention: the neural systems for directing attention to spatial locations and to time intervals as revealed by both PET and fMRI. *The Journal of Neuroscience,* **18**, 7426–35.

Coull, J. T., Nobre, A. C., and Frith, C. D. (2001). The noradrenergic alpha2 agonist clonidine modulates behavioural and neuroanatomical correlates of human attentional orienting and alerting. *Cerebral Cortex,* **11**, 73–84.

Coull, J. T., Frith, C. D., Büchel, C., and Nobre, A. C. (2000). Orienting attention in time: behavioural and neuroanatomical distinction between exogenous and endogenous shifts. *Neuropsychologia,* **38**, 808–19.

Desmedt, J. E. and Debecker, J. (1979). Wave form and neural mechanism of the decision P350 elicited without pre-stimulus cnv or readiness potential in random sequences of near-threshold auditory clicks and finger stimuli. *Electroencephalography and Clinical Neurophysiology,* **47**, 648–70.

Driver, J. and Spence, C. (2004). Crossmodal spatial attention: evidence from human performance. In C. Spence and J. Driver (Eds.) *Crossmodal Space and Crossmodal Attention,* pp.179–220. Oxford: Oxford University Press.

Eason, R. G. (1981). Visual evoked potential correlates of early neural filtering during selective attention. *Bulletin of the Psychonomic Society,* **18**, 203–6.

Eimer, M. (2001). Crossmodal links in spatial attention between vision, audition, and touch: evidence from event-related brain potentials. *Neuropsychologia,* **39**, 1292–303.

Eimer, M. (2004). Electrophysiology of human crossmodal spatial attention. In C. Spence and J. Driver (Eds.) *Crossmodal Space and Crossmodal Attention,* pp.221–45. Oxford: Oxford University Press.

Eimer, M. and Driver, J. (2000). An event-related brain potential study of cross-modal links in spatial attention between vision and touch. *Psychophysiology,* **37**, 697–705

Eimer, M. and Schröger, E. (1998). ERP effects of intermodal attention and cross-modal links in spatial attention. *Psychophysiology,* **35**, 313–27

Eimer, M., Van Velzen, J., and Driver, J. (2002). Crossmodal interactions between audition, touch, and vision in endogenous spatial attention: ERP evidence on preparatory states and sensory modulationS. *Journal of Cognitive Neuroscience,* **14**, 254–71.

Fabiani, M., Gratton, G., and Coles, M. G. H. (2000). Event-related brain potentials. Methods, theory, and applications. In J. T. Cacioppo, L. G. Tassinary and G. G. Berntson (Eds.) *Handbook of Psychophysiology,* pp.53–84. Cambridge: Cambridge University Press.

Frot, M., Rambaud, L., Guénot, M., and Mauguière, F. (1999). Intracortical recordings of early pain-related CO_2-laser evoked potentials in the human second somatosensory (SII) area. *Clinical Neurophyiology,* **110**, 133–45.

García-Larrea, L., Lukaszewicz, A. C., and Mauguière, F. (1995). Somatosensory response during selective spatial attention: The N120-to-N140 transition. *Psychophysiology,* **32**, 526–37.

Giard, M. H., Perrin, F., Pernier, J., and Peronnet, F. (1988). Several attention-related wave forms in auditory areas: a topographic study. *Electroencephalography and Clinical Neurophysiology,* **69**, 371–84.

Gougoux, F., Lepore, F., Lassonde, M., Voss, P., Zatorre, R. J., and Belin, P. (2004). Neuropsychology: pitch discrimination in the early blind. *Nature,* **430**, 309.

Griffin, I. C., Miniussi, C., and Nobre, A. C. (2001). Orienting Attention in Time. *Frontiers in Bioscience,* **6**, 660–71.

Griffin, I. C., Miniussi, C., and Nobre, A. C. (2002). Multiple mechanisms of selective attention: differential modulation of stimulus processing by attention to space or time. *Neuropsychologia,* **40**, 2325–40.

Grondin, S., Meilleur-Wells, G., Ouellette, C., and Macar, F. (1998). Sensory effects on judgements of short time-intervals. *Psychological Research,* **61**, 261–8.

Hansen, J. C. and Hillyard, S. A. (1980). Endogenous brain potentials associated with selective auditory attention. *Electroencephalography and Clinical Neurophysiology,* **49**, 277–90.

Hillyard, S. A. and Picton, T. W. (1987) Electrophysiology of cognition. In E. Plum (Ed.) *Handbook of Physiology: Sec. 1 The nervous system. V Higher functions of the brain: Part 2,* pp.519–84. Bethesda: American Physiology Society.

Hillyard, S. A., Hink, R., Schwent, V.L., and Picton, T. (1973). Electrical signs of selective attention in the human brain. *Science,* **162**, 177–80.

Hillyard, S. A., Simpson, G. V., Woods, D. L., Van Voorhis, S., and Münte, T. F. (1984). Event-related brain potentials and selective attention to different modalities. In F. Reinoso-Suarez and C. Ajmone-Marsan (Eds.) *Cortical Integration,* pp.395–414. New York: Raven Press.

Hötting, K., Rösler, F., and Röder, B. (2003). Crossmodal and Intermodal attention modulate event-related brain potentials to tactile and auditory stimuli. *Experimental Brain Research,* **148**, 26–37.

Johnson, R. (1986). A triarchic model of P300 amplitude. *Psychophysiology,* **23**, 367–84

Lange, K. (2009). Brain correlates of early auditory processing are attenuated by expectations for time and pitch. *Brain and Cognition,* **69**, 127–37.

Lange, K. and Heil, M. (2008). Temporal attention in the processing of short melodies: Evidence from event-related potentials. *Musicae Scientiae,* **12**, 27–48.

Lange, K. and Röder, B. (2006). Orienting attention to points in time improves stimulus processing both within and across modalities. *Journal of Cognitive Neuroscience,* **18**, 715–29.

Lange, K., Krämer, U. M., and Röder, B. (2006). Attending points in time and space. *Experimental Brain Research,* **173**, 130–40.

Lange, K., Rösler, F., and Röder, B. (2003). Early processing stages are modulated when auditory stimuli are presented at an attended moment in time: an event-related potential study. *Psychophysiology,* **40**, 806–17.

Mangun, G. R. (1995). Neural mechanisms of visual selective attention. *Psychophysiology,* **32**, 4–18.

Michie, P. T., Bearpark, H. M., Crawford, J. M., and Glue, L. C. T. (1987). The effects of spatial selective attention on the somatosensory event-related potential. *Psychophysiology,* **24**, 449–63.

Miniussi, C., Wilding, E.L., Coull, J. T., and Nobre, A.C. (1999). Orienting attention in time. Modulation of brain potentials. *Brain,* **122**, 1507–18.

Muchnik, C., Efrati, M., Nemeth, E., Malin, M., and Hildesheimer, M. (1991). Central auditory skills in blind and sighted subjects. *Scandinavian Audiology,* **20**, 19–23.

Näätänen, R. (1975). Selective attention and evoked potentials in humans – a critical review. *Biological Psychology,* **2**, 237–307.

Näätänen, R. (1982). Processing negativity: an evoked-potential reflection of selective attention. *Psychological Bulletin,* **92**, 605–40.

Näätänen, R. and Alho, K. (2004). Mechanisms of attention in audition as revealed by the event-related potentials of the brain. In M. I. Posner (Ed.) *Cognitive Neuroscience of Attention,* pp.194–206. New York: Guilford Press.

Näätänen, R. and Picton, T. (1987). The N1 wave of the human electric and magnetic response to sound: a review and an analysis of the component structure. *Psychophysiology,* **24**, 375–425.

Näätänen, R., Gaillard, A. W. K., and Mäntysalo, S. (1978). Early selective-attention effect on evoked potential reinterpreted. *Acta Psychologica,* **42**, 313–29

Nobre, A. C. (2001). Orienting attention to instants in time. *Neuropsychologia,* **39**, 1317–1328

Nobre, A. C. (2004). Probing the flexibility of attentional orienting in the human brain. In M. I. Posner (Ed.) *Cognitive Neuroscience of Attention,* pp.157–79. New York: The Guilford Press.

Picton, T. W., Alain, C., Woods, D. L., John, M. S., Scherg, M., Valdes-Sosa, P., et al. (1999). Intracerebral sources of human auditory-evoked potentials. *Audiology and Neuro-Otology,* **4**, 64–79.

Posner, M.I. (1980). Orienting of attention. *Quarterly Journal of Experimental Psychology,* **32**, 3–25.

Röder, B., Krämer, U. M., and Lange, K. (2007). Congenitally blind humans use different stimulus selection strategies in hearing: An ERP study of spatial and temporal attention. *Restorative Neurology and Neuroscience,* **25**, 311–22.

Röder, B., Spence, C., and Rösler, F. (2000). Inhibition of return and oculomotor control in the blind. *Neuroreport,* **11**, 3043–50.

Röder, B., Rösler, F., Hennighausen, E., and Nacker, F. (1996). Event-related potentials during auditory and somatosensory discrimination in sighted and blind human subjects. *Brain Research. Cognitive Brain Research,* **4**, 77–93.

Rousseau, R., Poirier, J., and Lemyre, L. (1983). Duration discrimination of empty time intervals marked by intermodal pulses. *Perception and Psychophysics*, **34**, 541–8.

Sanders, L. D. and Astheimer, L. B. (2008). Temporally selective attention modulates early perceptual processing: Event-related potential evidence. *Perception and Psychophysics*, **70**, 732–42.

Smith, D. B. D., Donchin, E., Cohen, L., and Starr, A. (1970). Auditory averaged evoked potentials in man during selective binaural listening. *Electroencephalography and Clinical Neurophysiology*, **28**, 146–52.

Spence, C. and Driver, J. (1996). Audiovisual links in endogenous covert spatial attention. *Journal of Experimental Psychology: Human Perception and Performance*, **22**, 1005–30.

Spence, C. and Driver, J. (Eds.) (2004). *Crossmodal Space and Crossmodal Attention*, Oxford, Oxford University Press.

Spence, C., Nicholls, M. E. R., Gillespie, N., and Driver, J. (1998). Cross-modal links in exogenous covert spatial orienting between touch, audition and vision. *Perception and Psychophysics*, **60**, 544–57.

Stevens, A. A. and Weaver, K. (2005). Auditory perceptual consolidation in early-onset blindness. *Neuropsychologia*, **43**, 1901–10.

Sutton, S., Tueting, P., Zubin, J., and John, E. R. (1967). Information delivery and the sensory evoked potential. *Science*, **155**, 1436–9.

Ulrich, R., Nitschke, J., and Rammsayer, T. (2006). Crossmodal temporal discrimination: Assessing the predictions of a general pacemaker-counter model. *Perception and Psychophysics*, **68**, 1140–52.

Van Voorhis, S. and Hillyard, S. A. (1977). Visual evoked potentials and attention to points in space. *Perception and Psychophysics*, **22**, 54–62.

Westheimer, G. (1999). Discrimination of short time intervals by the human observer. *Experimental Brain Research*, **129**, 121–6.

Woldorff, M. G. and Hillyard, S. A. (1991). Modulation of early auditory processing during selective listening to rapidly presented tones. *Electroencephalography and Clinical Neurophysiology*, **79**, 170–91.

Woods, D. L. (1990). The physiological basis of selective attention: implications of event-related potential studies, in J. W. Rohrbaugh, R. Parasuraman and J. Johnson (Eds.) *Event-related Brain Potentials: Basic Issues and Applications*, pp.178–209. New York: Oxford University Press.

Woods, D. L. (1995). The component structure of the N1 wave of the human auditory evoked potential. *Perspectives of Event-Related Potentials Research, EEG* (Supp.44), 102–9.

Woods, D. L. and Alain, C. (2001). Conjoining three auditory features: An event-related brainpotential study. *Journal of Cognitive Neuroscience*, **13**, 492–509.

Acknowledgements

The studies presented here were supported by the Deutsche Forschungsgemeinschaft (German Research Foundation), grants For 254/2-1, 2-2 and Ro 1226/4-1, 4-2, 4-3 to BR. We would like to thank our co-authors of the original papers Frank Rösler and Ulrike Krämer for their valuable contributions.

Chapter 29

Neurophysiology of temporal orienting in ventral visual stream

Britt Anderson and David L. Sheinberg

Knowing 'when' has practical consequences. In American football, quarterbacks alter the cadence of their snap counts in an effort to prevent the defence from estimating when a play will begin. Cricket bowlers know that they can be more successful by disguising their delivery to make the time of the arrival of the ball at the batsman less predictable (Renshaw and Fairweather, 2000). It is clear that a warning signal speeds your response (Niemi and Näätänen, 1981), but does it actually improve your perception of that event? Recent studies in cognitive neuroscience have confirmed these practical observations; knowing when something will happen can speed responses and improve perceptual discrimination. This chapter addresses which cellular events might underlie this enhanced perceptual performance.

Relatively few studies have recorded single neuron activity during *temporal* attention tasks, but there are several reports of studies that have examined the neural correlates of visual *spatial* attention. Therefore, we begin by summarizing the neurophysiological correlates of spatial attention before moving on to temporal attention. The most important observation is that, at the neural level, the correlates of spatial and temporal attention show several similarities. Whether a visual stimulus is cued spatially or temporally, there are increases in the spectral power of the local field potential (LFP), changes in neuronal firing rates, and increases in the gamma band spike field coherence (SFC). We therefore consider whether the practical partitioning of attention based on cue modality is respected at the neuronal level, and ask whether common neurophysiological mechanisms may mediate different categories of attention.

How might neurons respond to changing attentional state?

There are limited options for the effects of attention at the cellular level. Essentially, neurons can only change their spiking behaviour. We can measure this directly as changes in spiking activity or indirectly as modulation of the local field potential (LFP).[1] Action potentials, or 'spikes', are believed to be the information units of the central nervous system (Rieke et al., 1999; Gerstner and Kistler, 2002). In the visual centres of the brain, different neurons increase or decrease their firing rates to distinct stimuli. The nature and complexity of the stimuli that drive spiking vary with neuron type and brain area.

In addition to modulating spike rates, neurons can modulate the consistency of their spike responses. Neurons may show less variability in the number of spikes they fire or they may show

---

[1] LFP refers to low frequency oscillations recorded from electrodes implanted in, or on, the brain. If recorded extracranially, it is the same as the EEG. This electrical activity is presumed to reflect the summation of ongoing synaptic activity.

more consistent firing patterns. Another way that neurons change their responses is by modulating the degree to which they coordinate with neighbouring neurons. The term synchrony is used to characterize the extent to which spikes from two different neurons occur simultaneously or with a temporally consistent relationship. The physiological relevance of synchrony stems from the fact that when two spikes occur synchronously, they have the greatest effect on downstream neurons. There are various potential causes of synchrony, including coordination of activity by the LFP, sharing of common inputs, and direct cell–cell interactions.

Visual neurons change their activity patterns with attention. In the next two sections, we highlight a few of the many studies that have examined neuronal activity with changes in visual spatial attention. This will provide the background for a comparison with temporal attention.

Increased neuronal spiking with spatial and object attention

Spatial attention can cause neurons to increase or decrease their firing.[2] One of the earliest demonstrations of this effect in visual cortex was described by Moran and Desimone (1985). In a study of prestriate (area V4) visually responsive neurons in non-human primates, Moran and Desimone showed a strong effect of spatial attention on neuronal activity. If an effective stimulus for a neuron (e.g. a red bar) and a second ineffective stimulus (e.g. a green bar) were both present in the neuron's receptive field, the firing of the neuron was largely determined by the single stimulus that was relevant for the task. Control conditions showed that it was the spatial position of the stimulus and not the colour that was critical for modulating the neurons' responses.

This effect is not limited to simple stimuli like coloured bars, but can also be seen at the level of objects (Chelazzi et al., 1993, 1998, 2001). In a study of inferior temporal cortex, Chelazzi et al., (1998) used a memory-guided search task to manipulate object-based attention. Each trial began with a central fixation spot followed by the central presentation of one of twenty-four coloured images of complex objects (e.g. coffee mug, flower, cherries). The central image was then removed and, after a delay of 1500ms, during which the monkey had to maintain central fixation, an array of pictures was presented to the monkey. After the delay, the monkey was rewarded for moving his eyes to the picture matching the one presented just previously. This paradigm allowed the authors to compare trials in which the same images were on the screen, but where the identity of the target changed object-based attention.

Many neurons in inferior temporal (IT) cortex fire selectively and robustly to complex objects (see Figure 29.1). Chelazzi, et al. (1998) compared trials where a picture preferred by the neuron was the target image, to trials where a non-preferred image was the target; the choice array was the same. Regardless of which picture was the target, the neuron fired with an initial, transient response. If the target was the preferred image, the neuron's firing became more sustained. The difference in firing emerged well before the monkey had time to initiate an eye movement.

Chelazzi et al. (2001) performed a similar experiment, and obtained similar results, when the recording site was V4. Receptive field sizes of V4 neurons are smaller than those of IT neurons. The investigators were able to compare the effect of having an ineffective picture inside or outside a neuron's receptive field. When both an effective and an ineffective picture were in the receptive field of a V4 neuron, the firing of the cell was similar to the firing pattern observed when either image was presented alone. That is, if both images were in the receptive

---

[2] See Wurtz, Goldberg, and Robinson (1980) for a review of early studies on the superior colliculus and diverse cortical regions.

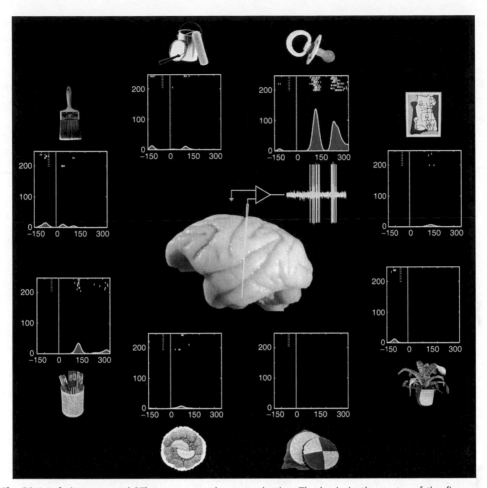

Fig. 29.1 Inferior temporal (IT) neurons can be very selective. The brain in the centre of the figure shows a lateral view of a macaque with a line indicating the approximate location of the recordings from this study. Encircling the brain are several pictures that the monkey viewed during the time that a single IT neuron was recorded. Below each picture are the 'rasters': plots that show for each trial, with that picture, the time of recorded spikes. Zero marks the time when the image appeared on the screen. At the bottom of each of the graphs is the average spiking response across all trials. Beneath the graph of the pacifier (baby's dummy) trials is the actual voltage trace for one trial. The large deflections are the spikes (action potentials). Note that the neuron fires robustly and consistently to the pacifier, and not to other round items or round items intersected by straight lines (the paint can to the left of the pacifier). However, the response of this cell is not all or none, because it does fire a few consistent spikes to the pencils (lower left).

field, and the neuron's effective image was the target, then the neuron responded robustly. If both images were in the receptive field, and the ineffective picture was the target, the firing rates were reduced. If the ineffective picture was outside the receptive field and only the effective image was in the receptive field, the neuron fired the same regardless of which image was the target. The authors interpreted their results as consistent with a biased competition model of attention (Desimone and Duncan, 1995; Desimone, 1998). In such a model, the stimuli compete to drive the output of a neuron and attention biases the competition in favour of the task relevant stimulus.

Visual neurons tend to be tuned; they fire more to some stimuli than others, and there often seems to be an optimal stimulus that evokes the maximal response. Firing decreases in a graded fashion as stimuli are changed from optimal, for example, by changing their orientation. Attention could alter the nature of this relationship in different ways. Most of the data on neuronal firing and attention have suggested that visual neurons either increase their baseline firing rates or increase their gain with attention. Both of these manipulations leave the shape of the stimulus-response tuning curve unchanged. Recently, it has been reported that feature-based attention can cause V4 neurons to alter the shape of their tuning curves to match the target better: the matched filter hypothesis (David et al., 2008).

Together, these results show that spatial, object-based, and feature-based attention are associated with increases in responses selectively associated with target stimuli or, alternatively, a filtering out of signals from non-attended items.

Increased neuronal coherence with spatial attention

Spatial attention has also been linked with increases in the strength of neuronal oscillations and the temporal coordination of spikes and LFP. The LFP is commonly divided into different 'bands' defined by the frequency of oscillation. The gamma band denotes oscillation frequencies in the range of about 20–70Hz. Taylor et al. (2005) used an innovative shape-tracking task to demonstrate that spatial attention affects gamma-band oscillations in area V4. The task presented two shapes, one each on the left and right sides of a computer display. Each shape independently morphed through a series of transitional shapes. The monkey was cued to attend to one side (and ignore the other side) and to indicate when the morph on the attended side returned to its initial form. Local electrical activity was recorded with an array of epidural electrodes. Computing current source density gave a spatially weighted sum of the essentially synchronous electrical activity from synaptic currents. As expected, there were changes in the power of gamma frequency range oscillations such that they increased when the stimulus was present, but in addition there was an increase in power in the gamma frequency range as a function of attentional condition. Increases in oscillation strength occurred at the times in the task when discrimination was required and showed a clear relationship to performance. When monkeys made errors, for example by responding to a repeated shape on the distractor side, the oscillation changes were qualitatively the opposite of what they were on correct trials.

One measure of the correlation between spikes and the LFP is called the spike field coherence (SFC). Fries et al. (2001) presented two orthogonally oriented luminance gratings, one inside and one outside the receptive field of a V4 recording site. The monkey's task was to maintain central fixation and report a colour change at a cued location. When attention was cued to a grating in one of the receptive fields, there was an increase in gamma-band oscillations (defined here as 35–60Hz) of the spike triggered average. Addressing whether these changes were more likely to be correlative or causal, Womelsdorf and Fries (2006) reanalysed these data and compared SFC magnitude with response time. The gamma-band SFC for recording sites in the receptive field of the attended stimulus was greater for trials with faster response times. On the other hand, the SFC for recording sites from the receptive field of the ignored stimulus was higher on trials with longer reaction times.

In their study of spike and LFP coherence, Bichot, Rossi, and Desimone (2005) employed a task where monkeys searched for targets defined by colour, shape, or both. The investigators reported that when monkeys fixated objects that shared features with a target, the coherence between the firing of V4 neurons and gamma-band oscillations of the LFP increased.

Synchrony may also increase at the single neuron level. In a study of visual grouping, Anderson, Harrison, and Sheinberg (2006) recorded simultaneously from pairs of IT neurons responsive to two different pictures. The monkey's task was to search for particular pairs of images in specific target configurations. When the monkey fixated a pair of pictures in the correct configuration, versus when he fixated the same pair of images in an incorrect figuration, the firing rates of both neurons increased and the number of coincident spikes was greater.

Neurophysiological changes with temporal attention

While single cell investigations of visual spatial attention are widespread, we know of only two studies that recorded from ventral visual neurons in monkeys while manipulating temporal aspects of attention (Ghose and Maunsell 2002; Anderson and Sheinberg 2008).[3] We review both studies and compare the results to the neurophysiological changes seen with visual spatial attention.

Firing rates and the hazard function

Ghose and Maunsell (2002) recorded from V4 neurons of macaque monkeys trained to detect changes in the orientation of contrast gratings. For each trial, the monkey was cued to attend to a particular location on the computer screen while maintaining central fixation. Drifting gratings were presented at two or four locations on the screen and occasionally one of the gratings would change orientation. When the drifting grating at the cued location changed orientation, and only when that grating changed, the monkey was to release a response lever. The time at which the test grating changed orientation was selected from a specified probability distribution. The form of the probability distribution determined the graph of the hazard function. A hazard function describes the probability of an event happening given that it has not already happened. Ghose and Maunsell (2002) recorded from eighty V4 neurons when the orientation change times were taken from a symmetric temporal probability distribution that was relatively flat between 1–2 seconds, and then tapered for shorter and longer times. This probability distribution leads to a gradually increasing hazard function with a peak at 2.25 seconds after stimulus onset.

The authors compared neuronal firing when the monkeys' attention was directed into the neuron's receptive field to neuronal firing when attention was directed away from the neuron's receptive field. In both cases, neurons showed a transient increase in firing with stimulus onset. With attention directed into the receptive field, firing gradually increased in parallel with the hazard function. To confirm the relation between neuronal firing and the stimulus hazard function, the authors designed a more arbitrary hazard function: there was high probability of the stimulus changing within the first 500ms of a trial, followed by a period of zero probability, followed by a period of positive probability. Ghose and Maunsell (2002) recorded from eighty-four additional neurons in monkeys trained on this schedule and confirmed that, with attention directed into the receptive field, the firing of neurons paralleled the shape of the hazard function. The rise in the attentional modulation lagged the hazard function by about 150ms. This study demonstrated that neuronal firing increased in parallel with temporal expectation (see also Kilavik and Riehle, Chapter 19, this volume) and suggests a potential mechanism for the behavioural benefits of temporal attention.

----

[3] It should be noted that other investigators have studied other cortical areas while manipulating a task's temporal aspects, e.g. Riehle, et al. (1997) motor cortex, and Janssen and Shadlen (2005) parietal cortex (lateral intraparietal area).

Changes with temporal expectation

To examine further the neurophysiological changes seen with temporal attention, we recorded from the IT cortex of two monkeys engaged in a temporal orienting task (Anderson and Sheinberg, 2008). The task employed a set of 100 pictures. Each picture was used both as a cue and as a target (examples of the pictures are shown in Figure 29.1, and Figure 29.2 provides a graphical overview

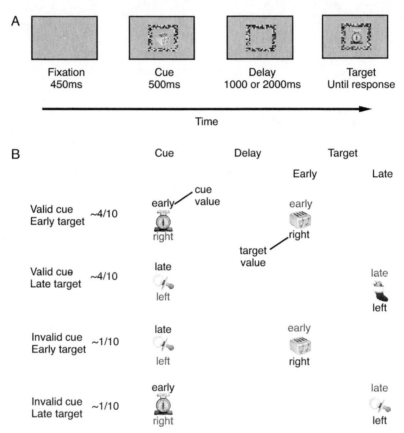

Fig. 29.2 An overview of the temporal attention task of Anderson and Sheinberg (2008). A) Outlines of the task. The monkey first acquired a central fixation point and then a cue image appeared encircled by a dynamic coloured frame. Following the cue image, the coloured frame (reproduced here in greyscale) appeared alone for either 1 or 2 seconds, depending on the cue value. Last, a target image appeared and the monkey had to press a button to obtain a juice reward. Each picture required a specific button press (left or right) that was consistent across all trials and all sessions. B) This gives more detail on the types of trials. Since each image was used as both a cue and a target, each image had two values: a cue value and a target value. Early cue values meant the target would appear in 1000ms and Late cue values meant 2000 ms. A target value of Left meant that when that image appeared as a target, the monkey was required to push the left response button to get his juice reward. Cues were valid 80% of the time. Examples of valid and invalid, early and late, trials are shown. Reprinted from Anderson, B. and Sheinberg, D. L. (2008). Effects of temporal context and temporal expectancy on neural activity in inferior temporal cortex. *Neuropsychologia*, **46**, 947–57, with permission of Elsevier.

of the paradigm). Each picture had two different meanings depending on whether it was the first or second image in a trial ('context'). When a picture appeared as the first image in a trial, it was a temporal cue and carried information about the delay until the target would appear. When a picture was the second image in a trial, it was the target and signalled the monkey to push a response button to acquire his reward. Each picture was assigned a specific cue value that was either 1 or 2 seconds. Each picture was also assigned a target value that was either right or left button press. When pictures appeared as cues they were valid 80% of the time.

In addition, all cues and targets were displayed centred in a dynamically modulating coloured frame that was centred on the display monitor. The intent was to keep the monkeys looking at the centre of the screen during the delay between pictures and to remove any spatial ambiguity about the target location. Pictures were scaled to span 3° of visual angle. The exterior border of the coloured frame spanned 4.5° with an interior opening of 3°. Each target could appear at one of four contrast levels. The progression from full to low contrast was implemented by averaging the colours of the image with the neutral grey background (from low contrast to high contrast the weightings for the image were: 0.015, 0.02, 0.1, and 1.0—full contrast).

The key components of the paradigm were the use of a cue to signal a temporal delay; this delay allowed the monkey to prepare a response, but since it only signalled when a target would appear, it did not permit the preparation of a specific motor action. Because cues were invalid 20% of the time, the sequence of a cue image, 1-second gap, and specific target image could occur with two different expectations. If the cue image signalled a 1-second delay, there was an 80% chance that the target would appear in 1 second. If the cue signalled a 2-second delay, there was a 20% chance the target would appear in 1 second. We hypothesized that different target probabilities would lead to differences of attention in time (Coull and Nobre, 1998). The response-time data support this interpretation (see Figure 29.3A). We could not analyse errors because both monkeys were nearly perfect at classifying the images. The recording sessions took place after several months of behavioural training.

The effect of cue validity was significant for trials with the 1-second delay. This is consistent with an attentional effect. For the trials with a 2-second delay, validity did not significantly affect response time. This is because there were only two time periods when the target pictures could appear. If the target did not appear after a 1-second delay, it had to appear after a 2-second delay.

The effects on neuronal firing parallel the results for response time. Figure 29.3B shows the peri-stimulus time histograms for the population of 50 neurons recorded from both monkeys. Typical of neurons in this region of the monkey brain, the response begins about 100ms after the picture appears on the computer screen. In Figure 29.3B, trials are divided into four groups depending on whether the target image appeared 1 (early) or 2 (late) seconds after the cue picture and whether the target delays had been validly or invalidly cued. For early trials, the effect on spiking activity parallels the response time data; a valid cue results in more spiking than an invalid cue. There is no effect of cue validity on the number of spikes seen with late trials. An effect of cue validity for both neuronal firing rate and behavioural response time, and for the early trials only, is consistent with the experimental effect being due to temporal expectation.

We also recorded the LFP and evaluated the effects of temporal attention on spectral power and the SFC. We computed the spectral power in a window from 550–1050ms after the cue was extinguished. Recall that target images could occur at 1000ms or 2000ms after the cue was extinguished. By comparing the LFP at this time, and separating trials based on cue value, we could compare sets of trials where the monkeys had different expectations about whether a target picture was imminent.

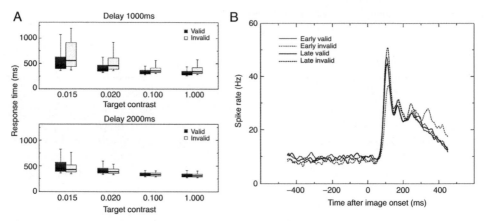

Fig. 29.3 Behavioural and neurophysiological results. A) Shows the response times of the temporal orienting task (data for both monkeys pooled). The upper portion of panel (A) shows the response times for trials when the target appeared after a 1000-ms delay. Target images appeared at one of four different contrast values, which are segmented along the x-axis. Black boxes indicate trials for which the cue was valid. The lower panel shows the same data for trials when the target appeared after a 2000-ms delay. Note that in the upper panel, invalidly cued trials are responded to more slowly and variably; indicating that the monkeys had learned the cue values and were using them to prepare for a response. B) Spiking responses of IT neurons are modulated by temporal attention. The data for 50 IT neurons are combined to show how spiking responses were modulated by temporal attention. All these data are for trials when the target image was shown at full contrast. Trials are divided by whether the cue was valid or invalid and whether the target image was shown early or late. The principal comparison is between the solid and dashed light grey lines, which shows that the early spiking response is diminished and slightly delayed when the monkey is not expecting the stimulus. Reprinted from Anderson, B. and Sheinberg, D. L. (2008). Effects of temporal context and temporal expectancy on neural activity in inferior temporal cortex. *Neuropsychologia*, **46**, 947–57, with permission of Elsevier.

Previously, changes in local field potential power have been found in humans using extracranial high density recordings (Fan et al., 2007, a posterior predominant 'orienting' network) or with subdural electrode arrays in subjects being evaluated for epilepsy surgery (Ray et al., 2008, prefrontal increases regardless of whether an auditory or somatosensory target). We, too, found an increase in spectral power of the LFP during epochs of increased temporal attention. The frequency range for which we observed this effect (16–24Hz) was somewhat lower than is usually reported for spatial attention. However, others have found changes in this frequency range. Tallon-Baudry et al. (2004) measured phase synchrony in monkeys performing a short-term memory task. A target image was presented and, after a variable delay, a comparison image was shown. Monkeys released a lever for matches and withheld the lever release for 800ms for non-matches. Synchrony between multiple electrode sites were compared in the 400-ms interval before presentation of the comparison image, and the strength of synchrony compared for incorrect and correct trials. The researchers observed significant changes restricted to the same sites near the superior temporal sulcus in both monkeys studied. The frequency band for which changes were observed was 15–20Hz (the beta frequency range). In addition to the changes we observed at 16–24Hz, we also observed an increase in the SFC in the lower gamma frequency range.

Similar neurophysiological consequences with spatial and temporal attention

The principal neurophysiological changes observed with *spatial* attention in higher order visual areas are: 1) target specific changes in spike rate; 2) increase in the power of oscillations measured from the LFP for the gamma frequency band while decreases for alpha frequency bands; and 3) an increase in gamma frequency band SFC. In our study of *temporal* attention, we found increases in spike rate, increases in oscillation power and increases in the SFC.

Is the critical difference the category of cue: temporal versus spatial, or the nature of the sensory modality? We would emphasize the similarities of the neural responses in ventral visual stream for spatial and temporal cues. There are at least two important caveats to this conclusion. First, the data from temporal attention tasks are limited. Further work will be needed to examine the extent to whether similarities rather than differences predominate. Secondly, the comparison of temporal and spatial cues has focused on the ventral visual stream. Conclusions might be different when 'spatial' areas are studied, for example, the lateral intraparietal area (LIP) (Gottlieb, Kusunoki, and Goldberg 1998; Janssen and Shadlen, 2005).

Are there types of attention?

We often label attention based on the sensory domain manipulated (visual, auditory, somatosensory) or the method of attentional manipulation (e.g. exogenous cues versus endogenous cues; predictive cues versus instructive cues). But these experimental partitions do not preclude attention from being functionally unitary. For instance, many different types of cues have been used to experimentally manipulate attention, but many of these different types of cues have a common connection: the cues explicitly or implicitly communicate information about the probability of where something will be seen (or heard or felt) or, in the case of temporal attention, when it will be seen (or heard or felt). Ideal observers use knowledge of stimulus probabilities to optimize where they set their decision criteria (Wickens, 2002). From this perspective, many different cue modalities can be argued to have a common effect: they influence a 'decider's' (Stolberg, 2006) subjective estimate of stimulus probabilities. At the level of a subject, a decision-criterion could be adjusted to optimize detection or maximize expected reward. This macro-level optimization may be implemented by changes at the neuronal level, changes in the magnitude and correlation of neuronal firing, which lead, in the aggregate to changes in a decision criterion.

Stüttgen and Schwarz (2008) give a concrete example of how this could work in their comparison of psychometric and neurometric functions for a rat whisker deflection paradigm. Sensitivity could be computed neurometrically, that is as a function of the activity of recorded neurons, or psychometrically, that is based on the actual report of the rats (measured as licks). For these studies the rats had their heads fixed and the stimulus used to deflect individual whiskers was transient and faint. The deflection was held briefly before slowly returning, by a cosine function, to baseline. Simultaneously with the whisker deflection the investigators recorded from single neurons in primary somatosensory cortex (barrel cortex). In a 25-ms window, determined to be optimal for decoding the stimulus from neuronal activity, most of the neurons fired either once or not at all. Computing the sensitivity of the neurons' firing with a standard signal-detection approach assumes a complete knowledge of when the stimulus will occur. This results in an upward biasing of the neurometric estimate. If, alternatively, one incorporates temporal imprecision into the neurometric estimate (which was accomplished in this report by jittering the observation windows), neurometric performance declines and becomes similar to the observed psychometric performance. Could attention in time be doing the inverse? Can a warning signal and the resulting change in temporal attention improve the alignment of the biological 'analysis window' thus improving perceptual performance? Neurophysiological results that show an increase in the SFC coherence with attention are consistent with improved synchronization and are consistent with the suggestion that a temporal cue might provide a cue useful for 'aligning' neural signals.

Conclusions

In contrast to the decades of work on spatial attention, neurophysiological studies of temporal orienting in the ventral visual stream are only just beginning. In our work on temporal orienting, we found, broadly, the same variety of changes in neuronal activity reported for spatial attention: changes in spike rate, LFP power, and SFC. For our temporal orienting task, spike rate changes were stimulus- and condition-specific. LFP power changes were primarily increases in the beta range. The SFC showed increases in the gamma range with lower frequency band decreases.

The division between spatial and temporal cueing is a natural one experimentally, but it may be more productive to look at what cues have in common as we seek to understand the neural bases for attention. Whether a cue communicates spatial or temporal information, it may be the magnitude of the information communicated by that cue which has the greatest correlation with the magnitude of neural and behavioural changes. Future research will be necessary to learn if indeed spatial and temporal orienting are similar neurophysiologically.

References

Anderson, B. and Sheinberg, D. L. (2008). Effects of temporal context and temporal expectancy on neural activity in inferior temporal cortex. *Neuropsychologia*, **46**, 947–57.

Anderson, B., Harrison, M., and Sheinberg, D. L. (2006). A multielectrode study of the inferotemporal cortex in the monkey: effects of grouping on spike rates and synchrony. *Neuroreport*, **17**, 407–11.

Bichot, N.P., Rossi, A. F. and Desimone, R. (2005). Parallel and serial neural mechanisms for visual search in macaque area V4. *Science*, **308**, 529–34.

Chelazzi, L., Miller, E. K., Duncan, J., and Desimone, R. (1993). A neural basis for visual search in inferior temporal cortex. *Nature*, **363**, 345–7.

Chelazzi, L., Duncan, J., Miller, E. K., and Desimone, R. (1998). Responses of neurons in inferior temporal cortex during memory-guided visual search. *J Neurophysiol*, **80**, 2918–40.

Chelazzi, L., Miller, E. K., Duncan, J., and Desimone, R. (2001). Responses of neurons in macaque area V4 during memory-guided visual search. *Cereb Cortex*, **11**, 761–72.

Coull, J. T. and Nobre, A. C. (1998). Where and when to pay attention: the neural systems for directing attention to spatial locations and to time intervals as revealed by both PET and fMRI. *Journal of Neuroscience*, **18**(18), 7426–35.

David, S. V. Hayden, B. Y., Mazer, J. A., and Gallant, J. L. (2008). Attention to stimulus features shifts spectral tuning of V4 neurons during natural vision. *Neuron*, **59**, 509–21.

Desimone, R. (1998). Visual attention mediated by biased competition in extrastriate visual cortex. *Philosophical Transactions of the Royal Society B: Biological Sciences*, **353**, 1245–55.

Desimone, R., and Duncan, J. (1995). Neural mechanisms of selective visual attention. *Annual Review Neuroscience*, **18**, 193–222.

Fan, J., Byrne, J., Worden, M. S., Guise, K. G., McCandliss, B. D., Fossella, J., et al. (2007). The relation of brain oscillations to attentional networks. *J Neurosci*, **27**, 6197–206.

Fries, P., Reynolds, J. H., Rorie, A. E., and Desimone, R. (2001). Modulation of oscillatory neuronal synchronization by selective visual attention. *Science*, **291**, 1560–3.

Gerstner, W. and Kistler, W. (2002). *Spiking Neuron Models: An Introduction*. Cambridge: Cambridge University Press.

Ghose, G.M. and Maunsell, J. H. R. (2002). Attentional modulation in visual cortex depends on task timing. *Nature*, **419**, 616–20.

Gottlieb, J.P., Kusunoki, M. and Goldberg, M. E. (1998). The representation of visual salience in monkey parietal cortex. *Nature*, **391**, 481–4.

Janssen, P. and Shadlen, M. N. (2005). A representation of the hazard rate of elapsed time in macaque area LIP. *Nature Neuroscience*, **8**(2), 234–41.

Moran, J. and Desimone, R. (1985). Selective attention gates visual processing in the extrastriate cortex. *Science*, **229**, 782–4

Niemi, P. and Näätänen, R. (1981). Foreperiod and simple reaction time. *Psychological Bulletin*, **89**, 133–62.

Ray, S., Niebur, E., Hsiao, S. S., Sinai, A., and Crone, N. E. (2008). High-frequency gamma activity (80-150Hz) is increased in human cortex during selective attention. *Clinical Neurophysiology*, **119**, 116–33.

Renshaw, I. and Fairweather, M. M. (2000). Cricket bowling deliveries and the discrimination ability of professional and amateur batters. *Journal of Sports Sciences*, **18**, 951–7.

Riehle, A., Grün, S., Diesmann, M., and Aertsen, A. (1997). Spike synchronization and rate modulation differentially involved in motor cortical function. *Science*, **278**, 1950–3.

Rieke, F. Warland, D., de Ruyter van Steveninck, R., and Bialek, W. (1999). *Spikes: Exploring the Neural Code.* Cambridge, MA: MIT Press.

Stolberg, S. G. (2006). The Decider. *The New York Times.* Available at: http://www.nytimes.com/2006/12/24/weekinreview/24stolberg.html

Stüttgen, M. C. and Schwarz, C. (2008). Psychophysical and neurometric detection performance under stimulus uncertainty. *Nat Neurosci*, **11**, 1091–9.

Tallon-Baudry, C. et al. (2004). Oscillatory synchrony in the monkey temporal lobe correlates with performance in a visual short-term memory task. *Cereb Cortex*, **14**, 713–20.

Taylor, K., Mandon, S., Freiwald, W. A., and Kreiter, A. K.(2005). Coherent oscillatory activity in monkey area V4 predicts successful allocation of attention. *Cerebral Cortex*, **15**, 1424–37.

Wickens, T. D. (2002). *Elementary Signal Detection Theory.* Oxford: Oxford University Press.

Womelsdorf, T. and Fries, P. (2006). Neuronal coherence during selective attentional processing and sensory-motor integration. *Journal of Physiology (Paris)*, **100**, 182–93.

Wurtz, R. H., Goldberg, M. E., and Robinson, D. L. (1980). Behavioral modulation of visual responses in the monkey: Stimulus selection for attention and movement. *Progress in Psychobiology and Physiological Psychology*, **9**, 43–83.

Acknowledgement

This work was supported by the James S McDonnell Foundation, NIH RO1-EY014681, and NSF CRCNS 0423031.

Chapter 30

Temporal prediction during duration perception

Viviane Pouthas and Micha Pfeuty

Neural correlates of time representations have been studied using both functional magnetic resonance imaging (fMRI) and electroencephalography (EEG). Event-related potentials (ERPs), reflecting the rapidly changing electrical activity in the brain evoked by external or internal events, enable different stages in the processing of these events to be differentiated. In this chapter, we will focus on the most familiar ERP correlate of time estimation, which can still be found in very recent literature, a slow brain potential called the contingent negative variation (CNV). It was initially described by Walter et al. (1964), using a paradigm that has now become standard. In this paradigm, subjects have to react as quickly as possible to an imperative stimulus that follows a warning stimulus presented a given time beforehand. When the time between the two stimuli is constant, a slow negative ERP component develops after the warning stimulus and slowly builds up to the imperative stimulus. The wave is therefore thought to reflect attention to the interval between the two stimuli, and expectancy for the stimulus to which one has to react. When the interval is variable, or when the imperative stimulus is omitted, the CNV amplitude decreases (Walter et al., 1964; Pouthas, 2003). Estimating the interval between the two stimuli is adaptive in that it allows the person to anticipate when the imperative stimulus will be delivered and to prepare to react at the appropriate time (Birbaumer et al., 1990; Rockstroh et al., 1993). However, although adaptive, the timing process remains implicit (Praamstra et al., 2006; Praamstra, Chapter 24, this volume). Consequently, the role of temporal preparation in the CNV is not necessarily time-locked to the time of onset of an imperative stimulus. Ruchkin and colleagues (1977) were the first to report correlations between the latency of CNV termination and temporal judgments. When the subject estimated the test duration to be either shorter or longer than the target (800ms), the CNV amplitude was observed to peak earlier (700ms) or later (900ms) respectively, than when the judgment was accurate. The covariation between the latency of CNV termination and duration estimation led the authors to suggest that the CNV reflects 'cognitive activity leading to the formation of the temporal judgments' (p.454). Following this seminal work, a major line of enquiry has been to determine when the CNV terminates or 'resolves', i.e. returns to baseline. Therefore, based mainly on our own studies, we will examine how CNV amplitude and time-course reflect temporal prediction for an external event during explicit timing tasks.

The memory trace of the target duration triggers the CNV resolution

Several decades after Ruchkin's pioneering work concerning the relationship between CNV time course and temporal judgments, a series of studies that delve further into this issue have been published (Pouthas et al., 2000; Macar and Vidal, 2003; Pfeuty et al., 2003, 2005). Using a matching-to-sample temporal discrimination task, in which five visual test durations (490–910ms) were to be judged equal or not equal to a previously memorized visual target duration (700ms), Pouthas et al. (2000) reported covariation between test duration and the latency at which the CNV crossed zero as it returned to baseline (or 'resolved'). Macar and Vidal (2003) criticized the use of this type of index, correctly arguing that it mixed two CNV characteristics, the amplitude peak and the slope of its return to baseline. In a later paper, we also stressed that the latency of the CNV peak seemed to be related to target duration when the current test duration was longer than the target (Pouthas, 2003). Following this observation, both teams provided evidence that the negative to positive shift of the CNV occurred only once the target interval had elapsed, even if the current test duration was already over, and irrespective of whether the stimulus modality was visual, tactile, or auditory (Macar and Vidal, 2003; Pfeuty et al., 2003).

Important additional and innovative findings emerged from further analyses performed by our team using a matching-to-sample temporal discrimination task, as in Pouthas et al. (2000), but with auditory stimuli (Pfeuty et al., 2003). Subjects had to determine whether the duration of a tone (490–910ms) matched that of a previously presented target (700ms). First, differences in CNV time-course over both hemispheres probably signalled differential brain activity in these regions. ERP analyses performed over the left and medial frontal electrode sites showed that for durations shorter than or identical to the target, CNV amplitude continued to increase until stimulus offset, whereas for durations longer than the target, the activity had already reached its maximum before stimulus offset (see also Kilavik and Riehle, Chapter 19, this volume). Statistical analyses confirmed that CNV amplitude increased significantly between short and target durations, but not between target and long durations. By contrast, right frontal activity was found to increase up to the end of the current test duration, even when the target duration had elapsed (Figure 30.1A). We hypothesized that left and medial frontal activity were linked to the memorized target duration and that right frontal activity subserved attention to current stimulus offset. Both processes would be necessary for explicit comparison of the current test duration with the memorized target duration. Secondly, a robust relationship was found between subjective target duration and the latency of the CNV peak, confirming that it was the duration stored in memory that internally triggered CNV resolution. Performance was assessed by calculating the percentage of 'equal to the target responses' for each test duration. On average, the highest percentage was obtained for the 'target test duration', which showed that subjects memorized the target duration accurately. Nevertheless, a large amount of inter-individual variability was found, the 'subjective target duration' of some subjects being significantly shorter or longer than the objective one. This large inter-individual variability gave us a useful means for revealing a correlation between subjective target duration and CNV peak latency over the left, but not the right, frontal region. The right CNV in fact displayed a pattern of slow rising negativity up to the end of the current test duration, which probably reflected a build-up of attentional resources towards the offset of the test duration that enabled the process of comparison to the signal given by the left hemisphere (Figure 30.1B). In other words, ERP effects were predictive of forthcoming behaviour: if there was a late resolution on left frontal sites, the judgment was likely to be 'equal to the target' for the longest test duration.

In a further study, we used a temporal discrimination task using two target durations (600ms and 800ms) and two ranges of test duration (450–800ms and 600–1050ms respectively) in different blocks (Pfeuty et al., 2005). The procedure was neatly controlled in that for half of the trial blocks the 800-ms test duration was the target duration, while in the other half it was the longest test duration for the 600-ms target. We compared CNVs between both conditions, i.e. when the 800-ms test duration was the target duration and when it was the longest test duration. The CNV over left and medial frontal electrode sites resolved earlier when 800ms corresponded to a test

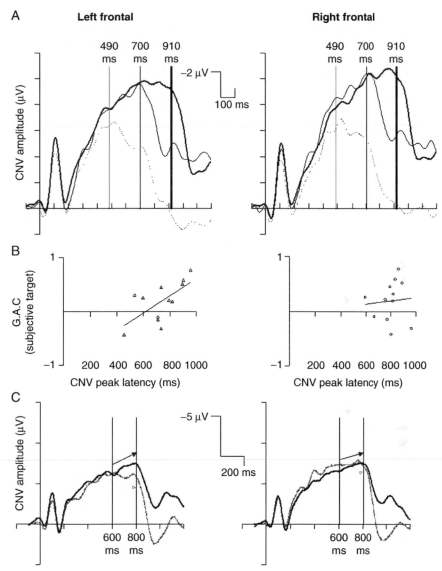

Fig. 30.1 Relationship between the left and right frontal CNV and the target and test durations, respectively. A) ERPs elicited over the left and right frontal areas during the comparison of three test tone durations (490ms, 700ms, and 910ms) to a memorized target tone (700ms). B) Scatter plots of the gradient asymmetry coefficient (g.a.c.) against the CNV peak latency, measured over the left and right frontal areas during the longest test duration (910ms). The g.a.c. value varied between −1 and +1. A positive/negative g.a.c. value indicated that the subjective target duration was above/below 700ms. C) ERPs elicited over the left and right frontal areas during the comparison of an 800-ms test tone duration with a memorized target tone of either 600ms (dashed line) or 800ms (bold line).

duration that was longer than the target duration (600ms) than when it was equal to the target duration (800ms). This demonstrated that the same duration was processed differently depending on the context of its estimation. By contrast, the effect of the memorized target duration on CNV time-course was not observed over the right frontal area (Figure 30.1C) (Pfeuty 2004). This confirms that the CNV reflects two different processes: temporal prediction for the end of target duration over left and medial frontal areas, and attention towards the end of current test duration over right frontal areas (see also Coull, Chapter 31, this volume).

The left and right frontal CNV as neural correlates of implicit and explicit timing

We hypothesized that the left and medial frontal CNV constituted an internal time reference corresponding to target duration. Once this reference has been formed, it may be used automatically, or implicitly. By contrast, the right frontal CNV subtends explicit timing of the current stimulus duration, which enables its comparison to the time reference held in memory (see also Vallesi, Chapter 22; Coull, Chapter 31, this volume). This explanation in some way parallels the distinction proposed by Coull and Nobre (2008) between the neural correlates of implicit and explicit timing.

Supporting this distinction, Praamstra et al. (2006) found analogous results in a paradigm in which timing was implicit (Praamstra, Chapter 24, this volume). They used a choice serial reaction-time task. In each series, the stimulus onset asynchrony (SOA) between successive stimuli was either 1.5 or 2.0 seconds, except the last SOA which was always equal to 1.75 seconds. Depending on the series, this final deviant SOA was either longer or shorter than the standard SOA. They observed that the CNV over left and right premotor cortex peaked before the end of the deviant SOA (1.75 seconds) when it occurred after a series of short SOAs (1.5 seconds), but not after a series of long SOAs (2 seconds). This effect was similar to that observed over left and medial frontal areas in our studies using explicit timing tasks (Pfeuty et al., 2003, 2005). The authors suggested that implicit and explicit interval timing rely on qualitatively similar mechanisms implemented in distinct cortical substrates. Interestingly, they did not report any difference in CNV time-course between the left and right hemispheres. In particular, when the deviant SOA (1.75 seconds) occurred after a series of short SOAs (1.5 seconds), the right frontal CNV was not maintained up until the end of the current SOA, as we had observed previously when the task required an explicit duration comparison (Pfeuty et al., 2003). Thus, in contrast to the left frontal CNV, which appears to be involved in both explicit and implicit tasks, the right frontal CNV appears to be involved specifically in explicit timing tasks.

An additional argument in favour of this hypothesis comes from a previous study (Pouthas et al., 2000) in which we contrasted CNV activity elicited by a visual stimulus, lasting 700ms and illuminated at $15cd/m^2$, during comparison of either stimulus duration or intensity to a previously memorized target duration (700ms) or intensity ($15cd/m^2$). A dipole analysis, performed to identify the generators of the frontal CNV activity, revealed that the activity time course of the left frontal dipole was similar in both discrimination tasks. This undoubtedly reflects the fact that implicit timing was engaged during the intensity task due to repeated exposures to the same 700-ms duration. By contrast, the activity time course of the right frontal CNV was very different in the two discrimination tasks. In the intensity task, the dipole did not show any activity, whereas in the duration task the activity was maintained up until the end of the current test duration. This is consistent with the fact that an explicit duration discrimination judgment was required in this task only.

The neural coding of the memory trace

A further question that has been raised concerns how the neural code of the target duration, or, in other words, the internal time reference, is established. Studies with animals have shown the existence of neurons with climbing activity. The characteristic of these neurons is that their spiking rate increases constantly during the interval separating a cue from a predicted reward. Interestingly, Komura et al. (2001) showed that when the interval is shortened (or lengthened), the slope of the climbing activity in thalamic neurons increases (or decreases), so that the same level of activity is reached earlier (or later), i.e. at the new reward time. Based on these results, we tested whether the activity time-course of the CNV recorded on the human scalp exhibits the same characteristics as *neural* climbing activity and may thus reflect the neural code of target duration. In the study described earlier (Pfeuty et al., 2005), in which two target durations were used (600ms and 800ms), the 800-ms test duration was compared with a target of either 600ms or 800ms. As shown earlier, the CNV resolved earlier in the first case, reflecting the end of the memorized target duration. Furthermore, the maximum level of activity did not differ between the two target durations, and the slope, which varied inversely with the length of the duration, was steeper for the shorter target duration (Figure 30.2). This effect was also reproduced by Praamstra et al. (2006) using an implicit timing task, which suggests that the neural coding of an internal time reference, probably based on the activity of climbing neurons, is similar for implicit and explicit timing tasks. It is proposed that a given level of activity in climbing neurons would signal the expected end of the target interval. If a temporal difference is detected between the expected and actual target end, the slope of the climbing activity would adjust so as to minimize this difference.

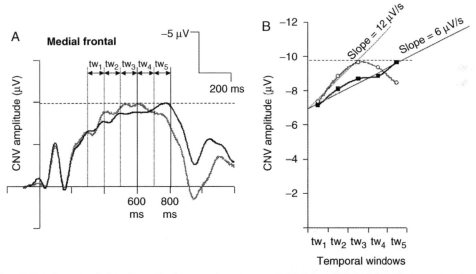

Fig. 30.2 Influence of the memorized target duration on CNV slope. A) ERPs elicited over medial frontal areas during the comparison of an 800-ms test tone duration with a memorized target tone of either 600ms (dashed line) or 800ms (bold line). B) Mean CNV amplitude over medial frontal areas for five successive temporal windows (tw) (defined from 300–800ms) for the 800ms test tone duration paired with short (empty circles and dashed line) versus long (filled squares and filled line) memorized targets. Mean CNV slopes are indicated for the short and long memorized targets.

The impact of sensory information on the neural coding of the memory trace

The findings described earlier suggest that, during an explicit timing task, there is a progressive build-up of the memory trace of the target against which test durations are compared. The steady CNV resulting from this build-up, which is a correlate of the subjective time reference, could be viewed as a 'conditioned brain response' (Walter et al., 1964; Los and Hesslenfeld 2005). This time reference and its neural correlate could then be used automatically in contexts similar to that in which it was memorized. But this raises the question of what happens for different contexts in which trace conditioning takes place. By comparing the global CNV waveform observed in different studies, it seems that CNV resolution reflects the end of target duration, irrespective of whether the stimulus modality is visual, tactile or auditory (Macar and Vidal, 2003; Pfeuty et al., 2003, 2005), or whether the interval is filled or empty (Praamstra et al., 2006). However, close examination of the study by Praamstra et al. (2006) reveals that when the deviant SOA (1.75 seconds) occurred at the end of a series of short SOAs (1.5 seconds), the CNV did not peak at 1.5 seconds (the end of the memorized target) but at 1.6 seconds (i.e. 100ms later). No such time lag was observed in the studies with filled intervals (Macar and Vidal, 2003; Pfeuty et al., 2003, 2005). This suggests that the neural marker of target duration may differ between filled and empty conditions. It is possible that the brain anticipates the offset of a current stimulus during filled intervals, whereas it anticipates the onset of a new stimulus during empty intervals.

In a recent study from our group, participants compared test durations (450–800ms) with a 600-ms target. Half the participants were tested with filled intervals and the other half with empty intervals (Pfeuty et al., 2008). The goal was to compare CNV amplitude and time-course elicited by filled versus empty intervals. The empty condition was associated with higher timing accuracy than the filled condition, in line with the results of previous studies (Grondin, 1993, Grondin et al., 1996, 1998). EEG data revealed higher CNV amplitude under the filled than the empty condition. One possibility is that there was a superimposition of timing-dependent activity and sustained sensory activity under the 'filled' condition, in line with previous EEG-MEG studies showing that the auditory cortex is involved in temporal processing with filled intervals (N'Diaye et al., 2004; Sieroka et al., 2003). Interestingly, the CNV time-course exhibited a marked difference between the two conditions for the long test duration (800ms). Under the 'filled' condition, the CNV amplitude increased up to the memorized target (600ms), and then decreased to the end of the test duration. Under the 'empty' condition, the CNV amplitude increased precisely concurrently with the end of the memorized target (Figure 30.3). Schubotz (2007; Schubotz, Chapter 25, this volume) has proposed that the prediction of future external events relies on the ability of our sensorimotor system to make simulations. We assume that participants simulated the memorized target interval during a test interval in order to predict its end. The different temporal profiles of the CNV observed between the two conditions would thus arise from the different temporal structures of the simulated sensory event. Under the 'filled' condition, the sensorimotor system would simulate a continuous tone whose offset occurs at 600ms, which is reflected by a continuous increase in the CNV up to 600ms (when the offset of the continuous tone is expected to occur) and then by a decrease. Under the 'empty' condition, the sensorimotor system would simulate a silent period finishing at 600ms with a brief tone, which is correlated with a clear-cut increase in the CNV at 600ms (when the onset of the brief tone is expected to occur). The involvement of sensory simulation in temporal processing has already been documented (Rao et al., 1997). In this study, haemodynamic activity was observed in auditory cortex when participants had to maintain the same tapping rate as an auditory tempo to which they had previously synchronized but which they no longer heard. This auditory activity indicates that participants

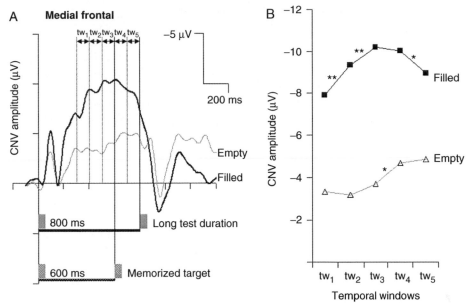

Fig. 30.3 Influence of the sensory structure of an interval on CNV amplitude and time course. A) ERPs elicited over medial frontal areas during the comparison of an 800-ms test duration with a memorized target of 600ms. Durations were represented by either filled (filled line) or empty (dashed line) intervals. B) Mean CNV amplitude over medial frontal areas for five successive temporal windows (tw) (defined from 300–800ms) for the 800-ms test duration under filled (black squares) or empty (empty triangles) conditions. The p-values indicate the significance, or lack thereof, of differences between adjacent temporal windows within the same condition (* p <0.05; ** p <0.01).

used a simulation of the auditory feedback to keep the tempo in memory. This hypothesis of a temporal representation by simulation helps explain the CNV waveform observed by Praamstra et al. (2006). In that study, the brain apparently simulated the arrival of a visual stimulus at 1.5 seconds, which was correlated with a specific increase in the CNV at 1.5 seconds.

To sum up, when a participant has to compare the duration of two tones explicitly (i.e. filled intervals), a memory trace of the first tone will be left in the sensorimotor system. At the second tone, the sensorimotor system simulates the trace of the first tone in order to anticipate its likely end. When a participant has to compare the duration of two empty intervals, the trace simulated during the second internal by the sensorimotor system is different, i.e. two short tones separated by a silent period. The temporal profile of the CNV reflects the temporal structure of the sensory information that is simulated. However, simulation would be efficient only when sensory information is similar for the two intervals to be compared. An interesting issue for future research would be to compare timing mechanisms in two situations: 1) when the sensory context between encoding and comparison is similar (filled/filled or empty/empty) and thus an implicit trace conditioning is available, and 2) when it is different (filled/empty or empty/filled).

Conclusions

Coull and Nobre (2008) suggest that explicit and implicit timing must be distinguished, arguing that fMRI studies demonstrate that discrete neural substrates are involved. However, this raises the question of whether this distinction is always clear, or whether the two types of timing pertain to the same continuum. We hypothesize that there is a progressive build-up of a time reference, i.e. that a sort of trace conditioning takes place either during the encoding phase of matching-to-sample (Pfeuty et al., 2003) comparison or reproduction tasks (Macar and Vidal, 2003; Pfeuty et al., 2005), or during the regular sequences of identical intervals in an oddball paradigm (Praamstra et al., 2006). Resolution of the CNV over left and medial frontal areas would be triggered by offset of the trace or, in other words, by the expected end of the target. However, unlike implicit timing tasks, explicit timing tasks require controlled cognitive processes to allow participants to detect consciously that the test duration is slightly shorter or longer than the target. These comparison mechanisms undoubtedly involve the right frontal areas where the CNV time course is related to the test duration rather than to the target (see Coull, Chapter 31 this volume, for a similar distinction).

A major challenge for future research is to clarify how the memory trace of target duration is coded. One possibility is that the slope of climbing activity in some thalamic, parietal or frontal neurons codes for the predicted end of target duration. An alternative, but not mutually exclusive, hypothesis is that trace conditioning occurs in the sensorimotor system. Predicting the end of the target interval would thus rely on the simulation of a memorized sensorimotor event.

References

Birbaumer, N., Elbert, T., Canavan, A.mG., and Rockstroh, B. (1990). Slow potentials of the cerebral cortex and behavior. *Physiological Review*, **70**, 1–41.

Coull, J. and Nobre, A. (2008). Dissociating explicit timing from temporal expectation with fMRI. *Current Opinion in Neurobiology*, **18**, 137–44.

Grondin, S. (1993). Duration discrimination of empty and filled intervals marked by auditory and visual signals. *Perception & Psychophysics*, **54**, 383–94.

Grondin, S., Ivry, R.mB., Frantz, E., Perreault, L., and Metthé, L. (1996). Marker's influence on the duration discrimination of intermodal intervals. *Perception & Psychophysics*, **58**, 424–33.

Grondin, S., Meilleur-Wells, G., Ouellette, C., and Macar, F. (1998). Sensory effects on judgments of short time-intervals. *Psychological Research*, **61**, 261–8.

Komura, Y., Tamura, R., Uwano, T., Nishijo, H., Kaga, K., and Ono, T. (2001). Retrospective and prospective coding for predicted reward in the sensory thalamus. *Nature*, **412**, 546–9.

Los, S. A. and Heslenfeld, D. J. (2005). Intentional and unintentional contributions to nonspecific preparation: electrophysiological evidence. *Journal of Experimental Psychology General*, **134**, 52–72.

Macar F. and Vidal F. (2003). The CNV peak: an index of decision making and temporal memory. *Psychophysiology*, 950–4.

N'Diaye, K., Ragot, R., Garnero, L., and Pouthas, V. (2004). What is common to brain activity evoked by the perception of visual and auditory filled durations? A study with MEG and EEG co-recordings. *Brain Research*, **21**, 250–68.

Pfeuty, M. (2004). 'Perception de la durée d' simples et séquentiels : étude comportementale et électrophysiologique.' [Duration perception of single and sequential intervals: a behavioral and electrophysiological study]. Unpublished doctoral dissertation, Paris, University Pierre et Marie Curie.

Pfeuty, M., Ragot, R., and Pouthas, V. (2003). When time is up: CNV time course differentiates the roles of the hemispheres in the discrimination of short tone durations. *Experimental Brain Research*, **151**, 372–9.

Pfeuty, M., Ragot, R., and Pouthas, V. (2005). Relationship between CNV and timing of an upcoming event. *Neuroscience Letters*, **382**(1–2), 106–11.

Pfeuty, M., Ragot, R., and Pouthas, V. (2008). Brain activity during interval timing depends on sensory structure. *Brain Research*, 112–17.

Pouthas, V. (2003). Electrophysiological evidence for specific processing of temporal information in humans. In W.H. Meck (ed.) *Functional and Neural Mechanisms of Interval Timing*, pp.439–56. Boca Raton: CRC Press.

Pouthas, V., Garnero, L., Ferrandez, A. M., and Renault, B. (2000). ERPs and PET analysis of time perception: spatial and temporal brain mapping during visual discrimination tasks. *Human Brain Mapping*, **10**(2), 49–60.

Praamstra, P., Kourtis, D., Kwok, H. F., and Oostenveld, R. (2006). Neurophysiology of implicit timing in serial choice reaction-time performance. *Journal of Neurosciences*, **26**, 5548–55.

Rao, S. M., Harrington, D. L., Haaland, K. Y., Bobholz, J. A., Cox, R. W., and Binder, J. R. (1997). Distributed neural systems underlying the timing of movements. *Journal of Neurosciences*, **17**, 5528–35.

Rockstroh, B., Müller, M., Wagner, M., Cohen, R., and Elbert, T. (1993). "Probing" the nature of the CNV. *Electroencephalography and Clinical Neurophysiology*, **87**, 235–41.

Ruchkin, D. S., McCalley, M. G., and Glaser, E. M. (1977). Event related potentials and time estimation. *Psychophysiology*, **14**, 451–5.

Schubotz, R. I. (2007). Prediction of external events with our motor system: towards a new framework. *Trends in Cognitive Science*, **11**, 211–18.

Sieroka, N., Dosch, H. G., Specht, H. J., and Rupp, A. (2003). Additional neuromagnetic source activity outside the auditory cortex in duration discrimination correlates with behavioural ability. *NeuroImage*, **20**, 1697–703.

Walter, W. G., Cooper, R., Aldridge, V. J., McCallum, W.C., and Winter, A.L. (1964). Contingent negative variation: an electric sign of sensori-motor association and expectancy in the human brain. *Nature*, **203**, 380–4.

Chapter 31

Neural substrates of temporal attentional orienting

Jennifer T. Coull

We are perpetually surrounded by a myriad of different stimuli in our spatially distributed and temporally dynamic world. The process of selective attention allows us to filter out information that is relevant for current action-perception goals. However, the process of selective attention is not restricted to the here and now, simply selecting relevant information 'on-line' from one moment to the next. To improve the efficiency of processing within our limited-capacity system, selected information can be collated in a dynamic way in order to build up expectancies of where and when relevant stimuli are likely to appear in the future. Such expectancy allows attentional resources to be directed, in an anticipatory way, to the location in space and/or the moment in time that a relevant stimulus is likely to appear. Anticipatory direction (or 'orienting') of attentional resources has a twofold effect: first, sensory perception of the stimulus is enhanced and second, motor responses to the stimulus are speeded.

To date, a vast number of studies have examined the psychophysical and neural bases of anticipatory orienting of attention in space, most notably using the paradigm developed by Posner et al. (1980; see also Lupiáñez, Chapter 2, this volume). These studies demonstrated that the locus of spatial attention can be directed, in an anticipatory manner by informative cues, to the most likely location of an upcoming stimulus in order to improve stimulus processing. Crucially, attention can be directed voluntarily and dynamically, such that the spatial locus of attention can shift from one location to another on a trial-by-trial basis. Within the temporal domain, it has been known since the beginning of the last century that maintaining a constant, or at least predictable, interval between warning and target stimuli (the 'foreperiod') across trials allows temporal expectancies to be implicitly established over time, thus speeding responses to target stimuli (Woodrow, 1914; (Niemi and Näätänen, 1981).

However, the foreperiod literature does not indicate whether these largely subconscious anticipatory processes can be harnessed and put under cognitive control. Nobre and myself have explored whether attention can be voluntarily directed to moments in time in a more flexible or dynamic manner, such that the temporal locus of attention can shift from one interval to another on a trial-by-trial basis (Nobre, Chapter 27, this volume). We hypothesized that subjects could be explicitly cued to direct attentional resources to discrete temporal intervals in order to enhance stimulus processing. With a grateful nod to the spatial orienting paradigm from which it was derived, we named this process 'temporal orienting of attention' (Coull and Nobre, 1998; Nobre, 2001). Two crucial points must be emphasized. First, temporal expectancies are proposed to change in a dynamic way, from one trial to the next. Expectation depends only upon the temporal cue presented within the current trial and is independent of all other trials in the experimental block. Second, temporal orienting is proposed to be voluntary and explicit, as compared to the more automatic or implicit nature of foreperiod effects. With temporal orienting, subjects are instructed to use informative cues consciously in order to direct attentional resources to a specific point in time. These cues, at least initially, were symbolic, or 'endogenous', in nature.

More recently however, we have also developed paradigms to examine how attention can be oriented in time through more stimulus-driven or 'exogenous' means. In these tasks, the temporally regular rhythmic movement of a dynamic visual stimulus entrains an expectation for the moment in time at which the next target stimulus should appear. In contrast to the endogenous temporal cueing task, there is no pre-learned association between an arbitrary cue and a particular delay. Moreover, subjects are not explicitly told to use the temporal information inherent in stimulus presentation to make predictions but, nevertheless, they appear to do so spontaneously in order to enhance performance. We have examined how the behavioural and neural signatures of endogenous temporal orienting compare to (and interact with) those of exogenous temporal orienting.

Endogenous temporal orienting with predictive pre-cues

The putative process of temporal orienting of attention is logically equivalent to the well-studied process of spatial orienting of attention, whereby attentional resources are directed to discrete locations in space in order to enhance stimulus processing. The basis of our experiments was an adaptation of the classic spatial orienting of attention task (Posner et al., 1980) in which subjects respond as quickly as possible to peripheral targets. In this task, a predictive pre-cue either correctly ('valid cue') or incorrectly ('invalid cue') predicts the location of an upcoming target. Target detection is faster for stimuli appearing at cued, rather than uncued, spatial locations due to a process of spatial attentional orienting. We hypothesized that target detection would also be faster for stimuli appearing at cued, rather than uncued, temporal intervals, due to a process of temporal attentional orienting.

Behavioural advantages of endogenous temporal orienting

In our temporal analogue of the Posner orienting task (hereafter 'endogenous temporal cueing task'), the subjects' task was to detect a target appearing in one of two peripheral locations after one of two inter-stimulus intervals (Coull and Nobre, 1998). Prior to target presentation, informative cues manipulated subjects' expectations of where *or when* the target would appear by predicting spatial location and/or temporal interval. The power of our 2 × 2 factorial design lay in the fact that we were able to examine both the well-established process of spatial orienting and the putative process of temporal orienting within the same experimental framework and within the same set of subjects. Target detection was consistently found to be faster when the target was preceded by a symbolic cue carrying temporally predictive information than when it was preceded by a neutral cue that carried no temporally precise information (e.g. Coull and Nobre, 1998; Coull et al., 2001; Griffin et al., 2001, 2002). This was also true when the incidental spatial component was removed from the task, and both cues and targets appeared within the same central position on the screen (Miniussi et al., 1999; Coull et al., 2000; Griffin et al., 2001).

Cues providing invalid temporal information (e.g. when the cue predicted a long delay but the target appeared unexpectedly after a short delay) led to significant slowing of RTs, otherwise known as the 'invalidity effect' (Coull and Nobre, 1998; Nobre et al., 1999; Coull et al., 2001; Griffin et al., 2001, 2002). Later experiments, seperately comparing valid or invalid trials to neutral trials, probed this effect further. It was shown that the behavioural advantages conferred

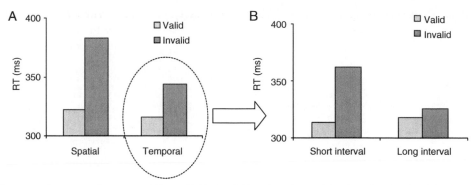

Fig. 31.1 A) Temporal cues providing reliable ('valid') rather than misleading ('invalid') information speed target detection in a way qualitatively similar to that of spatial cues, although the effect is smaller for temporal cues than for spatial ones (graphs drawn with data from Coull and Nobre, 1998). B) The smaller benefit of temporal (versus spatial) cueing is due to an interaction with changing conditional probabilities over time. If the temporal data are re-classified according to the length (short/long) of the interval between cue and target, the temporal orienting effect is significant only for invalidly cued targets appearing at the short interval (i.e. earlier than expected: 'premature' targets). Invalidly-cued targets appearing at the long interval (i.e. later than expected: 'delayed' targets) afford time for the response plan to be updated and for attention to be re-oriented to the later interval, thus negating the cost of having been invalidly cued (graphs drawn with data from Coull and Nobre, 1998).

by attending to a particular point in time were better conceptualized as benefits of temporally predictive information (valid trials were faster than neutral trials) than costs of temporally misleading information (invalid trials were no slower than neutral trials) (Coull et al., 2001; Griffin et al., 2001). Furthermore, it was shown that preparing for an imminent (short delay) target could have knock-on benefits for the detection of premature (invalid) probe stimuli that appeared as soon as 100ms after presentation of the temporal cue, with benefits increasing steadily the closer the probe was presented to the expected time (Griffin et al., 2001). These data illustrate that the preparatory processes initiated by the cue could start very soon after cue presentation but developed gradually over time to produce an optimal state of preparation for the expected point in time.

In sum, these results suggest that there is a behavioural advantage in knowing *when* to expect a target, which is qualitatively similar to that for knowing *where* to expect it (Figure 31.1A). Although the benefits of spatial cueing are extremely well known, this was the first time that such benefits had been shown to manifest themselves in the temporal domain. Moreover, later behavioural experiments, using choice, rather than simple, RT tasks, demonstrated the benefits of temporal orienting not just on the speed of motor detection but also on the speed of perceptual discrimination (Griffin et al., 2001). In other words, knowing when a stimulus is likely to appear improves processing of that stimulus, even when the type of response to be produced is unknown until the stimulus appears. This suggests that the processes underlying the orienting of attention in the temporal domain are not solely linked to preparation of a specific motor response, although effects on motor speed are greater than those on perceptual discrimination (see also Correa, Chapter 26, this volume) suggesting that the underlying functional mechanisms are more likely to be linked to motor, rather than perceptual, processing (Nobre, Chapter 27, this volume).

Neurophysiological mechanisms of endogenous temporal orienting

Event-related potentials (ERPs) are small voltage fluctuations, recorded from the scalp, which vary as a function of ongoing cognitive processes. Visual evoked potentials occurring soon after (~100ms) stimulus presentation reflect perceptual analysis of the stimulus, while later potentials reflect processes related to sensorimotor integration, memory retrieval, or response-preparation. To investigate the temporal dynamics of orienting attention in time, Miniussi et al. (1999), and later Griffin et al. (2002), examined ERPs elicited by temporally informative cues. Expectation that the target would appear after a short, rather than long, interval increased the negativity of the contingent negative variation (CNV) waveform. The CNV is linked to expectancies and motor preparation (Walter et al., 1964) and its pronounced negativity for short-cue trials is indicative of heightened expectancy for making an imminent response. The anatomical source of this CNV modulation was localized to supplementary motor area (Nobre, 2001), an area also linked to motor preparation, as well as to timing (Macar and Vidal, 2003; Pfeuty et al., 2005; Pouthas and Pfeuty, Chapter 30; Praamstra, Chapter 24, this volume). These results strongly suggest that temporal cueing enhances behaviour by encouraging preparation of a motor response at an expected time.

Sequential effects of foreperiod length have also been shown to modulate CNV amplitude (Los and Heslenfeld, 2005; Los, Chapter 21, this volume). Both sequential effects and temporally informative cues continually renew temporal expectancies on a trial-by-trial basis. However, while temporal cues regenerate temporal expectancies in an endogenous manner, the mechanism underlying sequential effects is likely to be more exogenous in nature. Specifically, the duration of the previous foreperiod may be used to predict (Requin et al., 1991) or condition (Los and van den Heuvel, 2001) the duration of the current foreperiod, resulting in longer RTs when there is a mismatch. That both temporal cueing and sequential effects modulate CNV amplitude could be taken as evidence for a common functional basis for exogenous (sequential effects) and endogenous (temporal cueing) forms of temporal expectancy (see also Pouthas and Pfeuty, Chapter 30, this volume). However, Los and Heslenfeld (2005) further report that presentation of temporally informative cues did not override the influence of sequential effects on CNV amplitude, suggesting that exogenous and endogenous temporal orienting processes can exist independently from one another.

Research from the field of spatial attention shows that the attentional state of the subject can modulate ERPs elicited by identical sensory stimuli. For example, if a target appears in an attended, compared to an unattended, spatial location both early visual-evoked potentials (P1, N1) and later response-related potentials are amplified (Hillyard et al., 1973; Mangun, 1995), suggesting that spatial orienting improves performance through facilitation of both perceptual and motor processing. By measuring ERPs during a temporal orienting of attention task the locus of the temporal expectation effect can be identified in a similar way. Specifically, it is possible to explore whether temporal orienting optimizes performance by enhancing early, perceptual processing, by facilitating later motor preparation, or by a combination of the two (Nobre, Chapter 27, this volume)? Temporal orienting (measured at the short interval) increased the amplitude of the P3 potential while also causing it to peak earlier (Miniussi et al., 1999; Griffin et al., 2002), reflecting modulation of decision-making and response preparation processes. Temporal orienting also attenuated amplitude of the N2 potential (Miniussi et al., 1999; Griffin et al., 2002), which is linked to response inhibition. In contrast to spatial orienting, temporal orienting did not modulate the P1 visual-evoked potential. However, when greater demands were made on stimulus discrimination (Griffin et al., 2002), temporal orienting enhanced the early N1 visual-evoked potential, albeit with a different scalp distribution to spatial orienting effects (see also Lange et al., 2006; Lange and Röder, Chapter 28, this volume for effects of temporal orienting on the N1 *auditory*-evoked potential). Considered together with the cue effects described above, these results suggest that temporal orienting enhances speed of target detection primarily by facilitating motor preparation rather than perceptual analysis.

Neuroanatomical substrates of endogenous temporal orienting

Despite localization techniques, the spatial resolution of ERP studies remains rather coarse. Functional neuroimaging, with either Positron Emission Tomography (PET) or, better yet, functional magnetic resonance imaging (fMRI), provides far greater anatomical precision. Furthermore, recent developments in event-related fMRI allow for a temporal resolution of around one second. Both PET and fMRI measure local changes in cerebral blood flow (coupled to neural activity), which vary as a function of ongoing cognitive processes. Regionally specific changes in the pattern of brain activity from one condition to another can index the anatomical and functional bases of experimental tasks.

The neuroanatomical correlates of directing attention in space versus time were compared using both PET and fMRI, in two independent subject groups (Coull and Nobre, 1998). Neuroimaging data revealed considerable overlap in activation of a fronto-parietal network for spatially and temporally informative cues as compared to a resting baseline. When compared to a neutral cue condition however, the only point of overlap was in posterior visual cortex. This suggests that while spatial and temporal orienting tasks engage identical perceptual and motor mechanisms, necessary for processing visual stimuli and preparing a motor response, their attentional orienting mechanisms may differ. Direct comparison of spatial to temporal orienting revealed a hemispheric lateralization in posterior parietal cortex (PPC). Spatial orienting preferentially activated right inferior parietal cortex, confirming many previous reports, whereas temporal orienting preferentially activated left parietal cortex (Figure 31.2A). When subjects made use of spatially and temporally informative cues simultaneously, both right and left parietal cortices were preferentially activated. In addition to the parietal activation, temporal orienting also selectively activated left ventral premotor cortex (vPMC) in the region of the frontal operculum.

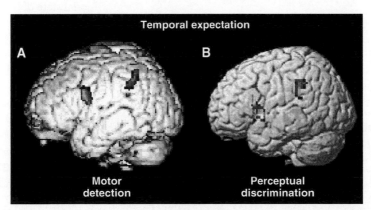

Fig. 31.2 (See also Plate 11) Using temporal expectancies to optimize behaviour activates a left fronto-parietal network, whether expectancies are established (A) endogenously by predictive pre-cues in a speeded motor detection task (Coull and Nobre, 1998) or (B) exogenously by predictable stimulus motion in a perceptual discrimination task (Coull et al., 2008).

Intriguingly, this premotor activity is unlikely to be a mere side-effect of the motor nature of the temporal orienting task since numerous reports by Schubotz and colleagues have demonstrated that ventral premotor cortex is activated by temporally predictable inter-stimulus intervals in purely *perceptual* prediction tasks (Schubotz, 2007; Schubotz and von Cramon, 2001; Schubotz et al., 2003; Schubotz, Chapter 25, this volume).

Left ventral premotor and, particularly, parietal cortex have also been implicated in motor orienting, whereby movement of a specific motor effector (e.g. index versus middle finger), rather than a spatial location or temporal interval, can be cued and therefore anticipated (Rushworth et al., 2001). The neuroanatomical overlap in left parietal-premotor cortices for temporal and motor orienting of attention is therefore suggestive of a corresponding functional overlap (Nobre, 2001). However, the left-lateralization for temporal orienting observed by Coull and Nobre (1998) cannot simply be dismissed as an incidental side effect of motor orienting since spatial and temporal orienting conditions were matched for the motor effector that would be used to register the response (index finger). Instead, spatial and temporal conditions differed in the predictability of *when* the response would be made.

Functionally dissociating the predictability of the time versus type of a future motor response has been a subject of investigation for many decades now. For example, in a cued choice reaction time (RT) paradigm, responses are speeded when a warning cue provides prior information about the type *or* timing of the impending motor response (Requin et al., 1991). To determine whether these two processes are *neurally*, as well as functionally, distinct, we could turn to functional imaging. However, one major drawback of the cued choice RT task, is the large number of trials needed to establish the temporal or motor expectancy, making its use in fMRI, or even ERP, paradigms rather unwieldy. We therefore decided to capitalize on the relative brevity of our cued orienting paradigm to investigate the neural overlap between temporal and motor orienting within a single experimental paradigm. Using a similar 2×2 factorial design to the temporal and spatial orienting paradigm described earlier (Coull and Nobre, 1998), visual cues informed subjects either when a motor response would be required (short/long delay) and/or which motor effector would be required to make the response (button-press/saccade). Subjects could therefore prepare to respond at a particular moment in time, but could not prepare the precise motor effector that would be required to execute the response. In other words, temporal orienting was disambiguated from motor orienting. Compared to neutral cues, both temporal and motor-effector cues independently speeded reaction times, confirming the behavioural utility of either type of cue. FMRI data revealed that left parietal cortex was consistently activated by temporal orienting, even when the motor effector that would be used to make the response was unknown (Cotti et al., 2009). Moreover, since blocks of trials contained an equal mixture of left- and right-sided responses, left-lateralized activation was not due simply to a predominance of right-sided responses. These data therefore confirm the fundamental role of left parietal cortex in temporal attentional orienting, and demonstrate that its activation is not simply due to incidental motor orienting mechanisms.

Exogenous temporal orienting by predictable stimulus motion

In all of the studies described thus far, endogenous symbolic cues were used to orient attention in time. Temporal expectancies can also be generated by more exogenous means, in which the temporal layout of the stimuli themselves generates the expectation. For example, in the auditory domain, musical rhythm generates temporal expectancies for when the next beat will fall

(Jones, Chapter 23, this volume), allowing us to clap along in time to the music. In the visual domain, the movement trajectory (direction and speed) of an oncoming car will generate an expectation for its location at some specified point in time, allowing us to take evasive action. Ecologically valid paradigms were therefore developed that were intended to mirror the way information is presented in real-world situations. Specifically, tasks were designed to investigate how dynamic trajectories could be used to deploy attentional resources to the expected moment that a transiently occluded target would appear, so as to enhance its processing.

Behavioural indices of exogenous temporal orienting

In the real world, we can predict the time at which a moving object is likely to reach a particular location, even if that object is temporarily hidden from view. To use a driving analogy, imagine a three-lane motorway on which you are overtaking a lorry that is itself overtaking a car set to exit the motorway up ahead. Despite the fact that the lorry is temporarily obscuring your vision of both the car and the motorway exit, you can use the car's speed to predict whether it will have exited the motorway by the time you have passed the lorry. This situation was mirrored in the laboratory by Doherty, Nobre, and colleagues (Doherty et al., 2005; Nobre, Chapter 27, this volume). They manipulated the predictability of stimulus direction and speed to generate expectations concerning the location and/or time of the stimulus' reappearance from behind a narrow occluding barrier. Spatial expectation was established by a constant directional angle of motion and temporal expectation was established by a constant rhythmic speed of motion. Erratic spatial trajectories and/or intermittent rhythmic speeds were used in the neutral expectation condition. The subject's task was to respond as quickly as possible to a target stimulus that could appear when or where expected as predicted by the object's trajectory prior to its occlusion. Two separate experiments confirmed that such exogenous temporal cues improved performance, whether the same visual rhythm was used to establish temporal expectancies across all temporal trials (Doherty et al., 2005) or whether different rhythms were used from one trial to the next (Correa and Nobre, 2008). Specifically, RTs were faster for targets that appeared at the time predicted by the rhythm of the pre-occlusion trajectory than for targets appearing before this time (Correa and Nobre, 2008) or for targets whose onset could not be predicted due to an erratic pre-occlusion trajectory (Doherty et al., 2005). Together, these results complement data from the endogenous temporal orienting task, described earlier, showing that attention can be tuned flexibly to different moments in time whether temporal expectations are derived endogenously or exogenously.

Neurophysiological mechanisms of exogenous temporal expectation

Using the rhythmic motion task described earlier, both Doherty et al. (2005) and Correa and Nobre (2008) showed that *exogenous* temporal expectation (induced by constant speed of motion) modulated the same late, response-related ERP components as *endogenous* temporal expectation (induced by informative pre-cues) (Miniussi et al., 1999; Griffin et al., 2002). Specifically, exogenous temporal expectation attenuated N2 amplitude and shortened P3 latency. Furthermore (and similar to previous endogenous temporal expectation studies) there were no effects of exogenous temporal expectation on P1 amplitude. However, when temporal expectation was combined with spatial expectation there were synergistic effects on P1 (Doherty et al., 2005). Specifically, knowing where *and* when the target was likely to appear enhanced P1 amplitude even more than simply knowing where it was likely to appear. This result suggests that temporal expectations can interact with and modulate spatial ones so as to enhance very early stages of perceptual analysis (Nobre, Chapter 27, this volume).

Neuroanatomical substrates of exogenous temporal expectation

Assmus et al. (2003, 2005) used predictable stimulus motion to identify the brain areas responsible for the perceptual integration of spatial and temporal information. Subjects estimated whether two moving objects would collide when their trajectories carried them behind an occluding mask. In other words, subjects made perceptual judgements about the predicted position of a stimulus at a particular moment in time. Left inferior parietal cortex and left ventral premotor cortex were activated by collision compared to size (control) judgements, the same areas that were found in our own study of endogenous temporal orienting (Coull and Nobre, 1998). More recently, Coull et al. (2008) have also found selective activation for left-lateralized inferior parietal and ventral premotor cortex in a perceptual collision judgement task, whether the stimuli were seen from a lateral (allocentric) or head-on (egocentric) perspective (Figure 31.2B). Collectively, these results suggest that left fronto-parietal areas may form a common network for temporal expectancies, whether the task is motor (speeded detection) or perceptual (delayed discrimination) in nature. Moreover, the same areas were activated whether the expectation had been established endogenously by a temporal pre-cue, or exogenously by the temporal dynamics of the stimulus itself. Note also that expectancies in these motion studies varied from trial to trial in a dynamic manner, just as in the endogenous temporal orienting task described above (Coull and Nobre, 1998) or for sequential effects in the variable foreperiod RT paradigm (Los, Chapter 21; Vallesi, Chapter 22, this volume).

However, O'Reilly et al. (2008) found preferential activation of a *right*-lateralized parietal-premotor network for spatiotemporal (velocity) judgements as compared to spatial (direction) ones. At face value, this paradigm appears very similar to those of Assmus and colleagues and Coull and colleagues, since all employed spatiotemporal trajectories, perceptual discriminations, and trial-to-trial variations in expectancies. However, the tasks performed by the subjects differed slightly across experiments. In the Assmus et al. and Coull et al. studies, subjects were required to make yes or no collision judgements. In the O'Reilly et al. study, subjects were required to judge whether the moving target had travelled further than expected or not far enough. It may be argued that this latter judgement makes more explicit demands on timing processes than do the collision judgement tasks since it relies on a bimodal *magnitude* response (shorter/longer). Coull and Nobre, (2008) have recently reviewed the functional imaging literature on timing and temporal expectations and found evidence to suggest that explicit timing tasks (in which subjects give overt estimates of stimulus duration) activate more right-sided brain areas, whereas implicit timing tasks (in which no estimate of duration is required, but the strict temporal structure inherent in the dynamics of stimulus presentation nevertheless enhance performance) activate more left-sided ones. This is, of course, a post-hoc explanation for the discrepancies in the O'Reilly et al. versus Coull et al. and Assmus et al. findings. Dedicated, controlled experiments would be required to test this hypothesis adequately.

Interestingly, O'Reilly et al. (2008) also observed selective activation of the cerebellum for spatiotemporal, but not spatial, expectancies. Cerebellar activity was not observed in either the Assmus et al. or Coull et al. studies. However, O' Reilly et al. examined temporal expectancies over a short duration (600ms) whereas the other two studies examined temporal expectancies over longer durations (approximately 1.5–3.5 seconds). Since recent transcranial magnetic stimulation (TMS) evidence (Koch et al., 2007; Lee et al., 2007) suggests that the cerebellum is particularly implicated in the timing of short (ms) durations, the differential activation of the cerebellum across these studies may simply be due to differences in the temporal range of intervals used. Notably, Coull and Nobre (1998) also observed preferential activation of the cerebellum with their endogenous temporal orienting paradigm, using intervals of 300ms and 1500ms.

Temporal re-orienting due to increasing conditional probabilities over time

Behavioural indices of temporal re-orienting

Valid trials in the endogenous temporal orienting paradigm index how attention is directed in time so as to benefit behaviour. By contrast, invalid trials index *shifts* in the direction of attention in time, and the resultant costs on behaviour. We have consistently found (Coull and Nobre, 1998; Coull et al., 2001; Griffin et al., 2002) that the cost of being invalidly cued is significantly smaller in temporal, compared to spatial, orienting tasks (Figure 31.1A). This is because temporal invalidity effects are negligible, or even absent, at long intervals, thus diluting the overall cost of invalid cueing (Figure 31.1B). Whether the stimulus display is spatial or foveal, significant RT costs have been observed for unexpectedly premature targets (the cue predicts a long foreperiod but the target appears after a short one) but not for unexpectedly delayed ones (the cue predicts a short foreperiod but the target appeared after a long one) (Coull and Nobre, 1998; Miniussi et al., 1999; Coull et al., 2000; Griffin et al., 2002). The temporal invalidity effect is therefore asymmetric, occurring only at short intervals but not at long ones. This is likely to be due to the bimodal nature of the cued interval: in these tasks, omission of the target at the short interval guaranteed that it had to occur at the longer one, reflecting the predictive information inherent in the passage of time itself. In other words, the *conditional probability* that the target will appear at the long interval, given that it did not appear after the short one, increases to 100% certitude.[1] Subjects can therefore voluntarily 're-orient' attentional resources to the long interval and so optimize responding at this later time point, effectively removing the behavioural cost of having been invalidly cued. This is akin to the 'strategic account' of the variable foreperiod effect (e.g. Niemi and Naatanen, 1981) in which RTs are monotonically faster for targets appearing after long rather than short foreperiods (see also Los, Chapter 21; Vallesi, Chapter 22, this volume). As time elapses, the conditional probability that a target will appear (given that it hasn't yet appeared) steadily increases (Figure 31.3b, inset), allowing for increasing levels of preparedness as time goes on, thus reducing RTs.

Correa and Nobre (2008) have recently investigated whether conditional probabilities interact with a more exogenous measure of temporal expectation, predictable stimulus movement (see also Nobre, Chapter 27, this volume). Using the rhythmic motion task described in the previous section, they manipulated whether the target appeared at the moment predicted by the pre-occlusion rhythmic motion (valid trials) or not (invalid trials). Crucially, this was measured for short, medium, or long occlusion times. As reported previously for endogenous temporal orienting tasks, RTs were faster for valid versus invalid trials at short, but not longer, occlusion times. In other words, and as suggested earlier in this chapter, the conditional probability effect counteracted the predictive capacity of rhythmic motion. In addition, the conditional probability effect (i.e. faster RTs at longer occlusion times) was significant for invalid trials but was abolished by valid trials, in which temporal expectations were fulfilled. In other words, the temporal expectation established by rhythmic motion counteracted the conditional probability effect.

---

[1] This dynamic change in the conditional probability of target occurrence over time is also known as the 'hazard function'.

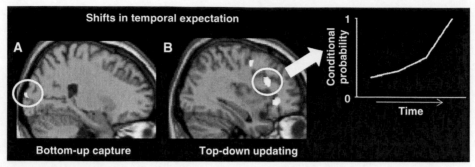

Fig. 31.3 Shifting attention in time to (A) premature versus (B) delayed targets differentially activates visual versus prefrontal brain areas (Coull et al., 2000), differentially reflecting bottom-up capture of attention versus top-down updating of the attentional focus. Right dorsolateral prefrontal cortex (DLPPFC) in particular has been shown to be engaged both by delayed targets in the temporal orienting paradigm (Coull et al., 2000) and by variable versus fixed intervals in the foreperiod reaction-time paradigm (Vallesi et al.2007, 2008, 2009; see also Vallesi, Chapter 22, this volume), implicating this area specifically in the *updating* of temporal expectancies as a function of evolving conditional probabilities over time (see graph inset).

The mutual interaction between these two factors suggests that a common mechanism for temporal expectation is involved in both types of effects.

Neurophysiological mechanisms of temporal re-orienting

When comparing ERPs across intervals of different lengths, it is important to rule out possible contributions from differential patterns of potential overlap from preceding events, which could lead to differences in baseline measures. To overcome this necessary limitation, Correa and Nobre (2008) used predictable rhythmic motion to modulate temporal expectations (as described in previous sections) and included a large range of intervals in each of their conditions. In addition, they manipulated the duration of the occlusion time in order to index the conditional probability effect.

First, they found that the conditional probability effect modulated similar ERP components to endogenous temporal cueing tasks and exogenous rhythmic motion tasks. Specifically, as occlusion time lengthened N2 amplitude and P3 latency decreased. The modulation of the same ERP waveforms by three distinct means of manipulating temporal predictability (endogenous temporal orienting, exogenous rhythmic motion, conditional probability effects) suggests shared neural substrates for temporal expectation. Second, they investigated the interaction between predictable rhythmic motion and the variable foreperiod effect. Echoing the behavioural results (described earlier), temporal expectation induced by rhythmic motion modulated ERP components at short, but not longer, occlusion times, and the conditional probability effect was significant for invalid, but not valid, trials. In other words, the temporal expectancies induced by rhythmic motion and by longer foreperiods were mutually interactive and influenced the same post-perceptual stages of information processing.

Neuroanatomical substrates of temporal re-orienting

The asymmetric invalidity effect for short versus long trials suggests the presence of distinct functional mechanisms for breaching expectations in these two trial-types. Trials in which targets appear later than predicted (i.e. delayed) afford time for subjects to re-orient attention, and may therefore invoke top-down, voluntary shifts of attention. By contrast, the sudden appearance of a target before expected (i.e. premature) interrupts the current focus of attention and captures the subject's attention reflexively, therefore emphasizing more bottom-up, automatic shifts of attention. We capitalized on the developing event-related fMRI methodology of the time to dissociate brain areas activated by unexpectedly (i.e. infrequent) premature versus delayed targets, in order to index these two distinct types of attentional shift (Coull et al., 2000). In addition, we used the opportunity to disambiguate the role of spatial attention in temporal orienting by designing a task in which all cues and targets were presented in a fixed (central) location. Although spatial location was task-irrelevant in the original temporal analogue of the Posner orienting task (Coull and Nobre, 1998), targets nevertheless appeared peripherally, thus potentially inducing reflexive shifts of spatial attention.

FMRI data (Figure 31.3) revealed distinct brain regions differentially sensitive to unexpectedly premature targets and unexpectedly delayed targets. Premature targets were accompanied by increased activation in visual cortex, suggesting the automatic capture of attention in time by unexpected sensory events (bottom-up attentional mechanism). Conversely, delayed targets were accompanied by activations in right ventrolateral and dorsolateral prefrontal cortex, suggestive of response inhibition and voluntary shifts of attention in time (top-down attentional mechanism). Specifically, we proposed (Coull et al., 2000) that a delayed target required subjects first to inhibit their prepared response at the early interval and then to update their response preparation plan for the later interval. This revised preparation plan would be held in working memory until the delayed target eventually appeared and allowed the potential behavioural costs of invalid cueing to be reduced. In agreement with our results, Vallesi et al. (2009) (see also Vallesi, Chapter 22, this volume) recently found activation of right dorsolateral prefrontal cortex during a variable versus fixed foreperiod paradigm. Moreover, the amplitude of prefrontal activation correlated with the magnitude of the behavioural benefit afforded by the variable foreperiod paradigm. Although both fixed and variable foreperiod paradigms create temporal expectancies for target onset time, expectancies in the variable foreperiod paradigm are also continually being updated within the course of a single trial as the conditional probability of target occurrence changes with elapsing time. Our results, together with those of Vallesi et al. (2009) suggest that right prefrontal cortex may be critical specifically for the *updating* of temporal expectancies, as conditional probabilities change over time throughout the course of a trial, rather than being critical for their implementation in the first place. By contrast, and as discussed previously, we have found evidence that the deployment of previously established, fixed temporal expectancies preferentially activates a left-lateralized fronto-parietal network.

Neurochemical modulation of temporal re-orienting

Indirect evidence in monkeys has suggested that exogenous temporal expectations, established through the use of a fixed foreperiod, may be particularly sensitive to noradrenergic (NA) manipulation (Witte and Marrocco, 1997). In a psychopharmacological fMRI study, we therefore investigated the NA modulation of endogenous temporal expectations in humans, using the cued temporal orienting paradigm, and compared it directly to that of spatial orienting (Coull et al., 2001). Healthy volunteers performed orienting tasks after administration of either placebo or the NA alpha-2 adrenoceptor agonist, clonidine, which impairs NA functioning. For the temporal orienting task, and as compared to placebo, clonidine slowed response times for unexpectedly delayed targets making them just as disruptive as unexpectedly premature targets, thus levelling out the asymmetric temporal orienting effect discussed earlier. This selective effect suggested that clonidine disrupted the benefit normally afforded by long foreperiods and the conditional probability effect. In other words, clonidine impaired voluntary (rather than reflexive) processes of temporal re-orienting.

Accompanying this behavioural effect was a drug-induced attenuation of activity in left insula, ventral premotor cortex, and prefrontal cortex. In other words, clonidine attenuated activity selectively in frontal components of the temporal orienting network. These anatomically selective effects are consistent with the behavioural effect of the drug on voluntary, rather than reflexive, processes of temporal re-orienting. Clonidine had a similarly specific behavioural effect during the spatial orienting condition. Compared to placebo, clonidine slowed detection of targets appearing in the left visual field, which is the side of space most sensitive to disruption in patients with clinical neglect (Mesulam, 1981). Accompanying this behavioural effect was a drug-induced attenuation of activity in right superior parietal cortex, an area that has been linked to spatial aspects of attention in innumerable studies (Marshall and Fink, 2001; Vandenberghe et al., 2001; Yantis et al., 2002). The anatomically-distinct effects of clonidine during temporal versus spatial orienting suggests that clonidine affected attentional orienting by modulating activity in functionally-specialised brain areas, rather than simply decreasing overall brain activity in a non-specific (sedative) manner.

Conclusions

Temporal orienting of attention depends upon temporal expectancies that have been established either with endogenous pre-cues or exogenous patterns of rhythmic stimulus presentation. Time is a unidirectional force, however, and these temporal expectancies can be further modulated by the predictive nature of time itself (Elithorn and Lawrence, 1955). Specifically, both endogenous (Coull et al., 2000) and exogenous (Correa and Nobre, 2008) temporal expectancies vary as a function of the increasing conditional probability of stimulus occurrence over time.

From a neural viewpoint, our electrophysiological and functional neuroimaging findings have demonstrated overlapping neural signatures for temporal expectancies generated either endogenously by temporal cues or exogenously by rhythmic motion. However, expectancies that are generated by the flow of time itself (as indexed by conditional probability effects) have quite distinct neural signatures. This neuroanatomical dissociation underlines the mechanistic differences between the initial implementation of a fixed temporal expectancy on the one hand (left parietal and premotor areas), and the updating of temporal expectancy as a function of the flow of time itself, on the other (right prefrontal areas).

Hemispheric lateralization of this sort is somewhat reminiscent of the hemispheric differences that have been observed in the control of action. Serrien et al. (2006) suggested that the left and right hemispheres differentially contribute to feedforward (planning of future limb dynamics) versus feedback (use of sensory input to control final limb position) aspects of motor control respectively. An analogous dissociation could be applied to the timing domain (see also Coull and Nobre, 2008), not only for tasks requiring a motor response but also those of a more perceptual nature.[2] Specifically, in the context of temporal expectancies, I propose that left-lateralized cortical areas make use of previously learned temporal information to predict future stimulus onset (i.e. feedforward mechanism) whereas right frontal areas compare current sensory input (presence or absence of the target) to the expected outcome (presence of the target at the predicted time) and update expectancies accordingly (i.e. feedback mechanism) (see also Pouthas and Pfeuty, Chapter 30, this volume).

---

[2] Schubotz (2007) has recently suggested that the feedforward characteristics of motor association areas can be used to predict not only future motor states, but also future perceptual states.

References

Assmus, A., Marshall, J. C., Ritzl, A., Noth, J., Zilles, K., and Fink, G.R. (2003). Left inferior parietal cortex integrates time and space during collision judgments. *Neuroimage*, **20**(Suppl 1), S82–88.

Assmus, A., Marshall, J. C., Noth, J., Zilles, K., and Fink, G.R. (2005). Difficulty of perceptual spatiotemporal integration modulates the neural activity of left inferior parietal cortex. *Neuroscience*, **132**, 923–7.

Correa, A. and Nobre, A. C. (2008). Neural modulation by regularity and passage of time. *J Neurophysiol*, **100**, 1649–55.

Cotti J., Rohenkohl G., Stokes M., Nobre A. C., and Coull J. T. (2009). Functional and neural dissociation of temporal versus motor expectations. *Neuroimage*, **47** (S1), S42.

Coull, J.T. and Nobre, A.C. (1998). Where and when to pay attention: the neural systems for directing attention to spatial locations and to time intervals as revealed by both PET and fMRI. *J Neurosci*, **18**, 7426–35.

Coull, J. and Nobre, A., 2008. Dissociating explicit timing from temporal expectation with fMRI. *Curr Opin Neurobiol*, **18**, 137–44.

Coull, J. T., Frith, C. D., Buchel, C., and Nobre, A. C. (2000). Orienting attention in time: behavioural and neuroanatomical distinction between exogenous and endogenous shifts. *Neuropsychologia*, **38**, 808–19.

Coull, J. T., Nobre, A. C., and Frith, C. D. (2001). The noradrenergic alpha2 agonist clonidine modulates behavioural and neuroanatomical correlates of human attentional orienting and alerting. *Cereb Cortex*, **11**, 73–84.

Coull, J. T., Vidal, F., Goulon, C., Nazarian, B., and Craig, C. (2008). Using time-to-contact information to assess potential collision modulates both visual and temporal prediction networks. *Front Hum Neurosci*, **2**, 10.

Doherty, J. R., Rao, A., Mesulam, M. M., and Nobre, A. C. (2005). Synergistic effect of combined temporal and spatial expectations on visual attention. *J Neurosci*, **25**, 8259–66.

Elithorn, A. and Lawrence, C. (1955). Central inhibition – some refractory observations. *Quart J Exp Psychol*, **11**, 211–20.

Griffin, I. C., Miniussi, C., and Nobre, A.C. (2001). Orienting attention in time. *Front Biosci*, **6**, D660–671.

Griffin, I. C., Miniussi, C., and Nobre, A.C. (2002). Multiple mechanisms of selective attention: differential modulation of stimulus processing by attention to space or time. *Neuropsychologia*, **40**, 2325–40.

Hillyard, S. A., Hink, R. F., Schwent, V. L., and Picton, T. W. (1973). Electrical signs of selective attention in the human brain. *Science*, **182**, 177–80.

Koch, G., Oliveri, M., Torriero, S., Salerno, S., Lo Gerfo, E., and Caltagirone, C. (2007). Repetitive TMS of cerebellum interferes with millisecond time processing. *Exp Brain Res*, **179**, 291–9.

Lange, K., Kramer, U. M., and Röder, B. (2006). Attending points in time and space. *Exp Brain Res*, **173**, 130–40.

Lee, K. H., Egleston, P. N., Brown, W. H., Gregory, A. N., Barker, A. T., and Woodruff, P. W. (2007). The role of the cerebellum in subsecond time perception: evidence from repetitive transcranial magnetic stimulation. *J Cogn Neurosci*, **19**, 147–57.

Los, S. A. and Heslenfeld, D. J. (2005). Intentional and unintentional contributions to nonspecific preparation: electrophysiological evidence. *J Exp Psychol Gen*, **134**, 52–72.

Los, S.A. and van den Heuvel, C. E. (2001). Intentional and unintentional contributions to nonspecific preparation during reaction time foreperiods. *J Exp Psychol Hum Percept Perform*, **27**, 370–86.

Macar, F. and Vidal, F. (2003). The CNV peak: an index of decision making and temporal memory. *Psychophysiology*, **40**, 950–4.

Mangun, G.R. (1995). Neural mechanisms of visual selective attention. *Psychophysiology*, **32**, 4–18.

Marshall, J.C. and Fink, G. R. (2001). Spatial cognition: where we were and where we are. *Neuroimage*, **14**, S2–7.

Mesulam, M. M. (1981). A cortical network for directed attention and unilateral neglect. *Ann Neurol*, **10**, 309–25.

Miniussi, C., Wilding, E. L., Coull, J. T., and Nobre, A. C. (1999). Orienting attention in time. Modulation of brain potentials. *Brain*, **122**(8), 1507–18.

Niemi, P. and Näätänen, R., 1981. Foreperiod and simple reaction time. *Psychol Bull*, **89**, 133–62.

Nobre, A. C. (2001). Orienting attention to instants in time. *Neuropsychologia*, **39**, 1317–28.

Nobre, A. C., Coull, J. T., Frith, C. D., and Mesulam, M. M. (1999). Orbitofrontal cortex is activated during breaches of expectation in tasks of visual attention. *Nat Neurosci*, **2**, 11–12.

O'Reilly, J. X., Mesulam, M. M., and Nobre, A. C. (2008). The cerebellum predicts the timing of perceptual events. *J Neurosci*, **28**, 2252–60.

Pfeuty, M., Ragot, R., and Pouthas, V. (2005). Relationship between CNV and timing of an upcoming event. *Neurosci Lett*, **382**, 106–11.

Posner, M. I., Snyder, C., and Davidson, B. J. (1980). Attention and the detection of signals. *J Exp Psychol*, **109**, 160–74.

Requin, J., Brener, J., and Ring, C. (1991). Preparation for action. In Jennings, J., Coles, M. (Eds.), *Handbook of Cognitive Psychophysiology: Central and Autonomic Nervous System Approaches*, pp.357–448. West Sussex: John Wiley and Sons.

Rushworth, M. F., Krams, M., and Passingham, R. E. (2001). The attentional role of the left parietal cortex: the distinct lateralization and localization of motor attention in the human brain. *J Cogn Neurosci*, **13**, 698–710.

Schubotz, R. I. (2007). Prediction of external events with our motor system: towards a new framework. *Trends Cogn Sci*, **11**, 211–18.

Schubotz, R. I. and von Cramon, D. Y. (2001). Functional organization of the lateral premotor cortex: fMRI reveals different regions activated by anticipation of object properties, location and speed. *Brain Res Cogn Brain Res*, **11**, 97–112.

Schubotz, R. I., von Cramon, D. Y., and Lohmann, G. (2003). Auditory what, where, and when: a sensory somatotopy in lateral premotor cortex. *Neuroimage*, **20**, 173–85.

Serrien, D. J., Ivry, R. B., and Swinnen, S. P. (2006). Dynamics of hemispheric specialization and integration in the context of motor control. *Nat Rev Neurosci*, **7**, 160–6.

Vallesi, A., McIntosh, A. R., Shallice, T., and Stuss, D. T. (2009). When time shapes behavior: FMRI evidence of brain correlates of temporal monitoring. *J Cogn Neurosci*, **21**, 1116–26.

Vandenberghe, R., Gitelman, D. R., Parrish, T. B., and Mesulam, M. M. (2001). Functional specificity of superior parietal mediation of spatial shifting. *Neuroimage*, **14**, 661–73.

Walter, W. G., Cooper, R., Aldridge, V. J., McCallum, W. C., and Winter, A.L. (1964). Contingent negative variation: an electric sign of sensorimotor association and expectancy in the human brain. *Nature*, **203**, 380–4.

Witte, E. A. and Marrocco, R. T. (1997). Alteration of brain noradrenergic activity in rhesus monkeys affects the alerting component of covert orienting. *Psychopharmacology (Berl)*, **132**, 315–23.

Woodrow, H., 1914. The measurement of attention. *Psychol Monogr*, **17**, 1–158.

Yantis, S., Schwarzbach, J., Serences, J. T., Carlson, R. L., Steinmetz, M. A., Pekar, J. J., et al. (2002). Transient neural activity in human parietal cortex during spatial attention shifts. *Nat Neurosci*, **5**, 995–1002.

Acknowledgements

I wish to thank the CNRS for financial support.

Index